MAY'S MANUAL

of the

Diseases of the Eye

First Edition, August, 1900.
Second Edition, September, 1901.
Third Edition, August, 1903.
Fourth Edition, August, 1905.
Fifth Edition, August, 1907.
Sixth Edition, August, 1909.
Seventh Edition, July, 1911.
Eighth Edition, August, 1914.
Ninth Edition, August, 1917.
Tenth Edition, April, 1922.
Eleventh Edition, August, 1924.
Twelfth Edition, August, 1927.
Thirteenth Edition, June, 1930.
Fourteenth Edition, August, 1934.
Fifteenth Edition, June, 1937.
Sixteenth Edition, June, 1939.
Seventeenth Edition, June, 1941.
Eighteenth Edition, December, 1943.
Nineteenth Edition, June, 1947.
Twentieth Edition, 1949.
Twenty-first Edition, 1953.
Twenty-second Edition, 1957.
Twenty-third Edition, 1963.
Twenty-fourth Edition, 1968.
British Edition by Mr. Claud Worth, Baillière, Tindall & Cox, London, 1906.
  Second Edition, May, 1908.
  Third Edition, October, 1911.
  Fourth Edition, November, 1914.
  Fifth Edition, September, 1924.
  Sixth Edition, December, 1929.
  Seventh Edition by Mr. Montague L. Hine, June, 1934
  Eighth Edition, June, 1939.
  Ninth Edition, May, 1944.
  Tenth Edition, 1949.
  Eleventh Edition by Mr. T. Keith Lyle, 1954.
Spanish Translation by Prof. C. E. Finlay; Salvat Editores, Barcelona, 1907.
  Second Edition, October, 1909.
  Third Edition, March, 1912.
  Fourth Edition, July, 1914.
  Fifth Edition, July, 1918.

Sixth Edition, May, 1921.
Seventh Edition, July, 1924.
Eighth Edition, October, 1927.
Ninth Edition, January, 1933.
Tenth Edition, Buenos Aires, 1943.
Eleventh Edition, Buenos Aires, 1948.
Twelfth Edition, 1952.
French Translation by Dr. Bouin: Steinhell, Paris, 1907.
  Second Edition, May, 1911.
  Third Edition, January, 1914.
  Fourth Edition, Masson et Cie., Paris, 1923.
  Fifth Edition, 1927.
  Sixth Edition, 1936.
Italian Translation by Prof. E. Trombetta, Unione Tipografico, Turin, 1905.
  Second Edition, January, 1909.
  Third Edition, January, 1916.
  Fourth Edition, December, 1920.
  Fifth Edition, March, 1925.
  Sixth Edition, March, 1934.
  Seventh Edition, 1953.
Dutch Translation by Dr. G. J. Schoute, Meulenhoff, Amsterdam, 1907.
  Second Edition, September, 1910; Third Edition, June, 1916; Fourth Edition, September, 1919; Fifth Edition, July, 1926; Sixth Edition, 1935.
German Translation by Dr. E. Oppenheimer; Hirschwald, Berlin, 1904.
  Second Edition, June, 1921.
Japanese Translation by Dr. T. Hidaka; Nankodo, Tokio, 1909.
  Second Edition, August, 1941.
Chinese Translation by Dr. T. M. Li; Presbyterian Mission Press, May, 1923.
  Second Edition, 1927; Third Edition, 1933; Fourth Edition, 1953.
Portuguese Translation by Prof. M. E. Alvaro; Spivak and Kersner. Rio de Janeiro.
  Second Edition, 1946; Third Edition, 1949; Fourth Edition, 1957.
Urdu (India) Translation, Osmania University, Hyderabad, India, 1940.

MAY'S MANUAL

of the

Diseases of the Eye

for Students and General Practitioners

TWENTY-FOURTH EDITION
REVISED AND EDITED BY

JAMES H. ALLEN, M.D.

Associate Dean, Tulane University Medical School; Professor and former Chairman, Department of Ophthalmology, Tulane University Medical School; Senior Surgeon, Section of Ophthalmology, Charity Hospital of New Orleans; Senior Surgeon in Ophthalmology, Eye, Ear, Nose and Throat Hospital; Consultant, U. S. Public Health Service Hospitals, Carville and New Orleans; Consultant, Veterans Hospital of New Orleans

With 258 illustrations
and 32 plates in color

ROBERT E. KRIEGER PUBLISHING COMPANY
HUNTINGTON, NEW YORK

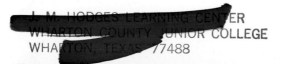

Original Edition 1968
Reprint 1974 — 1976

Printed and Published by
ROBERT E. KRIEGER PUBLISHING CO., INC.
645 NEW YORK AVENUE
HUNTINGTON, NEW YORK 11743

© Copyright 1968 by
THE WILLIAMS & WILKINS COMPANY
Reprinted by Arrangement

Library of Congress Catalog Card Number
ISBN Number 0-88275-190-5

Library of Congress Cataloging in Publication Data

May, Charles Henry, 1861-1943.
    May's Manual of the diseases of the eye for students and general practitioners.

    1. Eye--Diseases and defects. I. Allen, James Harrill, 1906-   ed. II. Title. III. Title: Manual of the diseases of the eye. [DNLM: 1. Eye movements. WW410 E97]
RE46.M4 1974   617.7'1   74-10746
ISBN 0-88275-190-5

Printed in U.S.A. by
NOBLE OFFSET PRINTERS, INC.
New York, N.Y. 10003

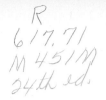
Preface to the Twenty-Fourth Edition

The twenty-fourth edition of *May's Manual of Diseases of the Eye* includes a number of revisions in structure as well as content. Some of these revisions were started with the twenty-third edition, but with the continuing rapid and extensive developments in ophthalmology, they will have to be continued with subsequent editions.

In this edition an attempt is made to obtain a better arrangement of the material; new material has been added; and some new illustrations have been provided.

The original purpose of presenting the material in a concise, practical and systematic manner for the use of the student and the general practitioner has been kept in mind. For this reason the section on the toxic effects on the eye of general medication has been added.

Again the editor respectfully dedicates this edition to the memory of the late author, Dr. Charles H. May; to the previous editor, Dr. Charles A. Perera, who maintained Dr. May's purposes and policies in continuation of publication of the *Manual;* to those dedicated physicians and scientists who made the publication of this material possible by their discoveries, practice and teaching, although neither time nor space has permitted specific citation of these contributions; to his confreres and associates who have suffered with and for him through this period of revision; and finally to the students of all stages who may find this material helpful.

JAMES H. ALLEN, M.D.

1430 Tulane Avenue
New Orleans, Louisiana 70112

Preface to the First Edition

In the following pages the author has endeavored to present a concise, practical, and systematic Manual of the Diseases of the Eye, intended for the student and the general practitioner of medicine. The great difficulty in preparing a book of this sort is to say enough but not too much. With this idea in view, the author has made the volume sufficiently comprehensive, up to date, and yet of limited size.

This restriction in size has been accomplished by omitting excessive detail, extensive discussion, and lengthy accounts of theories and rare conditions. The author has endeavored to give the fundamental facts of ophthalmology and to cover all that is essential in this branch of medicine, always keeping in mind that the book has been written for students and general practitioners. Space, therefore, has been allotted as the necessities of such readers require, estimated by an extended experience in teaching. Thus, rare conditions have merely been mentioned; uncommon affections, of interest chiefly to the specialist, have been dismissed with a few lines; and common diseases, which the general practitioner is most frequently called upon to treat, have been described with comparative fullness.

The book is not recommended as a substitute for the larger works, but as a means of supplying a foundation to which further knowledge may be added by reference to more extensive and comprehensive textbooks.

The illustrations, excepting a few cuts of instruments, are original, and have been inserted wherever it seemed that they would be of value in elucidating the text. The colored plates present the common external diseases of the eye and those changes in the fundus, the recognition of which is important in connection with general diseases including affections of the nervous system, as well as for ophthalmic diagnosis; hence the volume also supplies an atlas.

CHARLES H. MAY

August, 1900

Contents

Color Plates

Between pages 212–213

The old practice of dispersing color plates at intervals through the book has been abandoned. The text contains hundreds of references to these plates; to avoid frequent thumbing through the pages in search of the right one, they have all been grouped in a single easily-located spot in the center of the book.

1

External Examination of the Eye and Its Adnexa

Ophthalmology is a branch of general medicine and surgery from which, in practice, it cannot be separated. Thus examination of the eye does not mean merely the investigation of an isolated organ, but the examination of the *patient* with special reference to that organ and its functions.

Thorough examination of the eye requires the adoption of a definite *routine.* The history of the patient's complaint will lead the trained observer to concentrate his attention upon the affected part of the eye, but it is not safe to depart from a systematic plan of examination.

Examination of the eye may be divided into (1) objective, and (2) subjective or functional.

The *objective examination* may be subdivided into

(a) Examination of the face, the lids and the anterior portions of the eyeball by means of *inspection and palpation* using daylight or artificial light.

(b) Examination of the cornea and of the interior of the eyeball in the *darkroom,* with artificial light, by means of oblique illumination, the ophthalmoscope, transillumination, the slit lamp and biomicroscope.

Inspection. The patient should be seated facing a window or adequate source of artificial illumination. A *general inspection* will reveal any obvious abnormalities, such as asymmetry of the face or orbits, anomalies of movements of the lids or eyes, swelling, congestion, discharge, lacrimation, blepharospasm, etc.

The *lids* are observed for thickness, texture, color and position; the condition of their margins, whether reddened, swollen, crusted or ulcerated; the power of opening and closing; the size of the palpebral aperture; the condition, position and direction of the lashes; and the position and permeability of the lacrimal puncta. The region of the *tear sac* is examined for swelling and whether pressure with the tip of the index finger causes escape of secretion through the puncta.

Next the inner or *conjunctival surfaces of the lids* are inspected for any change in color, smoothness or thickness, and for the presence of secretion or foreign bodies.

A *headrest* is necessary in manipulations and treatment of the lids.

Exposure of the conjunctiva of the lower lid is accomplished by placing the thumb near the margin of the lid and pressing downward and backward while the patient looks upward (Fig. 1-1).

Eversion of the upper lid requires a little practice: The central lashes are grasped between the thumb and index finger of the right hand and the lid is drawn downward and away from the globe as the patient is directed to look downward (Fig. 1-2); the left index finger (or a probe held horizontally) is placed at the upper margin of the tarsus and pressed downward, at the same time quickly turning the lid. Unless the patient looks downward it is difficult to evert the upper lid. *Gentleness* is indicated; if the patient resists the attempt to evert the upper lid, it is wise to desist and to try again after assuring him that there will be no pain. After the lid has been turned, it can be kept everted by shifting the left thumb against the margin, the other fingers of

1

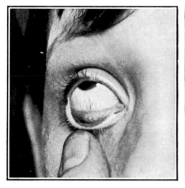

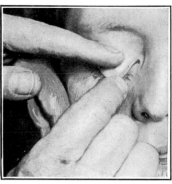

FIG. 1-1. Eversion of the lower lid.

FIG. 1-2. First step in eversion of the upper lid.

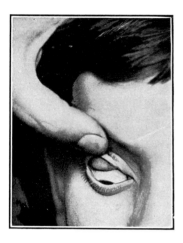

FIG. 1-3. Keeping the upper lid everted.

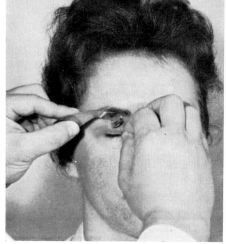

FIG. 1-4. Eversion of the lid to expose upper fornix. The blade tip of a double everter is placed at the upper border of the tarsus and, with the patient looking downward, the lashes are grasped between the thumb and index finger. Then by a combination of pressure downward with the everter and an outward and upward pull on the lashes, the lid is folded over the blade of the instrument.

the left hand being applied above the patient's forehead (Fig. 1-3). This exposes the tarsal portion of the conjunctiva.

To inspect the *retrotarsal fold* (upper fornix), a double everter or an applicator is placed at the upper border of the tarsus (Fig. 1-4) and pressed downward and forward; at the same time the tarsal portion of the lid is folded backward over the tip of the instrument (Fig. 1-5).

For the simultaneous exposure of the conjunctiva of both the upper and the lower lids, the index finger of the left hand replaces the thumb holding the everted upper lid, while the left thumb everts the lower lid by pressure upon its margin (Fig. 1-6).

The *eyeball* is examined to determine

its situation in the orbit, whether normal or whether the globe is pushed forward (exophthalmos, proptosis) or sunken (enophthalmos); this can be determined, roughly, by placing the 0 of a transparent millimeter rule at the outer margin of the orbit and observing the height of the summit of the cornea of each eye; a more precise measurement is obtained with a special instrument, the exophthalmometer (Fig. 1-7).

The small concave rest of each arm of the exophthalmometer is placed against the corresponding lateral orbital rim (Fig. 1-8) with patient's head resting steadily against a head rest. The separation of the lateral orbital margins is read off the front bar of the instrument. Then with the patient fixing the open left eye of the examiner, the position of the most prominent part of the cornea of the patient's right eye is observed in the reflecting mirror and the measurement read off the scale just above the mirror. Similarly, with the patient fixing the open right eye of the examiner, the position of the anterior surface of the patient's left cornea is measured. The results are recorded as O.D. 17 mm. O.S. 17 mm. at 98 mm. separation. In subsequent measurements the separation is set at 98 mm. in order to give accurately comparable results. Normally the corneas project 12 to 20 mm. anterior to the lateral orbital margin and the two eyes measure practically the same; however, any difference of more than 5 mm. between the positions of the two eyes needs an explanation (Chap. 16).

The *motility* of the eyeballs is assessed to determine whether the two eyes move together and whether the visual lines meet at the object of fixation. Any deviation is investigated to determine whether there is loss of motion in any direction (paralysis or paresis), or disturbance of muscle balance, either latent (heterophoria) or manifest (strabismus), as explained in Chapter 21. Oscillatory movements (nystagmus) should be classified (see Chap. 21).

The bulbar conjunctiva is examined for

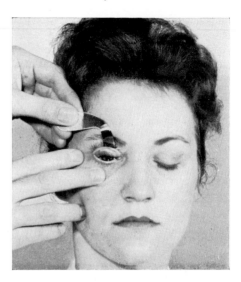

FIG. 1-5. Exposure of the upper fornix. By continuation of the pressure on the everter while the patient looks downward, the upper fornix is exposed.

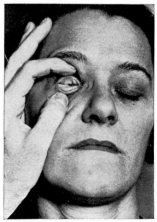

FIG. 1-6. Exposure of both upper and lower tarsal conjunctiva.

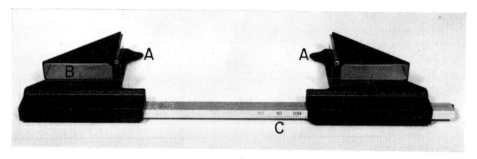

Fig. 1-7. Exophthalmometer. *A,* Concave rests for positioning against the lateral orbital rims; *B,* the reflecting prism containing the measuring scale; *C,* the scale for measuring separation of the orbital rims.

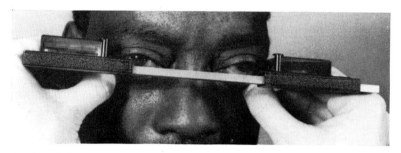

Fig. 1-8. Exophthalmometer in place, with right eye being measured. (Notice that the scale and the reflection of the eye are visible in the prism.)

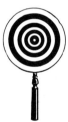

Fig. 1-9. Placido's keratoscope, one-tenth actual size.

edema (*chemosis*) or *congestion*. If the latter is present, its characteristics indicate the type of inflammation (Plate 8).

The *cornea* is inspected next, and may reveal dullness, ulceration, vascularization, opacities or foreign bodies. The *corneal light reflex* gives information concerning the curvature and smoothness of this part of the eye; by causing the patient to look in different directions, every part of the cornea is explored. Placido's keratoscope (Fig. 1-9), a target-like disk consisting of alternate black and white circles, may be useful for this purpose; distortion of the corneal reflection of the circles indicates an abnormality of curvature (Fig. 1-10).

For better illumination of the cornea a strong convex lens (13 to 15 diopters) may be used to concentrate the light of an electric bulb, placed to the side and slightly in front of the patient, by moving the apex of this cone of light over different parts of the cornea; or a flashlight with a concentrated and uniform beam of light may be used (Fig. 1-11). Greater details are observed if the illuminated area is inspected with a *binocular magnifier* (loupe, Fig. 1-12).

To bring an abrasion or ulcer of the cornea more clearly into view, we may instill a drop of 2 per cent solution of

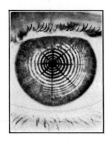

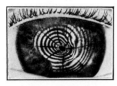

FIG. 1-10. Corneal reflection of Placido's disk, in a normal eye (*top*), and in keratoconus (*bottom*).

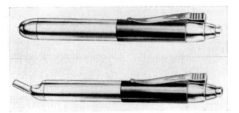

FIG. 1-11. *A*, Flashlight; *B*, flashlight which may be used as a flashlight or transilluminator.

fluorescein, washing off the excess with normal saline or boric acid solution. Wherever the corneal epithelium is abraded or the stroma exposed there will be a green stain.

Scars and opacities of the cornea are evidence of previous ulcerations or infiltrations.

When a corneal opacity is very faint and cloud-like, it is called a nebula; when denser, a macula, and when perfectly opaque and white, a leukoma (Fig. 7-7).

The sensitiveness of the cornea may be tested by touching it gently with a thread or a wisp of cotton, taking care not to touch the lids or lashes.

When there is much irritation, spasm of the lids (*blepharospasm*) prevents a proper examination. In such cases, the instillation of a local anesthetic will aid in exposing and examining the eyeball.

In infants or very young children, when blepharospasm, swelling, inflammation or obstinacy prevents inspection of the cornea in the usual way, the child is laid upon its back across the nurse's lap, after wrapping the upper part of its body in a large towel or sheet, and its head is

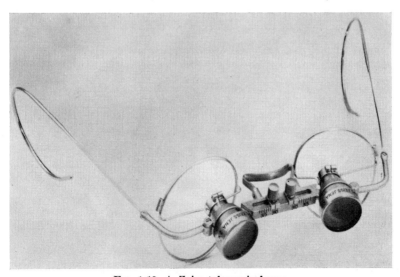

FIG. 1-12. A Zeiss telescopic loupe.

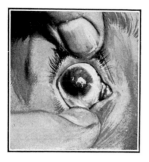

FIG. 1-13. Method of exposing the eyeball.

It is sometimes necessary to use *retractors* (Fig. 1-14) in order to separate the lids and with these the same caution is required against wounding the cornea or pressing upon the eyeball.

If the method of examining the eyes of infants just described should prove unsatisfactory, a general anesthetic must be employed.

steadied between the knees of the examiner, who sits facing the nurse. Holding the child's hands, the nurse steadies the patient's body with her arms, allowing the legs to remain free; thus when the child struggles it will expend its energy in motion of the feet while the head remains the fixed point. Under such circumstances the lids usually may be everted by pulling upon them at a little distance from the margin. To inspect the eyeball, the lids are opened by the thumbs placed at the edges, rolling in the latter somewhat and then separating, keeping close to the surface of the eyeball (Fig. 1-13). Having exposed the eyeball, the thumb of the right hand may be replaced by the index finger of the left, thus leaving the right hand free for other uses. The eye usually will be found turned upward, hence the cornea will be hidden from view; but after a minute it will appear in the palpebral aperture. Care must be taken not to scrape the cornea and cause an abrasion, nor to exert any pressure upon the eyeball, on account of the danger of perforation in case the cornea has become weakened by ulceration.

When the lids are separated forcibly, pent-up secretions are released suddenly and may squirt into the eyes of the examiner.

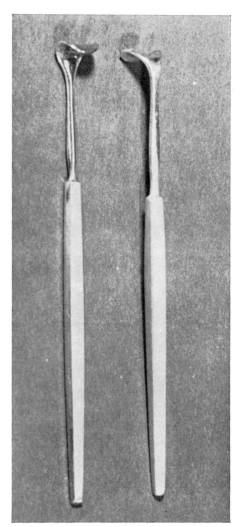

FIG. 1-14. Lid retractors.

The *anterior chamber* is examined for its depth and clarity of the *aqueous humor*. The chamber may be shallow in glaucoma or deep following dislocation of the lens or removal of a cataract. Normally the aqueous is clear but it may be diffusely cloudy with or without precipitates upon the posterior surface of the cornea (keratic precipitates) or it may be turbid with an accumulation of white blood cells (hypopyon) or of blood (hyphema) in the lower angle.

The *iris* is examined to determine its color, smoothness and thickness, whether its markings are clearly defined or blurred (*"muddy"*) and whether it is steady or tremulous during movements of the eyeball (iridodonesis). The latter condition is seen when the iris is not properly supported by the lens, *e.g.*, in the absence (aphakia), shrinkage or dislocation of the

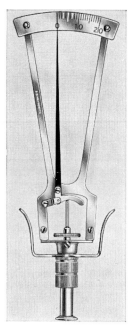

Fig. 1-16. Tonometer of Schiøtz.

lens. *Adhesions* to the cornea (anterior synechiae) or to the capsule of the lens (posterior synechiae) are looked for; these may require the instillation of a mydriatic for their detection.

Then the characteristics of the *pupil* are determined: size, shape and position. Its size is compared with that of its fellow; also its reaction to light, accommodation and convergence. The average size in health in daylight, at rest, is about 4 mm.; the size varies with exposure to light, accommodation and convergence; with age, being small in advanced years and wider in youth; and with the state of refraction, being smaller in hyperopes and larger in myopes.

Behind the pupil is the central part of the anterior surface of the *lens*. It is examined for clearness or any abnormality, such as cataract or deposits, making allowance for the gray reflex in the aged.

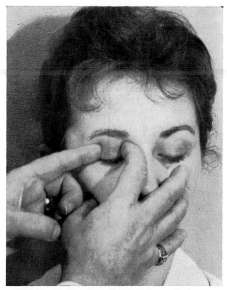

Fig. 1-15. Testing the tension of the eyeball. The globe is being fixed by the left index finger and pressure is being made on the globe with the right index finger. The pressure is being directed toward the left index finger.

To explore the lens fully, dilatation of the pupil and artificial illumination are required.

Palpation gives information concerning (1) tenderness in the ciliary region, (2) *tension* of the eyeball and (3) existence of tumors and swellings in and about the orbit.

Intraocular Pressure. The tension of

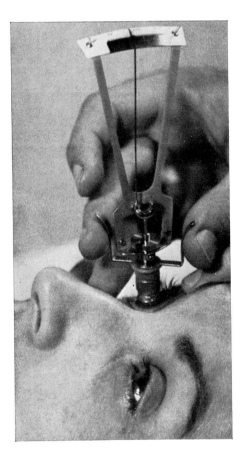

Fig. 1-17. Testing the tension of the eyeball with a Schiøtz tonometer. The lids are held away from the globe while the instrument is applied to the anesthetized cornea. The amount of indentation of the cornea is indicated by the needle. The scale reading is transposed into millimeters of mercury pressure (see Table 1-1).

TABLE 1-1

1955 Calibration Scale for Schiøtz Tonometers (Approved by the Committee on Standardization of Tonometers of the American Academy of Ophthalmology and Otolaryngology)

Tonometer Reading (R)	Plunger Load			
	5.5 gm.	7.5 gm.	10 gm.	15 gm.
0.0	41.5	59.1	81.7	127.5
0.5	37.8	54.2	75.1	117.9
1.0	34.5	49.8	69.3	109.3
1.5	31.6	45.8	64.0	101.4
2.0	29.0	42.1	59.1	94.3
2.5	26.6	38.8	54.7	88.0
3.0	24.4	35.8	50.6	81.8
3.5	22.4	33.0	46.9	76.2
4.0	20.6	30.4	43.4	71.0
4.5	18.9	28.0	40.2	66.2
5.0	17.3	25.8	37.2	61.8
5.5	15.9	23.8	34.4	57.6
6.0	14.6	21.9	31.8	53.6
6.5	13.4	20.1	29.4	49.9
7.0	12.2	18.5	27.2	46.5
7.5	11.2	17.0	25.1	43.2
8.0	10.2	15.6	23.1	40.2
8.5	9.4	14.3	21.3	38.1
9.0	8.5	13.1	19.6	34.6
9.5	7.8	12.0	18.0	32.0
10.0	7.1	10.9	16.5	29.6
10.5	6.5	10.0	15.1	27.4
11.0	5.9	9.0	13.8	25.3
11.5	5.3	8.3	12.6	23.3
12.0	4.9	7.5	11.5	21.4
12.5	4.4	6.8	10.5	19.7
13.0	4.0	6.2	9.5	18.1
13.5		5.6	8.6	16.5
14.0		5.0	7.8	15.1
14.5		4.5	7.1	13.7
15.0		4.0	6.4	12.6
15.5			5.8	11.4
16.0			5.2	10.4
16.5			4.7	9.4
17.0			4.2	8.5

the globe may be estimated by palpation. The patient is directed to look downward and then, with the index finger of one hand fixing the globe through the upper lid, pressure is made on the globe with the index finger of the other hand to determine the relative resistance. Comparable examinations should be made of the patient's other eye and the examiner's eyes (Fig. 1-15). Increase of tension is a prominent symptom of glaucoma; diminished tension (hypotony) often exists in degenerated eyeballs; alterations in tension are sometimes found in cyclitis.

For *accurate measurement* of the intraocular pressure an instrument, the *tonometer* of Schiøtz (Fig. 1-16), is in general use. The tonometer indicates, by movement of a needle upon a scale, the resistance offered to definite weights used to produce an indentation of the cornea. The eye is anesthetized with two instillations of Nupercaine or Pontocaine; cocaine is contraindicated since it may alter tension slightly and it softens the corneal epithelium so that an abrasion from contact with the tonometer may occur. The patient should lie on a couch, the eyes directed upward; the lids are separated with the fingers without pressing on the eyeball (Fig. 1-17); the tonometer is allowed to rest by its own weight on the center of the upturned cornea. Different weights are superimposed, depending on the degree of suspected alteration in tension; the needle of the instrument becomes deflected to a certain number which an accompanying scale translates into a definite number of millimeters of mercury (Table 1-1). The mean normal intraocular pressure with this instrument is 16.1 mm. of Hg with a standard deviation of ±2.8 mm.

For minute inspection of the cornea, anterior chamber, iris and lens, and for examination of the vitreous and fundus, the direct or indirect ophthalmoscope, the biomicroscope, with slit lamp illumination and transillumination, are used in a darkroom (Chap. 2).

2

Objective Examination of the Eye Conducted in the Darkroom

The Examination in the Darkroom comprises the following steps, which are best taken in the order given:

(1) *Oblique illumination,* for the physical examination of the anterior portions of the eyeball.

(2) *Examination with the ophthalmoscope at a distance,* for exploring all the media of the eyeball.

(3) *The direct method of ophthalmoscopy,* for examining the fundus, giving an erect picture greatly magnified.

(4) *The indirect method of ophthalmoscopy,* for examining the fundus, giving an inverted picture of low magnification.

(5) *Transillumination.*

(6) *Examination with the corneal microscope and slit lamp.*

The examining room should be dark. The patient should be seated; the examiner may either stand or be seated.

OBLIQUE ILLUMINATION

Oblique (lateral or focal) illumination furnishes a valuable means of exploring the cornea, anterior chamber, iris and lens. By means of a strong convex lens of 2- or 3-inch focus, light is concentrated upon the eye in such a manner that the apex of the cone of light corresponds to the part to be examined. The source of illumination is a frosted electric globe upon a "universal bracket," which can be swung to either side of the patient and raised or lowered; the light should be about 18 inches to the side of the patient, several inches in advance, on a level with the eye. The lens is grasped by its margin between the thumb and index finger, held so that its surfaces are at right angles to the direction from which the light proceeds, and steadied by means of the little finger placed against the side of the patient's face. After one eye has been examined, the supporting finger is kept in place, and the patient's head is turned slightly toward the light and the other eye illuminated. The light may be placed on either side; if the examiner is on the patient's right, the left hand holds the lens; if on the left, the right hand. After the cornea has been examined the lens is brought nearer to the eye so the apex of the cone of light corresponds to and explores the deeper structures.

With a second strong convex lens held at its focal distance (2 or 3 inches) in front of the patient's eye, the illuminated area can be magnified and examined in greater detail. Special combinations of convex lenses and prisms supported by a headband or a spectacle frame (binocular magnifier or loupe, Fig. 1-12) are more convenient for magnifying the illuminated area. The electric ophthalmoscope, with the head removed, and the convex lens capsule over the lamp, also may be used in the darkroom with good results in exploring the anterior structures. A pocket flashlight or a special illuminator attached to an ophthalmoscope battery handle (Fig. 2-1) serves the same purpose.

Opacities of the cornea, aqueous or lens, seen by oblique illumination, appear as *grayish or white spots* upon the background of the pupil (Plate 2*C, E, G, I*).

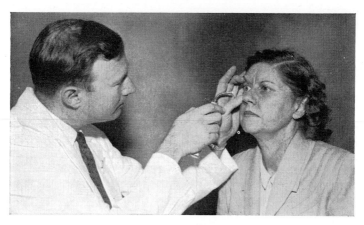

FIG. 2-1. Oblique illumination.

The Ophthalmoscope

The invention of the ophthalmoscope by Helmholtz in 1851 permitted an accurate study of the interior of the living eye, allowing recognition of changes in the fundus which give valuable information in the diagnosis of local, intracranial and systemic diseases. The original model of Helmholtz consisted of superimposed layers of glass which acted as a reflecting surface, with the source of illumination placed to the side of the eye under examination; subsequently a concave mirror was used for the reflector (Fig. 2-5C); later, Dennett introduced the electric ophthalmoscope, in which the source of illumination is within the instrument itself (Fig. 2-3); this made the examination much easier, especially with the improvement in the system of illumination now in general use.

The electric ophthalmoscope has superseded the old type of reflecting instrument, which is no longer in general use. But its occasional employment, especially for the indirect method of ophthalmoscopy, justifies the short description found later in this chapter.

The essential portion of the ophthalmoscope is a *reflector*. This is mounted upon a convenient handle and supplemented behind by a disk containing convex and concave lenses. The reflector serves to throw light into the interior of the eye, while the aperture in the lens disk, which is situated just above the level of the reflector, allows a portion of this light, after returning from the patient's eye, to pass into the eye of the observer. The *lens disk* is provided with a series of lenses which follow each other in regular order from weaker to stronger (Fig. 2-5B). This disk can be rotated by means of the finger applied to its milled edge so any lens can be placed behind the perforation; opposite each lens is an illuminated number indicating its strength in diopters.

The Electric Ophthalmoscope. A minature electric lamp with loop or coiled filament enclosed in the handle furnishes the light which passes through a convex condensing lens and a reflecting prism then into the patient's eyes. The indestructable prism reflector replaces the fragile mirror formerly employed. The lower end of the prism is convex and thus exerts additional convergence upon the rays. The prism is constructed so that it

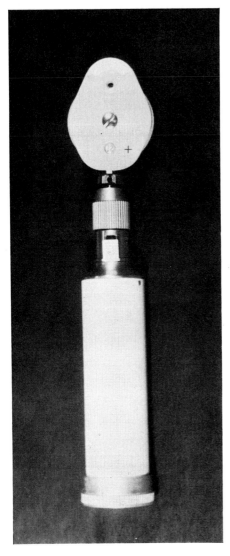

FIG. 2-2. The battery handle ophthalmoscope.

the eye of the observer receives the rays reflected from the background of the eye under examination. The illuminated portion of the fundus is a round area of equal intensity, free from shadows or lamp filament image, the intensity of illumination being controlled by a thumb rheostat. A removable pin-hole diaphragm cap can be fitted over the condensing lens; this addition reduces the size of the illuminated area, but permits more detailed study of any particular part of the fundus, and also is of advantage with small pupils. The lighting current is derived either from a dry cell battery in the handle (Fig. 2-2) or conducted by cords connected with the house current through a rheostat. For bedside ophthalmoscopic examinations the battery in the handle instrument is more convenient. It comes in various sizes any of which may be carried in the coat pocket but the cells in the smallest size naturally have to be replaced oftener than those in larger handles (Fig. 2-2).

There are a number of serviceable self-luminous ophthalmoscopes on the market; the simple ones are the best; complicated and very expensive varieties possess little advantage over the simpler forms for ordinary use.

The electric ophthalmoscope (with head removed) also is useful for illumination of the anterior structures of the eyeball, for transillumination and for muscle testing.

The reflecting ophthalmoscope. As stated above, the electric or self-luminous ophthalmoscope possesses so many advantages over the formerly used instrument (Fig. 2-5), in which the light is derived from an external source, that the old model has gone out of general use but the principles have been retained in the design of the Schepens binocular indirect ophthalmoscope (Fig. 2-9).

In the old type of instrument the source of illumination is on either side of

produces total reflection. This condensing and reflecting device is attached to the anterior surface of the lens disk of the ophthalmoscope in such a manner that the upper extremity covers only the lower portion of the sight hole; the upper portion is left free, and through this aperture the patient and on a level with his eyes (Figs. 2-7 and 2-9); when the direct method is employed the source of illumination must be on the side of the eye which is being examined. The old type of ophthalmoscope is provided with a concave mirror of about 10 inches' focus, having the form of a parallelogram, hinged so that it can be directed to the

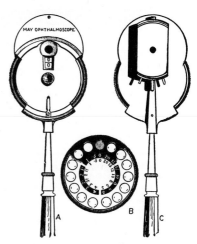

FIG. 2-5. The reflecting ophthalmoscope: *A*, rear side; *B*, lens disk; *C*, mirror side.

right or to the left according to the position of the light (Fig. 2-5*C*). Some experience is necessary in acquiring the technique, and annoying reflexes are more common than with the electric ophthalmoscope. It has the advantage, however, that a superior view of the fundus can be obtained when the *indirect method* is used, because of increased illumination furnished by the concave mirror.

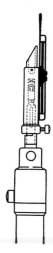

FIG. 2-3. The electric ophthalmoscope in section.

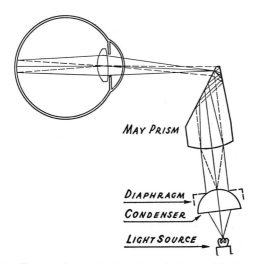

MAY PRISM

DIAPHRAGM
CONDENSER
LIGHT SOURCE

FIG. 2-4. Course of rays in the May electric ophthalmoscope.

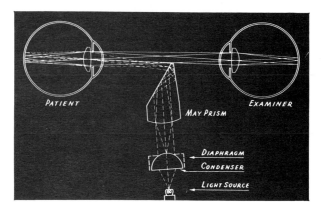

FIG. 2-6. Direct method of ophthalmoscopic examination with the electric ophthalmoscope.

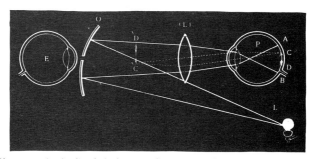

FIG. 2-7. Indirect method of ophthalmoscopic examination: formation of the image of the fundus with the old type of ophthalmoscope. This illustration will apply to the self-luminous ophthalmoscope if the external source of light (the electric bulb, *L*) is ignored and the electric ophthalmoscope itself is substituted for the mirror, *O*.

Principle of the Ophthalmoscope.

As ordinarily seen, the pupil appears black because the light which leaves it is necessarily reflected in the direction from which it came. If the eye of the observer is placed so as to intercept the returning rays, the interior of the observed eye will appear illuminated. With the ophthalmoscope, light is reflected into an eye under examination, and the observer's eye is placed in the path of the returning rays and receives some of these through the perforation in the lens disk.

Figure 2-6 illustrates the *direct method*. Rays proceeding from the totally reflecting prism pass into the examined eye,

lighting the fundus. From any portion of this illuminated area, rays are reflected, pass out of the eye under examination, above the level of the prism, through the perforation in the lens disk into the eye of the examiner; here they are brought to a focus on the retina; they are convergent and, being prolonged backward, form a magnified and erect image behind the eye of the patient.

Figure 2-7 explains the *indirect method*. From *L*, divergent rays proceed to the mirror *O*, are reflected and made convergent, passing into the examined eye *P*, crossing in the vitreous. They illuminate the fundus between *A* and *B*. From any portion of this illuminated area, *CD* for instance, rays are reflected and, passing out of the eye, are rendered parallel by its refracting apparatus. They fall upon the convex lens (*L*) and are brought to a focus at *C'D'*, forming an enlarged, inverted image in the air at the focus of the lens (*L*), which image can be seen by the eye of the examiner, *E*.

The Ophthalmoscopic Examination

Before attempting to see the fundus, the *media* must be examined. This step is important, since it will explain blurring or failure to see the fundus when changes in the media exist. One mode of obtaining such information, oblique illumination, has already been described; it is particularly applicable to the anterior media. A second method is the following.

Examination with the Ophthalmoscope at a Distance. This method explores *all the media*—cornea, aqueous, lens and vitreous. The light is reflected into the eye, and, returning from the background, traverses the media before reaching the eye of the examiner through the aperture in the lens disk. The ophthalmoscope is held in front of either eye of the observer, so that he can look through the perforation, and a +5.00 D. lens is rotated into the aperture of the lens disk; the instrument is steadied against the side of the examiner's nose and supraorbital margin. The distance between patient and examiner is about *15 inches*.

The light thrown into the eye of the patient reaches the background and is *colored orange-red* by contact with the choroidal vessels and retinal and choroidal pigment. This tinted light returns through the patient's eye and enters the eye of the examiner by means of the aperture in the lens disk. The tint varies with the color of the background of the individual, depending upon the abundance of choroidal and retinal pigment; hence it is brighter in persons of light complexion, and darker in others. It also is influenced by the amount of illumination, and consequently the reflex is brighter when the pupil has been artificially dilated. The patient is told to move the eyes in various directions, and in this manner different parts of the media are explored.

In the normal eye a homogeneous orange-red reflex (*fundus reflex*) is obtained (Plate 2*A*). If any details of the vessels of the fundus are seen, the eye is ametropic (Plate 2*B*). If, when the observer moves his head from side to side, these vessels appear to move in the same direction, the eye is hyperopic; if in the opposite direction, it is myopic.

If *opacities* exist in any of the media, they will appear as *dark* or black *spots* upon the colored background of the pupil. They are dark because they intercept a certain part of the light (Plate 2*D*, *F*, *H*, *J*). Opacities of the media may be either *fixed*, in which case they move only with the eye, or *movable* (floating), when they float about after the eye has been moved rapidly and then suddenly stopped; the latter occur only in abnormally fluid vitreous.

The exact *situation of opacities* of the media often can be estimated by oblique illumination. Another method (parallax) consists in observing the *displacement* of the opacity with regard to the *pupil*, when the observer's head is moved slowly from side to side. When there is no apparent motion of the opacity, it is in the plane of the iris; when it appears to move in the opposite direction, it is in front; and when in the same direction, it is behind this plane. A third method is based upon the *relationship of the motion* of the opacity to that of the *eyeball*. If, when the patient moves his eye, the opacity moves with (in the same direction as) the eye, it must be in front of the center of rotation of the globe (which corresponds to the anterior portion of the vitreous, about 10 mm. in front of the retina); if it moves in the opposite direction, it must be behind this point; if it has no motion, it must be exactly at the center. In both of these tests the greater the apparent motion, the more removed is the opacity from the plane of the iris and the center of rotation of the globe, respectively.

Additional details of changes in the media and iris may be obtained by placing *stronger convex lenses* in the sight hole of the ophthalmoscope. Thus a +12.00 is inserted in the sight hole and the examiner approaches the eye to bring the cornea, iris and lens into focus. Then by progressively reducing the strength of the lens in the sight hole, examining the media with each lens, the fundus eventually comes into focus and it is examined systematically. The expert may succeed with a pupil of natural size, but often it is necessary to *dilate the pupil*. Moderate dilatation is secured by instilling 1 drop of a 5 per cent solution of *cocaine* and waiting 30 minutes. A 5 per cent solution of *Euphthalmine* or *ephedrine,* or a 1 per cent solution of *Paredrine* or *Benzedrine,* or a 10 per cent emulsion of *Neo-Syn-*

ephrine acts more energetically. The effects pass off within a few hours. Greater dilatation follows the instillation of 1 drop of a 1 per cent solution of *homatropine;* this causes mydriasis in from 20 to 30 minutes, but the effects last from 24 to 36 hours.

Atropine should never be used to dilate the pupil only for ophthalmoscopic examination. Before using any mydriatic, one should be certain that none of the symptoms of glaucoma is present.

There are two methods of examining the fundus: (1) the *direct* and (2) the *indirect*.

The Direct Method of Ophthalmoscopic Examination is the one generally used; we obtain an erect image of the fundus *magnified about 15 diameters*.

The examiner sits or stands to the side of and facing the patient (Fig. 2-8). The ophthalmoscope is supported as in the previous method, and brought directly in front of the patient's eye *as close as possible*; the eye of the patient should not be more than 1 inch from that of the observer. For examination of the *right eye,* the examiner must be on the *right side,* and consequently the ophthalmoscope must be placed before the right eye of the

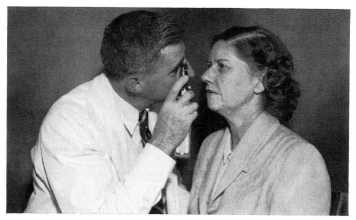

Fig. 2-8. Direct method of ophthalmoscopic examination.

observer. When the *left eye* is being examined, the examiner must be to the *left*, and use his left eye.

When both examiner and patient are emmetropic, and both relax their accomodation, the observer looks through the sight hole and obtains a clear view of the fundus without a lens. The patient is told to look at the opposite wall, directly forward, over the shoulder of the examiner, and not into the ophthalmoscope, as often he will be inclined to do. The anterior segment of the eye and the media are examined as described above, beginning with a +12.00 diopter lens in the ophthalmoscope and gradually focusing (turning the lens dial to progressively reduce the strength of the lens in the sight hole) until the fundus comes into view. If the patient has continued to look in the proper direction the optic nerve (*the disk* or *papilla*) usually will come into view, as it is a little to the inner or nasal side of the visual axis. Since it is the most prominent feature of the eye grounds, it is the best place to start the examination.

The parts around the disk are examined next, including the blood vessels and especially the macula. The *macular region* is found to the outer side of the disk, the distance corresponding to about twice the diameter of the papilla. When the pupil has been dilated artificially so it cannot contract in accommodation, the macula can be brought into view by directing the patient to look into the aperture of the lens disk. The extreme periphery of the eye grounds is brought into view when the patient looks up, down, to the right and to the left.

The *size* of any particular lesion is compared with that of the disk (*disk diameter*); this can be estimated more accurately by placing a cross-ruled graticule over the condensing lens in the ophthalmoscope, causing projection of cross squares 1° apart on the fundus. Changes in the *level* of the fundus (elevations, depressions, new growths) are measured in diopters; an elevation of 1 mm. corresponds to 3.00 D.

If *the observer is ametropic,* he either must wear his distance glasses, have a special correcting lens fitted to the aperture or rotate a correcting lens from one of those contained in the disk of the instrument into the aperture. *When the patient is considerably ametropic,* a suitable lens must be rotated into place behind the aperture; if he is myopic, this should be the weakest concave lens, and if hyperopic, the strongest convex lens which will give a distinct view; this gives an indication of how the direct method may furnish a *very rough* estimation of errors of refraction.

The emmetropic observer will be unable to obtain a distinct view of the fundus of a myopic eye, by the direct method, without putting behind the sight hole in the ophthalmoscope a concave lens of a strength at least sufficient to neutralize the myopia. He can examine a hyperopic eye either by putting up a convex lens or by using his accommodation. But in the direct method the observer should learn to *relax his accommodation.* The beginner often finds this difficult, since he cannot forget that he is looking at a very near object, and he accommodates accordingly. He is apt to place a concave lens of about 4.00 D. in the sight hole to neutralize his accommodation, even though the patient is not myopic, and with such a minus lens he will see the fundus distinctly. Relaxation of accommodation is encouraged by keeping both eyes open and looking in the distance with the uncovered eye.

The Indirect Method of Ophthalmoscopic Examination, although used much less than the direct method, has advantages in special cases. With the indirect method an *inverted image* of the fundus, *magnified about four diameters,* is

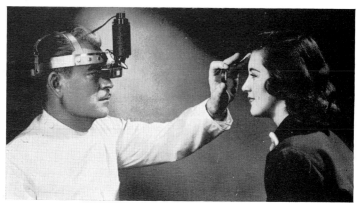

Fig. 2-9. Indirect method of ophthalmoscopic examination. The photograph shows the Schepens binocular ophthalmoscope manufactured by the American Optical Company.

obtained. A +4.00 D. *convex lens* is placed in the aperture of the ophthalmoscope; this enables the examiner to obtain a clear image with his accommodation at rest. By placing the ophthalmoscope before either eye, at a distance of about 15 inches from the patient, the fundus reflex is seen. A strong convex lens of 2 to 3 inches' focus (called the objective lens) now is held at about its focal distance in front of the eye to be examined. This lens is grasped at its edges by the thumb and index finger of the left hand and steadied by one of the other fingers against the forehead of the patient (Fig. 2-9). If a clear view of the fundus is not obtained, the objective lens is moved closer to or farther from the patient's eye, until a distinct image appears at a short distance in front of the lens, at its focus (Fig. 2-7).

After the right fundus has been seen, the examination of the left is made without any change in the position of ophthalmoscope, patient or examiner; only the objective lens is moved to cover the patient's left eye, being steadied by the middle finger placed upon the forehead; the little and ring fingers are flexed into the palm of the hand, so they will not obstruct the right or free eye of the patient and thus prevent him from gazing in any direction. In the examination of the left eye the ophthalmoscope may be held in the left hand and the lens in the right.

As in the direct method, the examination is begun by looking for the *entrance of the optic nerve*; the latter, situated a little to the inner or nasal side of the visual axis, is brought into view when the patient moves his eye somewhat inward, thus rotating the posterior pole of the eyeball outward; this is accomplished by having the patient look *over* the examiner's right *shoulder* on a level with the upper border of the ear, when examining the right eye, and over the left shoulder on a corresponding level for the left eye.

To see the *parts surrounding the disk,* the lens or the head is moved slightly in various directions, always remembering that the image is inverted, and that it moves with the lens, but in the opposite direction to that taken by the head. More peripheral parts are brought into view when the patient moves his eye up, down, to the right and to the left.

When the patient looks directly at the ophthalmoscope, the macula is brought into view, but since he must accommodate

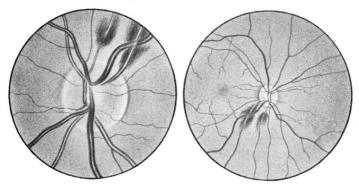

Fig. 2-10. The direct and indirect methods of ophthalmoscopy contrasted. The view of the fundus obtained by the direct method (*left*) is erect and highly magnified. That obtained by the indirect method (*right*) is inverted and less magnified, but a larger portion of the eye ground is seen at one time.

when fixing so near an object, the pupil will contract. On this account the pupil must be dilated to get a view of the macular region with the indirect method.

The beginner may encounter *difficulties*, in using the indirect method, which he will not have with the direct method. He may have trouble in bringing the disk into view, because the patient persists in watching the ophthalmoscope instead of looking across the examiner's shoulder. There may be an *annoying reflection* of the light from the cornea or from the surfaces of the lens before the patient's eye; such reflexes may be obviated by a slight inclination of the lens or a little variation in the position of the examiner which experience will soon indicate. *Confusing reflexes* from the margins of the sight hole indicate defects in the instrument, dust, or worn places in the black enamel, leaving a bright edge which reflects light into the examiner's eye.

The Direct and Indirect Methods Contrasted. The *direct method* (Fig. 2-10, *left*) gives an *erect* image which is highly magnified (about 15 ×), though a comparatively small portion of the field is seen at a time; hence it permits more *minute exploration* of particular parts.

The *indirect method* (Fig. 2-10, *right*) gives a larger field of view, though a smaller magnification (about 4 ×); *i.e.*, a larger portion of the background is seen at one time; hence it presents a *general view* of the background, which is *inverted*. It can be used successfully independent of errors of refraction in the patient's eye. On account of greater illumination details of the fundus often may be seen even when slight opacities of the media exist.

The Normal Fundus

The normal fundus exhibits a great many *variations* in details. It presents an *orange-red* surface, upon which the disk, the *blood vessels* and the *macula* are distinguished (Plates 3 to 6).

The Disk (*papilla*) represents the entrance or head of the optic nerve; it usually is circular, but sometimes oval in form. Its color is light pinkish, darker over the inner half, the outer portion being paler. The disk is much lighter in color than the rest of the fundus, and is separated from adjacent portions by a *sharply defined margin*, especially at the outer side. This margin often presents two *rings*: an inner, the *scleral* (Fig. 2-11),

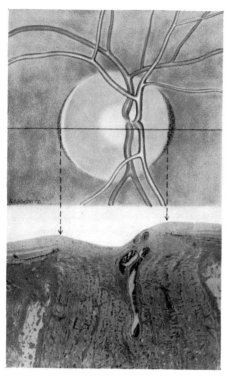

FIG. 2-11. Semidiagrammatic ophthalmoscopic view and longitudinal section of the disk. The horizontal line indicates the relative location of the section. The vertical lines indicate the corresponding points.

of white color, formed by exposure of the sclera when the opening in the choroid is larger than that in the sclera; and an external ring, the *choroidal* (Fig. 2-11), of dark color, formed by an accumulation of pigment at the margin of the aperture through which the optic nerve passes. This pigmented ring may be complete or incomplete; in the latter case it is generally found at the outer border. The margins of the normal disk occasionally are slightly indistinct, especially above and below; this appearance sometimes is seen in hyperopic eyes of young subjects, and must not be mistaken for optic neuritis (papillitis).

The center of the papilla presents a funnel-shaped depression (Fig. 2-11; Plate 6A) formed by the separation of the nerve fibers; this appears whiter than the rest of the disk and is known as the *physiologic depression or cup*. It may be comparatively large and occupy one-half or more of the disk, but never the entire papilla, in which respect it differs from the pathologic excavations of glaucoma and of optic nerve atrophy (Fig. 15-3). Grayish spots may be seen at the bottom of this physiologic excavation, when it is deep; these represent the openings in the lamina cribrosa, the connective tissue layer through which the fibers of the optic nerve pass (Plate 6A).

The Central Artery and Vein of the retina (Fig. 2-11) pass along the inner wall of the excavation, and upon reaching the surface of the disk usually divide into *superior and inferior divisions;* each of these soon divides and subdivides, giving off *nasal and temporal branches;* from these, smaller twigs are derived which become terminal and do not anastomose. Several small branches usually are given off from the main trunks and pass across the disk. The macular region is devoid of larger vessels, though finer branches are seen to approach this area. The retinal vessel wall is transparent, so only the stream of blood cells within the lumen is seen in the normal individual; however, the stream usually is referred to as if it were the entire vessel until visible pathologic changes occur in the vessel wall. The *arteries* are readily distinguished from the veins by their smaller diameter, bright red color and straighter course; they present a bright reflex running along the center. The *veins* are of greater thickness, of darker red color, more tortuous, and the light streak is fainter. Arteries and veins usually follow the same course. The blood vessels sometimes present visible pulsation, most easily seen in tortuous portions of their course. They are much more common in the veins than in the arteries; in the veins the pulsation is noticed especially where the central trunk appears on the disk; this pulsation is increased by pressure upon the eyeball. Easily visible pulsation in the retinal arteries is pathologic, occurring in glaucoma, cardiac disease and profound anemia. Sometimes a cilioretinal artery, derived from the ciliary system (circle of Zinn), is seen emerging near the temporal disk margin, forming a loop and then proceeding toward the macula; this may explain the preservation of function of a small part of the retina at or near the macula after obstruction of the central retinal artery.

The Retina itself is transparent. The *color* of the background is derived from the choroidal vessels, modified by the pigment-epithelial layer of the retina and the pigment of the choroid. It is bright *orange-red* in persons of fair complexion (Plate 3A), while in darker individuals it has a deeper, *brick red* color (Plate 4A); in Negroes it is brownish gray (Plate 5B). When the pigment-epithelial layer of the retina is well developed, the choroidal vessels cannot be seen. More often, considerable detail of the *vessels of the choroid* will be visible. This occurs under two conditions: In some cases there is no obscuration by the pigment layer of the retina, and the choroidal pigment is abundant and collected into the intervascular spaces presenting a granular or stippled appearance (tessellated fundus); these stand out as dark islands separating bright red lines and bands which anastomose freely, the choroidal vessels (Plate 4A). In other instances, there is little pigmentation in either retina or choroid, allowing the choroidal vessels to be seen plainly, now presenting a pattern of bright red anastomosing channels with ighter interspaces (Plate 3B). The choroidial vessels are most easily visible in the periphery, and are readily distinguished from retinal vessels by being less sharply defined, flat, having no light streak, by their free anastomosis and by occupying a plane posterior to the retina.

The Region of the Macula Lutea (Plate 6B), physiologically the most important part of the fundus, is situated less than two disk diameters to the temporal side of the entrance of the optic nerve, in the line of direct vision. Very often this region presents scarcely any distinctive feature. It is always *devoid of visible vessels*, and is somewhat *darker* than the rest of the fundus. Frequently a *bright spot* is seen in its center corresponding to the position of the fovea centralis, or there may be two or three of these bright spots. Sometimes the macular region is represented by a bright spot surrounded by an area of dark red color, about the size of the disk, oval horizontally, and this again encircled by a *bright halo*; this reflex is best seen in the indirect method and is most obvious in children of dark complexion, especially if they are hyperopic; it is especially evident in Negroes (Plate 5B).

Physiologic Variations. In children and adolescents of dark complexion the fundus frequently presents a bright luster, which changes its position with slight rotation of the ophthalmoscope, most apparent along the blood vessels; it resembles the shimmer of watered silk. Another peculiar but physiologic variation in appearance is sometimes produced by *opaque nerve fibers* (medullated nerve fibers); in such cases the axis cylinders of some of the optic nerve fibers retain their medullary sheath at the disk and continue in this condition for some distance, presenting whitish areas extending into the retina for a variable distance from the disk, terminating in brush-like extremities (Plate 4B). Occasionally the margin of the disk is indistinct and the papilla may even be slightly elevated; this condition, which is congenital, is called *pseudoneuritis* since it may be mistaken for optic neuritis by beginners (Plate 5*A*). Rarely a congenital anomaly characterized by tortuosity of the retinal vessels, especially the veins, may lead to the same error. The normal fundus presents *many minor variations;* hence experience is necessary to avoid regarding these as pathologic.

Ophthalmoscopy with red-free light. If the fundus is examined by light from which the red rays have been excluded by a suitable filter, the background will appear yellowish green in color, the macula standing out as a lemon-yellow area, the disk white, the fundus reflexes intense and the vessels almost black with sharply cut outlines. The nerve fibers become visible, those going to the macula running in a straight line, those more peripheral forming elliptical arches; thus disappearance of such fibers, for instance in optic nerve atrophy, may be seen. Slight alterations in the vessels, minute retinal hemorrhages, ill defined exudates and obscure changes at the macula become more apparent than with ordinary light. A disk having an aperture fitted with green glass is attached to some ophthalmoscopes, to be slid over the sight hole; this small addition gives only imperfect results as compared to those obtained with special instruments, since a much more intense light is needed than that produced by the ophthalmoscope. The method may be used for the detection of *minute changes* in the background when doubt exists with the ordinary examination.

Transillumination

This method of examination uses the passage of a beam of light through the sclera, from behind or the side, *lighting up the pupil;* anything which intercepts the light, such as a solid mass or dense opacity, will cause a shadow. The light also may be applied trans-sclerally to one part of the sclera so as to transilluminate the opposite portion of the sclera after transversing the vitreous; a dark area in the transilluminated sclera then indicates a pigmented tumor or the deposit of opaque material. Transillumination is used principally in the differential diagnosis between serous retinal detachment and an intraocular growth.

Instruments known as *transilluminators* are used; many electric ophthalmoscopes can be adapted for this purpose; with the May ophthalmoscope, the exposed electric bulb (Fig. 2-12) is applied to the sclera after local anesthesia, or merely to the external surface of the eyelids, and pressed firmly against the eyeball. Good results are obtained only when the examining room is absolutely dark.

The Slit Lamp and Biomicroscope

The slit lamp and biomicroscope (Fig. 2-13) furnish a combination for the study of *changes in the anterior portion of the eye.* The slit lamp supplies a brilliant light condensed into a beam which, traversing the parts to be examined, shows them in *optical section,* the remainder of the eye being in darkness. This illuminated area then is examined with the binocular microscope. This intense illumination and

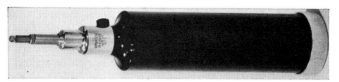

Fig. 2-12. The May electric ophthalmoscope arranged for transillumination.

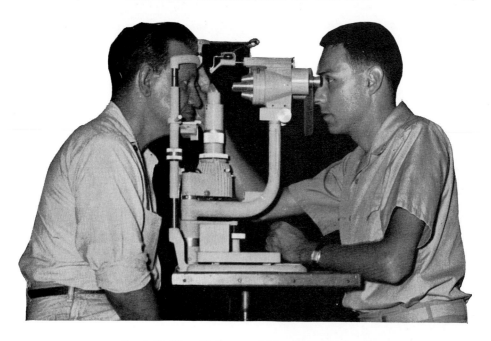

FIG. 2-13. The slit lamp and biomicroscope in use.

added magnification permit study of microscopic changes in the anterior portion of the eyeball. The successful use of this apparatus requires practice, and experience is necessary for interpretation of the findings; it often reveals important changes which otherwise would be overlooked.

The slit lamp projects a *sharply defined beam* which can be focused as desired. The microscope slides upon an adjustable table and the slit lamp is fitted to it in such a manner that the beam can be projected at any angle and can be transferred rapidly from one eye to the other. This versatility provides a variety of methods of examination. The beam may be focused directly upon an object such as a foreign body (*direct focal illumination*). The beam may be focused on a reflecting surface behind the object under examination, which is then viewed by transmitted light (*retroillumination*), or a bright secondary

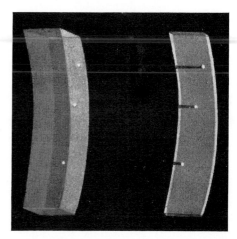

FIG. 2-14. Appearance of foreign bodies in the cornea, as seen with the broad beam of the slit lamp on the left and the narrow beam on the right.

source of light may be produced on the iris for examination of the cornea by transmitted light. If the cornea is vascu-

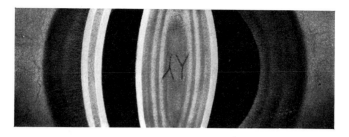

Fig. 2-15. Optical section of cornea and lens, as seen with the beam of the slit lamp (schematic).

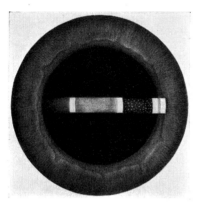

Fig. 2-16. Slit lamp beam appearance of an optical section of the anterior segment of the eye in iridocyclitis, showing aqueous flare and floaters.

larized, the actual circulation of the blood in the tenuous vessels is clearly visible. A third method makes use of the *zone of specular reflection*; the angle of the beam and the line of gaze of the patient are adjusted to the axis of the microscope so the light from a reflecting surface is received by the examiner. The endothelial cells lining the posterior surface of the cornea may be seen on the edge of the bright area, and the shagreen surface of the anterior and posterior lens capsules can be studied. The use of this *mirror light* gives valuable information regarding changes in the cornea and lens.

An examination with the slit lamp can

be made with either the broad or the narrow beam:

The broad beam is chosen mainly to gain information about the reflecting surfaces of the eye; these are the anterior surface of the cornea, Descemet's membrane, the posterior corneal surface, the anterior capsule of the lens, the surfaces of the various nuclei of the lens and the posterior capsule of the lens and, finally, the anterior third of the vitreous.

The narrow beam is used for examining the eye in *optical section* and has the advantage of giving a *third dimension,* permitting the estimation of the depth of structures; with this method the thickness of the cornea and the nature of its curvatures may be estimated. The site of a foreign body, the seat of a corneal infiltration or the depth of an ulcer may be determined (Fig. 2-14).

With the narrow beam the lens is divided into a series of concentric nuclei. The surfaces of these nuclei with their characteristic sutures, presenting anteriorly an erect Y and posteriorly an inverted Y (Fig. 2-15), may be examined with the broad beam; thus lens opacities can be located and their progress watched.

Clinically the slit lamp is of great value. The exact *localization* given by the apparatus often is important; thus it can be determined whether a foreign body has perforated the cornea and often whether there is a fragment of metal within the globe. The age of a corneal scar can be estimated, information sometimes of great value in medicolegal cases.

In Inflammatory Conditions of the Eye the slit lamp is indispensable. Particles consisting of cells or clumps of cells (conveniently termed *"floaters"*), or strands of fibrin, can be seen in the aqueous; or such exudates may be seen in the retrolental space and in the vitreous. Since the cornea is colder than the iris, there are convection currents in the anterior chamber; therefore, these particles circulate, rising on the iris side, falling behind the cornea. If the inflammation becomes more intense, the aqueous becomes albuminous, the convection currents cease and the particles are at rest. The beam of light now becomes visible as it traverses the anterior chamber, the so-called *flare* or Tyndall's phenomenon (Fig. 2-16). The finding of flare and the presence of particles in the aqueous humor often are the *earliest signs of serious inflammations,* such as uveitis or sympathetic ophthalmitis, and the use of the slit lamp permits detection of these formidable complications some days earlier than the ordinary methods of examination. The presence of cells in the anterior chamber may be an indication of choroiditis, and careful search with the ophthalmoscope then often will dislose a focus in the fundus.

Definite signs of inflammation found with the slit lamp may aid in the differential diagnosis between a malignant intraocular growth and an inflammatory lesion.

The *nature of corneal precipitates* elucidated with the slit lamp is of diagnostic value; frequently these cannot be seen with oblique illumination and the loupe. *Pellucid keratic precipitates* indicate serious inflammation of some portion of the uveal tract. The detection of these precipitates often is of great value in diagnosing a quiet uveitis and sometimes explains obscure cases of secondary glaucoma.

Examination of the vitreous and retina may be accomplished by the use of the slit lamp and biomicroscope with the addition of a special contact glass or a strong concave lens (Hruby lens) suspended in front of the patient's eye.

Gonioscopy. The angle of the anterior chamber can be seen in great detail by the use of a special contact glass placed upon the cornea, using strong illumination in combination with some form of magnifying device (loupe, corneal microscope or a special instrument known as the gonioscope). This method of examination is useful in patients with glaucoma, foreign bodies in the iris and tumors of the iris and ciliary body.

3

Subjective or Functional Examination of the Eye

The subjective examination, dependent upon the statements of the patient, comprises the testing of the function (vision or sight) of each eye separately. This function may be subdivided into (1) the form sense, (2) the color sense and (3) the light sense.

The *form sense* is the faculty which the eye possesses of perceiving the shape or form of objects, and is expressed as *acuteness of vision*. The *color sense* is the power which the eye has of distinguishing light of different wave lengths, *i.e.*, distinguishing colors. The *light sense* is the faculty of perceiving different degrees of intensity of illumination (brightness). Distinction is made between (a) *central or direct* and (b) *peripheral or indirect vision*.

THE ACUTENESS OF VISION

Central or Direct Vision. When a distinct image is required, the eye must be turned directly toward the object so the image falls upon the macula lutea, the portion of the retina which is adapted for the most acute vision; this constitutes *central or direct vision*. Acuteness is tested both for *distant* and for *near* vision.

Distant Vision. In testing for distance a range of 20 feet (6 meters) is selected, since rays of light from this distance are practically parallel. For this purpose use is made of *Snellen's test types*, which are constructed upon the following principle: Each letter is inscribed within a square (Fig. 3-1) which subtends a visual angle of 5′ at the distance at which the normal eye should distinguish the letter. The visual angle is included between two lines drawn from the extremities of the object through the nodal point of the eye, which is situated 15 mm. in front of the retina and 7 mm. behind the cornea (Fig. 3-2). Each side of the square is subdivided into five equal parts; the smaller squares thus formed subtend a visual angle of 1′, which is the minimum visual angle for the normal eye. If two black objects on a white ground are separated by a space subtending a smaller angle, they will no longer be seen separately, because the two images then will stimulate only a single sensory receptor unit in the layer of rods and cones of the retina. In order to subtend the same visual angle, the size of the letters must increase the farther they are removed from the eye (Fig. 3-2).

Snellen's Test Types consist of square-shaped letters arranged upon a chart, the size of the letters diminishing from above downward. The height of each letter subtends a visual angle of 5′, and the width of the component limbs a visual angle of 1′. The uppermost letter is of such a size that it can be read at 200 feet; then follow rows of letters which should be read at 100, 70, 50, 40, 30, 20, 15 and 10 feet, respectively (Fig. 3-3).

The acuteness of vision, or visual acuity, is expressed by a fraction, the numerator of which corresponds to the number of feet separating the patient from the chart (preferably 20 feet), and the denominator, to the number indicating the distance at which the smallest letters seen should be read by the normal eye. If the patient has average normal sight, his visual acuity will equal 20/20; this is expressed V.A. = 20/20 (or 6/6 by the

26

metric system). If he can see only the third line from the top, V.A. = 20/70. If he cannot read more than the top letter, V.A. = 20/200. If he reads some letters in the 50 line, but not all of this size, V.A. = 20/50 − or 20/70 +. Many persons, especially during youth, can read the line which should be read at 15 feet, or even 10 feet, when placed 20 feet from the

chart; the fractions in these cases would be 20/15 and 20/10.

If only 10 feet of space are available in the examining room, the effect of double this distance can be obtained by placing the test card back of the patient and having him read its reflection in a mirror 10 feet away. Or a test chart with smaller letters may be used; the numerator of the Snellen fraction then would be the distance from the chart and the denominator the distance at which the smallest letters read should be seen by the normal eye; in examinations at less than 20 feet, however, the effect of accommodation must be kept in mind.

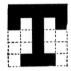

FIG. 3-1. Construction of Snellen's test types.

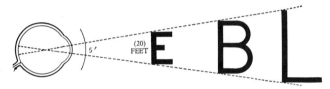

FIG. 3-2. Estimation of the size of Snellen's test types at various distances.

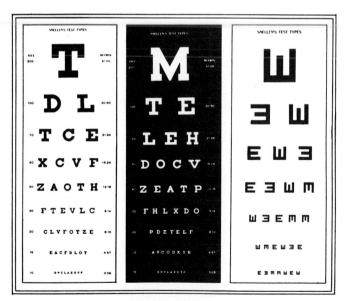

FIG. 3-3. Snellen's test types. *Left,* the usual style of chart; *center,* white letters on a black ground; *right,* test types for illiterates.

The Snellen figures do not represent the existing fraction of normal vision; the fraction is simply a record of the findings at a given distance; visual acuity of 20/40, for example, is not one-half of normal vision, but is merely a record of the ability to read, at 20 feet, letters which normally are seen at 40 feet. It is important to understand this distinction when visual disability is estimated as explained in Chapter 7.

If the patient's visual acuity is less than 20/200, the distance from the chart is reduced or larger test letters such as should be seen by the normal eye at 300 or 400 feet are used. If he can see only the 200-foot letter at 8 feet, V.A. = 8/200. If he cannot read the top letter at any distance, the distance in feet or inches at which he can correctly *count the examiner's extended fingers* held against a dark background is recorded; for example, V.A. = fingers at 1 foot or at 7 inches. If he has less sight than this, the hand is moved before the eye, and if he is capable of appreciating such movements, he has *"perception of hand movements"* at so many inches or feet. If vision is still further reduced, *perception of light* is tested by alternately shading and exposing the eye by means of the hand, or by throwing light upon the eye with the ophthalmoscope or flash light in the darkroom.

Each eye is tested separately, one eye being covered. Either daylight, or artificial light thrown directly upon the chart, may be used; the latter has the advantage of being more uniform. With daylight, the chart is hung opposite a window, at about the level of the patient's eyes, and the patient is placed with his back to the window. A *projection apparatus* may be employed to project the Snellen test letters upon a screen.

When the person is *illiterate,* a series of letters E, with sizes corresponding to those of the Snellen types, in which the openings point downward, upward and to the right and left (Fig. 3-3, *right*) may be used; the acuteness of vision then is determined by the smallest row of which the patient can correctly tell the direction in which the figures are open.

In the case of *children* who have not yet learned the alphabet, a chart presenting the pictures of common objects conforming in size to the standard angle is useful.

Near Vision. In a state of rest, the eye is adapted for parallel rays coming from a distant object. Thus, for divergent rays from a near object to be focused on the retina, there must be an increase in the refractive power of the eye; this change is known as *accommodation* and will be described more fully in Chapter 19.

The test types usually employed to determine near vision consist of different sizes of ordinary printer's types; the finest is numbered 1, successive numbers indicating coarser type. They are known as *Jaeger's test types* (Fig. 3-4). The patient should be placed with his back to the light, so the page is well illuminated, and each eye is tested separately. Acuity of near vision is expressed by J., followed by the number corresponding to the finest print which can be read; thus, J3 means that the patient is able to read the third paragraph.

THE FIELD OF VISION

Peripheral Vision (indirect vision) is exercised when the image falls upon some part of the retina outside the fovea centralis; such vision is indistinct, but of great importance for guidance and safety.

The Field of Vision represents the limits of peripheral or indirect vision; it is the space within which an object can be seen while the eye remains fixed upon some one point. It usually refers to one eye, the other being covered, and, when not otherwise stated, applies to a white

No. 1.

..Engaged in manual occupation of a coarser sort, the laborer has little opportunity either to try or to misuse his organ of vision; his sight, unless attacked by local inflam-

No. 2.

matory diseases or the consequences of constitutional disorders, remains good, though its acuteness lacks that extreme development

No. 3.

which follows abundant use in higher types of occupation. But with the literary worker it is differ-

No. 4.

ent : keeping pace more or less with mental activity, the eye is constantly called upon for

No. 5.

action, in reading for information and reference on the one hand, in recording the

No. 6.

fruits of such occupation on the other. Observation has shown that deteriora-

No. 7.

tion in eyesight and changes in the form, and hence in the dioptric

FIG. 3-4. Jaeger's test types for near vision.

object on a dark background. The field can be outlined roughly by the hand, by a lighted candle or the ophthalmoscope lamp in the dark room when vision is poor; but most exactly by means of a perimeter.

The confrontation test. The patient is placed with his back to the light, and the examiner faces him at a distance of 2 feet. After covering one eye, the patient is directed to fix that eye of the examiner which is opposite; the examiner closes his other eye. The hand, with fingers extended, is then moved from various parts of the periphery inward, midway between examiner and patient; the latter indicates when he sees the fingers. In this way the examiner can compare the patient's field with his own; if both are normal, patient and examiner must see the fingers simul-

taneously. This is a simple and rapid method and reveals any large defect in the field. Instead of the hand, a 1-cm. white knob on the end of a black rod may be used to measure the field in like manner.

Light projection. When the patient is no longer able to see the hand, a lighted candle or a small electric lamp may be used in the dark room; the eye under examination must be kept fixed directly forward and the other one well occluded; the light is moved about through the field of vision and the patient must tell not only when the light is exposed or shaded but also where he sees it.

The perimeter (Fig. 3–5) furnishes the most exact method for mapping and charting the field of vision. In its simplest form it consists of a metallic semicircle or quadrant, which can be revolved to take the direction of any meridian. This arc is

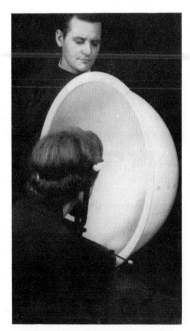

FIG. 3-5. Gams perimeter in use. The white spot is the test target.

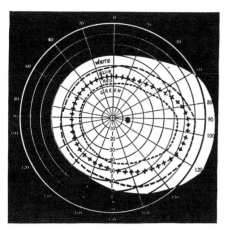

Fig. 3-6. Normal fields for white and colors (blue, red, green) with a 10-mm test object.

marked in degrees, 0 corresponding to the middle point and 90 to either extremity. The patient's head is supported on a chin rest; one eye is covered, and the other is fixed on a white spot located at the center of the arc, usually 13 inches distant. The test object, a white or colored disk or spere of varying size, is moved along the inner surface of the arc on an attached black movable carrier or on the end of a black rod. If the visual acuity is normal, an object 3 mm. or smaller is used; if vision is poor, a larger test object is substituted. The point at which the test object is first seen in each principal meridian is marked (automatically or by hand) upon a diagram of the normal field; a line connecting these points forms the boundary of the field.

The Extent of the Normal Form Field with a 3-mm. white test object at the usual distance of ⅓ meter is: outward, 90° (or more); upward, 55°; inward, 60°; downward, 70° (Fig. 3-6).

The restriction in the field upward and inward is due to interference from the nose and brow, and because the percipient layers of the retina do not extend as far forward on the temporal as on the nasal side.

The limits of the field vary according to the size and color of the test object, the intensity of illumination, contrast between test object and its background, state of adaptation of the eye and co-operation of the patient.

Perimetric readings are conveniently expressed by a fraction, the numerator of which states the size of the test object and the denominator its distance in millimeters; thus 5/330 indicates a 5-mm. test object used at the ordinary perimetric distance, ⅓ meter or 330 mm.

Pathologic Alterations in the Field of Vision consist of *limitation* and *defects*. Limitations may assume the form of contraction evenly in all directions (*concentric*), *irregular* contraction, or loss of part of the field on *one side* or the other.

Concentric contraction affects all parts of the periphery alike; when considerable, nothing but central vision may remain (Fig. 11-7); such contraction with preservation of good central visual function is met with, for instance, in retinitis pigmentosa. The contraction may affect only or especially one side of the periphery, for example, temporal or nasal contraction or upper or lower contraction. When one-half of the field is absent (Fig. 11-8), this constitutes *hemianopsia*. *Sector-shaped* contractions sometimes exist; the defect then has the shape of a triangle with a peripheral base. Certain affections produce characteristic contraction of the visual field; for instance, in atrophy of the optic nerve the contraction is concentric; in glaucoma it is usually greatest on the nasal side.

A scotoma is a defect within the visual field. A physiologic scotoma is the *blind spot* situated about 15° to the outside of the point of fixation, corresponding to the entrance of the optic nerve (the *black spot* in Fig. 3-6). According to their situations, scotomas are classified as central, paracentral, ring and peripheral. A *central scotoma* corresponds to the point of fixation (Figs. 11-1 and 11-2); when intense, it interferes with or abolishes central vision altogether; the scotoma accompanying hemorrhage at the macula furnishes an example. A *paracentral scotoma* is situated near the point of fixation, and a *ring or annular scotoma* encircles this point. *Peripheral scotomas* cause little disturbance of sight and may exist without the patient's knowledge, especially when situated far from the point of fixation; disseminated choroiditis furnishes examples of scotomas of this sort (Fig. 9-5).

Scotomas may be *positive*, when the patient sees them as black spots in his field, or *negative*, when they exist as defects in the visual field but are not perceived by the patient until the visual field is examined. Positive scotomas are due to changes in the media or in the retina. If the opacities exist in the vitreous, scotomas may be *motile*; muscae volitantes illustrate a defect of this sort. Negative scotomas may be *absolute*, when perception of light is entirely lost over the defective area, or *relative*, when there is only diminished perception of light or loss of perception of certain colors over this area. Toxic amblyopia gives an example of a scotoma which is central, relative and often negative.

For the detection of central and paracentral defects in the field within a radius of 30° and for estimating the size of the blind spot, 2-mm. white and colored test objects are used and the examination is conducted with a flat surface, in contradisinction to the perimeter arc. For this purpose the Bjerrum tangent screen or some modification such as the campimeter

is used. These instruments are known as *scotometers.*

The tangent screen consists of a large black curtain supported by a framework (Fig. 3-7). The patient is seated at a distance of 1 to 2 meters in front of the screen with his head supported so his eyes are level with the center of the screen. With one eye occluded, the patient fixes the other upon a white spot in the center of the screen. The test object, usually a 1- to 3-mm. white ball on the end of a long thin black rod, is moved from the periphery toward the center to determine the peripheral limits of the visual field. The target then is moved about systematically within these limits in an effort to locate defects in the field. If one or more are located, they are mapped by moving the target from the "blind" to the visible area marking the limits of the defect. Ordinarily the examination is made with the patient 1 meter away from the screen but the 2-meter distance between the eyes and the screen furnishes a larger projection of the defect and thus makes possible its early detection.

The campimeter slate supplies another method of outlining the blind spot and other scotomas.

THE COLOR SENSE

The color sense as a whole (*i.e.,* the faculty of distinguishing different colors) is investigated by a variety of methods. *Central perception of color* is tested by the use of color plates or the exhibition of samples of colored wool. *Peripheral perception of color* is tested by small objects, such as small colored disks 1 to 5 mm. in diameter, which are moved from the periphery toward the center, on the perimeter, the tangent screen or the campimeter (Fig. 3-6).

Tests for Central Color Perception are particularly useful in the examination

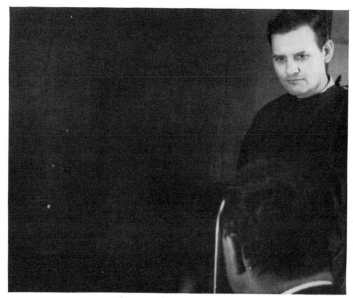

FIG. 3-7. Bjerrum tangent screen in use.

of employees in certain occupations in which perfect color perception is essential. This is important in railway, steamship and aviation services, as well as in automobile and truck driving, since the most commonly used signals are red and green, the colors in which most color-blind persons are defective.

Holmgren's test is used frequently and is convenient. It employs a large assortment of colored worsteds. This collection consists of (1) certain colors called *"test colors"* (a pale *green*, a light *pink* and a bright *red*), (2) lighter tints and darker shades of these colors (*"match colors"*) and (3) *"confusion colors"* (yellow, brown, gray, drab, fawn, mauve, pale blue, etc.), hues which experience has shown the color-blind individual will select as matching the test colors, but which appear entirely different to the normal eye. The test must be made in good daylight.

The pale green sample is given to the individual and he is required to select colors which match it; if he does this correctly, he has normal color sense. If he selects not only similar colors but also confusion colors, and in addition shows a certain hesitancy, his color sense is defective. Next a pink skein is selected and the person examined is asked to match this. If besides similar skeins he also selects blue or violet, he is *red-blind;* if he selects green or gray, he is *green-blind.* Finally, the bright red test skein is given to the individual for matching. If besides reds he chooses green and brown colors darker than the red, he is *red-blind;* if he selects shades of those colors lighter than the red, he is *green-blind.*

Stilling's test, Ishihara's test and Dvorine test (Plate 31) consist of plates upon which are figures made up of dots of the primary colors printed on a background of similar dots in confusion colors. While the figures composed of the primary colors are seen readily by a normal person, they are indistinguishable to the color-blind individual; this indicates color defect. The type of defect is determined by the plates on which he failed.

Other types of *polychromatic plates* (Rabkin, Hardy-Rand-Rittler) are valuable in screening individuals with defective color vision from normal observers, and in the diagnosis of the type and extent of the deficiency.

Color test lanterns often are used in the examination of railroad and steamship employees; colored disks are slid in front of an aperture in the lantern and smoked glass can be placed over these so as to imitate the appearance of signal lights under all conditions of weather and atmosphere.

The *anomaloscope* also is employed for testing the color sense.

The Field for Colors is smaller than that for white, but has the same general shape. It varies for different colors; that for blue is the largest, next comes red, while green has the smallest field. In rough dimensions the field for blue is 10° smaller than that for white; red 10° less than that for blue; and green contracted 10° as compared to red. The limits (given in Fig. 3-6) correspond to the points at which the *colors are recognized*, not to those points at which merely a moving object is perceived. The extent of the field for colors is influenced by the size, brightness and saturation of the test object as well as by the conditions affecting the limits of the form field.

Examination of the color fields is of considerable importance, since contraction of the field for colors frequently exists at an earlier period than that for white. It is a more delicate test. But one must not place too much dependence upon the accuracy of color fields, since the limits are rendered somewhat inconclusive by the fact that between the point at which the color is recognized and the point at which it disappears completely, there is a gap in which it appears modified in color or gray; with dull patients the estimation of the color fields is particularly unsatisfactory. On account of this unreliability of the estimation of color fields, many examiners find that more accurate results are obtained, when a limited restriction of field of vision is detected, by the use of minute white test objects (1 mm.) upon the tangent screen or perimeter.

THE LIGHT SENSE

The light sense is the ability to perceive gradations in intensity of illumination (brightness) and is tested by determining the lowest limit of illumination with which an object is still visible (*light minimum*), or the smallest difference in illumination which can be appreciated (*light difference*).

The accommodation of the sensitivity of the retina to the intensity of light is known as *adaptation*. In passing from a brightly lighted room to darkness, vision is much reduced at first; then the sensitivity of the eye to small intensities of light increases, usually reaching its maximum after 30 minutes; this adjustment is known as *dark adaptation*. It is measured by determining the minimum intensity of a small area of light which is just perceptible, after different time intervals, when all other light is excluded.

Conversely, when the eye is exposed to bright light, after having been kept in the dark, there is dazzling interference with vision; the adjustment which gradually diminishes this effect is known as *light adaptation*.

The estimation of dark adaptation is of practical value in occupations such as railway and steamship services, aeronautics and night driving. Defective dark adaptation is found in vitamin A deficiency, in some diseases of the retina and optic nerve and in glaucoma; severe reduction, constituting night blindness, is present in pigmentary degeneration of the retina (retinitis pigmentosa).

Tests for defective light sense, usually the estimation of dark adaptation by means of a special apparatus (adaptometer), do not form part of the generally employed routine examination of the visual function, such tests being indicated only in special cases.

4

The Lids

Anatomy and Physiology

The eyelids consist of movable folds formed, from before backward, of skin, loose connective tissue, muscular tissue, tarsus and fascia, and conjunctiva (Fig. 4-1). In addition, they present eyelashes, numerous glands, blood vessels, lymphatics and nerves.

The *skin* is thin and delicate, and joined to the subjacent muscles by loose areolar tissue. These characteristics explain the readiness with which extravasations of blood and edematous swellings occur in this region.

The *margin* of each lid presents a rounded anterior lip from which the *eyelashes* (cilia) spring; these form two or three rows of short, thick, curved hairs, their roots deeply embedded in the connective tissue and muscle; they are provided with sebaceous glands, known as glands of Zeis. In this situation also are modified sweat glands, the glands of Moll, which open into the hair follicles of the cilia, into the duct of a Zeis gland or on to the surface of the lid margin. The posterior border of the lid margin is a sharp lip, directly in front of which are the openings of the Meibomian glands. The surface between these two lips is known as the *intermarginal space*. The margins of the lids unite at an acute angle externally (*external canthus*). At the *internal canthus* the junction presents a rounded space which is occupied by a small, reddish elevation of modified skin, the *caruncle*.

In and behind the subcutaneous connective tissue are the *muscles* of the eyelids. The *levator palpebrae* is attached to the upper border and anterior surface of the tarsus and to the skin of the middle of the upper lid. The *orbicularis* muscle lies between tarsus and integument, being attached to the latter, but gliding loosely over the former; it forms a flat circle which surrounds the palpebral aperture; its function is to close the lids. A layer of unstriped muscular tissue also inserted into the proximal margins of the tarsal plates is known as the *palpebral involuntary muscle* (Müller's muscle).

The *tarsus* consists of a thin plate of dense fibrous tissue, giving to each lid its firmness; it is larger in the upper than in the lower lid. The tarsi are connected with the lateral walls of the orbit by means of the internal and external *tarsal ligaments*, and to the upper and lower margins by an aponeurotic layer of fibrous tissue known as the *palpebral* or *tarso-orbital fascia* or ligament. In the substance of the tarsus, occurring in parallel rows, are found the *Meibomian glands*, 30 to 40 in the upper and 20 to 30 in the lower lid. These are elongated sebaceous glands with blind extremities and numerous cecal appendages, filled with fatty secretion and opening on the free margin of the lid.

The palpebral *conjunctiva* is thin, vascular and closely adherent to the tarsus.

The *arteries* are derived from the ophthalmic and the facial; in the upper lid they form a superior arch running along the upper tarsal margin, and an inferior arch placed near the free border of the lid; in the lower lid there is merely one arch near the free edge. The *veins* empty into the ophthalmic, temporal and facial.

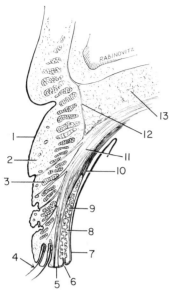

FIG. 4-1. Longitudinal section of the upper eyelid. *1.* Skin; *2,* areolar connective tissue; *3,* orbicularis muscle; *4,* cilia; *5,* white line of intermarginal space of lids; *6,* orifice of Meibomian gland; *7,* conjunctiva; *8,* tarsus; *9,* Meibomian gland; *10,* Müller's muscle. *11,* levator palpebrae superioris; *12,* orbital septum; *13,* orbital fat.

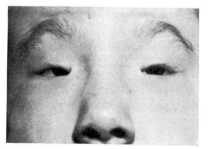

FIG. 4-2. Epicanthus and congenital ptosis.

The *lymphatics* pass to the preauricular, submaxillary and parotid lymphatic glands. The *third cranial nerve* supplies the levator, the *seventh (facial)* the orbicularis, and the *sympathetic* the palpebral involuntary muscles. The sensory supply is derived from the *fifth* nerve.

The lids *protect the eyes* from external injury, foreign bodies, undue exposure and excessive light. They serve to distribute the tears and the secretions from the various glands, thus lubricating the eyeball, keeping the surface of the cornea moist and transparent and washing away any dust which may have found its way into the eye.

Congenital Anomalies of the Lids

These include coloboma, epicanthus, distichiasis and ptosis.

Coloboma of the Lid is a triangular *notching* of the lid margin with absence of the lashes and glands in the affected area. The defect varies in extent and usually is situated at the junction of the inner and middle third of the upper lid. Damage to the cornea may result from exposure. Operative correction is necessary when the defect is extensive.

Epicanthus is a congenital condition, sometimes associated with ptosis, usually bilateral, in which a perpendicular fold of the skin extends from the root of the nose to the inner end of the brow, concealing the inner canthus and caruncle (Fig. 4-2). In Mongolians it is a racial characteristic. In slight degree it is seen in young children in association with a flattened bridge of the nose, often giving the appearance of convergent strabismus; it usually disappears with the development of the face. When sufficiently prominent to be a deformity, it can be relieved by operation.

Ptosis is a drooping of the upper lid caused by weakness or absence of the levator muscle. Congenital ptosis usually is bilateral and frequently is associated with paralysis of the superior rectus muscle. The condition is discussed more fully later.

The rare congenital anomalies include: *ablepharia*, absence of the eyelids; *ankyloblepharon*, partial or complete adhesion of the lids; *blepharophimosis* or blepharostenosis, a decrease in the size of the palpebral fissure, frequently familial and associated with epicanthus and ptosis; *cryptophthalmos*, absence of the palpebral fissure and usually accompanied by an underlying rudimentary eyeball; *distichiasis*, the presence of two rows of lashes, one of which usually is turned toward the cornea; *ectropion*, an outward turning of the margin of the lids; *entropion*, an inturning of the lid margins; *epitarsus*, a conjunctival fold running from the fornix to the lid margin; *microblepharia*, small eyelids; *symblepharon*, adhesions between the inner surface of the lid and the eyeball.

BLEPHARITIS

Hyperemia of the intermarginal space of the lids occurs frequently, especially in light-complected individuals and in persons suffering from ocular fatigue and loss of sleep. In addition, a number of other factors play contributing roles, such as dietary deficiencies; exposure to dust, smoke or other irritating atmospheres; general debility; general diseases and diseases of neighboring structures. In most of these, infection is not a factor so therapy must be directed toward finding and eliminating the source of the irritation. Local therapy should consist of hot and cold compresses and avoiding irritating topical medications, especially antibiotics, since infection seldom is a factor. In those instances in which hyperemia is simply a remission phase of a recurrent infectious process, other signs usually are present and a history will help in making the proper diagnosis.

Blepharitis marginalis or ciliaris is a common chronic inflammation of the intermarginal space of the lids which may consist only of reddening or thickening of the lid margins or, in its severest form, may include crust-covered ulcers of the lid margins with extension of the inflammatory process onto the skin and conjunctival surfaces of the lids associated with corneal complications. Several clinical forms of the disease have been described: *blepharitis oleosa* is an oily encrustation of the lid margins without ulceration; *blepharitis squamosa* is a dry encrustation of the lid margins by white or yellowish scales unaccompanied by ulceration; *blepharitis ulcerosa* is a yellowish encrustation with underlying ulcers of the lid margin; and *blepharitis angularis* is an inflammation of the lid margins associated with excoriations of the skin of the lateral and medial canthi.

Etiology. Blepharitis marginalis of the oleosa type is a part of the involvement of seborrheic dermatitis, whereas squamous and ulcerative blepharitis are usually due to staphylococcic infection, although frequently the staphylococcic infection is superimposed upon seborrheic blepharitis and rarely other bacteria may cause the disease. Blepharitis angularis typically is caused by infection of the lid margins by the Morax-Axenfeld bacillus, but it also may be caused by staphylococcic infection. In all cases, predisposing and ancillary factors play a contributing role in the development, maintenance or recurrence of blepharitis marginalis. These factors include all of those mentioned under hyperemia of the lid margins and, in addition, the exanthematous diseases, upper respiratory infections and parasitic infestation of the lashes (*phthiriasis palpebrarum*).

Seborrheic Blepharitis is characterized by mild hyperemia of the lid margins associated with grayish white, oily encrustations of the lashes and lid margins. Involvement of the lid margins is secondary to seborrheic dermatitis of the scalp (dandruff) and brow or face. Exacerbations and remissions of the ocular lesions parallel those of the lesion of the scalp.

Usually the ocular lesion is mild but, rarely, in severe exacerbations the lid margins show great redness and swelling associated with conjunctivitis and marginal corneal ulceration and infiltration. However, in most instances of this severe type of exacerbation there is a superimposed staphylococcic infection.

Treatment should be directed primarily toward control or elimination of the seborrheic dermatitis, for this is the only way in which the lid lesion can be eliminated. However, temporary improvement of the blepharitis may be obtained by mechanical cleansing of the lid margins followed by the application of an ointment containing 3 per cent ammoniated mercury. The patient can be instructed to do this for himself. In more obstinate lesions the physician should remove the crusts and apply an ointment of selenium oxide to the lid margins, being careful to prevent it from coming in contact with the conjunctiva and cornea and removing it after 2 minutes. This may be done daily if necessary in conjunction with ammoniated mercury ointment treatment by the patient at home.

Staphylococcic Blepharitis is a chronic and prolonged infection of the margins and glands of the lids by pathogenic staphylococci and is characterized by remissions and exacerbations. The process frequently begins in childhood and persists indefinitely. In the least active phases, the lid margins are slightly reddened and thickened (Plate 7-C), but with increased activity yellowish crusts form on the lid margins and become tightly adherent to the base of the lashes. In more severe lesions ulcers form on the lid margins under the crusts, and cracks and excoriations develop on the skin adjacent to the lid margins and at the canthi. Conjunctivitis, of some degree, always is associated with staphylococcic blepharitis (see Chap. 6). In the remissions, the conjunctiva is slightly hyperemic, especially over the lower lid and caruncle, but during exacerbations the entire conjunctiva is inflamed with the production of a mucopurulent or purulent discharge which may clot the lashes together during sleep, making it difficult to open the eyes on awakening. The cornea also may be involved in exacerbations by punctate epithelial erosions over the lower portion or by marginal ulcers.

The disease persists and runs its fluctuating course because of persistent infection of the glands of the lids, which usually is manifest as chronic inflammation but at times as acute abscesses of the Meibomian glands or the glands of the hair follicles. As a result, lashes are lost by destruction of the hair follicles, or at times the follicles are disturbed so the lashes are stunted and misdirected, sometimes rubbing and causing injury to the cornea.

Treatment should be directed toward elimination of the infection, especially the residual infection in the glands. The crusts are removed from the lid margins after warm, wet applications have softened them. The glands of the lids are expressed by gentle pressure and after the margins are cleansed, antibacterial agents may be applied. This treatment may be repeated by the physician daily or less frequently, but supplementary home treatment also is required. The patient is instructed to use hot, wet compresses for 15 minutes, three or four times a day, and is given a viscous solution of sodium sulfacetamide to use 1 drop in each eye every hour during the day, in the beginning. In more severe or complicated situations, one of the sulfonamides or an antibiotic which has been proven to be effective against the specific strain of staphylococci isolated from the patient may be given parenterally in addition to the local treatment. In situations in which periodic exacerbations occur in spite of such treatment, immunization with staphylococcus toxoid and vaccine mixtures (vatox) is of value in controlling the signs and symptoms of the inflammation.

Mixed Blepharitis, in which staphylococcic infection is superimposed upon seborrheic blepharitis, is encountered frequently. The signs and symptoms vary, depending somewhat upon which factor is most significant at the moment, but usually the staphylococcic is more evident; therefore, in general, treatment is directed against the seborrhea of the scalp and face and against the staphylococcic aspect of the blepharitis.

Blepharitis Angularis is characterized by reddened lid margins with cracks or excoriations of the skin of the lids at the external canthi and frequently at the medial canthi as well. A slight, foamy discharge or at times a slight mucoid discharge, or both, may cover part of the lid margins and the excoriations. Classically this lesion is caused by Morax-Axenfeld bacillus infection, but it also may be produced by staphylococcic infection; therefore an exact causative diagnosis requires the examination of cultures and scrapings made from the lesions.

The Morax-Axenfeld type of infection occurs most frequently in hot dry climates, and its treatment consists of the application of 0.5 per cent zinc sulfate ointment or 10 per cent sodium sulfacetamide ointment to the lid margins four times a day. A minimum of 1 month of treatment is required to eliminate the infection.

Sequelae occur especially in the staphylococcic form. There may be conjunctivitis, styes, permanent *loss of a greater or lesser number of lashes*, hypertrophy of the lid margin, trichiasis and ectropion.

The disfigurement is often an important symptom. After a long continued course there may be hypertrophy of the lid border, causing this part to become rounded and thick and to droop on account of its own weight, a condition which affects principally the upper lid, gives rise to a dull sleepy appearance and is known as *tylosis*. After a lengthy course all lashes may be lost except a few scattered fine ones, a condition to which the name *madarosis* is applied.

Edema of the Lids

This is a common symptom, favored by the structure of these parts. It may be (1) *inflammatory*, accompanying affections of the lids and adjacent parts, such as styes, dacryocystitis and infections of the orbit or the nasal accessory sinuses; it may be one of the signs of severe inflammation of the interior of the eye, such as iridocyclitis, acute glaucoma or panophthalmitis; (2) *traumatic* when due to injuries, including the sting of insects; (3) *systemic*, in renal, thyroid and cardiac disease and in trichinosis; and (4) *noninflammatory*, such as angioneurotic or allergic edema (Fig. 4-3).

Angioneurotic edema of the lids is a rapidly developing, recurrent swelling, frequently severe enough to close the lids. It is not accompanied by changes in the eyes and it disappears almost as quickly as it appears but causes much alarm to the patient. It is allied to urticaria and occurs most frequently in women, espe-

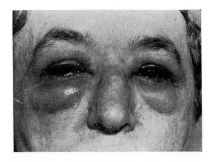

FIG. 4-3. Allergic edema of eyelids from sensitivity to a local anesthetic.

cially at the time of the menstrual period. Food is the most important causative factor and includes seasonal fruits, vegetables, shellfish, nuts, chocolate, eggs, wheat, milk and its products, pork and onions. Drugs frequently are responsible for chronic allergic edema of the lids; these include the antibiotics, especially penicillin and streptomycin; aspirin; barbiturates; phenolphthalein; bromides; acetopheneti- dine and injectants such as liver extracts, endocrine substances and foreign serums. In some instances angioneurotic edema is related to psychogenic factors. Cold compresses, applied for 10 minutes every hour or alternating every 10 minutes with hot compresses, usually decrease the edema temporarily. The use of a saline cathartic and sodium bicarbonate by mouth as well as avoidance of the allergens, when known, also are recommended. In severe or prolonged urticaria of the lid, topical or parenteral steroid therapy may be necessary.

Eczema is a nonspecific lesion characterized by vesicles, cracks and excoriations in a thin parchment-paper-like skin. It occurs in a variety of circumstances such as allergic and contact dermatitis, infectious dermatitis, dermatomycoses and localized neurodermatitis, any of which may affect the skin of the lids.

Contact dermatitis of the skin of the lids is a moist edematous eczema in the acute phase but may become dry in the chronic stage. Most frequently it is due to local allergic reaction to cosmetics such as fingernail polish, face powder, hair or lash dyes, etc., but almost as frequently drugs are responsible, especially antibiotics, atropine, eserine, topical anesthetics, etc. It also may be due to a variety of other agents, including poison ivy, primrose, oleander and a number of essential oils. Treatment consists of palliative measures such as cold compresses, and the topical or general administration of

steroids until the cause can be determined and eliminated.

A similar type of vesicular dermatitis is produced by the "id" reactions of allergy to bacteria, yeasts, fungi and their products. Elimination of the infectious process, which usually is a distant focus such as "athlete's foot," controls the lid lesion.

Atopic dermatitis, an hereditary eczema of the skin, frequently involves the lids and occasionally the cornea. Cataracts also occur during childhood in this disease and frequently require extraction during the second or third decade of life.

HORDEOLUM OR STYE

A stye is a circumscribed, acute inflammation at the edge of the lid, caused by *staphylococcus infection* of the glands of Zeis or of Moll, usually ending in suppuration.

Symptoms. A red *swelling* (Plate 7A) appears in the lash line of the *margin of the lid,* accompanied by pain, tenderness and often by considerable edema, especially when the stye is situated at the angles of the lids. Very soon a *yellowish summit* will be seen, indicating suppuration.

Etiology. Styes occur at all ages, but are most common in children and young adults. They often appear in *crops* or series. They frequently are associated with blepharitis, or a lowered state of health such as anemia or uncontrolled diabetes mellitus.

Treatment. At first *hot compresses* are indicated to hasten suppuration; as soon as a yellow spot is seen, the pus should be *evacuated* by a horizontal incision; the pain of such an incision is insignificant if a fine sharp knife is used and the incision limited to the yellow spot. To prevent the formation of others, the *general health* should be evaluated, the diet regulated with avoidance of an excess of sweets, anemia treated and tonsils and adenoids investigated. Cod liver oil or viosterol preparations often are indicated. The tendency to recur frequently is checked by treatment of the associated *blepharitis*.

Meibomitis, a fairly common, chronic infection of some of the Meibomian glands, causes red and swollen lid margins, sometimes with foamy secretion upon the conjunctiva; pressure upon the Meibomian ducts expels glairy, yellowish fluid; the disease explains some cases of multiple chalazia and some intractable examples of blepharitis and chronic conjunctivitis. Treatment consists of *expression of the ducts* by pressing the lid between a finger and a lid plate after topical anesthesia of the conjunctiva or by squeezing the lids against each other between the nails of the two thumbs of the surgeon; this is repeated every few days until no fluid can be forced out; at the same time the treatment of accompanying blepharitis is indicated.

CHALAZION

Chalazion is a *quiet chronic granulomatous enlargement* of one of the *Meibomian glands*, in consequence a stoppage of its duct, accompanied by involvement of the surrounding tissues. It occurs most frequently in *adults*. Very often several are found at the same time, and there is some tendency to recurrence in crops.

Symptoms. The process often develops slowly with insignificant or no symptoms until, after weeks or months, it has reached the size of a small or large pea. Then it presents a noticeable, circumscribed *swelling* (Plate 7B) which feels hard and is adherent to the tarsus, but not to the skin. On everting the lid its situation is usually shown by a red or purple (later gray) *discoloration* of the conjunctiva, and occasionally by a small mass of granulation tissue. Infrequently chalazia disappear spontaneously. Some-

times they suppurate (*suppurating chalazion* or *internal hordeolum*, to distinguish them from the more common external hordeolum or stye); this change is accompanied by acute inflammatory symptoms. Occasionally they form in the duct of the Meibomian gland and project from the edge of the lid in the form of a reddish gray nodule (*marginal chalazion*). Chalazia may be annoying either because of *disfigurement* or on account of conjunctival *irritation*.

Pathology. The Meibomian duct becomes obstructed through proliferation of its epithelium, and the surrounding tissues are infiltrated with lymphocytes and fixed connective tissue cells. Much of the gland tissue is replaced by small round cells (granulation tissue) containing giant cells (nontuberculous); the blood supply is cut off by the surrounding fibrous tissue and the contents then undergo degeneration, forming a jelly-like mass, which after longer duration becomes liquefied, the chalazion then forming a pseudocyst with thick fibrous walls.

Treatment. When small, chalazia need not be removed. Occasionally they disappear after applications of antibacterial ointments, followed by *massage* and *hot compresses*. When larger, they must be removed by *operation*, usually through the conjunctiva: The conjunctival sac is anesthetized with a topical anesthetic, the lid everted, the affected spot made prominant, a few drops of Novocain-Adrenalin solution injected, and a *vertical incision* made through the conjunctiva and wall of the chalazion with a small scalpel; the contents (Meibomian secretion, granulation tissue and mucilaginous fluid) are removed and the walls thoroughly *scraped* with a chalazion curette. Following the operation the cavity will be filled with a blood clot; this and the indurated walls cause a continuation of the disfigurement for a short time; absorption may be hastened by gentle massage for a few minutes twice a day.

Occasionally, when more accessible externally with no thinning or discoloration of tarsus to be seen upon everting the lid, the mass may be excised with forceps and curved scissors through a horizontal skin incision, after injecting Novocain-Adrenalin; the mass is encircled by the ring blade of the lid clamp (Fig. 4-4) or the chalazion forceps (Fig. 4-5), which is tightened to secure a bloodless field and to protect the eyeball; the wound is closed with fine silk sutures.

Marginal chalazia are difficult to get rid of except with the thermophore or by electrocoagulation.

LID ABSCESS

Both *abscess* and *furuncle* occur in the lids occasionally and, except for the greater amount of edema of the surrounding tissues, have the usual signs and symptoms.

They must be differentiated from three other inflammatory lesions—stye, acute dacryocystitis and orbital cellulitis. A

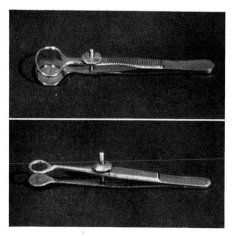

FIG. 4-4 (*upper*). Lid clamp (Desmarres chalazion forceps).
FIG. 4-5 (*lower*). Chalazion forceps (Lambert).

stye occurs only at the lid margin (Plate 7*A*), whereas an abscess or furuncle is located in the skin of the lid. *Acute dacryocystitis*, or inflammation of the lacrimal sac, lies behind the medial canthal ligament and pressure over the inflamed area may cause regurgitation of pus from the puncta, whereas a lid abscess or furuncle in that region lies superficial to but is limited above by the medial canthal ligament and pressure does not produce regurgitation of pus from the puncta. *Orbital cellulitis* produces exophthalmos, limited and painful eye movements and generalized edema of both lids, none of which occurs in lid abscess or furuncle.

Treatment of lid abscess or furuncle is application of heat to produce localization and fluctuation, then surgical drainage.

Eczema is a nonspecific lesion characterized by vesicles, cracks and excoriations arising in a thin parchment-paper-like skin. It occurs in a variety of circumstances, such as allergic and contact dermatitis, infectious dermatitis, dermatomycosis and localized neurodermatitis, any of which may affect the skin of the lids.

Erysipelas, an acute infection of the skin caused by any of several different types of group A hemolytic streptococci, is characterized by a glossy red, swollen, sharply demarcated patch accompanied by fever and malaise. It may occur sporadically as a primary lesion or may complicate other streptococcic diseases such as scarlet fever, otitis media, pharyngitis, membranous conjunctivitis, wound infections or puerperal sepsis. It is most often encountered in elderly or debilitated patients, but usually it responds to penicillin and general supportive therapy.

Gangrene, a severe necrotic lesion, rarely involves the lids but usually follows severe trauma, burns or freezing in debilitated or inebriated individuals. More rarely it may follow an exanthematous disease, *herpes zoster*, erysipelas, anthrax and diphtheritic conjunctivitis, but again usually in complicated circumstances such as superimposed trauma and superimposed infections. Treatment is directed against the infectious cause or causes while general supportive measures also are administered.

Anthrax, a highly infectious disease of warm-blooded animals, caused by *Bacillus anthracis,* is transmitted directly or indirectly to man. It is most prevalent in Europe and Asia but outbreaks in animals occur infrequently in the United States, and a small number of human cases arising from industrial uses of hides, wool and other animal products develop each year.

Involvement of the skin of the face and lids may occur without a macroscopic break in the skin. It occurs in the form of a malignant "pustule" or malignant edema.

The malignant pustule begins as a painless papulovesicular lesion which rapidly becomes hemorrhagic, ruptures and produces a deep ulcer which turns black and is surrounded by a brawny edema. Occasionally several lesions may coalesce to form a large irregular ulcer, and satellite lesions are not unusual. Regional lymphadenopathy, which may be painful and associated with inflammation of the surrounding tissues, develops early.

Malignant edema develops rapidly, involving the lids of both eyes, the face, the head and at times the neck and thorax. Multiple vesicles containing serosanguineous fluid soon develop, ulcerate and form ulcers with undermined bluish red edges.

If untreated, septicemia and death may follow either type of lesion. However 300,000 to 3,000,000 units of depot penicillin intramuscularly once or twice daily in association with 1 gm. of one of the sulfonamides orally every 4 to 6 hours and general supportive measures usually is followed by healing within 1 to 2 weeks.

Tuberculosis. The lids may be involved by a variety of clinical types of tuberculous lesions rarely, but the most common of these is *lupus vulgaris.* It can occur in any part of the skin but the face is the usual site. The primary lesion is a soft translucent brownish tubercle, the "apple butter" nodule surrounded by an erythematous base. Several of these lesions appear in childhood, slowly progress and extend into the lids as new nodules develop around the periphery. Ulceration and healing occur, but the process extends over many years with varying amounts of activity resulting in extensive tissue destruction and scarring. Ultimately all four lids may be destroyed with severe injury of the globes. In addition to the usual treatment of tuberculosis with isoniazid, *p*-aminosalicylic acid and streptomycin, vitamin D is beneficial in *lupus vulgaris.*

Syphilis of the Lids is occasionally seen as a primary sore, in the secondary stage or in the form of gummas. *Chancre* having the same characteristics as when found elsewhere occurs upon the lid margin, usually near the inner canthus, accompanied by enlargement of the preauricular and submaxillary lymph glands; it might be mistaken for stye, suppurating chalazion, dacryocystitis, vaccinia or epithelioma.

Tarsitis is a rare form of chronic inflammation, usually syphilitic (tertiary, gummatous infiltration of the tarsus), though it may be tuberculous or trachomatous, in which the lid is much thickened and its skin tense and reddened.

Phthiriasis Palpebrarum is an uncommon affection, usually found in children, in which the lashes are covered with the nits (Fig. 4-6) of the crab louse (*Pediculus pubis* or *capitis*). There are redness and itching of lid margins. The

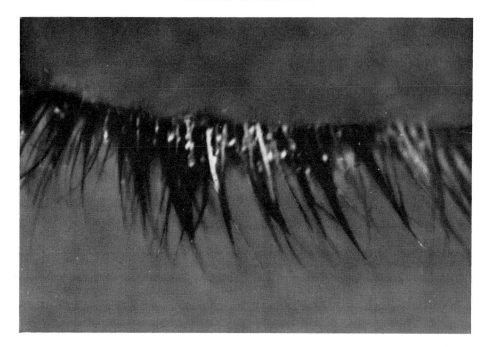

FIG. 4-6. Phthiriasis palpebrarum (pediculosis capitis), involving the lashes.

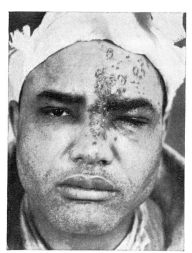

FIG. 4-7. Herpes zoster ophthalmicus.

parasites are destroyed with 3 per cent ointment of ammoniated mercury applied four times a day for 1 week. Other areas of infestation must be treated simultaneously.

Herpes Febrilis sometimes forms on the lids as well as on the lips and alae of the nose in the course of febrile affections, especially of the respiratory tract. Small vesicles, arising from a slightly reddened base, occur in groups, dry and heal in a few days without scarring. They may be associated with dendritic keratitis.

Herpes Zoster Ophthalmicus, a virus infection of the Gasserian ganglion or the trunk of the trigeminus, is characterized by a unilateral vesicular eruption sharply limited by the distribution of the second (ophthalmic) and frequently the first division of the fifth cranial nerve (Fig. 4-7). It rarely affects the third division. It begins with severe neuralgic *pain* on one side of the head and face, followed after several days by an eruption of *vesicles* upon inflamed bases. The vesicles at first are filled with clear fluid, but this soon becomes cloudy; then discolored crusts form and drop off, leaving permanent and disfiguring *scars*. The involved skin becomes red and swollen and this may be mistaken for erysipelas. In some cases the nasal branch also is attacked and then the eyeball becomes implicated; in such cases the cornea becomes insensitive and presents vesicles changing to ulcers, or there may be diffuse deep infiltration with involvement of the iris and ciliary body, leading to a serious ocular condition. It is most frequently observed in elderly, feeble patients but also may affect young adults occasionally, and children rarely. Its duration is from 3 weeks to several months. The *prognosis* usually is good, but is serious when the cornea and deeper parts are involved.

Treatment. At first *cooling* lotions are used; after vesicles have appeared, *bland dusting powders* (talcum, zinc oxide) or zinc oxide ointment with or without 10 per cent Ichthyol. For severe pain, sedatives; intramuscular injection of 0.5 to 1 cc. of Pituitrin, once or twice at 48-hour intervals, often relieves the pain. Steroids given after the acute phase have shortened the probable period of disability in some cases. If the eyeball is involved, treatment of corneal ulcer or iritis is indicated (see Chap. 7).

MOLLUSCUM CONTAGIOSUM

Molluscum Contagiosum, a virus infection of the skin, is characterized by the production of firm, flat-topped or umbilicated papillae arising from normal skin. A waxy material may be squeezed out of the papillus, or occasionally the lesion may rupture spontaneously and heal without scarring. The hypertrophic little tumors involve the skin, particularly of the chest, and sometimes the face and lids. When the tumor involves the intermarginal space of the lids, it is accompanied by chronic conjunctivitis and at times marginal keratitis, resulting in superficial vascularization of the cornea. The conjunctivitis and keratitis resist all efforts at treatment except removal of

the tumor. Microscopically the epithelial layers in the center of the tumor are greatly increased in number and the hypertrophied cells contain basophilic inclusion bodies (Fig. 4-8).

VERRUCA

Verruca, another virus-induced wart of the skin, may involve the skin of the lids and the intermarginal space of the lids. In the latter location they may produce chronic conjunctivitis and occasionally keratitis similar to that associated with *molluscum contagiosum*. The tumors are small, threadlike papillae (*verruca filiformis*), irregularly rounded elevations (*verruca vulgaris*), multiple filiform or dentate projections from a common base (*verruca digitala*) or irregular relatively flat warts (*verruca plana*). Inclusion bodies may be demonstrated in prickle cells on microscopic examination of sections. The tumors should be excised.

Vaccinia of the Lids occurs infrequently as the result of accidental inoculation, transfer of the virus from an inoculation, transfer of the virus from an inoculation site to the lids by the patient's fingers or as a result of localization of the virus in a pre-existing break in the skin during the period of viremia 2 to 6 days following vaccination. The lesion on the lid undergoes the same evolution and resolution as a primary inoculation, vesicle, pustule, crust and scar. The lesion usually affects the lower lid but sometimes both, and occasionally it involves the lid margin, endangering the cornea with ulceration, scarring and loss of vision. The lid usually is swollen and reddened around the lesion and, always, there is an associated lymphadenopathy of either the preauricular or the submaxillary lymph node or both.

TRICHIASIS

Trichiasis is an *inversion* of a varying number of *lashes,* so that they rub against

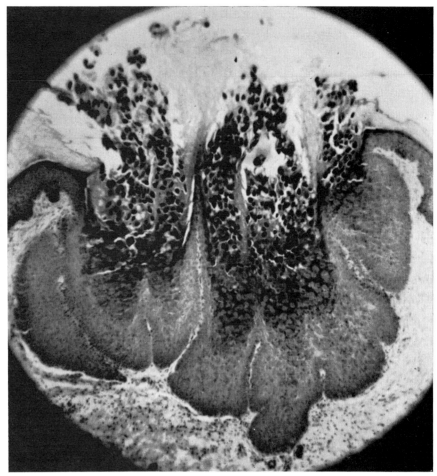

Fig. 4-8. Molloscum contagiosum. Section showing hyperplasia of epithelium and inclusion bodies in epithelial cells.

the cornea (Figs. 4-9, *second from left,* and 4-10). The margin of the lid may have a normal position, the displacement affecting only the lashes, or the margin may be turned inward as well as the lashes at times.

Symptoms. The misdirected lashes cause *mechanical irritation* and *injury to the cornea,* with ulceration, congestion, pain, lacrimation, photophobia, opacities and vascularization.

Etiology. The most frequent cause is *cicatricial contraction* of the conjunctiva and tarsus in old cases of *trachoma.* Other causes are blepharitis, burns, injuries to the lids and operation upon the lids.

Treatment. *Epilation.* When the misdirected lashes are few in number, they may be epilated with the cilia forceps, repeating this every few weeks, since the lashes grow again. The misdirected lashes are sometimes normal but often very fine, short, and of a pale color, and therefore not easily detected.

Electrolysis cures permanently. After Novocain infiltration of the lid margin, the sponge electrode of the positive pole is applied to the temple, and a fine platinum needle, corresponding to the negative pole, is introduced into the hair follicle; a weak galvanic current (2 milliamperes) is used. *Electrocoagulation* (diathermy) is equally effective and, after Novocain injection, painless.

Operation. When a great number or all of the lashes are misdirected, operations must be performed. These have for their object *correction of the faulty position* or *transplantation of the lashes.* Since trichiasis is frequently associated with entropion, these operations will be considered in connection with the latter disease.

ENTROPION

Entropion is *a rolling in of the margin of the lid* (and with it the lashes) (Figs. 4-9, *second from right,* and 4-10).

Varieties. There are two forms: (1)

cicatricial, due to cicatricial changes in the conjunctiva and tarsus, most commonly affecting the *upper lid,* and (2) *spastic,* due to spasm of the palpebral portion of the orbicularis muscle, most always occurring in the *lower lid* (Fig. 4-10). The second variety generally is found in old persons (*senile entropion*), who are predisposed through relaxation of the palpebral skin and the deep position of the eyeball resulting from the absence of fat.

Symptoms are due to *mechanical irritation* and *injury to the cornea* and consist of circumcorneal congestion, pain, lacrimation, photophobia, opacities, ulceration and vascularization of the cornea.

Etiology. The principal cause of the *cicatricial form* is the scarring resulting from burns and other injuries to the lids, operations upon the lids and trachoma, whereas the *spastic form* may be due to atrophy or absence of the eyeball, blepharospasm, inflammatory conditions of the lids and conjunctiva or the pro-

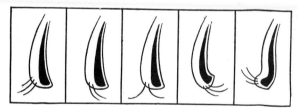

FIG. 4-9. Diagrammatic section of the upper lid, showing normal and abnormal positions of tarsus and lashes. From *left* to *right*: normal lid; trichiasis; distichiasis; entropion; ectropion.

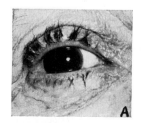
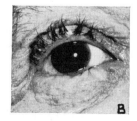

FIG. 4-10. Spastic entropion. *A*, Normal position of lids; *B*, lower lid stays rolled in after eyes are closed forcibly.

longed wearing of an ocular dressing especially in aged patients.

Treatment. *Nonoperative* treatment frequently is important in the spastic variety. Wearing an artificial eye over the stump left after enucleation, or over an atrophic globe (if tolerated), often relieves the symptoms. In other cases the cause should be removed whenever possible. The lid may be kept everted for a few days by *collodion* painted on the external surface, or by *adhesive plaster* passing from the margin of the lid to the cheek. If these simple means do not answer, an *operation* is indicated. In the cicatricial form, operation always is necessary.

Operations for Trichiasis and Entropion

The choice of an operation (there are a great many) is influenced by the peculiarities existing in the individual case.

The object of these operations is to remove the displaced lashes from contact with the eyeball either (1) by *changing the direction* of the lashes from a faulty to a correct one, (2) by *transplanting* the offending zone or (3) by *straightening* the curved tarsus.

In these operations either a plate (Fig. 4-11) or entropion forceps (Fig. 4-12) is used to protect the eyeball, check hemorrhage and give proper support to the lid. The plate is passed beneath the lid and pressed forward. If the entropion forceps are used, the solid blade is passed beneath the lid, and the latter secured by tightening the screw of the instrument. Subcutaneous injection of 2 per cent solution of Novocain in 1:20000 Adrenalin is sufficient to control pain and bleeding in most of these operations; occasionally general anesthesia is required.

The Jaesche-Arlt Operation *shortens the skin of the upper lid* by excision of a

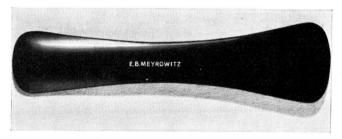

Fig. 4-11. Hard rubber plate.

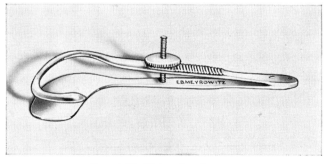

Fig. 4-12. Entropion forceps.

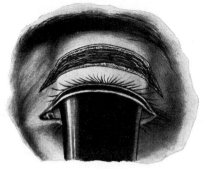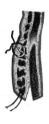

Fig. 4-13. The Jaesche-Arlt operation for entropion. *A (left)*, incisions; *B (right)*, completed.

horizontal strip, detaches the marginal zone of hair follicles and joins this part to the upper border of the skin defect, thus elevating the lashes and tilting them forward away from the cornea.

The lid is split throughout its entire length in the intermarginal space, so that the anterior lip contains the hair follicles. A second incision, dividing the skin down to the tarsus, is made 4 mm. from and parallel to the margin of the lid. A third incision extends upward in a curve between the two ends of the second incision. The elliptical piece of skin bounded by the second and third incisions is dissected away (Fig. 4-13*A*) without injury to the orbicularis, and the margins of the defect are united by fine silk sutures (Fig. 4-13*B*). The area from which the skin and lashes have been displaced may be allowed to cicatrize, or, better, is covered by a strip taken from mucous membrane of the mouth.

Hotz's Operation raises the zone of hair follicles and causes a curving forward of the lashes away from the cornea by *attaching* the lower border of a horizontal *skin* incision to the upper margin of the exposed *tarsus*.

A curved incision is made through the skin of the lid, following the upper border of the tarsus, from 2 mm. above one canthus to a corresponding distance above the other. A narrow strip of orbicularis along the upper border of the tarsus is excised. The sutures, three or more in number, then are passed through the upper wound margin, upper border of tarsus, returning through the orbitotarsal fascia and finally through the lower wound margin (Fig. 4-14*A* and *B*). This operation may be modified by the addition of an intermarginal incision, by grooving the tarsus, by excising a horizontal strip of integument or by removal of a marginal strip of orbicularis after undermining the skin down to the lid margin.

The Streatfield-Snellen Operation aims at straightening the inverted lid by *removal of a wedge-shaped piece from the tarsus*, the apex of the excised portion pointing toward the conjunctiva.

A transverse incision is made through the skin, 2 mm. above and parallel to the margin of the lid along its entire length. A strip of orbicularis and skin is excised, thus exposing the tarsus. A wedge-shaped piece, the apex of which is directed toward the conjunctiva, is removed from the tarsus along its entire length. The cut surfaces of the tarsus are brought into contact by three sutures, as shown in Figure 4-15.

Operations for Spastic (Senile) Entropion include:

(1) *Excision of a horizontal strip of*

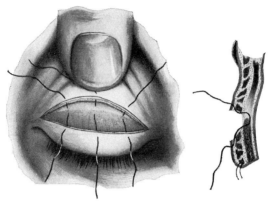

FIG. 4-14. The Hotz operation for entropion. *A* (*left*), front view; *B* (*right*), in section.

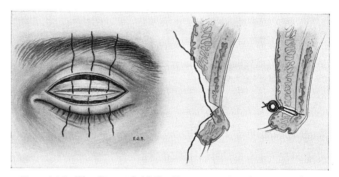

FIG. 4-15. The Streatfield-Snellen operation for entropion.

skin with the underlying orbicularis, the width being gauged so that when pinched up it causes the disappearance of entropion without producing ectropion; the margins of the wound then are united by silk sutures.

(2) *Hotz's operation.*

(3) *Operations upon the orbicularis muscle.* These aim at a tightening of the orbicularis overlying the lower border of the inferior tarsus, thus tending to produce eversion of the lid margin.

(4) *Canthoplasty.*

Canthoplasty consists of a *permanent enlargement of the palpebral fissure* by division of the external canthus. The indications are blepharospasm, spastic entropion and certain cases of trachomatous pannus.

The lids being separated and stretched at the external canthus with the fingers, one blade of blunt-pointed, straight scissors is introduced behind the external commissure as far as possible, and the entire thickness divided, the wound in the skin being made a little longer than that in the conjunctiva. This leaves a rhomboidal wound. The conjunctiva at the apex of the wound is loosened from underlying tissue and stitched to the center of the incision in the skin. A second suture is passed through the upper, and a third through the lower part of the wound, uniting conjunctiva to skin (Fig. 4-16).

Canthotomy is a *temporary enlargement of the palpebral aperture* by division of the external canthus as described in connection with canthoplasty; but since only a temporary effect is desired, sutures are omitted. This operation is indicated in some cases of acute purulent conjunctivitis, occasionally in phlyctenular keratitis and other affections when swelling of the lids exerts injurious pressure upon the eyeball, in blepharospasm, in the removal of an enlarged eyeball or orbital tumor and occasionally as a preliminary step in cataract extraction.

ECTROPION

Ectropion is an *eversion of the lid* with exposure of more or less conjunctival surface (Plate 7*D* and Fig. 4-9, *far right*). It may affect the upper or the lower lid, or both.

Symptoms. *Epiphora* (from eversion of punctum) causes excoriations and eczema of the lower lid, which in turn, through contraction, increase the deformity. The *exposed conjunctiva* becomes reddened and hypertrophied. In severe ectropion the cornea may suffer from exposure and drying as a result of imperfect closure of the lids.

Etiology. (1) *Cicatricial ectropion* is caused by contraction of scar tissue following wounds, operations, burns, ulcers and caries of the orbital margin or surrounding surfaces.

(2) *Mechanical ectropion* is caused by conjunctival hypertrophy from chronic inflammation of the conjunctiva or lid margins or both.

(3) *Senile ectropion* results from relaxation of the skin and orbicularis in old people and affects only the lower lid.

(4) *Paralytic ectropion* also affects only the lower lid, as a result of facial nerve paralysis.

(5) *Spastic ectropion* results from spasmodic contraction of the orbital portion of the orbicularis caused by irritation or swelling of the conjunctiva or staphylomatous lesions of the cornea, especially in children.

Treatment. *Nonoperative:* The spas-

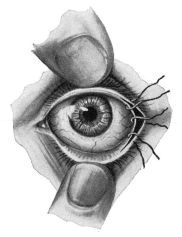

FIG. 4-16. Canthoplasty.

tic form frequently is relieved by a suitable retaining *dressing* applied after the lid has been properly placed. In the paralytic form a dressing may be applied, or a condensation shield (Figs. 4-17 and 4-18) may be used until the facial paralysis is relieved or, if the paralysis is permanent, until surgical correction can be made. In the senile form, during the early phases, a dressing may be applied at night and the patient is instructed to rub upward and inward, not downward and outward, in wiping away tears. In slight ectropion caused by hypertrophy of the conjunctiva, careful application of a superficial cauterizing agent, such as a 1 or 2 per cent solution of silver nitrate, may be of value; but the underlying conjunctivitis or blepharitis also must be treated. When these measures fail and in cicatricial ectropion, surgical correction is necessary.

Operations for Ectropion

In *senile and paralytic* forms of ectropion the lid may be replaced by (1) reduction of the length of the lid border and (2) tarsorrhaphy.

Shortening the Margin of the Lid, applicable when there is considerable elongation, may be produced by one of

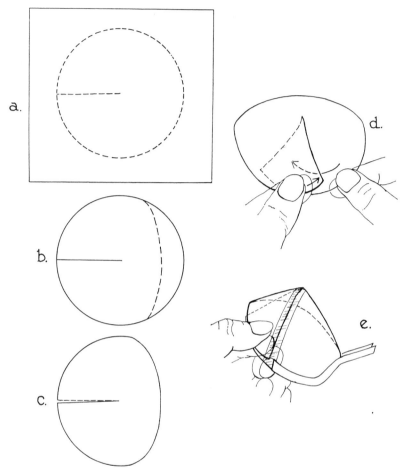

Fig. 4-17. Steps in preparation of a condensation shield. *a*, Outline of shield on transparent plastic or clear x-ray film; *b*, circular shield cut (3.5 inches in diameter), with *dotted line* indicating part to be removed for better fit against nose; *c*, plastic film ready to be folded to form conical shield as is being done in *d*; *e*, the edges of the cone are covered by adhesive tape.

several methods. A useful procedure of this type, *the Kuhnt-Szymanowski operation*, consists of the removal of a wedge-shaped piece from the posterior portion of the split lid, and a shortening of the anterior portion, together with excision of the cilia at the outer end of the lid (Figs. 4-19 and 4-20).

For *cicatricial ectropion* a great many operative procedures have been advo-cated. An essential condition for success is the thorough division of all cicatricial adhesions, so that the lid assumes a natural position, the object being to prevent recicatrization. If the ectropion is slight and but little skin has been lost, it may be sufficient to divide the cicatricial bands subcutaneously, or to cut out the scar and bring the margins of the wound together by sutures. In more extensive cicatricial ectropion a *reconstructive operation* (blepharoplasty) usually is required.

Blepharoplasty consists of covering the defect, formed by excision of a cicatrix, new growth or extensive ulceration, with *skin flaps with a pedicle*, taken from adjacent parts, or with *skin grafts*. In such operations it is necessary to produce firm lid adhesions for some time by the operation of median tarsorrhaphy to prevent contraction during the healing process, which jeopardizes the result of the operation.

There are many blepharoplastic operations with *pedunculate skin flaps*, the selection and modification depending upon the size and situation of the defect. The following represent the usual plans: (1) A lateral flap is detached on each side of

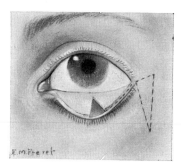

FIG. 4-19. Kuhnt-Szymanowski operation for ectropion; incisions.

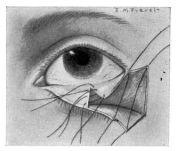

FIG. 4-20. Kuhnt-Szymanowski operation for ectropion; sutures in place.

the defect (lower lid only), freed from attachment, drawn over the part to be covered and united by a vertical row of sutures. (2) An adjacent quadrangular flap is taken from the cheek, slid inward over the defect (lower lid only) and sutured. (3) A tongue-shaped flap is dissected from the temple or cheek, the base of the flap adjoining the lid wound being the part which becomes twisted when the flap is transplanted and sutured into place.

Skin Grafting. The defect is filled in by a large piece of skin after the lids have been sutured together (median tarsorrhaphy). The area of the graft must be one-third larger than the defect to be covered, to allow for shrinkage. The graft may consist of the *entire thickness* of the skin (Wolfe's), or of only the *epidermis*

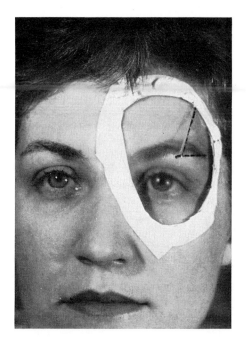

FIG. 4-18. Conical shield taped into place on eye; illustrates that condensation of moisture on inside of shield has already begun.

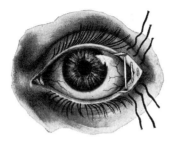

Fig. 4-21. Lateral tarsorraphy.

(Thiersch's). Entire thickness grafts are taken preferably from the opposite upper lid or from the region behind the ear, or if necessary, from the inner surface of the arm. If the entire thickness of skin is used, it is dissected free from subcutaneous connective tissue and fat. Thiersch grafts are best taken from the inner aspect of the arm or the outer surface of the thigh. The area to be covered must be clean and free from blood. When in place, the graft is covered with a layer of rubber tissue, next gauze, and then a firm dressing is applied for 4 or 5 days; the rubber tissue over the graft may be left in place still longer.

Skin grafting is used very extensively and with excellent results. If a portion of the graft should slough, it may be necessary to apply another graft later. Skin grafting causes less disfigurement than pedunculate flaps. Small defects are better covered with Wolfe grafts; when the skin is taken from the opposite upper lid or from behind the ear, the results are very satisfactory. When large surfaces are involved, Thiersch grafts must be used.

Tarsorrhaphy may be (1) lateral, or (2) median.

Lateral tarsorrhaphy. The object of this operation is to *reduce the width of the palpebral fissure* by uniting the edges of the lids at the outer commissure; it is indicated in lagophthalmos, especially in the exophthalmos of thyroid disease, and in some cases of senile and paralytic ectropion.

The edges of the lids are approximated at the outer canthus to the required extent, so as to give the operator exact knowledge as to how much union is desired. A lid plate is then passed behind the outer commissure, and the desired length of the border of each lid is excised, including the hair follicles. The length of the flap varies according to the effect desired (about 3 to 6 mm.); its breadth is about 1 mm. The denuded edges are brought together by silk sutures (Fig. 4-21).

Median tarsorrhaphy, a union of the lids by means of central intermarginal adhesions, is made when the lids are to be closed for some time but ultimately to be separated again; this operation is indicated in blepharoplasty to keep the lids in position during healing, and in neuroparalytic keratitis when the eye is to be kept covered for a lengthy period.

Areas of the posterior portion of the lid margins, opposite to each other, each having a width of 3 to 4 mm., are denuded on either side of the central third of the lids, and sutured together. When the lids are to be released, the adhesions are easily divided.

Ankyloblepharon is the adhesion of the margins of the two lids; it may be partial or complete, congenital or acquired; it often is associated with symblepharon.

Blepharophimosis is an apparent contraction of the palpebral fissure at its outer canthus owing to this angle being covered and hidden by a vertical fold of skin. It is seen in lengthy cases of chronic conjunctivitis in which, as a result of epiphora, irritating secretions and blepharospasm, eczema develops and draws the adjoining skin over the canthus.

Blepharochalasis, occasionally occurring in elderly persons, is a redundancy of the skin of the upper lid, causing a fold to hang down over the lid margin. If necessary, the excess skin may be excised.

Symblepharon, a cicatricial attachment between the conjunctiva of the lid and the eyeball, is described in Chapter 6.

PTOSIS (BLEPHAROPTOSIS)

Blepharoptosis is a *drooping of the upper lid* with narrowing of the palpebral fissure, smoothing of the lid and loss of the lid fold (Fig. 4-22). It may be unilateral or bilateral. All degrees of ptosis occur. When severe, it interferes with vision by covering the pupil. Patients attempt to raise the lid by forced action of the frontalis muscle, wrinkling the skin of the forehead and raising the brow (Figs. 4-2 and 4-22); when the condition is severe and bilateral, they favor exposure of the pupil by throwing the head backward; these actions are characteristic accompaniments of this anomaly. There often is associated defective upward movement of the eyes. Occasionally a curious elevation of the upper lid occurs, with movement of the jaw (Marcus Gunn jaw winking phenomenon).

Etiology. Ptosis may be congenital or acquired. When congenital it usually is bilateral and due to abnormalities of the oculomotor nerve. Ptosis may be the only involvement but most frequently it is associated with weakness or paralysis of the superior rectus muscle and rarely it is associated with paralysis of all of the extraocular muscles. It frequently is hereditary and dominant.

Acquired ptosis usually is unilateral. It may be due to neural, muscular or mechanical factors. When paralytic it usually is caused by a lesion of the oculomotor nerve and frequently is associated with paralysis of ocular muscles supplied by the

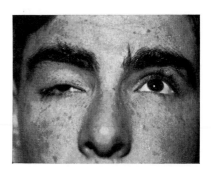

FIG. 4-22. Ptosis (right side).

third nerve and at times by the fourth and sixth nerves. Slight unilateral ptosis, miosis and anhidrosis due to paralysis of the sympathetic nerve supply is caused by lesions on the same side of the base of the neck affecting either the cervical sympathetic ganglia or fibers and is known as Horner's syndrome. Muscular factors are exemplified by the ptosis of myotonic dystrophy and of myasthenia gravis. The slowly progressive degenerative changes of the muscles eventually result in complete bilateral ptosis. The defect in myasthenia seems to be in humoral transmission at the myoneural junction. Unilateral or bilateral ptosis may be the first sign of myasthenia gravis. It eventually develops in more than 90 per cent of patients and in 80 per cent of these eventually is accompanied by transient or permanent diplopia. The ptosis increases with fatigue or toward the end of the day but usually is relieved by the injection of Prostigmin or tensilon.

Mechanical ptosis may be due to an injury of the lid or orbit; increased weight of the lid from a tumor or an inflammatory infiltration such as trachoma, tylosis, vernal conjunctivitis etc.; or lack of support of the lid as occurs with atrophy of the globe or following enucleation of the globe.

Treatment. The choice of treatment of blepharoptosis depends upon the cause, the extent of the ptosis, and the associated lesions.

In the congenital form treatment is surgical and the optimal time is determined by the severity of the droop. If the pupils are covered the operation should be done as early as possible to permit the development of normal visual function. The same applies when the child has to throw his head backward to an exaggerated degree, but if the pupils are adequately exposed surgery may be postponed to a convenient time, preferably between the ages of 3 and 5 years.

In acquired ptosis the cause should be determined and treated. Mechanical ptosis due to excess weight of the lid from a tumor or an inflammatory infiltration may be relieved by removal of the tumor or control of the inflammation. Luetic lesions of the lid or third nerve respond well to antisyphilitic therapy. Myasthenic ptosis usually is adequately controlled by medical therapy with Prostigmin or a similar drug. However, should such therapy fail after a thorough trial and in some of the mechanical cases operation is indicated. However a careful evaluation of the patient and of the associated lesions should be made before the surgical procedure is chosen or done. In those patients with associated paralysis of the superior rectus muscle or with absence of Bell's phenomenon (the eyes normally turn up and out on forcible closure of the lids) exposure keratitis may develop following correction of the ptosis, unless these defects also can be corrected. Other extraocular muscles may be paralytic or nonparalytic strabismus may exist in association with ptosis. Appropriate treatment should be planned for these problems either before, with or after ptosis surgery. The width of the palpebral fissure should be measured at its widest extent, usually at the middle of the lids, with the patient looking downward and upward. In making these measurements the effect of the frontalis muscle should be excluded by making pressure with a finger of one hand along the superior orbital margin. The difference in these widths indicates the relative activity of the levator palpebrae superioris. The normal variation is approximately 15 mm.

Operations for Ptosis

The aim of ptosis surgery is to lift the upper lid above the pupil to as near its normal position as possible in all directions of gaze of the eye without interferring with the lid covering the cornea when the eye is closed as in sleep. The various procedures seldom produce complete correction of the defect but satisfactory results usually can be attained. Numerous techniques have been developed but basically they fall into the following general methods.

(1) Resection or Resection and Advancement of the Levator Palpebrae Superioris Muscle. In ptosis due to weakness of the levator, excellent results are obtained by shortening this muscle, advancing its tarsal insertion, or doing both, but these methods are contraindicated in severe paresis or complete paralysis of the levator.

(a) *Resection operation.* The levator muscle is exposed either through a skin incision or through a conjunctival incision (Fig. 4-23). Sutures are placed through the belly of the muscle 10 to 20 mm. posterior to its insertion. The desired amount of muscle is resected and the stump of the muscle is attached to the upper border of the tarsus (Fig. 4-24). The skin or conjunctival incision is closed and the eye dressed to protect the cornea from exposure.

A modification of this, the Iliff procedure, designed for small amounts of ptosis or for improvement of small residual defects, consists of a block resection of conjunctiva and levator. An incision is made through conjunctiva and tarsus along its upper border (Fig. 4-25). At either end of the tarsus the incision is extended upward 6 to 8 mm. away from the tarsus. The conjunctiva and levator are elevated together, sutures placed through both 6 mm. from the tarsal incision and 5 mm. of the tissue resected (Fig. 4-26). The sutures are passed through the upper border of the tarsus pulling the levator and conjunctiva down to the tarsus closing the incision.

(b) Resection and advancement of the levator. The attachment of the levator muscle to the tarsus is exposed by a horizontal incision through the skin of the upper lid (Fig. 4-27). The anterior surface of the tarsus is exposed to within 1 to 2 mm. of the lid border. The levator is exposed anteriorly and posteriorly. Then double armed sutures are passed through the levator at the selected distance (10 to 20 mm.) above the tarsus. The levator muscle is resected and the sutures passed through the anterior surface of the tarsus (Fig. 4-28) pulling the levator down to and attaching it there.

(2) Use of the Superior Rectus Muscle to Elevate the Lid with Upward Rotations of the Eye. Several variations of this procedure have been used:

(a) Motais' operation employs the middle of the superior rectus tendon. It is freed and sutured to the anterior surface of the tarsus near the lid margin slightly nasal to its center (Fig. 4-29).

(b) Dickey makes use of a fascia lata sling beneath the superior rectus both ends of the strip being sutured to the tarsus.

(c) Berke in order to overcome the diplopia and hypotropia (lowering of the eye due to the added weight of the lid pulling on the muscle) shortens the superior rectus muscle leaving the excess tendon attached but splits it into three strips and attaches their distal ends to the an-

terior surface of the tarsus (Fig. 4-30). This technique is useful in ptosis associated with a weak superior rectus muscle or with the jaw winking syndrome; however, it does not overcome the inability to close the lids completely during sleep.

(3) Suspension of the Upper Lid from the Frontalis Muscle.

(a) Hess' operation. A 3-cm. incision in the brow permits undermining down to the lid margin. Three double armed sutures are introduced so as to form loops about 7 mm. from the lid border then are passed upward beneath the brow emerging 1 cm. above the incision where they are tied over rubber pegs or buttons and

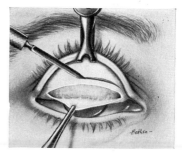

Fig. 4-23. Resection of the levator, conjunctival approach; conjunctiva has been incised and elevated away from the levator. The tarsus is being incised.

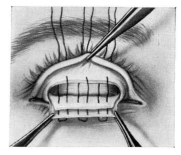

Fig. 4-24. Resection of the levator; the levator has been freed and a portion of it removed; sutures have been placed through conjunctiva levator muscle and tarsus then brought out through the skin of the lid prior to tying them.

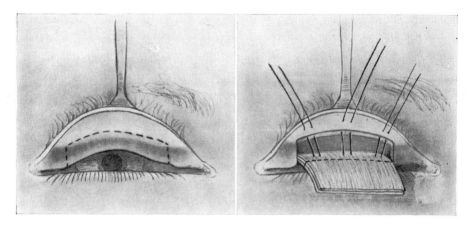

Fig. 4-25. Iliff procedure. Line of incision through upper border of tarsus with perpendicular incision through levator muscle and conjunctiva.

Fig. 4-26. Iliff procedure. Block dissection of conjunctiva and levator has been completed and sutures placed through both, 6 mm. posterior to the tarsal incision. The dotted line indicates the amount of conjunctiva and levator to be removed.

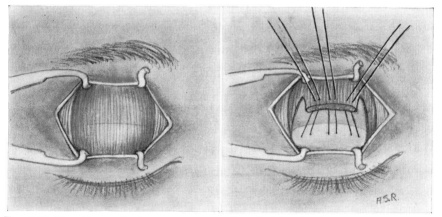

Fig. 4-27. Resection and advancement operation: incision has been made through skin and orbicularis, exposing the levator palpebrae superioris muscle.

Fig. 4-28. Resection and advancement operation: the desired amount of levator muscle has been resected. Double arm sutures have been brought out through the stump of the levator muscle. When tied, the sutures will advance the insertion of the levator onto the anterior face of the tarsus.

allowed to remain for 2 weeks. The skin incision is closed and the eye dressed to protect the cornea from exposure.

Modification of this have been made by several surgeons using fascia lata, stainless steel wire, gold chain and collagen tape instead of the sutures.

(b) **Reese's operation** depends upon the creation of lateral strips of orbicularis muscle over the tarsus leaving the medial 10 mm. attached. Each lateral strip is drawn up under the skin and attached to the frontalis muscle just above the brow.

A modification of this procedure makes

use of narrow strips of tarsus instead of orbicularis.

Blepharospasm, spasm of the orbicularis, closing the lids, is a symptom of ocular disease or of a neurosis. *The tonic form* (persistent) is present with foreign bodies, fissure at the outer canthus, corneal affections and inflammatory conditions of the eye in general; it is due to irritation of the terminal filaments of the trigeminus; rarely it is hysterical; treatment consists in removing the cause. The

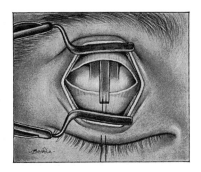

Fig. 4-29. Motais' operation; Kirby modification.

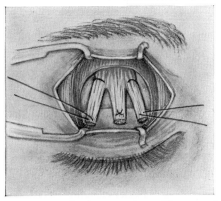

Fig. 4-30. Berke procedure. The superior rectus muscle has been disinserted and divided into three strips for a distance of approximately 5 mm. The muscle is reattached into its insertion on the globe, with the three strips extending through the lid and attached to the anterior surface of the tarsus.

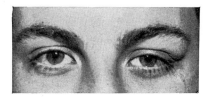

Fig. 4-31. Dermoid cyst below left outer eyebrow.

clonic variety (intermittent), often merely fibrillar twitchings, especially of the lower lid, unimportant although annoying, may depend upon errors of refraction, fatigue or conjunctivitis. Intermittent spasm may be a form of "habit chorea." Another variety, very obstinate, is sometimes seen in elderly persons, in whom the palpebral spasms are accompanied by similar movements of the neighboring facial muscles; this condition may be relieved for a variable period or even permanently by the injection of alcohol into the orbicularis.

Lagophthalmos, an incomplete closure of the palpebral fissure when the lids are shut, resulting in exposure and consequent injury to the cornea, may be due to congenital or acquired shortening of the lids, ectropion, paralysis of the orbicularis (facial paralysis), exophthalmic goiter and protrusion or enlargement of the eyeball; it is seen also in unconscious and moribund individuals. Tarsorrhaphy may be necessary to protect the cornea.

TUMORS OF THE LIDS

Benign Tumors include dermoid cyst, xanthelasma, milium, cyst and others.

Dermoid Cyst, a congenital tumor, forms a firm, round or oval, movable mass beneath the skin of the external canthus (Fig. 4-31) or of the medial portion of the upper lid. The tumor is excised.

Xanthelasma (xanthoma) is a flat or slightly raised, yellowish discoloration of the inner corium, found most frequently near the inner canthus in elderly women;

it is due to fatty degeneration of masses of connective tissue cells with yellowish pigment deposits (Plate 12*A*). Several of these tumors usually occur simultaneously. Xanthelasmas call for no interference except for cosmetic reasons; they may be removed by excision or by electrolysis.

Milium is a small, yellowish white elevation about the size of a pin's head, due to retention in a sebaceous gland, requiring merely puncture and expression.

Small Cysts (vesicles), with transparent contents, due to obstruction in the outlet of sweat glands, are often seen on the lid border; they give rise at times to irritation and should be punctured with the point of a Graefe knife.

The other benign tumors resemble those found in other parts of the body; they may be excised, the lids being very tolerant to considerable loss of skin; if too large an area of skin is involved or if the lid margin is implicated, a reconstructive operation may be required.

Malignant Tumors. Of these, sarcoma is rare, but carcinoma more common.

Carcinoma, when it attacks the lids, usually assumes that form known as *basal cell epithelioma* (Fig. 4-32). This occurs in elderly persons, especially at the inner end of the lower lid margin (Fig. 4-33). It begins as a small pimple or wart, covered by a crust, soon changes to an ulcer with indurated walls, and spreads, if unchecked, to neighboring parts. Its growth is slow, however, and many years may elapse before it assumes considerable size. The less frequent and more rapidly growing squamous cell epithelioma has greater malignancy and spreads to adjacent lymph nodes.

Treatment. The ideal treatment of

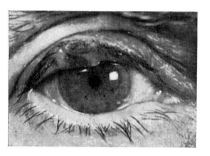

Fig. 4-32. Basal cell epithelioma of upper lid.

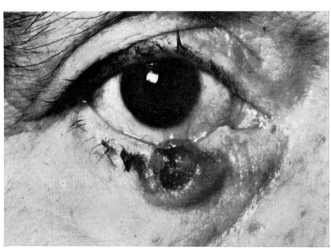

Fig. 4-33. Basal cell carcinoma of lower lid.

both varieties of epithelioma is complete and wide excision, with such reparative procedures as may be needed. Exposure to *x-rays or radium,* with sufficient protection to the eyeball, is effective, especially in the basal cell tumors, since this form is radiosensitive. Surgery and radiation often are combined. In the case of tumors which cannot be excised, radiotherapy or irradiation combined with chemotherapy offers the only chance of regression.

5

The Lacrimal Apparatus

Anatomy and Physiology

The lacrimal apparatus consists of a *secretory portion*, the lacrimal gland, and an *excretory portion*, which collects the tears and conducts them into the inferior meatus of the nose.

The lacrimal gland is a small, oblong body, placed in the upper and outer part of the orbit and divided into two portions. The upper part, the larger, about the size of a small almond, is situated in a depression in the orbital plate of the frontal bone, the lacrimal fossa, to which it is fixed by connective tissue; the lower division, the smaller, is known as the accessory lacrimal gland, and is placed just beneath the outer part of the conjunctiva of the fornix; there also are microscopic glands extending along the conjunctival fornix, especially laterally, forming Krause's glands. In structure the lacrimal resembles the salivary glands, consisting of acini containing cuboidal cells. The excretory ducts of both portions of the gland, the lacrimal ducts, 6 to 12 in number, pass downward and empty into the external half of the superior fornix conjunctivae by separate orifices.

The excretory portion of the lacrimal apparatus (Fig. 5-1) consists of the puncta, the canaliculi, the sac and the duct. The *puncta* are two minute openings, one of which is seen upon an elevation on each lid about 6 mm. from the inner canthus. They are the orifices of the *canaliculi*. The latter extend vertically for a short distance, then turn at right angles and pass horizontally inward in a curved course, to empty separately or joined into the lacrimal sac.

The lacrimal sac, situated at the inner side of the internal canthus, is the upper, dilated portion of the lacrimonasal duct, and is placed in a groove formed by the lacrimal bone and the frontal process of the maxillary bone; it measures 12 mm. in the vertical and 6 mm. in the horizontal and transverse diameters; its walls are thin; it is covered in front by the internal tarsal ligament and some fibers of the orbicularis muscle.

The nasal duct passes downward and slightly outward and backward in a canal formed by the maxillary, lacrimal and inferior turbinated bones, and terminates below in the forepart of the inferior meatus of the nose; its length varies from 15 to 24 mm., and its diameter from 4 to 6 mm.; it is somewhat contracted where it joins the sac and again at its lower extremity. The course of the duct is indicated by a line passing from a point just outside of the inner canthus along the groove between the ala of the nose and the cheek. Both sac and duct are formed of fibrous and elastic tissues and mucous membrane lined with columnar epithelium which may be ciliated; the duct is surrounded by a plexus of veins, densest around the lower part.

The lacrimal secretion is a slightly alkaline liquid containing a comparatively large amount of sodium chloride and an enzyme, *lysozyme*, which has an antibacterial function. Ordinarily the lacrimal gland secretes just enough to moisten the eyeball, and this is lost by evaporation. Tears are conveyed from the conjunctiva to the lacrimal sac by the act of winking, the lubrication of the margins of the lids by fatty material ordinarily preventing the tears from flowing over. Lacrimal secretion may be measured by Schirmer's test, using 5- by 25-mm. strips of filter paper; one end is placed in the inner angle of the lower cul-de-sac, covering the inferior punctum, the remainder of the strip protruding between the lids; when lacrimation is normal 10 to 15 mm. of the paper will be moistened in 5 minutes.

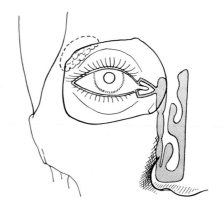

Fig. 5-1. Diagrammatic illustration of the lacrimal gland and the lacrimal apparatus.

THE LACRIMAL GLAND

Congenital Anomalies of the Lacrimal Gland

Congenital Absence of the lacrimal gland occurs only when there is failure of development of the conjunctiva and therefore always is accompanied by extensive anomalies such as cryptophthalmos or anophthalmos.

Congenital Cyst of the lacrimal gland is manifest as a tense fluctuant mass under the orbital margin. It may cause noninflammatory swelling of the lid, ptosis and proptosis as a result of a posterior extension which at times may reach the apex of the orbit. The cyst should be excised.

Congenital Prolapse may result from weakness of the orbital septum. A visible mass which is firm and lobular on palpation appears in the temporal portion of the upper lid. At times the gland may be replaced in the orbit by gentle manipulation.

Diseases of the Lacrimal Gland

Hyposecretion of Lacrimal Fluid results in dryness of the eyes and leads to corneal changes consisting of areas of superficial epithelial erosions which stain with fluorescein, and of epithelial threads at the borders (*filamentary keratitis*); in advanced cases the cornea may become opaque and vision much impaired. Deficiency in lacrimal secretion may result from extirpation of the lacrimal gland or scarring of the conjunctiva following trachoma, and exist in vitamin A deficiency (xerophthalmia or keratomalacia). Reduced production of lacrimal fluid is found in a condition known as *keratoconjunctivitis sicca*, often associated with defective secretion of the salivary glands and arthritis, Sjögren's syndrome. In vitamin A deficiency, the bulbar conjunctiva in the interpalpebral space may develop dry greasy areas (*Bitot's spots*).

Symptoms include a feeling of dryness and a burning, smarting sensation in the eyes, photophobia, stringy mucoid discharge and impairment of vision.

Treatment consists of the frequent instillation of a substitute for the scanty tears (Ringer's solution, Gifford's solution), increased vitamin A intake in the diet supplemented by vitamin A concentrates, and, if necessary, occlusion of the puncta (excision of the lining epithelium or its obliteration by diathermy or galvanocautery).

Lacrimation, an *excessive secretion of tears,* may result from psychic stimulation, exposure (facial paralysis), irritation of the end twigs of the trigeminus by foreign bodies, inflammations of the eye, wind and smoke, affections of the nose or irritation by bright light. It is common in old people, especially in the open air in cold weather, often without manifest lesion of the conjunctiva or tear passages.

Acute Dacryoadenitis produces swelling, redness and tenderness in the temporal portion of the upper lid associated with more or less ptosis, and at times a purulent discharge from the ductules or from rupture and drainage through the conjunctiva. The lesion may result from primary infection of the gland but usually is a metastatic complication of mumps, gonorrhea or one of the acute infectious systemic diseases such as scarlet fever or typhoid fever. Treatment in addition to that of the general disease consists of local application of heat and surgical drainage when fluctuation develops.

Chronic Dacryoadenitis causes a slow painless swelling of the lacrimal gland with some ptosis of the upper lid but without redness or tenderness. It occurs in the course of trachoma, as a result of hematogenous spread in tuberculosis and at times as a part of the involvement in sarcoid and Mikulicz's syndrome. Treatment is directed toward the cause but at times the enlarged gland may have to be excised.

Tumors of the Lacrimal Gland usually develop in the orbital portion, producing a firm or hard slowly growing mass in the upper temporal portion of the orbit, causing a downward and nasalward proptosis of the globe. The types include adenoma, adenocarcinoma, mixed tumor, lymphoma, lymphosarcoma and Hodgkin's disease. Treatment consists of excision and irradiation.

THE LACRIMAL PASSAGES

Congenital anomalies of the lacrimal passages include a variety of severe and rare malformations of the face and lids; however, the most common are *atresia of the lacrimal puncta,* a failure of the epithelium to perforate in an otherwise normal canaliculus; *supernumerary puncta and canaliculi,* reduplications of these structures, usually in the lower lid, which include multiple puncta in a single canaliculus as well as in multiple canaliculi; and *atresia of the nasolacrimal duct,* which most often is due to plugging of the duct by debris, but may be due to failure of the epithelial tube to open at the nasal end and, quite rarely, to bony obstruction.

Epiphora, an *interference with drainage of tears,* is a prominent symptom in all affections of the tear-conducting apparatus.

Investigation of the lacrimal passages includes digital or instrumental *pressure over the lacrimal sac* and *injection of normal saline* through the inferior punctum with the lacrimal syringe (Fig. 5-2). If fluid (watery, viscid, mucopurulent) escapes through the puncta upon pressure over the lacrimal sac, an obstruction in the nasolacrimal duct is indicated. The use of the lacrimal syringe should be preceded by instillations of a topical anesthetic into the conjunctival sac and by dilatation of the inferior punctum with the punctum dilator (Fig. 5-3). The lacrimal syringe is fitted with a cannula, the tip of which is passed vertically downward through the punctum and then horizontally into the canaliculus, and normal saline is gently injected; if the fluid passes freely into the nose and pharynx, no obstruction is present; if the solution returns through the superior punctum, obstruction must be present in either the nasolacrimal duct, the lacrimal sac or the junction of the

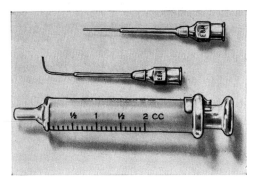

FIG. 5-2. Lacrimal syringe and cannulas.

common canaliculus with the lacrimal sac; if the saline returns through the lower punctum, there must be a block at the nasal end of the inferior canaliculus and injection through the superior canaliculus should be tried.

Eversion of the punctum. Normally, the lower punctum is directed backward and upward toward the eyeball. When everted, the lower punctum looks forward and away from the depression in which the tears accumulate, and the result is *epiphora.* The condition may be due to a relaxed state of the lids in old age and in facial palsy, to conjunctivitis, blepharitis and other conditions causing ectropion. It is remedied by correcting the ectropion.

Contraction and obliteration of the puncta and canaliculi may be congeni-

tal, or acquired from wounds and chronic inflammations of this region. Epiphora due to a narrowed inferior punctum may be relieved by dilatation of this structure with a punctum dilator (Fig. 5-3) or, in stubborn cases, by excision of a small triangular segment from the posterior aspect of the inferior punctum, separating the edges daily for several days until they remain open. Closure or stenosis of the nasal extremity of the inferior canaliculus is occasionally relieved by probing and dilatation of the stricture, or by intubation with a plastic tube.

Obstruction of the canaliculus may be caused by a cilium, which can be pulled out easily, or by concretions composed of yellowish white masses of Streptothrix or related organisms. When concretions are

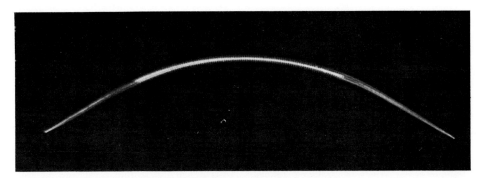

FIG. 5-3. Bowman's canaliculus dilator.

present in either or both canaliculi, these passages and the puncta become irregularly dilated in association with swelling of the tissues at the inner canthus; often concretions or yellowish white cheesy material can be expressed. Treatment consists of dilating the punctum and gently removing the foreign body, then irrigating the canaliculus.

Acute Dacryocystitis

Acute dacryocystitis is an acute purulent inflammation of the lacrimal sac due to obstruction of the nasolacrimal duct, resulting in stagnation of tears in the lacrimal sac followed by infection. The obstruction may be congenital or acquired.

Dacryocystitis in the Newborn. Approximately 1 out of 100 newborn infants has nasolacrimal obstruction. The majority of these, approximately 90 per cent, are due to debris retained in the nasolacrimal duct. Almost 10 per cent are due to failure of the epithelial tube to open completely, leaving thin valve-like membranous obstructions in the duct, the majority of which occur at the entrance of the lower end of the duct into the nose. In very few, less than 1 per cent, the obstruction is bony, owing to malformation of the nasal bones. Frequently the obstruction is bilateral.

In the newborn, tears are produced in appreciable amount only after the tenth to twelfth day of life and the usual secondary infection of the obstructed sac occurs about the same time, producing signs and symptoms of acute dacryocystitis between the twelfth and eighteenth days of life. Occasionally an obstructed sac becomes infected sooner when the infant develops an acute conjunctivitis in the first few days of life.

The most frequent cause of the infectious process in the newborn is pneumococcus, but *Streptococcus viridans* follows closely, then influenza bacilli, staphylococci

and, rarely, almost any pathogenic bacterium.

The signs and symptoms of acute dacryocystitis in the newborn usually consist of a purulent exudate on the conjunctiva of one or both eyes, associated with redness of the conjunctiva and epiphora. There may be swelling and redness of the medial portion of the lower lid, but induration and abscess formation of the sac and surrounding tissues seldom occur. Untreated, the inflammation subsides into a chronic phase with some purulent discharge and epiphora persisting indefinitely. The infection persists and is a constant threat to vision, for a slight injury of the epithelium of the cornea is all that is required to permit the infection to cause an ulcer, resulting in extensive scarring and loss of vision or even loss of the globe (see Hypopyon Ulcer of the Cornea, Chap. 7).

Treatment. Irrigation of the nasolacrimal passages daily or every other day will result in control of the purulent discharge within a few days. Then, with subsidence of the inflammation a few more irrigations will remove the obstruction in those 90 per cent due to retained debris. However, if the obstruction is not relieved by two or three daily irrigations after the purulent material has disappeared from the sac, the obstruction probably is due to a membranous obstruction, which will be opened by the passage of a probe (Fig. 5-4). In the very small group in which the obstruction is bony, a dacryocystorhinostomy will be necessary but should be delayed until the infant is approximately 1 year of age. During the period of treatment the parents may be instructed to instill 1 drop of a 15 per cent solution of sulfacetamide onto the conjunctiva eight times a day.

Acute Dacryocystitis in Children and Adults usually is unilateral and is the result of infection following an acquired

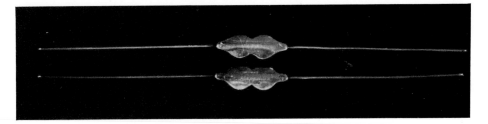

FIG. 5-4. Bowman's lacrimal probes.

obstruction of the nasolacrimal passages; it may arise quickly following the obstruction or occur as an exacerbation of a chronic dacryocystitis. The usual causes of acquired obstruction of the nasolacrimal passages are trauma, nasal or sinus infection, tuberculosis or luetic periostitis or, rarely, nasal tumors. Stagnation of the tears in the lacrimal sac is followed quickly by infection which, in order of frequency, is due to pneumococci, *S. viridans*, influenza bacilli, staphylococci and, rarely, almost any pathogenic bacterium.

Signs and symptoms. Epiphora occurs and is followed quickly by the development of redness, swelling, induration and tenderness over the medial portion of the lower lid and side of the nose. Pain also may occur. The conjunctiva becomes red and is covered over the lower portion by a purulent discharge. Pressure over the region of the sac may cause regurgitation of pus through the puncta; however, the pressure should be gentle to avoid rupture of the sac and extrusion of the infected material into the surrounding tissues. In some cases this occurs spontaneously and results in a cellulitis or an abscess, which may spread and rupture through the skin with drainage of the purulent material from the lacrimal sac onto the face. The acute process usually subsides quickly following the rupture and drainage, but unfortunately a fistula almost always persists with a constant flow

of tears onto the face. Even should the fistula heal, the process of abscess formation followed by reopening of the fistula and drainage may repeat itself indefinitely. In the majority of patients, even though untreated, the acute process subsides into a chronic dacryocystitis which may undergo an acute exacerbation at any time but persists indefinitely.

Treatment. Pressure over the sac and irrigation should be avoided, or accomplished gently and with care, in the very acute lesions. Cultures should be made from exudate taken from the punctum, and antibiotic sensitivity tests made on the infectious agents. In the interval, cold compresses may be applied for 10 to 15 minutes every hour to reduce the swelling and redness. Sulfonamides may be given by mouth, and, if improvement has not occurred by the time sensitivity tests have been made on the organisms isolated from the exudate, one of the effective antibiotics may be given orally or parenterally. Every effort should be made to prevent rupture and drainage of a lacrimal abscess.

After the acuteness has been controlled or in the less acute cases, the lacrimal sac should be irrigated daily or every other day until the infection subsides and the fluids return clear. During this period of treatment every effort should be made to determine the cause of the obstruction of the nasolacrimal passages. The nose and sinuses should be examined and any cause of obstruction removed if possible.

Unfortunately, in this form of dacryocystitis, permanent re-establishment of the flow of tears through the nasolacrimal duct is impossible in practically all instances; therefore, the usual treatment is to establish a new route for drainage of the tears from the lacrimal sac into the nose; that is, a dacryocystorhinostomy.

Chronic Dacryocystitis

Chronic dacryocystitis is a *chronic inflammation of the lacrimal sac*, usually due to an obstruction in the nasolacrimal duct, followed by infection of the lacrimal sac.

Etiology. *Obstruction of the nasolacrimal duct* either is of congenital origin (due to adhesion of the lining of the duct or to the persistence of a membrane in its lower end) or is the result of chronic nasal infection, trauma or ulceration (syphilitic or tuberculous). The congenital condition is known as *congenital impatency of the nasolacrimal duct*; this is seen in the newborn and in young infants.

Stagnation of the contents of the lacrimal sac is quickly followed by infection. As a result of contamination by micro-organisms from the conjunctiva, staphylococci, streptococci and pneumococci, a *purulent inflammation* of the lining of the sac is established. The secretion from the sac is most *infectious* and a constant source of danger to the eye, with the risk of hypopyon ulcer should an abrasion or ulcer of the cornea occur. The condition is an absolute contraindication to intraocular operations on account of the liability to infection.

Signs and Symptoms. The constant symptom is *epiphora* increased by exposure to cold, wind, dust, smoke, etc. There may be *fullness* in the region of the lacrimal sac; this distention is known as *mucocele* (Plate 7E). By pressing upon the distended sac, a *viscid fluid*, watery, or of

yellowish or slightly greenish color (depending upon the amount of pus), escapes from the puncta. A form of chronic conjunctivitis affecting chiefly the inner canthus (*lacrimal conjunctivitis*) and blepharitis always are present.

Course is chronic and extends over *years*; a long period may elapse before the patient seeks relief. After the mucopurulent material has filled the sac for a long time, there is atrophy of its mucous membrane and the character of the contents of the distended, atonic walls changes; the accumulation becomes more watery and consists principally of the tears contaminated with an abundance of micro-organisms. There exists constantly the danger of development of acute dacryocystitis (lacrimal abscess), occasionally followed by the formation of an external fistula.

Treatment consists of attention to nasal and conjunctival complications, massage, syringing, probing, dacryocystorhinostomy and extirpation of the sac. Simple measures should be tried first; only when these fail should probing or operation be tried.

Attention to any associated *conjunctivitis* and to any complicating *nasal disorder* is important.

Massage. The patient should be instructed to empty the sac by pressure several times a day.

Irrigation. The lacrimal syringe (Fig. 5-2) fitted with a moderately fine, straight or curved needle is employed, and a warm physiologic salt solution used; it may be necessary to dilate the lower punctum. The tip is passed vertically downward and then in the direction of the sac; the fluid often will escape from the upper punctum, but in many cases, when the swelling of the lining of the duct diminishes, it will pass into the nose and escape from the anterior nares when the patient inclines his head forward. Syringing should be repeated every few days. It should be preceded by instillations of a topical anesthetic into the conjunctival sac and sometimes also by the injection of a few drops through the inferior canaliculus.

Probing. If, however, the conservative treatment is unsuccessful, *dilatation with probes* is attempted, with use of Bowman's probes (Fig. 5-4). These are numbered from 1 to 8, the largest (No. 8) being about 2 mm. in thickness; they are curved before use. Probes generally can be passed through the natural opening after dilatation. Probing is facilitated and rendered less painful by the preliminary introduction of a few drops of a topical anesthetic into the sac and duct.

To pass probes into the lacrimal duct. Commencing with a small size, the surgeon passes the probe horizontally inward, standing behind (or in front of) the patient. When the probe reaches the inner wall of the sac, it is raised so that its lower end points toward the furrow between nose and cheek. It then is pushed downward *gently*, until it reaches the floor of the nasal fossa. If the probe does not pass readily, *force must not be used* for fear of injuring the wall of the duct or creating a false passage; it is withdrawn slightly and passed downward again, or a smaller or larger size is tried. When the probe is passed into the nose it is left in place for a few minutes and then re-

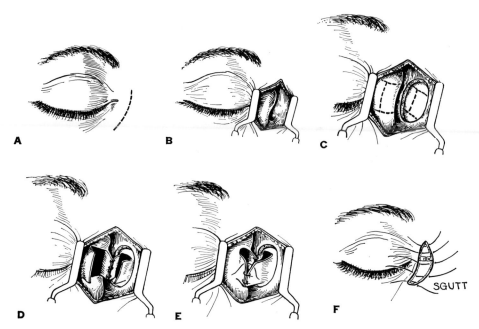

FIG. 5-5. Dacryocystorhinostomy. *A*, Skin incision for dacryocystorhinostomy or dacryocystectomy; *B*, lacrimal sac and lacrimal bone exposed; *C*, opening made in lacrimal bone and lacrimal crest, with *dotted lines* indicating the incision to be made in the wall of the sac and in the nasal periosteum and mucosa; *D*, posterior flap of the wall of the sac sutured to the posterior flap of the nasal mucosa; *E*, anterior flap of the wall of the sac sutured to the anterior flap of the nasal mucosa (drawing somewhat distorted for visualization of relative positions); *F*, reattachment of the medial canthal ligament and sutures in position for closure of skin incision.

moved. In infants this usually solves the problem.

Most cases of chronic dacryocystitis in adults, however, are obstinate, and conservative treatment gives only temporary relief. In such cases it usually is necessary to resort to operation, preferably a procedure to re-establish intranasal drainage by dacryocystorhinostomy.

Dacryocystorhinostomy is the operation of choice, since it restores the drainage of tears into the nose by joining the cavity of the lacrimal sac directly with the nasal fossa after removal of a segment of the intervening bone and periosteum.

Under local or general anesthesia, a curved incision is made through the skin, beginning 3 mm. above and nasal to the medial canthus and extending downward and outward 1.5 to 2 cm. (Fig. 5-5A). The medial palpebral ligament is cut and the lacrimal sac and anterior lacrimal crest are exposed. The dissection is continued posteriorly and laterally, separating the lacrimal sac from the floor of the lacrimal fossa (Fig. 5-5B). The lower portion of the anterior lacrimal crest is perforated with hammer and chisel or with a mechanically driven trephine, and the opening through the bone is enlarged with biting forceps or burr until it measures 1.2 to 1.5 cm. vertically and 1 cm. horizontally (Fig. 5-5C). Care must be taken to leave the nasal mucosa intact up to this point. The nasal mucosa and medial wall of the lacrimal sac are incised and united by fine sutures. Anterior and posterior flaps are created in the sac wall and nasal mucosa by making an I-shaped incision in each (Fig. 5-5C). The posterior nasal mucosal flap is sutured to the posterior flap of the sac wall (Fig. 5-5D) and the anterior flap of the nasal mucosa is joined to the anterior flap of the sac wall (Fig. 5-5E). The medial canthal ligament is sutured and the skin incision is closed with fine interrupted silk sutures (Fig. 5-5F). A pressure dressing is applied for 48 hours, and light dressings thereafter until the sutures are removed.

Dacryocystorhinostomy is contraindicated in cases in which the puncta and canaliculi are occluded, and in malignant or tuberculous involvement of the lacrimal sac.

Extirpation of the Lacrimal Sac (Dacryocystectomy) is indicated in patients in whom dacryocystorhinostomy is contraindicated.

Local anesthesia usually is sufficient; general anesthesia rarely is needed. The lacrimal sac is exposed as shown in Figure 5-5B. Using the anterior crest of the lacrimal groove as a guide, the sac is separated from periosteum with the aid of the handle of a scalpel and blunt scissors, beginning internally and then posteriorly, care being taken not to penetrate the wall; its upper extremity is freed and the canaliculi divided; it is cut off as low as possible. The excised sac is examined carefully to make sure that no portion has been left behind; if a portion of the sac is missing, it is located and excised or the suspicious area is curetted. The nasolacrimal canal is curetted. The medial canthal ligament is sutured and the skin incision is closed with interrupted fine silk sutures (Fig. 5-5F), and a firm dressing is applied for a few days. There usually is primary union with obliteration of the cavity. This operation abolishes the conduction of the tears, but often there is little annoyance from epiphora, probably through cure of the lacrimal conjunctivitis.

6

The Conjunctiva

Anatomy

The conjunctiva is a thin and transparent layer of mucous membrane which lines the eyelids and is reflected on to the eyeball, forming a sac, the *conjunctival sac.* There are three divisions: (1) the *palpebral* conjunctiva, covering the under surface of the lids; (2) the *ocular* or *bulbar* conjunctiva, coating the anterior portion of the eyeball, and (3) the *fornix,* the transition portion, forming a fold between lid and globe. The conjunctiva differs somewhat in structure in each of these portions.

The palpebral conjunctiva, in the greater part of its extent, is closely adherent to the subjacent tarsus, allowing the Meibomian glands to show through. Its surface is smooth, but presents a number of minute projections, or *papillae.* It is covered with cylindrical epithelium. Its stroma is of an adenoid character, containing a large number of lymph corpuscles, which sometimes project as small round masses (*lymphoid follicles*).

The conjunctiva of the fornix is similar in structure to that of the lids. It constitutes a very loose fold (*retrotarsal fold*), insuring great freedom of movement to the eyeball. It is richly supplied with blood vessels. This and its lax condition explain its liability to great swelling in inflammations of the conjunctiva. Opening into it are the lacrimal ducts and the accessory lacrimal glands.

The bulbar conjunctiva covers the anterior surface of the eyeball, being loosely attached to the sclera by connective tissue (*episcleral tissue*), with the exception of the margin representing the boundary between cornea and sclera (*limbus*), where it is firmly adherent. In structure it resembles the rest of the conjunctiva but contains no glands. It is covered with laminated pavement epithelium which is continued uninterruptedly over the cornea and constitutes its outer layer. Near the inner canthus it forms a crescentic fold (plica semilunaris), the rudiment of the nictitating membrane or third eyelid of the lower animals.

The vascular supply of the conjunctiva is derived from the blood vessels of the fornix—the *posterior conjunctival* (derived from the palpebral) and the *anterior ciliary.* The latter pass forward along the rectus muscles and pierce the sclera near the limbus to reach the interior of the eye, giving off one set of branches which form vascular loops surrounding the cornea and supply it with nourishment, and another set (*anterior conjunctival*), which pass backward in the conjunctiva and anastomose with the posterior conjunctival. This arrangement, together with the posterior ciliary arteries and the retinal system of vessels, constitutes the entire vascular system of the eye. Thus the bulbar conjunctiva presents *two vascular systems*—the posterior conjunctival and the anterior ciliary. The nature of the injection in any given case is of some value in locating the seat of the congestion.

The *nerves* of the conjunctiva, branches of the fifth, terminate in free ends or in tactile corpuscles, especially in the palpebral portion. Lymphatic vessels are found in considerable numbers.

Congenital and Developmental Anomalies

Congenital and developmental anomalies of the conjunctiva are rare. The more extensive and serious ones are associated with severe anomalies of adjacent structures, such as total failure of development of the conjunctiva in cryptophthalmia. However, less severe ones include *epitarsus*, which consists of apron-like folds of conjunctiva attached to the inner tarsal surface of the lid, almost always the upper lid; *congenital xerosis*, a drying and opacification of the conjunctiva, usually acquired and rarely congenital; *pterygium*, a triangular overgrowth of conjunctiva (see p. 91) onto the cornea which may be both congenital and hereditary; *failure of development of the caruncle* or *reduplication of the caruncle*, which occurs rarely; and *dermoid cysts*, which involve the conjunctiva and caruncle occasionally.

Chemosis is an edematous swelling of the bulbar conjunctiva (Fig. 6-1); it results from trauma, local irritants, dionine instillations, allergic reaction and trichinosis; it often accompanies severe conjunctival inflammations and exophthalmos. In severe examples, ballooning folds of edematous conjunctiva may overlap the cornea, a condition seen frequently in gonorrheal conjunctivitis.

Emphysema of the Conjunctiva results from infiltration of the tissues of the orbit and subconjunctival tissues by air following fracture or necrosis of the bones of the medial orbital wall. The spongy distention of the tissues usually occurs suddenly after blowing the nose, and resembles chemosis, but palpation of the lids or conjunctiva will reveal crepitation. Cold compresses and pressure dressings should be applied and the patient instructed to refrain from blowing his nose.

Subconjunctival Hemorrhage occurs frequently and results in bright or dark red patches, of greater or lesser size, involving more or less of the bulbar conjunctiva (Plate 8D), unaccompanied by inflammatory symptoms. This condition (*ecchymosis*) is seen often after injuries, operations, the blood dyscrasias and inflammations of the conjunctiva. It is observed frequently in persons with brittle blood vessels, as a result of various straining efforts, such as sneezing, and in children after whooping cough. Sometimes the hemorrhage occurs without apparent ex-

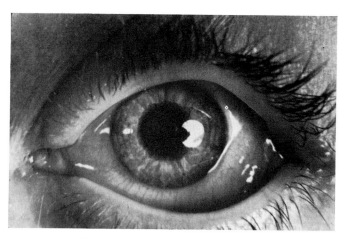

Fig. 6-1. Chemosis of the conjunctiva.

citing cause, the subject being unaware of its existence until he notices the discoloration. The hemorrhage itself is of *no importance* and the blood becomes *absorbed* within a week or two; the disappearance of the discoloration can, however, be hastened by the use of hot, moist compresses for 10 minutes at a time several times a day.

Hyperemia of the Conjunctiva (Plate 8*A*) is a very common condition which manifests itself in a congestion affecting chiefly the conjunctiva of the lids and fornices. It may be only a *transitory* condition or it may exist in *chronic* form, but often it is the first stage of chronic catarrhal conjunctivitis. However, it must be distinguished from hyperemia of the ciliary vessels or ciliary injection (Plate 8*B* and *C*), which is a sign of corneal or intraocular disease. Actually, because of intercommunication of the conjunctival and scleral or ciliary vessels, injection of both groups of vessels occurs, although there is predominant congestion of one group so differentiation usually may be made even in severe conditions. Table 6-1 indicates the differences between the two types of congestion in typical examples.

Etiology. The transitory form often is caused by local *irritants* such as foreign bodies, dust, wind, smoke, exposure to bright light or to glare such as exists at the seashore or on the water, or it ac-

TABLE 6-1

Comparison between Conjunctival and Ciliary Injection.

	Conjunctival Injection	Ciliary Injection
Cause	Conjunctival irritation	Keratitis, iritis, iridocyclitis or glaucoma
Location	Most intense in fornices; fades toward cornea	Most intense near cornea; fades toward fornices
Color	Bright brick red	Dull purplish red
Vessels	Individual vessels seen; they move with conjunctiva	Vessels not seen; injection not changed by movement of conjunctiva
Effect of 1:1000 Adrenalin	Injection disappears temporarily	Injection persists
Discharge	Mucopurulent or purulent	Lacrimation only
Photophobia	None	Usually present
Tenderness	None	Circumcorneal
Pain	Scratchy sensation	Deep pain or ache
Pupil	Normal size; reacts normally	Small in keratitis and iritis, dilated in glaucoma; reacts sluggishly

companies acute coryza and hay fever. The chronic form frequently is the result of uncorrected *errors of refraction* or the use of *faulty glasses*, misplaced lashes, vitiated or smoky atmosphere, *alcoholism*, overuse or *abuse of the eyes*, especially with insufficient illumination, or it accompanies nasal catarrh, blepharitis, lacrimal obstruction, plethoric states and congestive heart disease. A recurrent form is caused by gout.

Symptoms. There is *congestion* of the palpebral conjunctiva with slight swelling and roughness and little or no discharge. The patient complains of a dry, hot, gritty, *smarting sensation*, the eyes feel *tired*, water easily and are *uncomfortable* when exposed to light, and the lids feel *heavy*. These symptoms are most intense with near use of the eyes, especially with artificial illumination.

Treatment consists of *removal of the exciting cause*, especially correction of the errors of refraction. Use of zinc sulfate in 0.2 per cent solution two or three times a day often affords relief.

CONJUNCTIVITIS

Inflammation of the Conjunctiva is known as *conjunctivitis* or *ophthalmia*. The common varieties are:

(1) Catarrhal; (a) acute, (b) chronic.

(2) Purulent; (a) ophthalmia neonatorum, (b) gonorrheal.

(3) Membranous; (a) diphtheritic, (b) nondiphtheritic.

(4) Follicular; (a) acute, (b) chronic.

Acute Catarrhal Conjunctivitis

Acute catarrhal conjunctivitis is inflammation of the conjunctiva accompanied by *mucoid* or *mucopurulent discharge*. It also is known as acute mucopurulent and *acute simple conjunctivitis*.

Signs. The palpebral conjunctiva and that of the fornix are brilliant *red* and are *swollen* (Plate 10*A*). There usually is but slight congestion of the bulbar conjunctiva, but in severe cases it may become intense, and edema of the bulbar conjunctiva (chemosis, Fig. 6-1), small conjunctival hemorrhages and edema of the lids may be added. The *secretion* varies according to the severity of the affection; it is at first *watery* with some flakes of mucus, later *mucoid*; but in severer forms, it is *mucopurulent;* in very severe examples, the amount of pus may be so considerable that the character of the discharge, together with the severity of the objective signs, may leave doubt for 24 hours whether the disease is not the beginning of a purulent inflammation. The secretion accumulates during the night and dries upon the edges of the lids during sleep.

Symptoms. There are scratching, burning and *smarting* sensations referred to the lids; the latter feel hot, heavy and as if sand or a foreign body were underneath. There is more or less photophobia. There may be some blurring of sight when the altered secretion lies upon the cornea. The symptoms usually are worse toward evening; they vary in severity with the degree of inflammation. The affection may be limited to one eye, but usually *both eyes* are implicated, either from the start or after 2 or 3 days.

Course. Untreated acute simple conjunctivitis usually reaches its height in 3 to 6 days and heals in 10 to 14 days. Sometimes the acute symptoms subside and a subacute or chronic catarrhal conjunctivitis remains. Blepharitis may be present. In severe cases small, grayish infiltrations (catarrhal ulcers, Plate 12*E*) may form at the corneal margin. The coalescence of a number of these may cause a marginal ulcer, which usually is superficial and heals readily, but occasionally becomes deep and serious.

Etiology. The micro-organisms most frequently responsible for acute catarrhal conjunctivitis include *Diplococcus pneumoniae, Streptococcus viridans, Hemophilus influenzae* and *Hemophilus conjunctivitidis* (Koch - Weeks bacillus) (Plates 9 and 11). Mixed infections may occur. However, many other organisms may produce acute catarrhal conjunctivitis less frequently, such as *Hemophilus hemolyticus, Streptococcus hemolyticus, Klebsiella pneumoniae, Proteus vulgaris, Proteus ammoniae, Escherichia coli, Shigella dysenteriae,* Vincent's organisms, *Neisseria catarrhalis, Staphylococcus aureus* and *Salmonella typhi.* Examination of secretion smears stained by Gram's method during the height of the inflammation, as well as cultures, usually will permit exact identification of the causative agent. Organisms isolated in culture should be tested for sensitivity to the various antibiotics.

The disease occurs at *all ages* and at all times during the year, but is most common in the spring and autumn, in childen and young adults. Infection frequently is spread through droplet infection and contact with fingers, towels, handkerchiefs, etc., of patients suffering from the disease. The discharge is *contagious,* especially when it is abundant and when it contains much pus; hence the affection often presents a number of examples in the same household or school. Some are associated with coryza, rose cold, hay fever and grippe; others are associated with the exanthemas, accompanying or following measles or, less frequently, scarlet fever, smallpox and others.

Treatment. Careful determination of the causes of chronic catarrhal conjunctivitis is essential for successful treatment. Irritative factors should be eliminated, ocular disabilities corrected, systemic diseases or metabolic problems treated and the infectious element controlled. Sulfacetamide (drops or ointment), because it is broadly effective against the common causes of this type of infection, may be used while other factors are being determined and controlled. One drop of a 15 per cent solution of sodium sulfacetamide containing a viscous substance such as methylcellulose should be instilled onto the conjunctiva every hour during the day, and a small amount of 10 per cent sulfacetamide ointment or 1:3000 bichloride of mercury ointment instilled each night at bed time. Antibiotic preparations are not necessary in the usual acute catarrhal conjunctivitis and should be avoided because of the high incidence of induction of sensitivity on topical application to the conjunctiva, especially in ointment vehicles. However, when needed for unusually severe, prolonged or complicated infections, the antibiotic should be selected on the basis of sensitivity tests made with the infecting bacterial strain and it should be administered orally or parenterally rather than topically.

Though the disease may disappear without interference, treatment reduces its duration, adds to the patient's comfort and prevents the change into subacute or chronic conjunctivitis. *Iced compresses* applied for 15 minutes from three times a day to once every hour reduce edema and congestion and frequently promote comfort.

Special Clinical Varieties. *Traumatic conjunctivitis* is the name given to acute catarrhal conjunctivitis when excited by the presence of a foreign body or by traumatism.

Conjunctivitis due to intense light is seen in *electric ophthalmia* (photophthalmia) following undue exposure to the electric arc used in welding and the bright arc lights employed in motion picture studios, and also after dazzling caused by reflection from snow (*snow blindness*) or following the use of a sun lamp if the eyes are not properly protected; in all of these cases the condition is caused by the ultraviolet rays. The symptoms are apt to be delayed for 12 hours or more after exposure; they consist of those present in acute conjunctivitis, but there is apt to be more pain, photophobia, lacrimation and smarting of the lids, the pupils are contracted and there may be superficial epithelial ulceration of the cornea. The affection disappears in a few days, during which the patient can be made more comfortable by cold compresses and the instillation of a cycloplegic.

Acute conjunctivitis may follow prolonged applications of *x-rays* or *radium* to parts adjacent to the eyes without sufficient protection to the latter; the symptoms are similar to those produced by intense light.

Lacrimal conjunctivitis accompanies dacryocystitis; it is generally limited to the inner third of the palpebral and ocular conjunctiva, is caused by infection from the germ-laden secretion of the diseased lacrimal sac and usually is unilateral.

Exanthematous conjunctivitis is the name given to that variety which is associated with the exanthemas; this form is seen most commonly in measles and often also in scarlatina.

Acute epidemic conjunctivitis, popularly known as *"pink eye,"* is a very *contagious* form of acute catarrhal conjunctivitis occurring most often in spring and autumn, presenting *intense symptoms* and *profuse discharge* and excited by the pneumococcus or, much less frequently, by the Koch-Weeks bacillus (*Hemophilus conjunctivilidis,* Plate 9A). This is the variety which sometimes gives rise to very severe signs of swelling and redness of the lids, subconjunctival hemorrhages and copious discharge, leading one to suspect the purulent form of conjunctivitis. It always is advisable to examine a smear and culture of the conjunctival secretion and to identify the responsible organism before deciding definitely upon the nature of the infection.

Chronic Catarrhal Conjunctivitis

Chronic catarrhal conjunctivitis is a chronic inflammation of the conjunctiva, presenting symptoms somewhat similar to those found in the acute form but milder in degree, and associated with only *slight* mucoid or mucopurulent secretion. It is known also as *chronic simple conjunctivitis.*

Signs. The conjunctiva of the lids is *reddened* and smooth; in old cases it may be *hypertrophied* and *velvety.* The secretion usually is mucoid and slight, often presenting a minimal crusting along the lid margins or at the inner canthus upon awakening. There may be some *excoriation* at the outer angle.

Symptoms, although less severe, are of the same kind as in the acute form: *burning* and *smarting* sensations, a feeling of dryness, an annoyance as from a foreign body, a *heavy, sleepy feeling* that causes some difficulty in keeping the lids open; the eyes water and tire easily. The symptoms generally are *worse at night.*

Course. The disease probably is the most *common* of ocular affections. It usually occurs in *adults,* and frequently in old persons. It is apt to be of *lengthy* duration, lasting months and even years.

Complications. *Blepharitis* frequently is present. Eczema of the lower lid, and eversion of the inferior punctum producing epiphora, are not uncommon; sometimes ectropion and corneal ulceration occur.

Etiology. Chronic catarrhal conjunctivitis may be the sequel of acute catarrh or may be caused by improper hygienic *surroundings, irritating atmosphere* (smoke, dust), continuous exposure to wind, insufficient sleep, alcoholic excesses, exposure of the conjunctiva in ectropion, *eye strain,* overuse or local irritation (trichiasis, etc.). It usually is *bilateral,* but when due to local irritants or dacryocystitis it may be unilateral. Cultures from the conjunctiva may show almost any pathogenic organism, but those most frequently responsible for the infection are *Staphylococcus aureus, Moraxella lacunata, Streptococcus viridans* and *Diplococcus pneumoniae.*

Angular Conjunctivitis, a variety of chronic catarrhal conjunctivitis caused by the Morax-Axenfeld bacillus (*Hemophilus duplex,* Plate 9*B*), is *subacute or chronic,* often tedious in its course and usually occurs in adults. There is moderate redness and swelling of the palpebral conjunctiva, the lid margins and the skin of the lids, which frequently shows excoriations especially at the *angles.* The symptoms include *smarting* and a feeling of foreign body in the eye. There is slight, grayish foamy *discharge* along the lid margins at the angles of the lids and over the excoriations of the skin. Rarely there is a complicating marginal corneal ulcer. Treatment of the blepharitis and conjunctivitis is satisfactorily accomplished by frequent applications of sulfacetamide drops or ointment. One of the tetracycline antibiotics, given orally or parenterally, should be added when corneal ulcerations occurs.

Follicular Conjunctivitis

Certain types of inflammation of the conjunctiva are characterized by hyperplasia of the subconjunctival lymphoid tissue with the production of follicles (Plate 10*C*). Normally the lymphoid layer is thin, with several accumulations which resemble follicles of adenoid tissue elsewhere in the body except that they have no connective tissue supporting structure. Three to six of these follicles normally are found over either end of the upper tarsus and adjacent fornix, and a similar number occur in the lower fornix. In individuals with a constitutional lymphoid hyperplasia, an asymptomatic folliculosis of the conjunctiva occurs along with hypertrophied tonsils, adenoids and lymphadenoid tissue generally, but subsides and disappears between the ages of 18 and 22 years as the constitutional lymphoid hyperplasia subsides. In some individuals this type of conjunctival folliculosis may be quite extensive. In follicular conjunctivitis, similar follicles appear in increasing number in the fornices and under the palpebral conjunctiva. In most instances the lower fornix shows more involvement than the upper.

Follicular conjunctivitis may be acute or chronic. The acute form occurs in virus infections and with the onset of inclusion blennorrhea and trachoma, whereas chronic follicular conjunctivitis occurs in chronic conjunctival irritation and in the prolonged phase of trachoma and inclusion blennorrhea.

Acute Follicular Conjunctivitis

Epidemic Keratoconjunctivitis is an acute, moderately infectious disease of the conjunctiva caused by adenovirus type 8. It frequently begins in one eye but usually is followed by involvement of the other eye within 3 to 5 days. Edema and redness appear abruptly in the lower fornix and lid, spreading rapidly upward onto the globe and into the upper fornix and lid. Follicles develop in the fornices quickly but are more numerous below. Preauricular (Fig. 6-2) and submental lymphadenopathy occur at the onset. Lacrimation occurs at the onset but changes quickly to a mucopurulent or purulent discharge. Small subepithelial infiltrates appear in the cornea several days after the onset, producing photophobia and some disturbance of vision. They usually disappear as the conjunctivitis subsides, but occasionally tiny residual

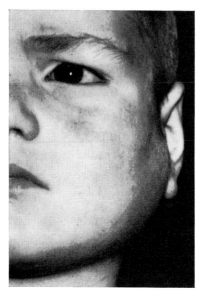

FIG. 6-2. Preauricular lymphadenopathy.

scars persist; however, these usually cause little or no disturbance of vision. The diagnosis is made on the history and clinical manifestations and is supported by secretion smears or scrapings from the conjunctiva which show a preponderance of lymphocytes and mononuclear cells, without bacteria or inclusion bodies. The disease usually is epidemic, occurring in employees of factories or other associated groups, but also is endemic in many localities.

Acute Follicular Conjunctivitis, Type Béal; Pharyngoconjunctival Fever; Greely Disease. Similar forms of acute follicular conjunctivitis with regional lymphadenopathy, but less severe and without corneal infiltrates, although superficial epithelial opacities of the cornea sometimes appear, occur epidemically, usually in the warmer months of the year, as the result of infection with other types of adenovirus. In some of these there is an associated mild pharyngitis and mild fever

but all are self-limited, usually running a course of 14 to 21 days. Secretion smears and scrapings are identical with those from epidemic keratoconjunctivitis, so the diagnosis is based on the clinical findings.

Treatment of all adenovirus infections of the conjunctiva is palliative since the viruses are not affected by the antibacterial drugs. Therefore cold compresses are applied for 15 minutes several times a day, and irritating topical applications are avoided. A cycloplegic (0.2 per cent scopolamine, 1.0 per cent atropine or 5.0 per cent homatropine) may be used to control photophobia, and bed rest and force fluids in those patients with fever and pharyngitis.

Purulent Conjunctivitis

Acute purulent inflammation of the conjunctiva may be caused at times by any organism capable of producing an acute catarrhal conjunctivitis, but usually is caused by the gonococcus in the form of (1) adult gonorrheal ophthalmia or conjunctivitis or (2) infantile purulent conjunctivitis or ophthalmia neonatorum.

Adult Gonorrheal Ophthalmia

Symptoms. *First stage: infiltration.* After a period of incubation varying from 12 hours to 3 days (short in severe cases), there occur great *swelling, redness and tenseness of the lids,* so that the latter cannot be opened voluntarily and can be separated only with difficulty. The *conjunctiva* of the lids and fornix is intensely *swollen, reddened* and uneven, and in severe cases it may be covered by a pseudomembrane; there are *chemosis* (Fig. 6-1) and infiltration. The *secretion* is at first *serous,* somewhat colored with blood and containing a little pus. The eye is tender to touch. The patient complains of a hot, smarting pain in the eye and a dull aching in the brow and temple. As a rule only *one eye* is affected. There may be slight fever and some swelling of the preauricular gland. This stage lasts about 2 days and is followed by the second stage.

Second stage: purulent discharge. The swelling of the lids and conjunctiva and the chemosis *diminish* and the eye becomes less tender. A *profuse purulent discharge* escapes continually from between the lids. This condition continues for 2 or 3 weeks, all symptoms gradually diminishing.

Third stage: convalescence or papillary swelling. The eye may return to normal in 2 or 3 weeks. More frequently, however, there is a stage of *papillary swelling*, a chronic inflammation of the lids; the palpebral and retrotarsal conjunctiva remains thickened and red and presents, especially over the tarsus, an uneven granular or velvety appearance, with hyperemia of the ocular conjunctiva, lasting several weeks.

Course. The disease always is a *serious* one, but exhibits various degrees of severity. Cases in which there is slight infection, or in which the disease has been contracted from a chronic gonorrhea, are the mildest. The very intense cases probably have been acquired through contagion from the secretion of a very virulent gonorrhea, and especially from contamination during the early stages of venereal infection.

Etiology. The disease is always acquired through infection from *gonorrheal secretion*, either *directly*, the fingers of the patient transferring the bacteria from the genitals, or *indirectly* by means of contaminated towels, etc. It is, fortunately, not very common.

Complications. A frequent and important complication is *corneal ulceration.* This begins with a circumscribed grayish infiltration, which becomes yellow and breaks down, so that ulcers are formed.

The ulcers vary in situation, size and course. They may be central or marginal; the latter may be confluent, so as to form an annular ulcer. The ulcers may *perforate*, and this may be followed by cicatrization with or without incarceration of the iris, staphyloma and other sequelae of corneal ulceration. Panophthalmitis may result. Severe and early involvement of the cornea is most common in intense attacks; in such cases, *serious* and permanent damage or loss of the eye is to be feared.

Prognosis depends, to a certain extent, upon the severity of the case and the behavior of the cornea. Since the introduction of sulfonamide and penicillin therapy, most cases are cured without complications, provided that the patient receives adequate and proper treatment before corneal ulceration occurs.

Treatment. The advent of the antibiotic drugs has revolutionized the management and prognosis of gonococcal conjunctivitis. However, the patient should be separated from other ocular patients and isolation techniques employed in his care. Cap, mask, gown, gloves and protective glasses should be worn by attendants while examining or treating the patient.

Intramuscular penicillin combined with oral administration of sulfonamides should be started as soon as secretion smears show Gram-negative intracellular biscuit-shaped diplococci. Depot-type penicillin in doses of 300,000 units should be given twice a day. An initial dose of 1 gm. of one of the sulfonamides should be followed by a 0.5-gm. maintenance dose four times a day. Treatment should be continued for a minimum of 72 hours or until two consecutive daily scrapings fail to show gonococci.

The rapid action of this treatment has eliminated the necessity of many of the formerly important local therapeutic measures, such as irrigation of the conjunctiva and shielding of the uninfected eye. However, cold compresses may be used to reduce the congestion and edema of the lids and to promote the comfort of the patient. They may be used continuously at first, but as the swelling is reduced they should be used intermittently, and they should not be used in treatment of actual corneal ulceration. Cycloplegia should be established and maintained when corneal involvement occurs.

Prophylactic treatment. Attendants should protect their own eyes from contamination when exposed to gonorrheal patients; if contamination does occur the eye should be irrigated thoroughly as quickly as possible. The conjunctiva is gently irrigated with saline, after the instillation a drop of 10 per cent solution of Argyrol, until no trace of color remains. Thereafter one drop of a 15 per cent solution of sulfacetamide may be instilled every hour for 3 days with daily examination for evidence of infection.

Metastatic Gonorrheal Conjunctivitis is an uncommon form of inflammation of the conjunctiva excited by the localization of gonococci in the subconjunctival tissue from a gonorrheal bacteremia and, like gonorrheal arthritis, which is apt to be present at the same time, is a complication of gonorrhea. The symptoms resemble those of severe catarrhal conjunctivitis, consisting of swelling and redness of the lids and conjunctiva with episcleral congestion, slight pain and limited discharge which is free from gonococci. The affection occurs in adults, is usually bilateral and runs its course in 2 or 3 weeks. It frequently is associated with metastatic gonorrheal iritis, and occasionally metastatic keratitis. There is a tendency to relapses, but combined penicillin and sulfonamide therapy as described above reduces this possibility.

Ophthalmia Neonatorum or Infantile Purulent Conjunctivitis

Ophthalmia neonatorum is an *acute purulent gonorrheal conjunctivitis occurring in the newborn,* presenting similar symptoms, complications and course, and requiring treatment similar to gonorrheal ophthalmia of adults. However, the incubation period may vary from 12 hours to 5 days.

The symptoms (Plate 10*B*) are the *same in kind as in the adult form,* but often less severe and more apt to be limited to the palpebral and retrotarsal conjunctiva. *Both eyes* usually are involved, though one generally is worse than the other; however, the disease may be monocular. The cornea is implicated less frequently, especially if the affection is treated from the start. If seen early, before the cornea is affected, and properly managed, this part very often escapes damage.

Prognosis, with proper treatment, is *generally favorable.*

Etiology. Infection usually occurs from contamination of the conjunctiva during passage through the infected cervix of the mother. Occasionally the infection may occur before birth as a result of spread of infection into the conjunctival sac following premature rupture of the membranes. Under these circumstances the infection usually is evident at birth and is more severe than usual, and frequently corneal ulceration is present. Occasionally the infection occurs as a result of contamination from infected debris on the skin of the lids, face or hands shortly after birth, but when the infection develops later than the fifth day of life the contamination has occurred after delivery, from napkins, towels or fingers which have been in contact with the genitals of the mother.

Many cases of conjunctivitis of the newborn are due to other infectious agents such as *Staphylococcus aureus, Diplococcus pneumoniae, Streptococcus viridans* or *hemolyticus, Hemophilus influenzae* and, rarely, a large number of other bacteria, but most of these develop later than the fifth day of life and rarely produce frankly purulent conjunctivitis. Inclusion blennorrhea, on the other hand, frequently has an acute purulent onset in the newborn, but it usually begins between the 6th and 21st days of life with an average incubation period of 7 days. Chemical conjunctivitis from Credé prophylaxis usually is mild, begins within 12 to 24 hours after delivery and disappears by the 3rd or 4th day after birth. Secretion smears and cultures, however, should be made in all cases in order to confirm the diagnosis.

Treatment is similar to that employed in adult purulent conjunctivitis, systemic treatment with suitable doses of *penicillin* and *sulfonamides.*

When lid retractors are used for inspection of the cornea, great care must be exercised not to injure the cornea, a possibility which is increased by the struggles of the infant.

The general health of the infant must be looked after, since enfeebled conditions render treatment unsatisfactory and favor corneal complications.

Credé's Method of Prophylaxis consists of *cleansing* the lids immediately after birth and instilling 1 drop of a 2 per cent solution of *nitrate of silver*, thus destroying any gonococci which may have entered the conjunctival sac. This causes redness of the conjunctiva for a day or two (chemical conjunctivitis); a *1 per cent solution* of silver nitrate frequently is substituted and is less irritating but equally efficacious.

Ophthalmia neonatorum is much less common now than formerly; the first great reduction in frequency followed the employment of Credé's method of prophylaxis, but recently the *antepartum*

treatment of the birth canal of the mother has reduced the incidence even further. Institutions for the blind now report many fewer cases of blindness following ophthalmia neonatorum since the employment of these two prophylactic measures. Because of this and because of the great effectiveness of combined penicillin and sulfonamide therapy, the necessity of prophylactic treatment of the eyes of the newborn is diminishing. This also probably accounts for the apparent success of a number of substitutes for the silver salts.

Purulent Conjunctivitis of Young Girls, due to contamination, directly or indirectly, from gonorrheal vaginitis in themselves or gonorrheal cervicitis from older girls with whom they live, is encountered in asylums, hospitals and in poor and crowded living conditions. The symptoms resemble those of purulent conjunctivitis but are much less severe, the cornea seldom is involved and the prognosis is good with proper treatment.

Membranous Conjunctivitis

Under this heading are included the *uncommon* examples of conjunctivitis in which an exudate forms a *membrane* on the surface of the conjunctiva. In true membranous conjunctivitis the membrane penetrates the substance of the conjunctiva and can not be removed without leaving a raw bleeding surface (Fig. 6-3) but in pseudomembranous conjunctivitis the membrane forms on the surface of the epithelium and is easily detached without leaving bleeding points.

Diphtheritic Membranous Conjunctivitis is a rare disease, usually associated with nasopharyngeal diphtheria, and due to the *Klebs-Loeffler bacillus*, which is found in the smears and cultures of the exudate. The disease begins acutely with edema of the lids, intense inflammation of the conjunctiva and the formation of a grayish yellow infiltrating true membrane.

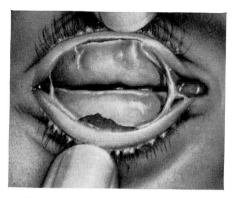

Fig. 6-3. Membraneous conjunctivitis.

The lids become hard and there is a tendency to necrosis of the involved areas of conjunctiva. Corneal ulceration may develop if the bulbar conjunctiva is involved. The *constitutional symptoms* of diphtheria also are present. In the healing process, cicatricial deformities result if there has been much necrosis. Treatment includes large doses of *antitoxin* and local and systemic use of penicillin. Precautions should be observed against laryngeal obstruction for diphtheritic conjunctivitis always is accompanied by at least nasopharyngeal diphtheria. Corneal ulceration must be treated as described in the next chapter. Some cases of diphtheritic conjunctivitis are mild and may be pseudomembranous, purulent or rarely catarrhal. In these types the patient usually has some immunity to diphtheria toxin but treatment should be the same as in the membranous lesion. Diagnosis in all types is based on the demonstration of *C. diphtheriae* in smears and cultures.

True membranous conjunctivitis also may be produced at times by mixed infections, severe chemical injury and as a complication of erythema multiforme.

Pseudomembranous Conjunctivitis includes all types in which an easily removable membrane forms on the conjunctiva. This occurs in occasional in-

stances of purulent and mucopurulent conjunctivitis due to gonococcus, streptococcus, or pneumococcus, especially in mixed infections, vernal conjunctivitis, chemical injuries and thermal burns. Smears and cultures always should be made. Treatment in the infective cases is that of purulent and catarrhal conjunctivitis; the examples resulting from burns should be handled as described under injuries of the conjunctiva.

Inclusion Blennorrhea

Inclusion blennorrhea, an oculogenital disease affecting the conjunctiva of adults and infants, the urethra of the adult male and the cervix of the adult female, is caused by a Rickettsia-like organism, *Chlamydia oculogenitalis*. In the adult the disease usually is the result of bathing in contaminated swimming pools (swimming bath conjunctivitis) but occasionally is caused by accidental contamination in obstetricians, ophthalmologists and nurses, whereas in the infant the infection usually is the result of contamination of the conjunctiva during birth.

In the adult, after an average incubation period of 7 days, an acute follicular conjunctivitis with swelling and redness of the conjunctiva, more intense in the lower fornix, and mucopurulent to purulent discharge appears in one eye and frequently involves the other eye within a few days. There is an associated regional lymphadenopathy in approximately half of the cases. Without treatment, the acute phase lasts 21 to 30 days and subsides into a chronic follicular conjunctivitis of 3 to 6 months' duration. The cornea never is affected.

In the infant the lesion becomes follicular in character only after 4 to 6 weeks, as the lymphoid layer of the conjunctiva is not developed until about that time. In other respects the disease is similar to the adult variety.

The diagnosis is made on the basis of the clinical appearance of the conjunctiva, the lack of corneal involvement and the demonstration of cytoplasmic inclusion bodies in epithelial cells in scraping preparations from the conjunctiva stained by Giemsa's method (Plate 11*B*).

Treatment. Oral administration of sulfonamides for 10 days is the treatment of choice. In the adult the usual dosage is 0.5 gm. four times a day, and in the infant 0.25 gm. four times a day. In those cases in which sulfonamides may not be used one of the tetracycline antibiotics may be used.

Trachoma

Trachoma is a chronic follicular keratoconjunctivitis (Plate 10*E* and *F*) of infectious origin occurring at all ages. It is widely distributed throughout the world, being most prevalent in the Orient, the Middle East and the Mediterranean area, but with persistent foci in the Americas. It is common in Russia, Poland, Hungary, Japan and China, prevalent in Italy, Prussia, Ireland and Northern Brazil, but especially frequent in Arabia and Egypt. It is endemic in the latter country, and a majority of the natives are afflicted. It is supposed that Napoleon's soldiers increased the prevalence of the disease, Egyptian ophthalmia as they called it, upon their return to Europe. In Europe it occurs much more extensively in the east than the west and much more frequently in low lands (Belgium, Holland, Hungary) than in elevated countries (Switzerland). In America it was common among immigrants from eastern Europe until the U. S. Immigration Service began strict exclusion of affected individuals, and it was fairly common among native Americans in certain sections of the United States, including the mountainous regions of Tennessee, Virginia and West Virginia, the Carolinas, southern Illinois, Indiana and Missouri. It also was frequent among American Indians, 10 per cent of the entire Indian population of the United States being affected, but since the introduction and widespread use of the sulfonamide drugs there has been a drastic reduction in the numbers of infectious cases. Negroes are rather immune but not entirely exempt.

Etiology. Trachoma is an *infectious* disease caused by a Rickettsia-like organism, *Chlamydia trachomatis*. It is most contagious during the early stages. It is transmitted by contaminated fingers, towels, handkerchiefs, etc., used in common by many persons. *Predisposing factors* are crowded living quarters and uncleanliness; hence the disease is found most often among the *poorer classes*. Districts with an insufficient supply of water often are the seat of *bad hygienic conditions* favoring the spread of trachoma.

Microscopic examination of the conjunctival scrapings in trachoma reveals the presence of *cytoplasmic inclusion bodies* (Plate 11*B*) in the epithelial cells. The bodies are similar to those found in inclusion blennorrhea.

Symptoms. More or less photophobia, blepharospasm, lacrimation and burning sensations, feeling of foreign body, pain and visual disturbance. In some cases there may be no subjective symptoms. There is a variable amount of mucopurulent discharge. The course of the disease on the conjunctiva can be divided into *four stages*.

Stage I (insidious) trachoma may exist for some time before the development of symptoms of *slight conjunctivitis*, thickening, edema and congestion of the conjunctiva, and the formation of *minute follicles and papillae in the upper tarsal conjunctiva*. Microscopic examination of conjunctival scrapings shows epithelial cell *inclusion bodies* which are indistinguishable from those of inclusion conjunctivitis. This stage lasts several weeks to several months, sometimes passing imperceptibly into Stage III but at others developing into acute trachoma.

Stage II (acute). Occasionally the disease begins acutely (*acute trachoma*) and is accompanied by intense inflammatory symptoms and profuse purulent discharge, in which case conjunctival smears and cultures are studied to determine whether the disease is acute pure trachoma or whether there is superimposed bacterial infection. Acute pure trachoma usually shows a predominance of follicular development although there also are many papillae, whereas in acute trachoma with secondary bacterial infection papillary hypertrophy is predominant. As the secondary infection subsides the follicles become more prominent and at times they may develop on the semilunar folds and at the limbus. The subconjunctival infiltration, by increasing the weight of the lid, causes it to droop and produces trachomatous ptosis, which may persist into Stage III. Acute trachoma may persist for many weeks to many months, gradually passing over into the cicatricial stage.

Stage III (cicatricial) trachoma is characterized by the appearance of *scar tissue*, leading eventually to cure of the disease. The *papillae and follicles gradually disappear*, but the cicatricial changes and contraction lead to certain *sequelae*; the seriousness of which depends upon the severity of the process. In the tarsal conjunctiva the cicatricial process causes a narrow, whitish band parallel with the lid margin, the white line of Arlt (Plate 10E), sometimes a network; in advanced and severe cases the entire surface may be replaced by a pale, smooth *cicatricial membrane*. In the fornix, cicatrization changes the conjunctiva into a pale, bluish white membrane, and as a result of contraction the *transition fold is shortened* or disappears.

Stage IV represents healed trachoma. Infiltration of the conjunctiva and tarsus will have disappeared, but *scar tissue* remains and this frequently causes various *sequelae*.

Trachoma does not always progress uninterruptedly; there often are *intermissions and exacerbations. Relapses* are quite frequent, especially when treatment has been discontinued too soon.

Corneal Involvement. A characteristic finding is the development of *trachomatous pannus* (Plate 10F), consisting of loops of vessels extending into the cornea between the epithelium and Bowman's membrane occurring first at the upper limbus.

Trachomatous pannus invades the cornea all around the periphery but always is most advanced into the cornea above, least below and to an intermediate extent nasally and temporally. The affected part of the cornea presents a *cloudy* appearance, and is grayish and translucent; its surface is *uneven and vascularized*, the blood vessels springing from the conjunctival vessels at the limbus. The process advances until it covers the *upper half* of the cornea; in severe cases the entire cornea may be covered and *vision may be reduced* to perception of light, the final visual acuity depending upon the extent of corneal opacification and unevenness. In severe cases, iritis is apt to develop. Pannus is not produced by the mechanical irritation of the upper lid rubbing against the cornea, but is due to a change similar to that which occurs in the conjunctiva; it is an infiltration with the addition of new blood vessels between Bowman's membrane and the corneal epithelial layer. Small superficial corneal *ulcers* often are found near the margin of the advancing pannus. The patient complains of *photophobia and pain*.

Sequelae. Complete cure occurs usually in the mildest cases only, or in some of the moderate examples when they are subjected to early treatment. Sequelae are very common, affect the conjunctiva, cornea and lids, and produce permanent disability of the eye. They are:

(1) *Trichiasis and entropion* resulting from cicatricial contraction of the conjunctiva with curving of the tarsus; they are worse in the upper lid. As a result of this distortion of the lid with consequent changes in the position of the cilia, there is mechanical interference with the cornea, causing ulceration.

(2) *Ectropion* (usually of the lower lid), which sometimes follows as a result of hypertrophy of the conjunctiva and contraction of the orbicularis.

(3) *Symblepharon*, resulting from cicatricial contraction of the conjunctiva; when considerable, there is obliteration of the fornix. This condition restricts the movements of the eyeball.

(4) *Corneal opacities* caused by pannus and corneal ulcers. After lasting some time, pannus changes into a thin, permanent layer of connective tissue.

(5) *Staphyloma of the cornea* in some cases, after threatened or actual perforation of corneal ulcers.

(6) *Xerosis*, a dry, scaly state of the conjunctiva, with similar changes in the cornea; it may occur in severe forms.

Treatment. Oral sulfonamide therapy is the treatment of choice. In adults 0.5 to 1 gm. of one of the absorbable sulfonamides usually is given four times a day for 10 to 14 days, and in children 0.25 to 0.5 gm. four times a day for the same period. In those patients in whom sulfonamides cannot be used one of the tetracycline antibiotics may be substituted. For example, tetracycline may be given in 250-mg. doses every 6 hours for 10 to 12 days. Topical application of these drugs is much less effective and requires a much longer period of treatment; therefore it is used generally only as a supplementary measure.

Palliative measures include cold compresses to control the inflammatory symptoms and cycloplegics to control the photophobia associated with the corneal lesions.

Treatment of Complications. The operation of *peritomy*, the excision of a narrow strip of conjunctiva surrounding the cornea, is occasionally performed for the relief of severe cases of pannus after the active inflammatory reaction has subsided. The object of this operation is to cut off the vascular supply. This procedure may be modified by insertion of a strip of mucous membrane from the lip into the circumcorneal denuded area.

Trichiasis demands surgical correction if extensive, or either epilation or electrolysis if only a few cilia are involved.

Xerosis is an indication for median tarsorrhaphy to prevent drying of the cornea.

General treatment must not be neglected. *Hygienic surroundings* should be as perfect as possible, with cleanliness and proper ventilation. Outdoor employment, good food and attention to the general health are important aids to a cure.

Prophylaxis is very important. The patient must be warned of the *contagiousness* of the secretion, and the necessity for keeping his handkerchiefs, towels, wash basin, etc., apart from those of other persons. In schools, asylums, institutions and barracks the *prevention of epidemics* of trachoma is a matter requiring vigilance, inspection of every new inmate and *isolation* of trachoma cases so long as the latter are capable of conveying the disease.

Tuberculosis of the Conjunctiva, both primary and secondary, is rare, usually unilateral, and presents granulations with ulceration and involvement of the preauricular and submaxillary glands; it may be mistaken for trachoma, tularemia or Parinaud's conjunctivitis. The diagnosis is established by finding tubercle bacilli in an excised portion, or by the evidence obtained after placing a fragment into the anterior chamber of a rabbit. Treatment comprises excision, or scraping with subsequent cauterization, and general treatment of tuberculosis, with isoniazid, p-aminosalicylic acid and streptomycin.

Parinaud's Conjunctivitis is a rare disease of the conjunctiva due to infection with a leptothrix. It usually is limited to one eye. Inflammatory nodules develop with numerous pinpoint gray or yellowish areas beneath the conjunctival epithelium, representing infiltration of the tissues with large mononuclear cells surrounding tissue necrosis, but there is no ulceration. Accompanying these conjunctival changes is considerable inflammatory enlargement of the preauricular gland with no tendency to suppurate. There is only slight constitutional disturbance, no pain and little discomfort. Prognosis is favorable and cure results within several weeks. Diagnosis is confirmed by excision and biopsy of one of the nodules, which will show the organisms in the pinpoint foci of necrosis. This seems to have a favorable effect on the disease. Iodides given by mouth also are beneficial.

Tularemic Conjunctivitis is rare except in certain parts of the southwestern United States, and is due to infection with *Bacillus tularense* usually transmitted from infected rabbits or other rodents. It is accompanied by serious constitutional symptoms with enlargement of the preauricular gland. The conjunctiva is chemotic and there is diffuse purulent infiltration accompanied by necrotic foci, resulting in the formation of several discrete ulcers.

Acne Rosacea Conjunctivitis and Blepharoconjunctivitis occur in adults with acne rosacea. There are recurrent attacks of minute corneal infiltrations or ulcers at or near the limbus with an increase of symptoms and the addition of pain and photophobia. This variety of conjunctivitis is intractable; it has been thought to be associated with deficiency of vitamin B_2 but nearly always shows a superimposed chronic *Staphylococcus aureus* infection.

Thus oral administration of riboflavin in a 5-mg. dose, one to three times a day, should be supplemented by treatment of the infectious element.

Allergic Conjunctivitis

Allergy enters into the production of a number of clinical affections of the conjunctiva, the chief of which are atopic conjunctivitis, contact conjunctivitis, phlyctenular conjunctivitis and vernal conjunctivitis. In addition angioneurotic edema at times involves the conjunctiva as well as the lids.

Atopic Conjunctivitis

Atopic conjunctivitis is a variety of acute catarrhal conjunctivitis usually due to sensitivity to pollens in individuals showing other allergic lesions such as rose colds, hay fever, or occasionally asthma. The onset is acute with infection, edema or chemosis, lacrimation changing to a watery mucoid discharge and intense itching. Scrapings from the conjunctiva contain numerous eosinophils (Plate 11A). Treatment consists of the detection and removal of the sensitizing substance or desensitization to it and relief of the discomfort by the use of Adrenalin and iced compresses. Benefit also has been obtained from the topical use of steroid solutions and occasionally from the general use of antihistaminics. Topical use of antihistamine solutions, however, frequently produces contact conjunctivitis.

Contact Conjunctivitis

Contact conjunctivitis is an allergic reaction to topically applied drugs and chemical substances. It is an acute catarrhal type of conjunctivitis and nearly always is accompanied by contact dermatitis of the skin of the lids. Itching, redness and chemosis with lacrimation characterize the conjunctival lesion. Scrapings occasionally contain eosinophils. Although practically every drug used on the conjunctiva has produced contact conjunctivitis, on occasion, the more common offending agents are butyn, atropine, eserine, pilocarpine, the antihistamines and the antibiotic agents. Treatment consists of the elimination of the cause, with local use of vasoconstrictors, cold compresses, and occasionally topical application of one of the steroid solutions.

Phlyctenular Conjunctivitis

This disease, also known as *eczematous conjunctivitis*, is a *circumscribed* inflammation of the conjunctiva, accompanied by the formation of one or more small bleb-like projections called *phlyctenules*. The latter consist of accumulations of lymphoid cells, which rapidly soften at their apices and form small *ulcers*. The phlyctenules may appear upon the conjunctiva, and then the disease is called phlyctenular *conjunctivitis*; they may be found upon the cornea, when the affection constitutes phlyctenular *keratitis*; or they may occur, and most frequently do occur, at the *limbus*, producing phlyctenular *keratoconjunctivitis*. Very frequently they occur in all three situations in the same individual. The pathology, symptoms and treatment being the same in all cases, it is convenient to describe the three varieties collectively under the title of *phlyctenular ophthalmia*, whether the phlyctenules occur in the epithelial layer of the ocular conjunctiva or its extension on the cornea.

Signs. The essential sign is the occurrence of one or more small, gray or yellow *elevations* or nodules (1 or 2 mm.), at some part of the conjunctiva or cornea, frequently at the limbus. The phlyctenule is surrounded by a localized conjunctival *hyperemia* (Plate 13*E*). The nonaffected parts of the ocular conjunctiva are but slightly changed from the normal but there may be an associated catarrhal conjunctivitis of mild type. The phlyctenule rapidly develops a small *ulceration* at its apex. It heals without leaving any changes in the conjunctiva. The entire process lasts from a few days to 2 weeks.

Occasionally one or more phlyctenules are of large size with purulent contents; such cases have been called *pustular ophthalmia*.

Occasionally, a number of phlyctenules appear at the same time; in this manner the entire ocular conjunctiva may be reddened, and in such cases the palpebral conjunctiva will be congested. The nodules may become absorbed without going through the stage of ulceration.

When the phlyctenule appears upon the *cornea*, the infiltration and subsequent ulcer occasionally are *superficial* and heal without the production of lasting changes in the cornea. But often they spread into the corneal substance, and then leave a permanent *opacity*. Very rarely, the ulcer perforates the cornea; or a number of ulcers may, by confluence, spread along the surface of the cornea.

Fascicular keratitis. The ulcer resulting from the phlyctenule may advance from the margin to the center of the cornea, drawing after it a fascicle of blood vessels. In this manner there is formed a narrow, red band of vessels, extending some distance over the cornea; at the apex of this fascicle is a small, gray crescent, corresponding to the advancing margin of the ulcer, which has healed in the peripheral parts. This form of ulceration always remains superficial; when the process terminates, the blood vessels gradually cease carrying blood and a superficial linear opacity remains.

Occasionally, as a result of persistent recurrence of phlyctenules, the cornea becomes clouded, uneven and covered by superficial vessels; this condition is known as *phlyctenular pannus.*

The phlyctenule, in severe cases, may involve the deep layers of the cornea, forming a deep infiltration; this either becomes absorbed completely or leaves an opacity of the cornea; or, rarely, it may become purulent and a deep ulcer may result.

There is considerable *lacrimation*; if there is any discharge, it is mucous or mucopurulent ·but not abundant. As a result of constant lacrimation, frequently there are added *blepharitis,* excoriations at the external angle and *eczema* of the lids, ectropion of the lower lid and occasionally blepharophimosis.

Symptoms. *Blepharospasm,* and with this also *photophobia,* are severe when the cornea is involved, but slight or absent in conjunctival cases. When the cornea is involved, the child will remain in a dark corner or bury its face in a pillow, and the eyes can be examined only with difficulty. There is intense discomfort, but usually not much pain.

Pathology. Phlyctenules begin with an infiltration of the subepithelial layer of the conjunctiva and of the cornea, respectively, with leukocytes which soon invade the epithelial covering; this forms a nodule somewhat raised above the surface. Necrosis takes place, the nodule bursts and an ulcer is formed. In many cases, when the infiltration is superficial, the defect is replaced with epithelium; in cases of deeper involvement, with scar tissue.

Course. The phlyctenules usually occur in *crops*; before one is completely cured another is apt to appear. In this way the course may become *protracted* and may extend over weeks. Each phlyctenule lasts from a few days to a week or two. *Relapses* are very common. Phlyctenules occur most frequently in *children*; they are uncommon in adults; in the latter, a single large phlyctenule may present the local appearance of episcleritis.

Etiology. The disease is *common.* Allergy to tuberculous products is an etiologic factor in most cases, but allergy to other bacterial products also may be a cause. Poor diet and unsanitary conditions in general are contributory factors and predisposing causes. It is common in children debilitated from disease and in those recovering from the exanthemas, especially measles. Other manifestations of the predisposing diathesis are swelling of the cervical lymphatic glands, eczema, rhinitis, blepharitis, otitis media, etc. Sometimes, however, the affection occurs in children apparently in good health, although close inquiry usually discloses a dietary or constitutional factor.

Prognosis is *favorable*; serious results are uncommon. The phlyctenules often leave no traces. In corneal cases opacities of greater or lesser density remain, and if these are central, sight will be affected. Frequent recurrences may result in a number of cloud-like opacities of the cornea.

Treatment. Since this disease represents a manifestation of bacterial allergy, resembling tuberculids of the skin, any therapy which controls the exudative and inflammatory reaction of the tissues is of value, permitting the process to subside and healing to take place. The topical use of *cortisone*, in the form of 0.5 per cent or 2.5 per cent solution instilled every hour or two, or in 1.5 per cent ointment three or four times a day, has proved beneficial. Cortisone blocks the tissue response to the acute allergic trauma and minimizes the permanent scarring of the cornea in patients with keratitis.

Tuberculin therapy is valuable in patients manifesting a hypersensitivity to tuberculin and in the prevention of recurrences.

For prominent symptoms of irritation it is advisable to apply *cold pads* if the phlyctenules involve the conjunctiva, and *hot compresses* if they form upon the cornea.

In corneal cases, the *photophobia and blepharospasm* often are very annoying symptoms, but these can be controlled by placing the iris and ciliary body at rest with adequate cycloplegia. For this purpose 0.2 per cent scopolamine or 1 per cent atropine may need to be instilled one to three times a day.

General treatment is of great importance. Correction of faulty diet and elimination of secondary bacterial infections of the conjunctiva and lid margins are important therapeutic procedures. The *nose* and nasopharynx should receive proper treatment. These patients should not be allowed to remain in the house and in the dark, as they are inclined to do on account of the photophobia. *Smoked glasses* with side protection and adequate cycloplegia relieve this symptom. Internally, *cod liver oil* or vitamins A and D are of great benefit. *Sun baths* and artificial sun irradiation of the body (with proper protection of the eyes) may be of some value.

Vernal Conjunctivitis

Vernal conjunctivitis or spring catarrh is an allergic disease of the conjunctiva, of *chronic* course, lasting for years, recurring during *warm weather* and disappearing entirely or to a great extent in winter. It affects *both eyes* and occurs chiefly in children, most frequently in *boys*. It attacks either the tarsal or the limbic conjunctiva, or occasionally both.

Signs. In the *palpebral form*, the upper palpebral conjunctiva presents hard, flattened papillae, separated by furrows, giving a *cobblestone* appearance (Plate 12*C*). Both upper and lower palpebral conjunctivae are *bluish white* in color, as if covered with a thin layer of milk. In the *limbic form*, the conjunctiva adjacent to the inner and outer portions of the cornea presents *gelatinous hypertrophies* (Plate 12*D*), sometimes slightly pigmented; these may involve the cornea for a short distance; occasionally the hypertrophy surrounds the cornea. There are conjunctival *congestion*, mucoid, *stringy secretion* and thin pseudomembranes in the most acute phases. During winter these changes become less intense or almost disappear; they return with warm weather.

Symptoms include a feeling of *heat, lacrimation, intense itching* and *photophobia*; these become worse in warm weather and disappear in the winter.

Pathology. The papillae consist of dense fibrous material in the subconjunctival tissue, later undergoing hyaline degeneration; the epithelium is greatly thickened and sends short prolongations into the fibrous deposits; the hypertrophied epithelium and the pseudomembranes account for the milky appearance. *Eosinophilic* leukocytes are abundant in the secretion (Plate 11*A*) and the subconjunctival tissue. The gelatinous limbic lesion consists principally of greatly thickened epithelium.

Course. The disease continues in this intermittent way for several years or longer, finally becoming extinct and leaving no traces or very slight changes behind. Occasionally a grayish line concentric with the limbus but with a clear area between the linear opacity and the limbus, thus resembling the arcus senilis, is left and also there may be slight thickening, discoloration and irregularity in the palpebral conjunctiva. The diagnosis is evident; it scarcely can be mistaken for trachoma, since the type of individual, the milky appearance, recurrence in hot weather, freedom of fornix involvement and absence of complications will prevent error.

Treatment. Topical therapy with *cortisone* has proved valuable. The subjective symptoms can be made less annoying by the use of 1 per cent monohydrated sodium carbonate solution. This is slightly alkaline and dissolves the stringy mucous secretion, which seems to be quite irritating.

Temporary relief from the distressing subjective symptoms may be obtained by the instillation of 1:10,000 *Adrenalin*, the use of *cold compresses* and the wearing of *smoked glasses*. Exposure to *radium* or beta-irradiation, when the papillae are of large size, results in some improvement; however, this remedy must be used cautiously, since cataract has followed such applications.

Symblepharon

Symblepharon is a *cicatricial attachment* between the conjunctiva of the lid and the eyeball (Fig. 6-4). It may affect both lids, but usually the *lower*; some-

times it includes part of the cornea. It is called *anterior or partial*, when extending bridge-like from lid to globe, leaving a free portion of conjunctiva corresponding to the fornix; *posterior*, when it involves only the fornix; and *total*, when the lids are adherent to the globe throughout.

Etiology. It is caused by the junction of two opposing granulating surfaces; hence, it occurs after *injuries*, especially *burns* from lime, acids and molten metal; also after operations, and sometimes it follows *trachoma* or, rarely, diphtheritic conjunctivitis.

Symptoms. Symblepharon often *interferes* with the movement of the eyeball, and this may cause diplopia. Traction upon the adherent parts excites *irritation*. In extensive cases the cornea is included and sight affected, or, if there is inability to close the lids, lagophthalmos and its sequelae may be present. There is apt to be disfigurement.

Treatment. If anterior and not extensive, the band is divided and the two raw surfaces kept from uniting by *separating* them daily with a probe, interposing a roll of absorbent cotton saturated with some bland oil or ointment or a symblepharon ring.

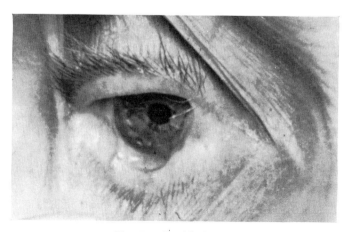

Fig. 6-4. Symblepharon.

In more *severe forms*, and in posterior and total symblepharon, the separated raw surfaces must be *covered with conjunctiva* or with *grafts* of mucous membrane to keep them from uniting. This may be done by loosening the adjacent bulbar conjunctiva and suturing it over the defect or by transplanting pieces of mucous membrane from the lip.

Conjunctival Concretions are seen often, especially in elderly persons, appearing as small, bright yellow points beneath the conjunctiva; they consist of accumulations in the spaces formed from sealing off of the surface in the presence of papillary hypertrophy. The condition is sometimes called *lithiasis conjunctivae,* but the concretions do not contain calcium. Sometimes they change into tiny hard masses which project, acting like foreign bodies and causing discomfort; under such circumstances they should be picked out with the point of a needle or knife after surface anesthesia.

Pinguecula is a small, slightly raised *yellowish* spot situated to the inner and outer sides of the cornea, where the conjunctiva is most exposed to wind, dust, etc., especially in *old people* and most conspicuous when the conjunctiva is reddened. It is not formed of fat as its name implies, but of thickening of the conjunctiva owing to excessive development of yellow elastic tissue and hyalin. When conspicuous it may attract attention and cause worry until its nature is explained, but it rarely calls for excision.

Pterygium

Pterygium is a triangular fold of membrane, occupying the interpalpebral fissure, extending from the inner or outer part of the bulbar conjunctiva to the cornea (Fig. 6-5); the apex is immovably united to the cornea and is usually blunt; the base spreads out and merges with the conjunctiva.

When recent, pterygium is rich in blood vessels and hence of a red color; later it changes into a white, tendinous *membrane,* and becomes stationary. The central portion is firmly attached to the sclera but above and below its margin it is represented by a fold of conjunctiva. It grows slowly toward the center of the cornea, giving rise to moderate symptoms of *conjunctival irritation* and disfigurement, and when it encroaches upon the pupillary area it interferes with vision. It generally is situated to the inner side of the cornea, less frequently to the outer side or in both situations. It may occur in one or both eyes.

Etiology. It usually occurs in persons who are exposed to *wind* or *dust* (farmers, coachmen, masons, sailors).

Pathology. The affection is thought to consist of a degenerative process due to long continued irritation; vascularized connective tissue grows forward beneath the corneal epithelium and there is destruction of Bowman's membrane.

Treatment consists of *removal* by one of a number of different *operative* methods. The pterygium may be dissected away and cut off, the conjunctival defect closed by uniting upper and lower borders, undermining to bring the edges together. The *apex* of the pterygium must be thoroughly excised from the cornea, and its attachment scraped or *cauterized* with the electrocautery, to prevent recurrence. Instead of cutting off the pterygium, it may

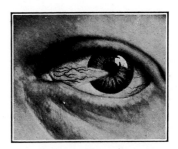

FIG. 6-5. Pterygium.

be dissected from the cornea and underlying sclera, and the apex sutured underneath the detached conjunctiva, either above or below; or it may be divided into halves, of which one is *transplanted* above and the other below, being held in the conjunctival pocket by a suture. There is a tendency to recurrence.

Pseudopterygium is an attachment of a fold of conjunctiva to any part of the cornea as a result of ulceration of the latter; it occurs occasionally after ulcers, gonorrheal and diphtheritic conjunctivitis, burns and other injuries. A fine probe can be passed under the conjunctival attachment at the limbus; this distinguishes it from a true pterygium. When separated from its corneal attachment the conjunctival fold retracts to its normal position.

Pigmentation of the Conjunctiva

In addition to the variations of the normal pigmentation associated with variations in general pigmentation of the individual, the conjunctiva exhibits abnormal pigmentation under a number of circumstances. Such pigmentation is especially noticeable because of the normal transparency of the conjunctiva and the white background afforded the bulbar conjunctiva by the sclera, which also becomes pigmented at times, however, in some of the same conditions.

Hematogenous pigmentation is the most frequent form of conjunctival discoloration. It follows subconjunctival hemorrhage, especially when extensive, multiple or repeated, and may be idiopathic; traumatic, the result of general diseases such as the blood dyscrasias, scurvy, malignant malaria or blackwater fever, yellow fever and vascular disease; or the result of local infectious diseases such as hemorrhagic conjunctivitis (pink eye).

Bile pigments produce a yellowish discoloration of the conjunctiva and sclera

as the earliest manifestation of generalized icterus in obstructive jaundice, icterus neonatorum and hepatitis.

Melanin pigmentation, in addition to variations of the normal and that associated with nevi and melanotic tumors, is increased in Addison's disease, ochronosis, keratomalacia, certain inflammatory lesions and certain drugs. In *Addison's disease* a gradually developing diffuse pigmentation involves the conjunctiva as well as other epithelial and subepithelial tissues exposed to light. Intensification of the pigmentation may occur around the limbus, producing a black circle around the cornea. In *ochronosis* the pigment occurs as sharply delimited sepia-colored depositions in the conjunctiva and sclera, usually in the palpebral fissure area on both sides of the cornea. In *keratomalacia* pigmentation may involve both the conjunctiva and cornea. Pigmentation of the conjunctiva also is likely to occur in *chronic trachoma,* repeated attacks of vernal conjunctivitis and other chronic irritative lesions of the conjunctiva. Prolonged use of *Adrenalin* or contact with *carbolic acid,* either as a medication or in the chemical industry, leads to increased melanin in the conjunctiva.

Amyloid, hyaline and *lipoid* deposits in and under the conjunctiva in various degenerative diseases and processes give the conjunctiva a yellowish tinge.

Metallic discoloration is the result of medication or foreign bodies. *Argyrosis* resulting from general or topical use of silver salts (Plate 12B) produces a grayish discoloration which becomes brown or brownish black with continued use of the medicine.

Siderosis produces a rust-colored granular spot around the sight of an iron foreign body. *Arsenic* and *gold* may at times result in the deposition of dark granules in the conjunctiva and periphery of the cornea.

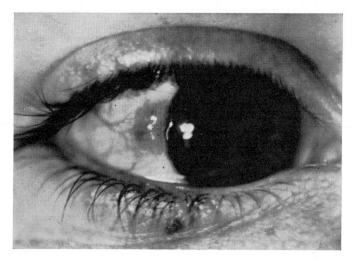

FIG. 6-6. Papilloma of the limbus.

Temporary staining associated with more or less irritation of the conjunctiva follows the application of various dyes to the conjunctiva. The aniline dyes are the most frequent, probably because of their wide usage in the chemical industry where there is greater chance of accidental contamination. However, a severe form of conjunctival inflammation, often leading to local and sometimes to diffuse necrosis, follows the accidental or purposeful insertion of a piece of an indelible or copying pencil under the conjunctiva. The purple dye (methyl violet) diffuses fairly rapidly into the surrounding tissues, producing inflammation which may involve the cornea. The foreign body should be removed as quickly as possible.

Conjunctival cysts. Epithelial implantation cysts of the conjunctiva result from entrapment and proliferation of epithelium following a wound. A single cyst or several cysts may occur. Other epithelial cysts may follow inflammation of the conjunctiva or arise from unknown causes.

Retention cysts arise as a result of blockage of the duct of an excretory gland by inspissated secretion, inflammation or scar tissue. They usually develop in the upper or lower fornix.

Lymphatic cysts develop as ectasias of the lymph vessels of the conjunctiva. They are superficial, thin-walled, circumscribed and filled with a clear fluid. They occur more frequently than epithelial cysts.

Epithelial tumors. Papillomas arise from the limbus, the caruncle and the lid margin. Limbic papillomas usually arise from a broad base and extend as flat masses (Fig. 6-6) onto the conjunctiva

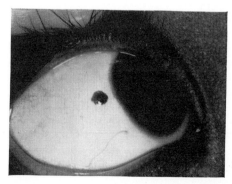

FIG. 6-7. Heavily pigmented nevus.

and cornea whereas those arising from the caruncle and lid margin usually are red, fleshy cauliflower-like or irregular projections. They frequently recur following excision.

Leucoplakia occurs at the limbus in the form of slow growing opaque white plagues composed of epithelium showing varying degrees of acanthosis, dyskeratosis and hyperkeratosis.

Intra-epithelial epithelioma produces a similar appearing lesion at the limbus, but it occurs less frequently. Microscopically there is some acanthosis, more dyskeratosis pleomorphism, multinucleated giant cells, vacuolated cells with pyknotic nuclei surrounded by clear halos and mitotic figures throughout the affected epithelium, but the basement membrane remains intact.

Squamous cell carcinoma may develop from any of these epithelial lesions but usually it becomes papillomatous and spreads to involve the corneal epithelium. It remains superficial for a long time and when invasion does occur it is late and usually is limited to minute extensions into the substantia propria. Penetration of the sclera and intraocular involvement is quite rare.

All of the epithelial tumors may be cured by local excision especially if done early. Simple papillomas tend to recur more commonly, probably, because they frequently are infectious in orgin.

Vascular tumors. All types of hemangiomas and lymphangiomas may occur in the conjunctiva. They usually are congenital and include telangiectatic lesions in association with nevus flammeous or port wine stain of the lids and face which usually remains stationary in size; capillary and cavernous hemangiomas which frequently become sclerosed and shrink or disappear, and lymphangiectasis or cavernous lymphangiomas.

Nevus. Nevi are the most common tumors of the conjunctiva and usually are junctional or compound in type. They are similar to nevi of the skin except they have a large number of epithelial inclusions in the form of solid nests, adenomatous structures or cysts. Pigmentation varies greatly from nonpigmented fleshy pink to dense black (Fig. 6-7).

Melanoma. Melanomas usually occur in the bulbar conjunctiva or at the limbus and arise from nevi. They usually are black or brownish gray and richly vascularized. Limbus melanomas often are bulky pedunculated masses. Microscopically these tumors are epitheloid or mixed epitheloid and spindle cell in type but they are much less malignant than similar lesions of the skin.

Precancerous and cancerous melanosis. Precancerous melanosis of the conjunctiva consists of diffuse and wide spread pigmentation of varying degrees of the epithelium beginning in the basal layer associated with a subepithelial inflammatory infiltration with pigment phagocytosis.

Cancerous melanosis, a very malignant neoplasm, develops quite frequently from precancerous melanosis. Multiple nodular lesions appear and spread into the orbit relatively quickly. Distant metastasis also may occur.

Lymphomas. Lymphomas of the conjunctiva may occur alone, in conjunction with generalized lymphosarcoma or with one of the leukemias. The usual lesion is a smooth pink elevated tumor of the fornix or of the caruncle but may be extensive. It subsides rapidly after small doses of x-ray therapy.

7

The Cornea

Anatomy

The cornea is the clear, transparent, anterior portion of the external coat of the eyeball. It is nearly circular, but is slightly wider in the transverse (12 mm.) than in the vertical direction; its radius of curvature is somewhat shorter than that of the sclera. The junction of the two is known as the *limbus*, but their tissues are in complete continuity. The cornea, approximately 1.0 mm. in thickness, has five layers (Fig. 7-1), from without inward: (1) layer of epithelial cells, (2) Bowman's membrane, (3) stroma, (4) Descemet's membrane and (5) a layer of endothelium.

The epithelium covering the front of the cornea is of the stratified variety, formed of flattened epithelial cells superficially, of polygonal cells beneath these and of columnar cells most deeply. Practically it is part of the bulbar conjunctiva.

Bowman's membrane is a thin, homogeneous membrane which separates the corneal epithelium from the stroma of the cornea. Although usually described as a separate membrane, it is really a part of the corneal stroma, and when highly magnified is seen to be composed of fine fibers which are intimately connected with the subjacent layer.

The corneal stroma, the thickest layer, is formed of connective tissue arranged in *lamellae,* the planes of which are parallel to the surface of the cornea; these lamellae are connected with one another. The ultimate fibrils of which the lamellae are composed, as well as the different bundles of fibrils forming the lamellae, are held together by means of a transparent *cement* substance. The corneal substance is traversed by a system of spaces or *lacunae,* situated in the cement substance separating the laminae, and sending off prolongations in every direction; these form small *canals* by means of which the lacunae of the same plane and those placed above and below communicate. The spaces are filled with branching cells (*corneal corpuscles*), the branches of the cells passing into the small canals and communicating with adjoining cells. These cells are known as the *fixed corpuscles* in contradistinction to the leukocytes, which move about and are called the *wandering cells* of the cornea. The stroma of the cornea passes uninterruptedly into the sclera.

Descemet's membrane (the posterior elastic lamina) is a thin, firm, structureless, transparent and highly *elastic* layer, placed posterior to the corneal stroma; at the periphery of the cornea it passes over into radiating bundles of elastic fibers which form the meshwork of the angle of the anterior chamber.

Posteriorly, next to the anterior chamber, is a single layer of flattened, hexagonal cells, the *endothelium.*

The cornea is not provided with blood vessels. The *capillary loops* from the anterior ciliary vessels form a ring around the circumference of the cornea. Its nutrition is provided for by the system of lymph canals just described. It is richly supplied with *nerves* derived from the ciliary nerves (trigeminus).

The line between cornea and sclera is known as the *limbus.*

Congenital and Developmental Anomalies

Congenital and developmental anomalies of the cornea involve aberrations in size, shape, curvature and clarity. In rare instances the cornea may not be developed, but this usually occurs only with other severe abnormalities of the eye and orbit. The more common anomalies in size are microcornea and megalocornea.

Microcornea is a small cornea, 10 mm. or less in diameter, occurring in an otherwise relatively normal eye. Vision is unaffected but there is a definite tendency toward the development of glaucoma with increasing age. Even though small cornea occurs as a part of the generally diminished size of the eye in microphthalmos and other deformities of the globe, it should not be designated as microcornea.

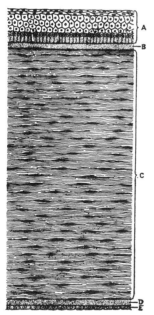

Fig. 7-1. Vertical section of the cornea, showing minute anatomy. *A*, Layer of epithelial cells; *B*, Bowman's membrane; *C*, stroma; *D*, Descemet's membrane; *E*, layer of endothelium.

Megalocornea (anterior keratoglobus) is a bilateral enlargement of the anterior segment of the eye in the absence of an increased intraocular pressure, occurring almost exclusively in males. Although the enlargement of the cornea (diameter always more than 13.5 mm.) is the most prominent feature, the anterior chamber is deep, the lens usually is large and frequently there is some atrophy of the iris stroma. Dislocation of the lens, leading to secondary glaucoma, or cataract or both, may occur in adult life. Occasionally embryotoxon also is present.

Anomalies in Shape of the cornea are rare but consist of encroachment of the sclera in the horizontal or vertical diameter, causing pear-shaped or oddly outlined clear cornea.

Anomalies in Curvature

These include cornea plana, keratoconus and posterior keratoconus.

Cornea Plana is a rare failure in development of the average curvature of the cornea, with the result that the cornea is flatter and smaller and corneoscleral junction is less distinct than usual.

Keratoconus or Conical Cornea is a noninflammatory *conical protrusion* of the center of the cornea (Fig. 7-2*b*) due to gradual *thinning*, with the apex being displaced slightly downward and nasally. It is a late developmental anomaly frequently but not always hereditary. Its onset and course may be hastened by malnutrition, the general disability associated with acute infectious diseases or in endocrine imbalance.

It is of *infrequent* occurrence, usually bilateral, more common in females and begins to develop at puberty. When well developed it is seen easily by viewing the eye from the side or by raising the upper lid and noticing the bulge as the patient looks downward. It also is recognized by the distortion of the light reflex during

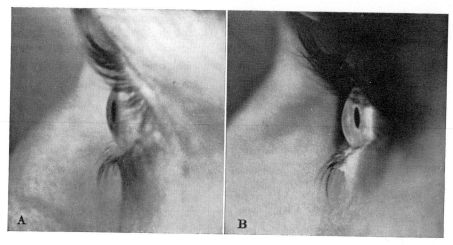

FIG. 7-2A. Lateral view of the normal eye.
FIG. 7-2B. Keratoconus.

retinoscopy and the distortion of the ophthalmoscopic appearance of the nervehead and vessels of the fundus, as well as by the shape of the corneal light reflex with Placido's keratoscope (Figs. 1-9 and 1-10). The thinning of the cornea produces an irregular astigmatism which progressively becomes worse for many years before becoming relatively stationary. As the thinning progresses an opacity develops at the apex of the cone and a gray, yellow, brown or olive green pigmented line, forming an incomplete ring (Fleischer's ring), develops around the base of the cone. Early the astigmatism may be corrected with strong spherocylindrical lenses, but better visual acuity usually can be attained with contact lenses. In addition the wearing of scleral contact lenses (Fig. 7-3) may slow the progress of the lesion.

Posterior keratoconus is an extremely rare anomaly of curvature of the posterior surface of the cornea which usually does not affect vision.

Congenital opacities of minute or microscopic character occur frequently, but larger ones are rare. They may be the result of anomalous development or occasionally the result of intrauterine disease.

Congenital anterior staphyloma. A corneal staphyloma is an opaque bulging cornea which has a bluish grape-like appearance caused by adherence of uveal tissue to its posterior surface. A congenital anterior staphyloma, due either to maldevelopment or to intrauterine inflammation, may be limited to the cornea or include anterior sclera. It is present at birth, frequently ulcerates, may perforate and usually requires enucleation or removal of the eye.

Embryotoxon is an annular opacity situated in the deep layers of the periphery of the cornea continuous with the sclera. It occurs frequently in association with blue sclera (see Chap. 8).

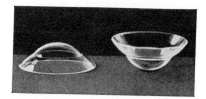

FIG. 7-3. Ground contact lenses.

Hyaline membranes on the posterior surface of the cornea occur rarely and stretch across the anterior chamber close to the posterior surface of the cornea.

Corneal dermoid. See Tumors, p. 114.

Birth injuries of the cornea are seen occasionally in the form of temporary edema, diffuse opacification or linear ruptures of Descemet's membrane.

Degenerations of the Cornea

Arcus Senilis is an opaque white or grayish ring or part of a ring, situated just within the sclerocorneal junction and separated from the sclera by a thin clear zone (Fig. 7-4). It is due to a deposit of lipoid material and occurs most frequently in elderly persons, although it is seen occasionally in younger individuals in whom it is diagnosed as *arcus juvenilis.*

Band-shaped Opacity (*transverse calcareous film of the cornea,* band or zonular keratopathy) is a whitish or grayish band which extends across the cornea in the palpebral aperture and often contains calcium salts. It is due to disturbed nutrition of the cornea and occurs in eyes with extensive scarring of the cornea, in patients with chronic uveitis as in Still's disease in children, in patients with hypercalcemia and in degenerating globes.

In eyes which retain vision, the treatment consists in gently scraping away the band or removing the epithelium and dis-

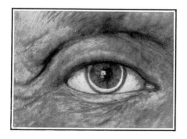

Fig. 7-4. Arcus senilis.

solving the opaque material by repeated instillations or a continuous bath of a 0.01 M solution of edathamil (ethylenediaminetetraacetate, EDTA) buffered to pH 8.0.

Corneal Dystrophies

Dystrophic lesions may affect primarily the endothelium or the stroma.

Endothelial Dystrophy (epithelial and endothelial dystrophy of Fuchs) is a bilateral chronic affection of the cornea in adults which begins as an endothelial degeneration followed by stromal edema, then epithelial edema, and the formation of vesicles, bullae and epithelial erosions, accompanied by blurring of vision, photophobia and pain. Eventually scarring and vascularization of the cornea occur. Hypertonic solutions produce temporary reduction in the edema early in the disease, but more permanent dehydration of the cornea may be obtained at times by irradiation of the lacrimal gland or section of the superficial petrosal nerve.

The Stromal or Familial Dystrophies are hereditary bilateral lesions characterized by hyalin-like deposits in the superficial stroma in the central or axial portion of the cornea. The deposits, which may appear as granular, macular or reticular (lattice-like) opacities, usually become manifest about puberty and progress slowly throughout the rest of life. Symptoms are limited to slight blurring of vision for many years, but later epithelial erosions occur over the elevated opacities and are accompanied by photophobia and pain, which at times may become moderately severe. Palliative therapy, including superficial keratectomy, may relieve moderate symptoms but eventually corneal transplantation becomes necessary.

Salzmann's nodular dystrophy is composed of superficial stromal opacities of varying size and shape which follow some inflammatory lesions of the cornea. If the nodules involve the central portion of the cornea considerable disturbance of vision occurs and is relieved only by corneal transplantation.

INFLAMMATIONS OF THE CORNEA

Inflammations of the cornea (keratitis) in general present the following.

Signs: (1) *Infiltration,* with dullness of surface and diminution of transparency; this may be followed by (a) complete absorption of the infiltration, (b) incomplete absorption, leaving opacities, (c) suppuration, with formation of an ulcer, and (d) cicatrization (repair).

(2) Limited or general *vascularization,* an extension of the limbic vessels into the cornea between the epithelium and Bowman's membrane, produces *pannus,* whereas extension of scleral vessels into the stromal layers of the cornea produces *interstitial vascularization;* either may be limited or involve the entire circumference of the cornea. Occasionally both pannus and interstitial vascularization occur in the same cornea.

(3) *Circumcorneal injection.*

(4) Often complicating *conjunctivitis.*

(5) Always congestion of neighboring deep parts (*iris* and *ciliary body*), resulting in photophobia (pain on movement of the inflamed iris stimulated by exposure to light), and at times exudation into the anterior chamber.

Symptoms are *pain, photophobia, blepharospasm, lacrimation* and *interference with vision.*

Varieties. Inflammations of the cornea may be divided into (1) *ulcers, superficial keratitis,* and (2) *deep keratitis.*

Ulcer of the Cornea

Ulcer of the cornea occurs *commonly* after trauma or lowered resistance of the corneal epithelium. There is *infiltration* of the involved region with *loss of substance.*

Symptoms are pain, photophobia, lacrimation and blepharospasm. Sometimes these symptoms are slight and yet the ulcer may be extensive and serious.

Signs. An ulcer begins with a dull, grayish or grayish yellow *infiltration* of a circumscribed portion of the cornea (Plate 13*A* and *B*); *suppuration* takes place in this area, the superficial layers are cast off, and thus there is *loss of substance.* The process may progress in two directions: either it may travel over the cornea so as to involve a greater *area,* or it may become *deeper;* it may extend both in area and in depth. Very often the advance takes place in one direction, across the cornea, sometimes with a tendency to heal at the opposite side, so the ulcer merely changes in situation (creeping or serpiginous ulcer). There nearly always is more or less grayish *infiltration* of the cornea immediately *surrounding* the loss of substance or in advance of the creeping border, and considerable ciliary *injection.*

If the ulcer is small and superficial, it will cleanse itself in the course of a few days, the infiltrated border will become clear, and repair set in; this may be accompanied by the appearance of blood vessels which spring from the limbus; the process terminates in cicatrization. When the ulcer is very superficial the cornea may remain perfectly transparent. But when Bowman's membrane and some of the stroma of the cornea have been destroyed, new connective tissue takes their place, resulting in a scar which is always more or less *opaque;* however, it may clear to a certain extent, especially in young patients. The previous seat of the ulcer also may be marked by a slight depression (*corneal facet*).

When the ulcer is deeper, both subjective and objective symptoms are more severe, and the complications and sequelae are more serious. Neighboring structures give evidences of inflammation; conjunctivitis, congestion of the iris, even *iritis and cyclitis* with their signs and symptoms, including hypopyon. The suppurative process may spread to the interior of the eye, setting up *purulent iridocyclitis* or panophthalmitis with destruction of the eye, especially if the process is virulent.

Hypopyon is a collection of pus in the anterior chamber, consisting of polymorphonuclear leukocytes. The pus is not derived from the ulcer, but is an exudation from the iris and ciliary body when these parts participate in the inflammation. It collects at the bottom of the anterior chamber (Plate 13*B*), or it may partially or completely fill this space. Very often it is fluid, but after existing for a time it is apt to have the addition of fibrin and then it becomes less fluid and forms a semisolid, globular mass. It remains sterile as long as there is no perforation of the cornea and may disappear and reappear repeatedly in the course of the affection.

A deep ulcer may heal with no other permanent injury except dense corneal *opacity*, or bulging (*keratectasia*) may be added. Deep ulcers frequently have their course modified by the occurrence of *perforation* of the cornea, which, in healing, affects the usefulness and safety of the eye in various ways.

Perforation of the Cornea may occur rapidly or may be preceded by a protrusion of Descemet's membrane through the floor of the ulcer, forming a small, transparent vesicle (*keratocele, descemetocele*). Perforation may be spontaneous, or it may be caused by increased pressure resulting from blepharospasm, from various straining efforts, such as crying, sneezing or coughing, or occasionally by force exerted in examining the eye. The aqueous humor escapes, often carrying the

iris into the wound; the eye feels soft; the anterior chamber is obliterated, the pupil contracts even though there has been previous dilatation from atropine, and iris and lens are in apposition with the cornea. Although perforation of the cornea is an unfavorable development and exposes the eye to the risk of infection of deeper parts, sometimes leading to iridocyclitis and even panophthalmitis, it frequently initiates a favorable effect upon the course of the affection; the symptoms are relieved, and the ulcer tends to heal.

When the opening closes by cicatrization, the iris may regain its normal position. But frequently it continues entangled in the perforation, or remains *prolapsed*, and becomes incorporated within the scar. Such a condition is called *anterior synechia*; the dense, white cicatrix to which the iris is attached is known as *adherent leukoma* (Plate 13*C*). Most frequently only a portion of the iris is drawn into the scar; the pupil then is more or less pear-shaped. Occasionally the entire pupillary margin may be adherent, causing both seclusion and occlusion of the pupil. If the iris remains fastened to a bulging cicatrix of the cornea, the condition is known as *corneal staphyloma*.

At the time of perforation, the *lens* may become dislocated, and occasionally it escapes. When it is pushed forward and lies in apposition with the margins of the opening and then recedes after the anterior chamber is re-established, it frequently presents a proliferation of the subcapsular epithelium which has become irritated by the pressure of the lens upon the cornea, forming a white spot upon the center of its anterior surface (Fig. 17-1), known as *anterior polar cataract*.

Occasionally the perforation fails to close and a *fistula* of the cornea results; this condition exposes the eye to subsequent serious inflammation and jeopardzes its safety. *Intraocular hemorrhage* may follow a sudden perforation of the cornea and destroy sight.

Pathology. The changes accompanying corneal ulcer comprise infection, infiltration, necrosis and repair. The infection is exogenous and is caused by the entrance of pyogenic organisms through some defect in the corneal epithelium. There is at first *infiltration* of the epithelium and, if deeper, also corneal lamellae with leukocytes. Then follows *necrosis* of the affected parts; the slough is cast off in part, leaving an excavation. Finally *repair* sets in, assisted by superficial blood vessels (pannus), which extend from the limbus and supply the material which replaces the loss of substance; this replacement may consist entirely of epithelial cells growing in from the edges of the ulcer, provided that the latter has been superficial. But if Bowman's membrane and the lamellae have been destroyed the defect is filled in with fibrous tissue devoid of the transparency, and a more or less opaque *scar* results.

Etiology. Ulcers of the cornea usually are found in *adult* and *aged* individuals; phlyctenular ulcers are the only ones which are common in children. Ulcers are much more frequent among individuals in whom *general health is poor*.

The process essentially is an *infection* by various micro-organisms (pneumococci, streptococci, staphylococci, etc.), frequently introduced by the secretion of chronic *conjunctivitis*, and especially by that of *dacryocystitis*, when the protecting corneal epithelium has been lost at some spot.

The exciting causes are: (1) trauma which is the most frequent cause and consists of injury by foreign body, fingernail scratch, misplaced cilia, etc.; (2) lacrimal sac infection; (3) conjunctival inflammation (purulent, membranous, trachoma-tous); (4) disturbance in nutrition of cornea (paralysis of trigeminus, keratomalacia, glaucoma); (5) exposure of the cornea; (6) infection during operation; (7) acute infectious disease.

Diagnosis is made by the demonstration of a loss of substance of epithelium or deeper structures by examination with magnification such as is obtained with a loupe or slit lamp and corneal biomicroscope. This can be facilitated by the instillation of fluorescein stain onto the conjunctiva and cornea. After removal of the excess by irrigation with normal saline solution the injured epithelium and the exposed stroma of the cornea retains a bright green color for a short time.

Treatment may be divided into (1) constitutional, (2) treatment of pre-existing local conditions and (3) local treatment of the ulcerative process.

Constitutional. The general condition of the patient should be examined and treatment instituted for any general disease, debility or deficiency which could be partially responsible for or could delay healing of the corneal lesion.

Foreign protein. In virulent forms of ulcers, such as ulcus serpens, typhoid vaccine is employed intravenously. Polyvalent serum, antipneumococcus serum and diphtheria antitoxin (2000 units) are used by subcutaneous injections. These agents often act favorably. Sulfonamides orally, or antibiotics orally or parenterally, may be of value in certain types of infection.

Treatment of pre-existing local conditions. Foreign bodies must be removed and other local irritating conditions remedied. Even the smallest abrasion of the cornea should not be regarded lightly. Conjunctivitis and dacryocystitis must receive careful attention; infections of the respiratory passages and the nasal sinuses should be eliminated.

Local Treatment includes local or general treatment for the specific infectious agent (sulfonamides, antibiotics, etc.) atropine or scopolamine, hot compresses, scraping, cauterization, thermophore and paracentesis of the anterior chamber. Topical cortisone has value in marginal keratitis, phlyctenular keratitis and sclerosing keratitis, by reducing the inflammatory reaction but is contraindicated in infectious ulcers.

Atropine or scopolamine must be instilled in sufficient quantity to keep the pupil dilated; it has a sedative effect and acts favorably upon the ulcer by putting the iris and ciliary body at rest.

Topical anesthetics must not be used by the physician more often than absolutely necessary and should never be prescribed for home use because of their deleterious effect on the cornea.

Ointments should not be used in the treatment of corneal ulcers or abrasions because they delay healing and at times may be the cause of recurrent corneal erosions.

Dressings should not be used on infectious suppurative lesions since they not only prevent the free flow of discharge but also produce more favorable conditions for bacterial multiplication. In superficial epithelial erosions and in clean wounds and abrasions of the cornea, dressings may be of value at times.

Hot compresses may be applied for half an hour at a time, several times a day; they favor healing of the ulcer.

To limit spread of an infected ulcer the advancing border may be scraped and cauterized or treated by thermophore. *Cauterization* may be effected by heat or by chemicals. Cautery by heat is applied by an electrocautery or by an actual cautery. With either instrument the hot tip may be applied directly to the margin of the ulcer or held close to the ulcer (chauffage) until it shows the desired amount of whitening. A less intense but more accurately controlled application of heat can be made with the *thermophore,* an instrument which develops and maintains a set temperature below the cauterization level, at the tip of the instrument. *Chemical cauterization* may be effected by tincture of iodine, pure liquid carbolic acid or pure trichloracetic acid, but caution must be exercised to limit the action of the chemical to the ulcer and avoid its spread to clear cornea.

Paracentesis of the anterior chamber, made with a Wheeler knife after topical anesthesia, is of value in limiting the spread of an ulcer, at times, or in preventing a threatened perforation. After a slanting perforation of the cornea the knife blade is twisted slightly to allow aqueous to drain out slowly. The chamber refills with secondary aqueous, which contains a higher concentration of proteins and antibodies.

After spontaneous perforation of an ulcer, atropine is instilled, a firm dressing applied, and complete *rest* insisted upon with avoidance of all straining efforts. If there is a recent *prolapse* of the iris, no attempt to return this membrane to its normal position should be made; the prolapsed iris should be seized and *excised* close to the cornea; if there are adhesions to the margins of the opening, these should be freed with an iris repositor. The operation has the effect of an iridectomy. Sometimes the perforation is covered by a flap made from the adjacent bulbar conjunctiva. Iridectomy also may be indicated if, during the process of healing of a perforation, there is an increase of tension, causing a bulge of the cicatrix. But if the prolapse has existed for some days it must be allowed to remain for subsequent operative correction.

After the healing process has become fairly initiated, hot compresses are used to hasten cicatrization and to clear the cornea as much as possible.

Clinical Forms. Certain variations in the course of corneal ulcers have already been considered. The nomenclature of ulcers of the cornea is quite extensive and founded upon peculiarities in the symptoms or course. The following warrant special mention:

Simple ulcer is the name often given to the form which is small and superficial with symptoms of slight or severe irritation, no tendency to perforation, terminating in uncomplicated healing; phlyctenules and slight injuries often cause such ulcers.

Catarrhal ulcer may complicate catarrhal conjunctivitis in adults. With increase in symptoms, peripheral punctate infiltrations appear, concentric with and just within the limbus, and later form minute superficial ulcers (*marginal ulcers*); or several combine to form a thin crescent at the limbus (Plate 12*E*). The course usually is favorable and healing prompt; if opacities remain, they do not reduce vision, being outside of the pupillary area. Occasionally this type of ulcer is due to a vascular or connective tissue disease.

Deep ulcer is one which shows a tendency to involve the deeper layers and to perforate rather than to spread over the cornea. The symptoms are apt to be severe and hypopyon often is present; hence the results frequently are serious.

Serpent ulcer (hypopyon ulcer, pneumococcus ulcer) is a *virulent* form in which the process *spreads* over a considerable portion of the cornea and at the same time also into its depth. It is quite *common*, especially in warm weather; it occurs almost exclusively in adults, particularly in individuals with chronic dacryocystitis and in elderly, debilitated individuals; it may be found in eyes suffering from absolute glaucoma. The cause is an *injury*, often a slight one, such as a foreign body or a scratch with the fingernail, and the infecting agent is the *pneumococcus* to which sometimes other micro-organisms are added. The symptoms usually are severe. Accompanied by some swelling of the lids and severe conjunctival and ciliary congestion, a grayish yellow infiltration appears near the center of the cornea; this changes rapidly to an ulcer with *sloughing margins*; the advancing edge presents a yellowish crescent (Plate 13*B*). Surrounding the ulcer is a cloudy area made up of fine lines; the rest of the cornea often is dull and gray. The ulcer spreads very rapidly in size and depth and advances in the direction of the yellowish edge, and in this manner much of the cornea becomes destroyed; then *perforation* takes place. There is early and intense *iritis*, and *hypopyon* almost always is present. Owing to the virulence of the process and the accompanying iritis, much *damage* results to the eye: adhesion and prolapse of the iris are frequent, the pupil often is occluded and iridocyclitis and panophthalmitis are common; even in favorable cases there will be dense opacity of the cornea and often staphyloma; therefore serious *impairment of vision* results. However, early and intensive treatment with sulfonamides orally and penicillin intramuscularly will prevent many of the serious sequelae.

Diplobacillary ulcer is a milder type of hypopyon ulcer caused by the diplobacillus of Morax-Axenfeld (*Moraxella lacunata*) or the diplobacillus of Petit (*Moraxella liquefaciens*). It has a much more favorable course than the ordinary form of hypopyon ulcer, having a tendency to spread laterally, but is less apt to perforate. Topical and general treatment with a sulfonamide or tetracycline antibiotic or both act favorably.

Rodent ulcer (Mooren's ulcer, chronic serpiginous ulcer) is a rare, superficial form, never perforating, which occurs in elderly, enfeebled subjects, sometimes bilaterally, of lengthy duration and unknown cause. It commences by a gray infiltration, soon changing to an ulcer which spreads by a gray rim; the latter undermines the epithelium and superficial lamellae, thus presenting an *overhanging edge at the advancing border*; this feature is characteristic. There may be moderate or intense irritative symptoms, including severe pain. As soon as cicatrization begins there will be a relapse and an advance on the cornea; thus a succession of extensions and remissions follow each other and, unless the process is arrested by cauterization, the entire cornea becomes covered and sight is permanently and seriously impaired. Treatment consists of the application of the electrocautery to the entire ulcer and especially to the advancing edge, but is rarely effective.

Marginal ring ulcer (annular ulcer) is one which encircles the periphery of the cornea and, if deep, interferes with its nourishment. Examples of superficial ulcers of this sort are seen in phlyctenular keratoconjunctivitis as the result of the coalescence of marginal phlyctenules; also in elderly, gouty individuals in whom a number of small superficial ulcers form more or less of a circle but, although accompanied by much irritation and a tendency to relapse, cause little damage. A more serious type is observed occasionally in debilitated subjects in whom the ulcers are deeper, form a groove encircling the cornea and tend to perforate; this also may happen as a complication of gonorrheal ophthalmia and rarely in severe staphylococcic and other virulent infections.

Central ulcer (indolent ulcer) is the name given to a simple ulcer when its base is transparent or but faintly gray, this peculiarity being due to defective corneal nutrition. It is usually small, superficial, central, devoid of symptoms of irritation, shows no tendency to spread or to per-forate, occurs chiefly in weak children or in trachoma and is followed by little or no opacity, but often by a small pit (*facet*) which easily escapes detection, but which causes much reduction in vision on account of irregular astigmatism. Attention to the general health is an important aid to local treatment of the ulcer.

Atheromatous ulcer is one which develops in old degenerated scars of the cornea. Having subnormal vitality, such scars become infected easily; the ulcer then spreads rapidly and perforates; panophthalmitis usually follows. Such eyes often are blind, and enucleation is indicated.

Abscess of the cornea is a purulent infiltration in the substance of the cornea covered both anteriorly and posteriorly by sound tissue.

The term *ring abscess of the cornea* refers to an infection following perforating wounds (rarely operations), in which a yellow ring of deep infiltration develops a few millimeters within the limbus, soon followed by necrosis of the whole cornea and panophthalmitis. A frequent cause is *Pseudomonas aeruginosa*.

Keratitis e lagophthalmo (desiccation keratitis) is due to *exposure of the cornea* from defective closure of the lids (lagophthalmos). Under such circumstances the epithelium of the exposed cornea becomes desiccated and is cast off, leaving vulnerable areas which become infected; ulceration follows. The lower portion of the cornea is affected most frequently, because this part is left uncovered during sleep when the eyeball turns upward. The causes are paralysis of the orbicularis (*facial paralysis*), exophthalmos, various deformities of the lids and long continued exhausting illness. Treatment consists in relieving the lagophthalmos if possible, application of a condensation shield or closure of the lids by a dressing or by median tarsorrhaphy; in slight cases it may be sufficient to apply a dressing at night.

Neuroparalytic keratitis is a form of infiltration and ulceration observed after *paralysis of the trigeminus*, in some cases of intracranial disease involving the Gasserian ganglion or after radical treatment for the relief of trigeminal neuralgia, whether by section of the sensory division of the ganglion or by injection of alcohol into the fifth nerve. The disease is considered by some to be trophic, and by others to be due to exposure and lodgment of foreign bodies upon the insensitive cornea, which is vulnerable from dryness owing to the absence of reflex closure of the lids. Its course is chronic and begins with a large central infiltration of the cornea with characteristic exfoliation of the epithelium, followed by ulceration and, in severe cases, by hypopyon and perforation; there is ciliary congestion but no pain, the cornea being anesthetic, and no lacrimation. In mild cases, with proper protection of the cornea, the course may be more favorable; but even in these, there are apt to be relapses and in the end the cornea often is flattened and covered with a large leukoma. Treatment, besides that of corneal ulcer, consists in *keeping the lids closed* by a dressing, or median tarsorrhaphy.

Keratomalacia (xerotic keratitis) is a rare affection due to lack of nutrition of the cornea. It is an uncommon disease occurring in badly nourished infants and young children suffering from *lack of vitamin A* in the diet, and in the course of greatly debilitating diseases; the latter class of patients are so ill that they allow the lids to remain open constantly and the cornea to be exposed. The process begins with dryness of the conjunctiva of both eyes; soon the cornea becomes cloudy, dull and greasy looking, then ulcerates and often perforates. There is an absence of inflammatory symptoms. In those patients who are old enough to complain of this symptom, night blindness is present. Most of the cases occur during the first year of life and these generally die; in older children the affection may be less severe, but dense corneal opacities persist. Treatment consists in measures to increase the general strength (vitamin A-rich diet, cod liver oil, etc.); locally, the usual measures for corneal ulcers, especially warm, moist compresses and protective dressings, are used.

Keratitis sicca or drying of the cornea is due to a disturbance in the precorneal film or a diminution in the production of tears. It may result from temporary drying of the cornea by prolonged opening of the lids or from the application of topical anesthetics and other surface-tension-reducing agents. This type of drying is quickly reversible by closure of the lids and wetting by tears. However, prolonged states of dryness of the cornea are encountered in vitamin A deficiency states as a forerunner of keratomalacia or in dacryosialoadenopathy atrophicians (Sjögren's syndrome).

In temporary drying of the cornea the epithelium loses its luster and multiple superficial fine gray opacities appear in the epithelium. These disappear rapidly by wetting with tears. However in Sjögren's syndrome, which is a general disease characterized by dryness of the eyes, mouth and throat associated with polyarthritis, the punctate opacities of the lusterless cornea progress to the development of fine epithelial filaments on the cornea, associated with moderate chronic conjunctival injection and a slight mucoid discharge in the lower fornix. In addition, the saliva is scanty, the parotid gland may be palpable and usually several joints are enlarged. The patient complains of dry eyes, slight diminution in vision, stringy discharge, a scratchy or slightly painful sensation upon opening the lids after sleeping, dryness of the mouth and throat and stiffness or pain and some swelling, usually of several joints.

Although dryness of the eyes is observed readily in advanced stages of the syndrome, diminished tear production can be detected quite early by use of the Schirmer test. A strip of filter paper 5 mm. broad and 30 mm. or more long is bent at right angles 5 mm. from one end. The short end is placed on the conjunctiva of the lower lid with the long end projecting out over the margin of the lower lid. With average filter paper the normal production of tears will wet 15 mm. or more of the projecting strip in 5 minutes, whereas the reduced production in Sjögren's usually wets 10 mm. or less of the strip. An electrophoretic analysis of the tears reveals no lysozyme.

The epithelial opacities and filaments stain with fluorescein solution or with a 1 per cent aqueous solution of rose bengal.

Treatment consists of the use of drops of various solutions as a substitute for tears, or, occasionally, of closure of the puncta lacrimalis in an effort to retain the tears on the conjunctiva and cornea. Among the solutions which are used as artificial tears are 1 per cent monohydrated sodium carbonate, 0.5 per cent methylcellulose solution or Gifford's artificial tear solution (gelatin, 1.0 per cent; chlorobutanol, 1.0 per cent; sodium chloride, 0.9 per cent; potassium chloride, 0.024 per cent; calcium chloride, 0.042 per cent; dextrose, 0.1 per cent; sodium bicarbonate, 0.02 per cent; distilled water, 100.0 cc.)

Superficial Keratitis

Phlyctenular Keratitis (Plate 13*E*) is a superficial involvement of the cornea in the course of phlyctenular conjunctivitis (keratoconjunctivitis). The special symptoms arising when the cornea is involved

have been described in the previous chapter.

Superficial Punctate Keratitis occasionally complicates acute affections of the respiratory tract. It begins with the symptoms of acute conjunctivitis. Numerous small gray spots, slightly elevated, appear in the superficial layers of the cornea, beneath Bowman's membrane; these are accompanied by gray radiating lines and by some general clouding. The disease resembles herpes, but there are no vesicles. It occurs in young persons, affects one or both eyes and lasts several months, after which there is complete absorption. Treatment comprises attention to the conjunctivitis and the bronchial affection, atropine, hot compresses, smoked glasses and later mildly stimulating applications.

A punctate type of epithelial keratitis frequently occurs in staphylococcic and pneumococcic conjunctivitis and occasionally in other severe conjunctival infections.

Dendritic Keratitis (Herpetic Keratitis) is an acute recurrent form of superficial corneal ulcer (Plate 12*F*) due to the herpes virus, normally affecting only one eye. The primary infection usually occurs in infancy or early childhood either as a subclinical infection or as an acute follicular keratoconjunctivitis which may at times be associated with extensive vesicular lesions of the skin of the lids, fever and malaise. A circulating antiviral immunity develops during the primary attack and persists throughout life. Apparently as a result of the primary infection the virus becomes established in the corneal epithelium and, under the influence of a "trigger mechanism" such as fever, upper respiratory infection, general disease, foreign bodies on the cornea, minor injuries of the epithelium, exposure to excess sunlight or local contact with irritants, produces a recurrent episode of keratitis. This takes the form of a line of epithelial edema and opacification which quickly develops into an ulcer which sends out lateral branches ending in knob-like extremities. Immediately the patient experiences a scratchy or foreign body sensation in the eye, photophobia, lacrimation and, at times, pain. With repeated attacks superficial opacities appear and the sensitivity of the cornea becomes diminished. The individual attack varies in duration but the average length of the untreated attack is 21 days. In some attacks the dendritic figure becomes broadened and develops into a large epithelial ulceration called a geographic ulcer because its irregular margin resembles the ragged outline of an island on a map. In severe or prolonged attacks the ulceration may spread into the stroma, or secondary infection may produce extensive stromal ulceration with hypopyon. In rare instances dendritic keratitis is followed by a diffuse infiltrative lesion of the cornea, diskiform keratitis (see below).

Treatment of the epithelial types of involvement with 0.1 per cent solution of 5-iodo-2′-desoxyuridine in a dosage of 1 drop every hour during the day and every 2 hours at night until the ulcer heals, then 1 drop every 2 hours during the day for 5 additional days, is effective in a high percentage of cases. In resistant cases sodium iodide (1 grain per 10 pounds of body weight orally three times a day) or application of tincture of iodine to the corneal surface after the epithelium has been removed, followed by a firm dressing until there is no further staining with fluorescein, or a combination of the two is of value. *Corticosteroids are contraindicated.*

Vesicular Keratitis and Bullous Keratitis are varieties which occur in *blind eyes with increased tension* in absolute glaucoma and in damaged eyes with opaque and insensitive corneas; the dis-tinguishing feature is the occurrence of small, clear *vesicles*, or large transparent *blebs*, accompanied by intense symptoms of *irritation* and a tendency to *recur*. Vesicles also are seen on the cornea in the course of acute febrile diseases, especially pneumonia and influenza, in herpetic keratitis and in the keratitis complicating herpes zoster ophthalmicus. A special type of bullous keratitis, recurrent corneal erosion, frequently follows abrasion of the cornea, such as a fingernail scratch, which is treated with ointment. The epithelium heals over a thin film of ointment, then breaks down, probably from movements of the lids. This may recur repeatedly until the use of ointments is discontinued.

Pannus, a superficial vascularization and growth of scar tissue into the cornea between the epithelium and Bowman's membrane or replacing Bowman's membrane, occurs in chronic marginal ulceration of the cornea, trachoma, phlyctenular and serpiginous keratitis, acne rosacea keratitis, leprotic keratitis and in degeneration of the eyeball. A limited superficial vascularization of the cornea of the pannus type also occurs locally in the limbic type of vernal conjunctivitis.

Deep Keratitis; Interstitial or Parenchymatous Keratitis

This disease represents the principal form belonging to the group of deep keratitis. It is essentially a *cellular infiltration of the deep layers of the cornea,* without ulceration, of frequent occurrence in childhood, chronic in its course and associated with inflammation of the uveal tract; the keratitis is merely a part of a *uveitis,* participation of the uveal tract being hidden during the stage of opaque cornea.

Signs. The affection begins either in the center or at the margin of the cornea. If it starts in the center, this part will present a *grayish infiltration,* the superficial layers at first retaining their normal luster; this central patch soon spreads so that the whole cornea becomes implicated. If it commences at the periphery, one or more grayish spots are seen, which soon spread toward the center and involve all the cornea. After the infiltration has become general, the cornea becomes *softened*, of a dense grayish or sometimes yellowish gray color, so that the iris can be seen only with difficulty, and visual acuity is reduced to little more than perception of light. The surface of the cornea now is *steamy* and resembles ground glass. At this period, or even before, thin, deep-seated blood vessels (derived from the anterior ciliary) make their appearance and pervade more or less of the cornea (Plate 13*F*). The advent of the blood vessels gives the limbus a red and swollen appearance which circumscribes either sectors of the periphery or the whole cornea, giving rise to a dirty red or yellowish red discoloration, which is known as the *salmon patch*. The lesion is accompanied by intense photophobia and ciliary congestion, which last for 1 or 2 months.

The inflammation then begins to subside. The cornea *clears* irregularly, the blood vessels become smaller and quit carrying blood, the irritative symptoms disappear and *vision improves*. Several months or even a longer period are consumed in this process. In favorable cases, after a year or more the cornea will have cleared almost completely or a faint central opacity will remain. Evidence of the previous occurrence of the disease, however, can be obtained in later years, for slit lamp and biomicroscope examination will reveal delicate opaque lines representing obliterated blood vessels in the deep layers of the cornea. Not all cases, however, run such a benign course.

The anterior portion of the uveal tract is regularly involved. In mild cases, this consists merely of congestion of the iris. But in more serious types there are *iritis, choroiditis, cyclitis* and changes in the *vitreous*; in such cases, after the cornea becomes less opaque, adhesions of the iris to the lens (posterior synechiae), changes in the iris and choroid, opacities of the vitreous and even seclusion and occlusion of the pupil become visible. In some severe cases keratectasia may follow. Hence more or less serious *impairment of sight* may result from these inflammatory processes. Furthermore, the clearing process in the cornea may come to a standstill, leaving a dense *opacity*.

Symptoms. During the period of infiltration and vascularization there are *photophobia, blepharospasm, lacrimation, pain* and *interference with vision,* the intensity varies to a certain extent but usually is severe. The symptoms gradually subside during the progress of absorption.

Both eyes usually are involved; frequently the inflammation in the second eye commences after that in the first has existed for some weeks or months. In the exceptional cases that occur in adults, the disease is more apt to be unilateral.

Pathology. The disease essentially is a *deep keratitis with involvement of the uvea.* Between the laminae of the stroma, especially those placed most posteriorly, there is cellular infiltration, gathered chiefly around capillary vascularization and causing thickening of the cornea. There is irregular thickening and haziness of the corneal epithelium. Bowman's membrane is wavy and irregular and beneath it are found minute capillaries. Descemet's membrane is wrinkled. The endothelium usually is missing from the posterior surface of the cornea and is replaced by an accumulation of lymphocytes. During resolution there is thinning of the cornea. The changes in the uvea are described under Uveitis.

Etiology. The disease usually occurs *between the 5th and 15th years,* less commonly after this period and rarely after 30. The great majority of cases are due to *inherited syphilis;* in few instances it is tuberculous or the two conditions may be associated. It is rarely the result of acquired syphilis; it then is unilateral and can be precipitated or activated by trauma. In many cases there will be other *signs of inherited syphilis* (Fig. 7-5), such as characteristic physiognomy, peculiar conformation of the skull (square forehead, prominent frontal eminences, depressed bridge of nose), radiating scars at angles of mouth, scars in the mouth and pharynx, ozena, enlarged cervical lymphatic glands, nodes on the bones and more or less impairment of hearing. The permanent teeth are ill-developed; the most characteristic dental changes are seen in the upper central incisors, which have a vertical notch in the free margin; their angles are rounded off and there is abnormal separation between the two teeth *(Hutchinsonian teeth,* Fig. 7-5).

Treatment. In luetic interstitial keratitis active antiluetic treatment with intramuscular injections of 300,000 to 1,200,000 units of penicillin per day should be started at once. After 2 days cortisone drops may be used six to eight times a day. In those rare cases due to tuberculosis, treatment with isoniazid, *p*-aminosalicylic acid and streptomycin should be started as soon as possible.

During the active inflammation of all types, atropine or scopolamine drops must be used several times a day to keep the iris and ciliary body at rest and control the photophobia. Dark glasses are used to overcome glare. After the activity has subsided, irritants such as dionine solution or yellow oxide of mercury ointment may be used to improve fluid exchange in the cornea and perhaps aid in the resolution of the residual opacities.

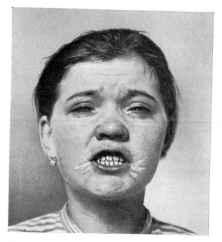

FIG. 7-5. From a photograph of a patient, the subject of interstitial keratitis, exhibiting the signs of inherited syphilis, including Hutchinsonian teeth.

Cogan's oculo-vestibulo-auditory syndrome is a nonsyphilitic interstitial keratitis usually affecting young adult males and characterized by an abrupt onset with vertigo and tinnitus followed by deafness. The cause is unknown, but the disease has developed shortly after smallpox vaccination in several patients and in others has been associated with periarteritis nodosa.

Keratitis diskiformis is an uncommon unilateral stromal keratitis occurring in adults. A gray disk-shaped opacity develops in the middle layers of the cornea with a denser spot in the center and sometimes concentric lines at the circumference, but there is no ulceration. The duration is several months. It clears from the periphery but always leaves a permanent central opacity of the cornea. It follows severe herpes simplex keratitis and may occur in other virus diseases of the cornea. The treatment of keratitis in general is indicated but generally is ineffective. Some cases are tuberculous and respond to tuberculin therapy.

Keratitis profunda is a form of inflammation of the cornea occurring in adults, in which a gray, central opacity of the cornea, composed of dots and striae, develops in the middle and deep layers accompanied by moderate symptoms of irritation; it usually becomes entirely absorbed in a few weeks, but may leave some permanent opacity. In most cases the cause is unknown; it may occur after contusion of the eye and then it clears promptly; it also has been ascribed to exposure to cold and to malaria. The treatment should be similar to that of interstitial keratitis.

Sclerosing keratitis is the name given to the corneal complication of scleritis. The portion of the cornea adjacent to the scleritic nodule participates in the process, and presents a triangular opacity with apex toward the center of the cornea; the whole margin of the cornea may participate, but the pupillary area usually remains clear or only slightly involved. The symptoms and treatment correspond to those of the causative scleritis.

Protrusions of the Cornea

Staphyloma of the Cornea (*anterior staphyloma*) is a bulging *cicatrix lined by adherent iris*. It is one of the sequelae of perforation of corneal ulcer. It may be *total*, when it replaces the entire cornea, or *partial*, when it occupies only a portion of this area. In shape it may be globular, conical or lobulated (Fig. 7-6). Its color is whitish with bluish areas representing spots where pigment shows through the thin cicatrix; it may be all white or all bluish. Most of the cornea is replaced by connective tissue. Blood vessels frequently are seen on the surface. It varies in size, being small in some cases and so large in others that the lids cannot close.

Symptoms. Besides the signs just mentioned, there are changes in the eyeball, in the staphyloma and in the lids. There almost always is *increased tension,* often due to seclusion of the pupil; this secondary glaucoma causes *pain,* produces changes in the interior of the eye which lead to *blindness,* results in an increase in the size of the bulging and is responsible

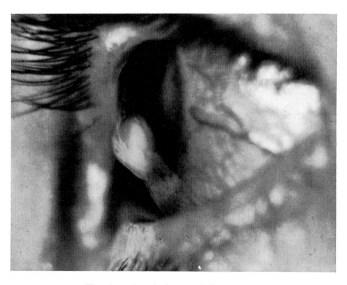

Fig. 7-6. Staphyloma of the cornea.

for staphyloma of the sclera. The conjunctiva becomes the seat of inflammation from mechanical irritation. The summit of the protrusion becomes dry and ulcerated and frequently ruptures, after which the opening heals; this process may be repeated a number of times, until the eye is lost and a shrunken globe remains.

Even before these secondary changes have taken place, there is considerable *deformity* and *sight* is very much *reduced.* In total staphyloma there merely is perception of light; in the partial form the amount of sight depends upon the condition of the cornea which is preserved, the position of the pupil and the extent to which the curvature of the cornea is altered.

Treatment. In *partial staphyloma,* an *iridectomy* should be performed for the purpose of reducing tension, flattening the protrusion and preventing its increase, and to serve for optical purposes. The part of the iris corresponding to the most clear portion of the cornea is selected. If there is no anterior chamber and the iris lies against the posterior surface of the cornea, this operation is impossible. In such cases, a portion of the staphyloma may be excised, the wound closed with sutures and a pressure dressing applied for a considerable period of time.

In *total staphyloma,* enucleation usually is necessary. *Enucleation,* or one of its substitutes, is indicated in certain cases in which the staphyloma is very large, painful or disfiguring; enucleation usually is the wisest procedure since excision of partial staphyloma is not entirely free from the danger of causing sympathetic ophthalmitis.

Keratectasia is a protrusion of the cornea devoid of iris following inflammation with perforation; the bulging portion is opaque. It may follow thinning from an ulcer which has not perforated or it may be due to softening of the cornea after pannus and interstitial keratitis. There always is great reduction of vision. When fully developed, treatment is of no avail.

Opacities of the Cornea

This term refers to a lack of transparency of the cornea resulting from inflammation, ulceration or injury. According to density, the corneal opacity is called *nebula* (Fig. 7-7, *left*) when faint and cloud-like, often overlooked until examined by oblique illumination; *macula* (Fig. 7-7, *center*) when large enough to be appreciated as a gray spot in daylight; and *leukoma* (Fig. 7-7, *right*) when dense and white. When the iris is attached to the scar tissue, the condition is spoken of as *adherent leukoma* (Plate 13C).

Opacities of the cornea reduce vision when they encroach upon the pupillary area. Even slight opacities cause much *visual disturbance* because of the resulting diffusion and irregular refraction of light; a nebula over the pupillary area will interfere with vision more than a circumscribed leukoma covering only a part of the pupil. Dense opacities cause *disfigurement.*

Treatment. *Hot compresses,* used to reduce the density of *recent* corneal

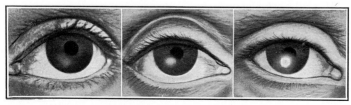

FIG. 7-7. *Left,* corneal nebula; *center,* corneal macula; *right,* corneal leukoma.

opacities, act most successfully in children and when the opacity is superficial. *Dionine* (1 to 10 per cent) is useful; 1 per cent is instilled every other day at first but the strength is increased when the reaction (chemosis, congestion, swelling of lids, burning sensation) becomes negligible.

In suitable cases of superficial corneal opacity, vision often can be improved by removal of the opaque corneal layers (superficial keratectomy). When the leukoma entirely occludes the pupillary area, iridectomy for *artificial pupil* may be performed, the coloboma being made opposite a clear part of the cornea; when there is no clear portion of the cornea and vision is much reduced, the operation of *corneal transplantation* is used in suitable cases.

Corneal transplantation (lamellar or penetrating keratoplasty) consists of the replacement of a portion of the anterior layers or of the entire thickness of the leukomatous cornea by a corresponding segment of a clear human cornea obtained from a fetus, a fresh cadaver or an eye freshly removed because of choroidal tumor or other cause. Ideal results are obtained in cases with normal anterior chambers; the transplants remain transparent in a large portion of such cases but they are less likely to remain transparent when the host cornea is covered by pannus.

Tattooing and coloring. To remove the disfigurement in cases of leukoma, tattooing and coloring occasionally are used. *Tattooing:* the eye is anesthetized and the leukoma is covered with a thick paste of India ink which is introduced obliquely into the corneal substance, either by means of an instrument consisting of a row or bundle of round needles or with a grooved needle (Fig. 7-8); the

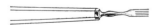

FIG. 7-8. Tattooing needles.

color fades in the course of a few years and then the operation may be repeated. *Coloring:* the epithelium is scraped from the desired area and a neutral 4 per cent solution of gold chloride is applied repeatedly by means of a cotton applicator and allowed to soak in for 4 minutes, followed by Adrenalin for the latter's reducing effect; a dark brown or almost black spot of greater or lesser permanence results.

When the opacity covers only a part of the pupillary area, tattooing and coloring are useful in preventing the diffusion of light from the edges, which is so annoying to the patient and reduces the acuteness of vision; these procedures cut off the irregularly refracted rays and thus improve vision.

Tattooing and coloring operations are contraindicated when the cornea is very thin or when likely to increase intraocular disease by irritation, such as may happen when the iris is extensively attached to the leukoma; even in quiet eyes these procedures are not entirely devoid of danger.

Pigmentation of the Cornea may be due to melanin, blood, metals or drugs.

Melanin occurs normally in the epithelium of the limbus and periphery of the cornea in variable amounts in highly pigmented individuals, but develops in some patients as a result of chronic infectious processes of the cornea and conjunctiva or in association with a melanoma of the limbus. Melanin granules are deposited on the posterior surface of the cornea in small amounts as the result of increasing age and in myopia, but in larger amounts in inflammatory processes of the iris and ciliary body, in diabetes mellitus, in pigmentary glaucoma and at times in pigmented tumors of the uvea. Frequently the pigment granules are fine and scattered but at times, because of convection currents in the aqueous, they may form a vertical line (Ehrlick-Turk line) or a vertical spindle (Kruckenberg's spindle) on the endothelial surface.

Blood staining of the cornea usually follows hemorrhage in the anterior chamber associated with increased intraocular pressure. The hemorrhage always results from trauma or surgery but usually represents continuous or repeated bleeding into the anterior chamber. The cornea becomes rusty brown, greenish black or greenish yellow either throughout its extent or in the axial portion. The staining persists for many months, slowly clearing from the periphery toward the center.

A superficial pigmented line (Hudson-Stähli line, superficial senile line), due to hemosiderin deposition in breaks in Bowman's membrane, occurs as a horizontal brown or gray slightly wavy line at about the junction of the middle and lower third of the cornea in a high percentage of persons over 50 years of age and in younger

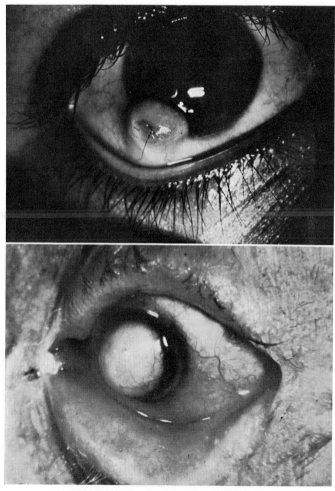

FIG. 7-9 (*upper*). Dermoid of limbus.
FIG. 7-10 (*lower*). Dermoid of cornea.

individuals following injuries and inflammatory lesions. A similar type of pigmentation is seen in the Fleischer ring around the base of the conical protrusion of the cornea in keratoconus.

Metallic pigmentation of the cornea occurs from excessive general or local use of silver salts, local application of copper salts or from foreign bodies of copper or iron imbedded in or near the cornea.

Pigmentation of the posterior peripheral layers of the cornea occurs in Wilson's hepatolenticular degeneration. The pigmentation produces an interplay of bright red to green or blue color in a ring around the periphery of the cornea, the Kayser-Fleischer ring. This ring is thought to be due to deposition of copper in the cornea as a result of faulty metabolism.

Tumors of the Cornea

Since the majority of tumors involving the cornea arise from the conjunctiva or limbus (Fig. 7-9), these have already been described (p. 93). However, rarely a dermoid may occur in the cornea with clear corneal tissue completely surrounding it (Fig. 7-10). The tumor is identical with dermoids arising elsewhere. Removal with transplantation of clear cornea into the defect is the treatment of choice.

8

The Sclera

Anatomy

The *sclerotic* coat (sclera) is the tunic which, with the cornea, forms the external fibrous layer of the eyeball; it is strong, opaque and inelastic, and serves to maintain the form of the globe. Its thickness is about 1 mm., but varies at different points, being thinnest posterior to the insertions of the rectus muscles. Its structure resembles that of the cornea, being composed of bundles of *connective tissue* with some elastic fibers, disposed in both longitudinal and transverse layers, between which are a few flat cells; these parts, however, are arranged much less regularly than in the cornea. Anteriorly, the structure of the sclera is continuous with that of the cornea. In the child, the sclera often has a bluish white color, owing to its being thinner and allowing the dark pigment of the choroid to show through. The sclera is pierced about 2.5 mm. internal to the posterior pole of the eye by the optic nerve; here it has blended with it the external fibrous sheath of the nerve. The part through which the nerve passes is known as the *lamina cribrosa*.

The outer surface of the sclera is white and smooth, covered by *Tenon's capsule* and the conjunctiva, to which it is joined by *loose connective tissue (episcleral)*; in front, it presents the insertions of the extrinsic muscles of the eyeball. Its inner surface, brown and rough (*lamina fusca*), is united by filaments of pigmented connective tissue to the choroid, forming the outer wall of the *suprachoroidal space;* where it is pierced by vessels and nerves, a communication between the capsule of Tenon and the suprachoroidea is established. The points of emergence of the anterior ciliary veins are often marked by small brown dots; and the anterior portion of the sclera sometimes presents slate-colored or violet spots of pigmentation, especially in Negroes. Though traversed by many blood vessels, the sclera itself has a very scant vascular supply; but the episcleral tissue contains numerous vessels.

Congenital Anomalies of the Sclera

Blue sclera (Plate 8E) is an hereditary congenital anomaly in which the sclera appears uniformly light blue in color owing either to thinning or to increased transparency. It is associated with abnormal fragility of the bones, osteogenesis imperfecta, resulting in multiple or repeated fractures from minor trauma or at times almost spontaneous fractures; weakness of the supporting tissues of the joints, resulting in frequent dislocations and subluxations, and deafness, which usually comes on after the age of 20. Other associated anomalies include embryotoxon megalocornea, keratoconus, zonular cataract, late development of the teeth, cleft palate, spina bifida, congenital heart disease, hemophilia and atrophy of the skin. The cause is unknown and therefore no specific treatment is available; however, protective and palliative methods should be used.

Dermoid cysts or tumors occasionally develop in the sclera especially at the limbus (Fig. 7-9). Cartilagenous plaques also may occur either alone or as a part of a dermoid.

Clear cysts in the sclera at the limbus occur rarely as a developmental anomaly. They usually are continuous with the anterior chamber of the eye.

Inflammation of the Sclera may be either superficial or deep. The *superficial form,* called *episcleritis,* is limited to the superficial layers of the sclera and the episcleral tissue and is relatively harmless. The *deep* form, known as *scleritis,* involves the sclera itself and extends to subjacent and contiguous parts, causing serious consequences. There often is an absence of a sharp line of division between the two forms.

Episcleritis

Episcleritis is an uncommon inflammation of the episcleral tissue, including the superficial layers of the sclera.

Symptoms. There are slight to moderate *discomfort,* lacrimation, pain and photophobia. A flat or slightly raised hard and immovable *nodule* in a patch of dark red or purple color is seen in the ciliary region (Plate 10*D*), usually on the temporal side, associated with conjunctival or *episcleral congestion;* it is tender on pressure. After 1 or more weeks, the nodule will disappear; it never ulcerates; absorption usually being complete. Occasionally some discoloration of the sclera remains but others are apt to take its place; in this way the process may encircle the cornea. Owing to this tendency to relapses, the disease often lasts many months. One or both eyes may be involved. Rarely the cornea and iris are implicated. The disease may resemble a severe case of phylctenular conjunctivitis; it may merge gradually into scleritis.

Pathology. There are edema and infiltration with leukocytes in the episcleral tissue and in the superficial layers of the sclera.

Etiology. It usually is observed in *adults,* especially in women; often in those with connective tissue disease and in *rheumatic* and gouty individuals. Tuberculosis, allergy, syphilis and rarely leprosy have been implicated as causes at times. It is the first sign of general toxic reaction to some of the sulfonamides, especially sulfathiazole (Fig. 8-1).

Treatment. Systemic disorders such as syphilis, tuberculosis or connective tissue diseases should be treated. Topical or systemic steroid therapy is valuable in allergic lesions.

Transient periodic episcleritis is a

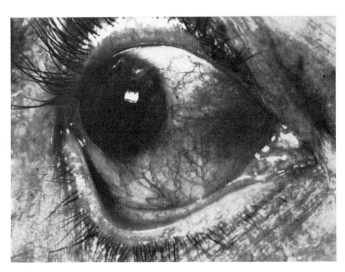

FIG. 8-1. Episcleritis.

fairly common variety of episcleritis which appears in sudden attacks lasting several days and reappears at intervals of several weeks or months; it may recur for years. It is seen in gouty and rheumatic adults. Treatment is that recommended for episcleritis.

Scleritis

Scleritis is an infrequent inflammation of the entire thickness of the sclera of *lengthy* duration and often is *serious* in consequences. *Both eyes* usually are involved. *Relapses* are very common.

Symptoms are *pain*, usually severe, and frequently radiating to neighboring regions, *tenderness* over the ciliary region, lacrimation and photophobia; secondary glaucoma often ensues.

There are dark red or *violet patches* adjacent to the cornea; in some cases this is circumscribed; in others the involvement may extend to the equator or surround the limbus forming *annular scleritis;* sometimes small, while, hard nodules develop in the inflamed area beneath the conjunctiva. After subsidence of the inflammation the affected area often is marked by pale violet discoloration. The sclera at first is softened in the affected areas; the weakened sclera, unable to withstand intraocular pressure, bulges and *ectasia,* violet in color, results.

Complications. The *cornea* is implicated frequently and sclerosing keratitis follows. Secondary glaucoma often results. As a rule the uvea is involved and then the signs and symptoms of uveitis are present. As a result of these changes, vision often is seriously affected and sometimes lost.

Pathology. The middle layers of the sclera become edematous; between the lamellae there is an infiltration of lymphocytes. The swollen lamellae break down and become necrotic; they may be replaced by fibrous tissue. The infiltration extends into the cornea and uveal tract. Later there is thinning of the sclera.

Etiology. The disease is most common in *young adults*, especially in women. *Tuberculosis* is considered a frequent predisposing cause; other etiologic factors are rheumatoid disease, connective tissue diseases, gout, disorders of menstruation and syphilis. An especially resistant form of the disease associated with rheumatoid lesions elsewhere frequently is referred to as scleromalacia perforans.

Treatment. The cause should be de-

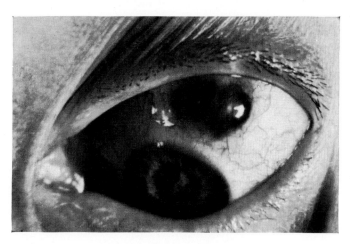

FIG. 8-2. Ciliary staphyloma.

termined and treated, or any related general disease should be treated by general measures such as intensive antiluetic or antituberculosis therapy. Steroid therapy alone or in combination with salicylates is valuable at times in rheumatoid scleritis, whereas some of the new antimalarial drugs may be valuable in the connective tissue disorders. Topical application of cycloplegics and hot or cold compresses relieve photophobia and make the patient more comfortable.

Hyaline degeneration of the sclera, a misnomer, consists of asymptomatic, small, round, translucent, gray areas 2–3 mm. in diameter located slightly anterior to the insertions of the recti muscles in persons over 60 years of age. The spots actually are due to the deposition of calcium oxalate crystals in the scleral fibers.

Staphyloma (Ectasia) of the Sclera

A *thinning and bulging* of the sclera which, when partial, occurs either at the anterior portion (*ciliary*), the equator (*equatorial*) or the posterior portion of the eyeball (*posterior*); when total it involves the entire globe (congenital glaucoma).

Ciliary and Equatorial Staphylomas are caused by a disturbed relationship between the resistance of the sclera and the intraocular tension; such conditions are found after chronic glaucoma, iridocyclitis, ectasia and staphyloma of the cornea, scleritis and injuries of the sclera. They present a *bluish gray or violet* bulging, (Fig. 8-2) which may be limited or extend all around the cornea. This bulging shows a tendency to increase; occasionally it ruptures. The distinction is made between true ciliary staphyloma, in which the sclera over the ciliary body gives way, and *intercalary* staphyloma, in which the bulging part is at the limbus.

In some cases control of increased intraocular pressure by drugs or surgery may prevent further enlargement of the bulge. Occasionally the staphylomatous sclera may be excised and the defect closed. In some cases, when the enlarged eyeball causes much discomfort or disfigurement and is sightless, *enucleation* or evisceration is advisable.

Posterior Staphyloma, situated at the posterior pole of the eyeball, is of common occurrence and is associated with high myopia and myopic degenerative changes of the choroid and retina.

9

The Uvea

Anatomy

The second or vascular coat of the eye (*uvea or uveal tract*) lies immediately beneath the sclera; it provides for the nourishment of the eyeball, and it is formed of three parts, which from before backward are known as the *iris*, the *ciliary body* and the *choroid*. These three portions are so *intimately associated* that when one part becomes diseased, the others frequently participate.

Iris

The *iris* is a colored membrane, circular in form, hanging behind the cornea immediately in front of the lens, and perforated in its center by an aperture of variable size, the *pupil*; it serves to regulate the amount of light admitted to the interior of the eye, and cuts off the marginal rays which would interfere with the sharpness of the retinal image. Its peripheral border springs from the ciliary body. Its free inner edge, the boundary of the pupil, lies upon the anterior capsule of the lens when the pupil is contracted or moderately dilated; with maximum dilatation it hangs free in the anterior chamber. The iris separates the *anterior* from the *posterior chamber* of the eyeball. Its anterior surface presents great variation in color in different eyes, and is marked in the peripheral or ciliary portion by radially directed, wavy lines, converging toward the circle of irregular elevations and small depressions (crypts) situated in the pupillary portion. Other finer lines are seen extending from this ring, the collarette, to the pupil; this appearance is produced by the subjacent blood vessels.

In *structure*, the iris consists of a delicate, spongy connective tissue stroma, containing branched pigmented cells, muscular fibers and an abundance of vessels and nerves. It is covered anteriorly by endothelium except at the crypts, where the stroma of the blood vessel layer communicates directly with the anterior chamber—an arrangement which permits rapid exchange from iris to anterior chamber and *vice versa*; posteriorly it presents the posterior limiting membrane and the retinal pigment layers.

The *color* of the iris depends partly upon the pigment in the stromal cells, which is variable, and partly on that in the cells of the retinal layers, which is constant.

The muscle tissue, of neuroectodermal origin, consists of (1) the *sphincter pupillae*, a narrow band about 1 mm. wide, situated close to and encircling the pupil posteriorly and supplied by the *third nerve*, and (2) the *dilator pupillae*, consisting of long spindle-shaped cells arranged meridionally, which extends along the posterior surface of the blood vessel layer from the sphincter pupillae to the root of the iris and is supplied by the *sympathetic*.

The *posterior surface* of the iris is covered by two strata of pigmented cells, the *pigment epithelium*, which extends to the free border around which it turns a little, forming the black fringe of the pupillary margin.

The *vessels* of the iris come from the two branches of the ophthalmic known as the long posterior ciliary arteries; each artery divides into an upper and a lower branch; these anastomose with the corresponding vessels of the opposite side and with the anterior ciliary, and form a vascular ring just behind the attached margin of the iris, the *greater arterial circle* of the iris. This gives off branches to the ciliary body and iris; the iris branches converge toward the pupil and here form by anastomosis a smaller vascular circle, the *lesser arterial circle* of the iris, just beneath the collarette, the juncture of the ciliary and pupillary portions of the iris. The veins of the iris follow the arrangement of arteries just described; they chiefly pass backward to the venae vorticosae.

The *nerves* are given off from the plexus in the ciliary body, and are derived from the third, the nasal branch of the ophthalmic and the sympathetic.

Ciliary Body

The ciliary body is that part of the tunica vasculosa which extends backward from the base of the iris to the anterior part of the choroid; it consists of the *ciliary processes* and of the *ciliary muscle*. A longitudinal section is of triangular shape, with a narrow base directed forward, giving origin to the iris. The outer side of the triangle is formed by the ciliary muscle; the inner side is divided into two parts: an anterior, which bears the ciliary processes (corona ciliaris), and a posterior portion (orbiculus ciliaris), which is smooth.

The *ciliary muscle* (the muscle of *accommodation*) consists of nonstriated muscular fibers arranged in bundles running in three different directions—meridional, radial and circular; the first two sets are attached anteriorly to the scleral spur. The proportion between circular and longitudinal fibers varies according to the re-fractive condition of the eye; the circular set is well developed in hyperopia (Fig. 20-3, *center*), but atrophied in myopia (Fig. 20-3, *right*). When the ciliary muscle contracts, it draws the ciliary processes and choroid forward and inward, thus relaxing the suspensory ligament and allowing the lens to become more convex.

The *ciliary processes* consist of about 70 folds arranged meridionally so as to form a circle; they are extremely vascular. They serve to *secrete the nutrient fluids* in the interior of the eye which nourish neighboring parts, especially the cornea, lens and part of the vitreous. The inner surface of the ciliary body is covered by two layers of epithelium: externally, pigment epithelium, and internally, next to the vitreous, a layer of cylindrical nonpigmented cells.

The *ciliary body* is supplied by branches from the greater circle of the iris and by the anterior ciliary *arteries*. The *veins*, constituting the greater part of the ciliary processes, pass backward to the vortex veins of the choroid. Some of the veins from the ciliary muscle pass backward, pierce the sclera and run beneath the conjunctiva with the anterior ciliary arteries. These constitute the violet subconjunctival vessels seen running backward in ciliary injection and in deeper congestion (glaucoma). They anastomose with the conjunctival veins, and communicate with Schlemm's canal. The ciliary body is richly supplied with *nerves*, especially the ciliary muscle, in which there is a nerve plexus with ganglion cells.

Choroid

The choroid is a *dark brown membrane* placed between the sclera and the retina, extending from the ora serrata to the opening for the optic nerve. It consists mainly of *blood vessels*, united by delicate connective tissue containing numerous *pig-*

mented cells; these vessels are arranged according to their caliber into three superimposed layers.

This vascular structure is bounded on either side by a nonvascular membrane; accordingly, the choroid can be divided into *five layers*: (1) externally, the *suprachoroid*, connected with the sclera by loose connective tissue; the long posterior ciliary arteries and the long ciliary nerves course in this layer; (2) the layer of *large vessels*, chiefly anastomosing veins, the spaces between which are filled with connective tissue and pigment cells; the arteries are derived from the short ciliary; the veins are arranged in curves converging to four principal trunks (*vortex veins*) which pierce the sclera behind the equator of the eyeball; (3) the layer of *medium-sized vessels*; (4) the layer of *capillaries* (choriocapillaris); (5) the *lamina vitrea* (membrane of Bruch), a homogeneous membrane which is placed next to the pigment layer of the retina.

The *function* of the choroid is to serve chiefly as a *nutrient organ* for the retina, vitreous and lens.

Pupil

The normal pupil is circular and regular in outline. It is larger in the young than in advanced life. Its size should equal that of its fellow; both should respond alike when one is subjected to a change in intensity of illumination. The movements of the pupil are contraction and dilatation.

The contracting fibers of the iris (*sphincter pupillae*) are supplied by the *third nerve*. The dilating fibers (*dilator pupillae*) are supplied by the *sympathetic*. Changes in the size of the pupil also depend upon variations in the caliber of its *blood vessels*, which also are supplied by the sympathetic.

Contraction of the pupil is effected by stimulation of the oculomotor nerve and by paralysis of the sympathetic. *Dilatation* follows paralysis of the third nerve or stimulation of the sympathetic.

The *oculomotor nerve fibers* are conveyed through the ciliary ganglion and short ciliary nerves. The nucleus of origin of the third nerve concerned in the movements of the iris is in the floor of the aqueduct of Sylvius, and can be divided into three portions: (1) that giving rise to the sphincter fibers of the *iris*, (2) *accommodation* (ciliary muscle) and (3) *convergence* (internal rectus). The *sympathetic or dilating fibers* are given off from the ciliospinal center of the lower cervical spinal cord; thence the impulses pass to the two long ciliary nerves by way of the superior cervical ganglion, the carotid plexus and the first division of the fifth nerve.

The *pupil contracts* upon exposure to light, with accommodation and with convergence. The light contraction may be direct or consensual. The *direct light reflex* is obtained by exposing one eye to increased illumination and observing the contraction of the pupil of this eye. The *consensual or indirect light reflex* is obtained by throwing light into one eye and observing the contraction of the pupil of the other eye. The direct and consensual reactions are equal. The *accommodation and convergence reflex* is obtained by directing the patient to look at an object held several inches in front of the face in the midline; the pupils will be seen to contract. These three actions are *associated*.

The *dilatation reflexes* of the pupil are seen upon shading the eye (both direct and consensual) and upon looking at a distant object. In addition there is a *sensory reflex:* when sensory nerves are stimulated, as by scratching or tickling the skin, both pupils dilate.

The consensual contraction is explained

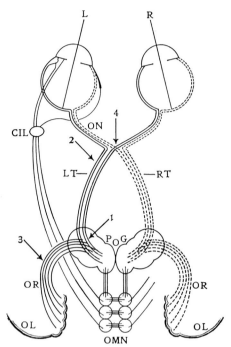

FIG. 9-1. Visual and pupillary reflex paths. *L*, left eye; *R*, right eye; *ON*, optic nerve; *LT*, left optic tract; *RT*, right optic tract; *POG*, primary optic ganglia; *OMN*, oculomotor nuclei; *OR*, optic radiations; *OL*, occipital lobe; *CIL*, ciliary ganglion. Division of the fibers at *1* abolishes the reaction of the pupil to light when the left half of either retina is illuminated; at *2*, the same result with right homonymous hemianopia; at *3*, right homonymous hemianopia with preservation of the reaction of the pupil to light.

by the fact that the light stimulus in one eye is carried by the optic nerve and passes to both optic tracts and in this way to the nucleus of the third nerve of each side (Fig. 9-1). Blindness in one eye abolishes the direct reflex in this eye, but its consensual reflex is preserved.

In certain disease conditions, there may be loss of light reflex, without interference with sight; this is seen, for example, in paralysis of the iris as a result of the use of a mydriatic or in oculomotor

paralysis. The *Argyll-Robertson pupil* (reflex iridoplegia), frequently a symptom of syphilis of the central nervous system, especially in tabes, contracts with accommodation and convergence, but does not respond to light; it usually is accompanied by miosis. It is explained by an interruption in the path from the optic nerve to the oculomotor nucleus, the connections of the centers for accommodation and convergence remaining unaffected, *i.e.*, a lesion in the connecting neuron which runs from the afferent pupillomotor fibers to the sphincter nucleus.

The characteristics of the pupils—size, equality and reflexes—are of great value in the diagnosis of various affections of the nervous system and in the localization of cerebral lesions. Hence it is important to be familiar with the afferent and efferent routes which control the movements of the pupil (Fig. 9-1; Plate 32).

The course of the *afferent impulse* is retina, optic nerve, both optic tracts, corpora quadrigemina, nuclei of origin of the third nerve in the floor of aqueduct of Sylvius (there being a communication between the two sides). The *efferent impulse* travels on either side from these nuclei to the third nerve, the ciliary ganglion, short ciliary nerves, to the iris.

When the pupil diminishes in size as a result of exposure to light, its contraction is not perfectly continuous; there are a number of minute oscillations during the contracting period. When these oscillations are large and noticeable, independent of illumination, the condition is known as *hippus*; it is bilateral and of central origin, but its cause and significance are unknown.

Adie's syndrome or tonic pupil is an anomaly in which there is one myotonic pupil, often associated with absent tendon reflexes. The condition generally is unilateral but may be bilateral. The defective pupil is larger than its fellow and is slightly irregular. The affected pupil reacts poorly or hardly at all to light but on near fixation shows a delayed and sometimes accentuated constriction which persists for some time after the normal pupil dilates. The cause is unknown. There should be no difficulty in distinguishing this condition from the Argyll-Robertson pupil.

Hemiopic pupillary reaction, Wernicke's sign, occurs in association with hemianopsia caused by lesions of the visual pathways anterior to the lateral geniculate body. Light thrown obliquely onto the seeing half of the retina produces a pupillary constriction but when thrown onto the blind half of the retina fails to produce this reaction (Fig. 9-1). In hemianopsia resulting from lesions lying behind the primary optic ganglia the pupillary reaction occurs when either half of the retina is illuminated since the afferent pupillary fibers have left the visual fibers at the ganglia and so are not affected. This test is difficult to perform.

Miosis, anhidrosis and slight ptosis of one eye, **Horner's syndrome,** results from interuption of the ipsilateral sympathetic nerve supply of the dilator pupillae muscle, the sweat gland of the side of the face and neck and Müller's involuntary levator muscle of the upper lid by a lesion of the cervical sympathetic trunk or the lower cervical and upper thoracic anterior spinal roots. Among the causes are mediastinal tumors, adenomas of the thyroid gland, neurofibromatosis, multiple sclerosis, syringomyelia, tumors of the cervical cord, occlusion of the posterior inferior cerebellar artery, trauma, and rarely lesions of the apex of the lung. A congenital form of Horner's syndrome occurs and is associated with decreased pigmentation of the affected eye. In Horner's syndrome the pupil of the affected eye does not dilate with 4 or 5 per cent cocaine solution whereas the normal pupil does. In cases of Horner's syndrome due to lesions of the sympathetic fibers above the superior cervical ganglion, the affected pupil is hypersensitive to adrenaline and dilates on the instillation of 1 drop of 1:1000 epinephrine hydrochloride whereas the normal pupil does not.

Drugs which cause dilatation of the pupil are *mydiatics*. These include cocaine, Euphthalmine, Paredrine, Benzedrine, ephedrine, and Neo-Synephrine. Drugs which in addition to dilating the pupil produce paralysis of accommodation are *cycloplegics*. The commonly used cycloplegics are atropine, scopolamine and homatropine. Drugs which cause constriction of the pupil are *miotics*. These include eserine, pilocarpine, Prostigmin, Carcholin, diisopropylflurophosphate (DFP), Phospholine iodide, and demecarium bromide.

Congenital Anomalies

Congenital anomalies of the uvea include persistent pupillary membrane, aniridia, heterochromia, albinism and colobomata.

Persistent pupillary membrane. In the fetus the pupil is closed by a thin, transparent, delicate vascular membrane, the capsulopupillary membrane. The membrane and its vessels are absorbed gradually in the seventh or eighth month of fetal life. A few shreds frequently remain at birth but occasionally a larger part of the membrane persists and becomes pigmented along with the iris.

Aniridia usually is a dominant, bilateral, hereditary anomaly in which the anterior portion of the embryonic optic cup develops only a rudimentary iris which ordinarily is not visible. Thus the blackness of the pupil fills the entire area usually occupied by iris and pupil. Visual acuity is reduced to 20/80 or less and is not improved by the creation of an artificial iris (use of pinhole lenses, contact lens with an iris painted on or by tatooing of the cornea). Glaucoma frequently develops during youth and is difficult to treat. Photophobia is a frequent complaint.

Heterochromia. Occasionally, the two irides are different in color, pigment occurs in spots or blotches (piebald iris) in some eyes, or a part of one iris, usually a sector, has a different color from the rest. This is known as heterochromia iridis and may occur as a simple localized developmental defect sometimes with dominant heredity or it may occur in association with three systemic abiotrophic dominant disorders: Waardenburg's syndrome; Romberg's syndrome or facial hemiatrophy; and status dysraphicus. In addition heterochromia may result from trauma, inflammation or degeneration of the iris, or from surgery or injury to the cervical sympathetic nerves in association with Horner's syndrome (p. 123). Finally all of these must be distinguished from heterochromic iridocyclitis which develops as a chronic inflammation in adult life (p. 149).

Albinism is a congenital and hereditary deficiency of pigment associated with lowered visual acuity, nystagmus and photophobia and often accompanied by refractive errors. The condition may be complete or partial. The lashes and brow as well as other hairs are white, the iris white or pinkish and the choroidal vessels are abnormally prominent against the white background of the sclera (Plate 3*B*).

Coloboma is a congenital defect resulting from complete closure of the fetal fissure. Since the fetal fissure closes near the equatorial portion of the optic cup and proceeds both anteriorly and posteriorly, various types of defect may result from arrest of closure occurring at various stages of fetal development. Thus a notching of the iris, usually present in the inferior portion, may occur alone or there may be a defect involving the entire iris and ciliary body. The defect may extend all the way back to the optic nerve or

only the posterior portion of the uvea may be involved. In the latter instance the defect in the choroid and retina appears as a large white patch bordered with more or less pigment situated below the disk. The whiteness is due to the exposed sclera but retinal vessels may be seen running across this area (Plate 17*A*). There is a scotoma corresponding to the defect. Other congenital anomalies frequently are associated.

UVEITIS

Inflammatory lesions of the uvea are caused by a wide variety of factors and infectious agents thus producing diverse manifestations. For example the inflammation may involve the anterior uvea, the posterior uvea or may diffusely involve the entire tract. Either one of these may be acute or chronic and severe or mild. The inflammatory reaction may be serous, purulent, plastic or granulomatous but several of these tend to merge thus it is more practical to classify them as purulent, serous or nongranulomatous and granulomatous uveitis.

Purulent inflammation of the uvea usually arises from exogenous or metastatic infection by pyogenic bacteria or occasionally by fungi which involve the entire tract producing suppuration and abscess formation. When limited to the internal portions of the eye it is classified as endophthalmitis but when it extends into the sclera and surrounding structures it is panophthalmitis (Chap. 17).

Nonpurulent inflammation of the uvea seldom involves the entire tract usually showing a greater intensity in one portion, for example iritis, cyclitis, iridocyclitis or choroiditis. However, in every case there is some extension of the inflammatory reaction into adjacent segments, but since posterior choroidal lesions tend to remain more localized than iris and ciliary body lesions, it has become more practical to

divide these affections into anterior uveitis
and posterior uveitis.

ANTERIOR UVEITIS

According to its course, anterior uveitis
may be acute or chronic and according to
its characteristics either granulomatous or
nongranulomatous.

Signs. The signs of anterior uveitis include circumcorneal or ciliary injection,
inflammation of the iris and exudation into
the anterior chamber. These vary with the
acuteness of the inflammation and with
the granulomatous or nongranulomatous
character of the process.

Circumcorneal injection is diffuse, purplish red, more intense immediately around
the cornea fading toward the fornices and
does not blanch after the instillation of
1:1000 epinephrine solution. In addition
there also is some congestion of the conjunctival vessels and in severe acute or
prolonged inflammation both types of
congestion may become intense, but in
mild serous or granulomatous lesions congestion may be minimal.

The iris looks altered. In acute anterior
uveitis it appears swollen and dull. Its
markings become indistinct and its color
changes, becoming greenish in blue or
gray irides and muddy in darker varieties.
At times radial vessels become visible.
These changes are due to congestion and
edema of the iris and exudation of fibrin
and cells into its substance and into the
anterior chamber. In granulomatous lesions soft gray globular accumulations of
exudate may occur at the pupillary border
(Gilbert-Koeppe nodules) or on the surface of the iris (Busacca nodules) and in
some types large or small nodular infiltrations may develop in the iris stroma.

The pupil, because of the congestion and
infiltration of the iris, is contracted and
sluggish in action. Adhesions form between
the posterior surface of the iris and the
anterior capsule of the lens producing

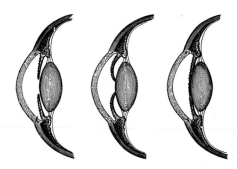

FIG. 9-2. Section of the anterior portion
of the eyeball, showing, *left*, the iris in its
normal relations; *center*, annular posterior
synechia (seclusion of the pupil), *right*,
total posterior synechia and occlusion of the
pupil.

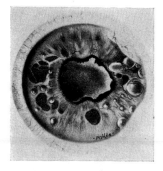

FIG. 9-3 Nodular iritis in sarcoidosis,
with posterior synechiae causing irregular
pupil.

posterior synechiae (Figs. 9-2 and 9-3).
These cause irregularities in the shape of
the pupil especially after the instillation
of atropine but when they continue to
develop they may bind the entire pupillary margin to the lens capsule, a condition referred to as seclusio pupillae (Fig.
9-2). Exudate may form in the pupil
and after organization and extension of
vessels from the iris result in an inflammatory membrane occluding the pupil,
occlusio pupillae. As a result of either or
both of these changes aqueous cannot pass
through the pupil into the anterior chamber and so pushes the peripheral portion

of the iris forward against the posterior surface of the cornea producing iris bombé. As a consequence the intraocular pressure rises producing secondary glaucoma. Unless the iris bombé is corrected quickly peripheral anterior synechiae form between the peripheral iris and the posterior surface of the cornea, increasing the severity of the secondary glaucoma. The character of the aqueous humor is changed. The protein content is increased so it becomes plasmoid in character. Along with this, fibrin and cells accumulate in the anterior chamber but as a result of the thermal circulation of the aqueous humor they are kept in suspension floating upward along the anterior surface of the iris and downward just behind the cornea. These give a turbid appearance to the aqueous humor so that a thin beam of light which is not seen in its passage through normal aqueous humor becomes visible in plasmoid aqueous humor (Tyndall's phenomenon, Fig. 2-16). Some cells and fibrin may be deposited on the posterior surface of the cornea forming keratic precipitates (KPs). They usually involve the lower part of the cornea first and to a greater extent but in severe inflammation they may affect the entire surface of the cornea giving it a cloudy appearance. In acute lesions the precipitates are fine and dust-like but in chronic uveitis pigment granules and large, greasy, gray, mutton fat-like precipitates develop among the fine deposits. In acute inflammation the exudate may contain so many cells they tend to accumulate into a yellowish pool of pus in the lower angle of the anterior chamber (hypopyon). In acute or chronic inflammation with an exudate rich in fibrin (plastic uveitis) a grayish fibrin clot may form in or completely fill the anterior chamber. In recurrent inflammation blood may accumulate in the chamber (hyphema). In some instances the anterior chamber may be deeper than normal.

In severe anterior uveitis especially affecting the ciliary body the upper lid may be swollen, vision diminished more than can be explained by the visible opacities and tenderness over the ciliary body greater than in other types of uveitis.

The intraocular pressure generally is normal or lower than normal but occasionally the increased viscosity of the aqueous humor resulting from its increased protein content (plasmoid aqueous) hinders its passage through the regular outflow channels thus producing an elevation of the intraocular pressure. This may be accentuated by obstruction of these channels by fibrinous and cellular exudate into the anterior chamber. Unless controlled these changes may stimulate the development of peripheral anterior synechiae which increase the severity of the secondary glaucoma.

The anterior capsule of the lens may present evidences of exudation similar to those on the posterior surface of the cornea as a result of deposits from the slow upward thermal circulation of the aqueous humor. In addition small deposits of iris pigment may be seen where posterior synechiae have been torn away.

Inflammation of the ciliary body produces similar transudation and exudation into the aqueous humor of the posterior chamber which when severe may become organized forming an opaque cyclitic membrane which in infants and young children may simulate a tumor of the eye and sometimes is referred to as pseudoglioma (Chap. 14). Both extensive exudation and cyclitic membrane formation interfere seriously with metabolism of the lens which may result in cataractous changes.

Symptoms. The symptoms of anterior uveitis consist of photophobia, pain, lacrimation and interference with vision.

Photophobia results from pain produced by movement of an inflamed iris on exposure of the eye to light. In acute inflammation photophobia can be severe but can be controlled by keeping the iris at rest by the adequate use of cycloplegic drops (atropine, scopolamine, etc.).

Lacrimation usually accompanies photophobia but is not completely eliminated by the use of cycloplegic drugs.

Pain in acute anterior uveitis frequently is severe and often is described as a throbbing ache located in the eyeball and radiating to the forehead and temple. It usually is worse at night. It is accompanied by tenderness of the eyeball when there is involvement of the ciliary body. This pain is in addition to photophobia; it is likely to be especially severe in viral uveitis (herpes simplex and zoster) and is not relieved by cycloplegic drugs but requires analgesics or at times stronger medications. Pain seldom occurs in chronic anterior uveitis and then usually is mild.

The diminution in acuteness of vision depends upon turbidity of the anterior chamber, deposits on the pupillary portion of the lens and the posterior surface of the cornea and inflammatory inhibition of the ciliary muscles reducing the focusing activity of the eye. When the visual loss is great it may indicate severe exudation and pupillary or cyclitic membrane formation or involvement of the posterior uvea.

Differential diagnosis. Anterior uveitis most frequently is mistaken for acute catarrhal *conjunctivitis,* an unfortunate error because it delays the prompt instillation of atropine. Diagnosing glaucoma as anterior uveitis, however, is most serious since the use of atropine is disastrous in glaucoma but necessary in anterior uveitis. The differential points given in Table 9-1 ought to prevent such errors.

Course. Anterior uveitis may be *acute* and run its course in several weeks; or it may be chronic and last a number of months. A great many attacks terminate *favorably,* especially when subjected early

to proper treatment; the exudation becomes absorbed, and the iris returns to a normal condition with no evidence or mere traces of former inflammation. On the other hand, *serious complications* and disastrous sequelae may arise; hence the prognosis should be guarded. Chronic cases present very mild or almost no inflammatory symptoms. Most forms of anterior uveitis have a tendency to recur (*recurrent anterior uveitis*); relapses are common, partly because of the irritating effects of synechiae, but probably more as a result of failure to eliminate the causative factor. Anterior uveitis may involve *one or both eyes;* when both eyes are attacked, the second usually is affected a short time after the first.

Complications. Posterior synechiae are the most common complications of anterior uveitis but may be prevented entirely or broken if adequate mydriatic and cycloplegic treatment is started early enough and maintained until all inflammation has subsided. However, if allowed to form, posterior synechiae leave some pigmented remnants attached to the lens when broken away by treatment but if not properly controlled, the synechiae may extend round the circumference of the pupil producing seclusio pupillae or they may result in adhesion of all of the posterior surface of the iris to the adjacent lens (Fig. 9-2). In either case the aqueous humor is unable to pass from the posterior chamber through the pupil into the anterior chamber. Thus with continued production of aqueous humor by the ciliary body, the peripheral portion of the iris is pushed forward (iris bombé) unless this is relieved either by iridectomy or transfixation of the iris, the chamber angle becomes occluded by the bulging peripheral iris with the result that it becomes adherent to the posterior surface of the cornea (peripheral anterior synechiae). With continued production and accumulation of the

TABLE 9-1

Differential Diagnosis of Anterior Uveitis, Acute Conjunctivitis and Acute Glaucoma

Diagnostic Point	Anterior Uveitis	Acute Conjunctivitis	Acute Glaucoma
Iris	Swollen, dull and discolored	No change	Congested, discolored, dull, pushed forward
Pupil	Small, sluggish; irregular after use of atropine	Normal	Dilated, oval, immobile
Anterior chamber	Normal depth, presents exudation	Normal	Shallow
Cornea	Transparent and sensitive (may present deposits on posterior surface)	Transparent	Steamy and insensitive
Injection	Ciliary (circumcorneal); dull red zone surrounding cornea and fading toward fornix	Conjunctival; coarse meshes, most pronounced in fornix and fading toward cornea	Ciliary and episcleral; also conjunctival
Conjunctiva	Usually transparent	Reddened and opaque	Congested and chemotic
Lacrimation and discharge	Lacrimation but no discharge	Mucous or mucopurulent discharge	Lacrimation but no discharge
Tension	Usually normal or low	Normal	Increased
Ciliary tenderness	Some	None	Some
Pain	Radiating to forehead and temple, worse at night	Discomfort, hot gritty feeling, but no real pain	Severe in and about eyes, with headache
Photophobia	Severe	None	None
Vision	Dimness	No interference with vision, except blurring caused by discharge smeared over surface of cornea	Greatly reduced

aqueous humor the intraocular pressure increases (glaucoma). In plastic anterior uveitis, the pupil may become occluded by the development of an inflammatory pupillary membrane (occlusio pupillae) which then is followed by the development of iris bombé and secondary glaucoma.

Rubeosis iridis rarely may result from prolonged chronic anterior uveitis.

Plastic inflammation of the ciliary body resulting in a fibrin-rich exudative reaction in the posterior chamber may result in the production of an inflammatory membrane extending from the ciliary body across the posterior chamber and either passing behind or surrounding the lens (cyclitic membrane).

Retinal detachment may accompany the active phase of Vogt-Koyanagi-Harada uveitis or may develop as a late complication following contraction of a cyclitic membrane.

Band-shaped keratopathy, a horizontal band of opacity and calcium deposition in the superficial layers of the cornea which frequently occurs in anterior uveitis associated with Still's disease in children also occurs rarely in children and adults suffering from other forms of uveitis. In addition disciform keratitis (Chap. 7) vascularization of the posterior layers of the cornea, endothelial dystrophy, stromal edema and bullous keratopathy rarely complicate anterior uveitis.

Opacities of the lens occur at the sites of attachment of posterior synechiae probably as a result of disturbance in metabolism locally. Similar but more extensive opacities develop from long standing inflammatory deposits on the lens, from inflammatory pupillary membranes, and from cyclitic membranes. Occasionally, secondary cataract develops in uveitis without any of these other complications.

Secondary glaucoma may develop in anterior uveitis without seclusio or occlusio pupillae; the plasmoid aqueous humor apparently does not escape adequately through the outflow channels. This may be accentuated when these channels also are partially or completely occluded by fibrinous or cellular exudate. These patients also usually develop peripheral anterior synechiae sooner or later and these increase the severity of the secondary glaucoma. Ciliary staphyloma may follow long standing glaucoma.

In severe inflammation or in often repeated inflammation, atrophy of the iris and ciliary body may occur. With this there is diminished production of aqueous humor which eventually leads to hypertension and when severe, is followed by extensive degeneration of the eye ending in phthisis bulbi.

Etiology. Anterior uveitis can arise from inflammatory processes involving the anterior segment of the eye, from systemic disorders, and from unknown causes (idiopathic).

Local causes. Anterior uveal irritation results from even slight trauma or injury to the cornea or sclera since the vascular supply of the anterior sclera and cornea is derived from the anterior ciliary vessels which after perforating the sclera and entering the ciliary body anastomose with the long posterior ciliary vessels to form the great arterial circle of the iris and supply the iris and ciliary body. More severe trauma, of course, produces more intense uveitis and injury involving the anterior uvea and sclera may result in sympathetic uveitis. Traumatic anterior uveitis also may occur with a foreign body in the cornea, anterior chamber, iris or ciliary body. Occasionally relatively inert foreign bodies retained in the anterior chamber angle may be responsible for recurrent attacks of mild to moderate serous anterior uveitis.

Bacterial, viral and fungal infections of the conjunctiva producing keratitis, and infected epithelial or ulcerative lesions of the cornea produce anterior uveitis of varying intensity. In mild infections, and early in more serious lesions of the cornea, the uveitis is sterile resulting either from reflex vascular stimuli or from direct action of chemical stimuli which reach the uvea from the site of the infection. In some instances as in pneumococcic ulcer a sterile hypopyon may result. Later the organisms, especially the fungi, may invade the anterior chamber even before corneal perforation occurs. The viruses of herpes simplex and zoster also frequently produce severe and prolonged uveitis occasionally accompanied by hypopyon, consequent to severe keratitis.

Episcleritis, although usually due to systemic diseases, may be a limited local ocular inflammation but if located at or near the limbus frequently is associated with anterior uveal irritation.

Diseases of the lens also may produce anterior uveitis. Release of soluble degeneration products of hypermature cataract through the intact or broken lens capsule produce a toxic reaction and inflammation of the anterior uvea. A somewhat similar clinical anterior uveitis resulting from an autoimmune reaction to lens substance may develop after lens injury or extracapsular cataract extraction (p. 146).

Other local causes of anterior uveitis include idiopathic disease of the iris (heterochromic cyclitis) inflammatory products of intraocular tumor and degenerative lesions of the eye (phthisis bulbi).

Systemic causes. Anterior uveitis occurs in the course of a number of systemic diseases. Acute infectious diseases of childhood such as mumps, varicella, rubella and rubeola frequently are accompanied by mild to moderately acute anterior uveitis. Other infectious diseases which affect adults as well as children and which are accompanied by various types of anterior uveitis are gonorrhea, syphilis, yaws, tuberculosis, leptospirosis, relapsing fever, bacillary dysentery, actinomycosis, blastomycosis, coccidiomycosis, and, rarely, many others. Systemic diseases which may have an infectious origin include, sarcoid, ileitis, ulcerative colitis and Behçet's syndrome. Other systemic diseases which have an associated anterior uveitis at times include rheumatoid arthritis, ankylosing spondylitis or Marie-Strümpell syndrome (15 to 20 per cent of patients), Still's disease, gout, psoriasis and Reiter's syndrome.

Hypersensitivity may play a considerable role in the production of anterior uveitis particularly of the acute recurrent type. Both the immediate and the delayed types of hypersensitivity appear to be implicated at times as well as autoimmune processes.

Idiopathic anterior uveitis. In spite of the numerous local and systemic factors enumerated above, the specific cause of anterior uveitis cannot be determined in a little over 50 per cent of the cases.

Pathology. Inflammation of the iris presents changes similar to those occurring in other connective tissue, modified by the great vascularity of this membrane and the looseness of its stroma. There are dilatation of the blood vessels and changes in the capillary walls, transudation of protein-rich lymph into the stroma and into the anterior chamber, and exudation of leukocytes, lymphocytes (Fig. 9-4) and fibrin into the stroma and anterior chamber. The cells which find their way into the anterior chamber cause cloudiness of the aqueous humor and adhere to the posterior surface of the cornea, forming keratic precipitates and also deposits upon the anterior lens capsule. All of these products of inflammation may be completely absorbed or they may become organized, forming adhesions between the iris and the anterior capsule of the lens. In chronic iritis and after repeated attacks of acute iritis, the iris may become atrophic. Similar changes occur in the ciliary body. In both structures the cellular infiltration is characteristic of acute or chronic inflammatory reactions in other tissues. In acute purulent or suppurative lesions the characteristic cell is the polymorphonuclear leukocyte. In acute serous or nongranulomatous uveitis, lymphocytes predominate. In chronic granulomatous uveitis lymphocytes, mononuclear cells, plasma cells and epitheloid cells with occasional giant cells produce the characteristic nodular lesions.

Treatment consists of (1) cycloplegia, (2) treatment of causative factor or factors, (3) foreign protein or steroid therapy and (4) local heat, general rest and supportive measures.

Cycloplegic therapy (1 per cent atropine or 0.2 per cent scopolamine either in solution or in ointment) puts the iris and ciliary body at rest, thus relieving photophobia, diminishes congestion of the iris and ciliary body, prevents the formation of synechiae or tends to break those already formed.

Sufficient should be instilled to keep

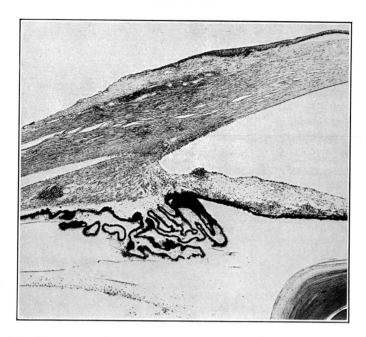

Fig. 9-4. Section of anterior segment of eyeball in iridocyclitis, showing nodule of lymphocytes in ciliary body and on the root of the iris.

the pupil widely dilated; 1 drop every 2 hours at first, and later, after the pupil is well dilated, three or four times a day. Atropine ointment may be found preferable to the solution; a small portion (half the size of a small pea) is placed in the conjunctival sac either on the end of a glass rod or delivered from a collapsible metal tube; it is sometimes easier to use, especially with children, and in the latter it is less likely to produce atropine poisoning. When the inflammation is very severe, the pupil will not dilate readily. Under these circumstances the action of the cycloplegic drug may be made more effective by the instillation of 1 drop of a 5 per cent solution of cocaine followed in 1 minute by 1 drop of 2.5 per cent Neo-Synephrine and in another minute by the cycloplegic. Another drop of cycloplegic 15 minutes later, when the decongesting action of the Neo-Synephrine is reaching its maximum, gives additional effectiveness.

This combination of drops sometimes is used to break synechiae which resist simple cycloplegic therapy, but greater effect can be obtained by injecting 0.05 to 0.1 cc. of the cycloplegic subconjunctivally at the limbus, at the point nearest the synechiae. Either of these procedures is effective only if the adhesion is fresh. In some instances intoxication or sensitivity may develop to the cycloplegic being used. This is more frequent with atropine than scopolamine but may happen with either. In such a case the other drug is substituted.

In some cases of iridocyclitis the intraocular pressure is increased; however, cycloplegic therapy should be maintained, for the rise in pressure is due to the inflammatory process, which is controlled most effectively by keeping the eye at rest. The increased intraocular pressure, however, usually can be controlled by the use of a carbonic anhydrase-inhibiting agent such as acetazolamide (Diamox) in doses of 125, 250, or 500 mg. by mouth every 6 hours or dichlorphenamide in doses of 25 mg. orally every 6 hours.

Treatment of causative factor or factors. Although immediate attention is given to putting the eye at rest, every attempt should be made as quickly as possible to determine any factors which may be responsible for or contribute to the inflammation. General infectious disease (syphilis, gonorrhea, etc.) should be treated and local infectious processes should be treated or eliminated (teeth, sinus, tonsils, etc.). Whether these are actual causes is incidental, for they at least contribute to the lowered general resistance of the patient. More specific recommendations are made under the various clinical types described below.

Foreign protein or steroid therapy. Where specific causative factors are not obvious, nonspecific foreign protein therapy often is of great value and is beneficial in either infectious or allergenic inflammations. Typhoid H antigen, given intravenously in stimulating doses of 5 to 10 million organisms in elderly or debilitated individuals or in "shock" doses of 25 to 50 million organisms in vigorous adults, stimulates all of the defense mechanisms of the individual and the larger doses usually produce a rise in temperature of several degrees for a few hours. When repeated the doses must be increased 2 or sometimes 3 times in order to obtain the same reaction produced by the previous dose. Children should not be treated by intravenous foreign protein injections because of the lability of their heat regulation mechanisms; however, stimulation of the defense mechanism can be accomplished by intramuscular injection of typhoid vaccine in doses of 0.5 cc., gradually increasing to 2.0 cc.

Steroids, by blocking defense reactions, are especially valuable in allergic and un-infected traumatic inflammatory processes, and thus frequently are valuable topically or by general administration in allergic or traumatic iritis or iridocyclitis. They should not be used either topically or generally in uveitis of an infectious origin either of the acute purulent or chronic infectious type or in conjunction with or before foreign protein therapy. Steroids may result in an increase in intraocular pressure; therefore, when used this must be kept in mind.

Local heat, general rest and supportive measures. Moist, hot compresses for several hours each day diminish the pain and the inflammation. It is only in traumatic iritis that cold compresses may be of service for the first day or two.

Other important indications are *absolute rest* in bed in the early stages, light diet, abstinence from alcohol, a brisk *purge* and avoidance of use of the eyes. *Aspirin* often gives relief from pain even in nontraumatic cases.

Paracentesis occasionally is made in certain obstinate cases to produce a favorable effect upon the course of the disease; but as a rule, operative procedures are indicated only after inflammatory symptoms have subsided, for the purpose of remedying sequelae and preventing recurrences; for instance, when iris bombé has resulted, increase of tension is likely and requires iridectomy or transfixation of the iris.

POSTERIOR UVEITIS

Inflammation of the posterior portion of the uvea may have an insidious or an acute onset but eventually develops into a chronic granulomatous process. In either the acute or chronic phase the overlying retina is involved in the inflammatory process.

Signs. There are no external signs of posterior uveitis. Ophthalmoscopic examination made early or at the onset of the disease reveals diffuse or patchy indefinite thickening and slight elevation of the choroid. These elevations have a yellow or grayish white color fading indistinctly into the surrounding choroid. Retinal vessels are elevated as they pass over these areas. In mild cases these lesions disappear leaving little or no visible change in the choroid but usually after several weeks or months the infiltrates and edema subside and the affected choroid and retina atrophy and adhere to each other. These atrophic areas are of various sizes and shapes, whitish in color due to thinning of the choroid permitting the sclera to show through; often they present visible choroidal vessels and are characterized by the irregular deposition of more or less black pigment especially at their margins. In mild lesions cellular exudate may be limited to the choroid and retina. However in the usual chorioretinitis inflammatory cells pass into and appear in the vitreous humor as fine floaters and increase slowly or rapidly until the vitreous humor at times becomes so hazy that details of the fundus are obscured. In severe or prolonged chorioretinitis the floaters sooner or later appear in small numbers in the aqueous humor of the anterior chamber along with a slight Tyndall's phenomenon. Some of the floaters become deposited on the posterior surface of the cornea and slowly aggregate to form mutton fat precipitates on the lower portion of the cornea. The optic disk may be hyperemic at first but later becomes dirty yellowish red with blurred margins, a condition known as choroiditic atrophy. The visual field examination may show slight peripheral contraction and scotomas corresponding to the inflammatory or atrophic areas.

Symptoms. The patient complains of disturbances of sight. Vision is blurred and diminished due to the opacities in the vitreous humor and the areas of inflammation of the choroid. Because of the elevation of the retina over these areas there is distortion of objects (metamorphopsia), either micropsia, when objects appear too small or macropsia when objects appear too large. If the inflammatory areas are located peripherally, the visual field defects they produce (Fig. 9-5) may not be noticed but if the macula is involved there is great reduction in or loss of central vision. Often the patient complains of seeing a black spot, the expression of a positive scotoma. Frequently the patient sees flashes of light, sparks, or bright circles (photopsiae) before the eyes. There is no pain unless the iris or ciliary body is involved.

Complications. The retina and vitreous humor always are involved to a greater or lesser extent and other neighboring structures may be implicated in posterior uveal inflammation (ciliary body, iris, optic nerve, and sclera). Posterior uveitis also may cause posterior polar cataract.

Etiology. Acute posterior uveitis may be caused by infection resulting from a perforating injury or by metastatic pyogenic infection. In either case the entire uveal tract becomes involved rapidly leading either to endophthalmitis or panophthalmitis (Chap. 17).

Exudative or nonsuppurative posterior uveitis frequently is due to a systemic or constitutional disease. This may be an infectious disease such as congenital or ac-

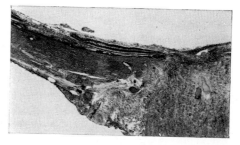

FIG. 9-5. Section of posterior segment of eyeball in severe uveitis, showing chorioretinitis with exudate lying on the internal surface of the retina and optic nervehead.

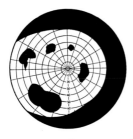

Fig. 9-6. Peripheral scotomas in exudative choroiditis.

quired syphilis, acute infectious diseases of childhood, tuberculosis, brucellosis, histoplasmosis, mucormycosis, cytomegalic inclusion disease and others. Posterior uveitis also may be associated with the connective tissue diseases or the immunogenic disorders, i.e., immediate or delayed hypersensitivity or autoimmune disease. However, one of the more common causes of inflammatory lesions of the posterior segment of the eye, at the present time, *Toxoplasma gondii*, actually invades the retina primarily and produces uveitis secondary to the necrotic retinitis (Chap. 10). Rarely proliferative nodular chorioretinal lesions are caused by infestation with *Toxocara canis* and other parasites.

Pathology. In the early stages there are congestion and infiltration of polymorphonuclear leukocytes, lymphocytes and fibrin in the affected part of the choroid and overlying retina. This explains the appearance of the soft fluffy areas seen with the ophthalmoscope. In purulent lesions the polymorphonuclear leukocytes continue to accumulate until suppuration occurs but in serous or nongranulomatous uveitis lymphocytes become predominant. As the inflammation increases, the lamina vitrea is broken through and the leukocytes increase in the retina and invade the vitreous humor producing opacities floating in the vitreous body (Fig. 9-6). In chronic granulomatous uveitis, mononuclear cells, epithelioid cells and giant cells appear in the inflammatory foci producing typical granulomatous nodules. Later the exudates diminish and usually disappear with atrophy of the choroid and retina with fusion of the two layers over the involved areas. In some instances the exudate is replaced by scar tissue. Pigment granules are released by necrosis or atrophy of the chromatophores and pigment epithelial cells. Then they are phagocytosed by macrophages which become concentrated at the margins of the lesion to a lesser extent within the scarred or atrophic areas.

Prognosis is dependent upon the *position of the patches* of exudation with subsequent atrophy. A single patch involving the macular region will seriously impair vision. On the other hand, the process may extend over a considerable part of the fundus and yet central vision remains good, if the macula escapes.

Treatment. *Removal of the etiologic factor* is the most important indication; *antisyphilitic treatment* in syphilitic cases; isoniazid, *p*-aminosalicylic acid and streptomycin in tuberculous cases; or special treatment in other specific cases; attention to the general health. Injections of *foreign protein* sometimes are useful. Atropine may be indicated to rest the eyes.

Clinical Varieties of Posterior Uveitis

Several different clinical varieties of posterior uveitis occur but they do not represent distinct etiologic entities.

Diffuse choroiditis (Plate 16A). In this form there are patches of exudation, each gradually shading into the surrounding portions of the choroid. They spread and coalesce so that later, when atrophy has taken place, a *large part of the fundus* appears white or yellowish white between retained islands of unaltered fundus; in these atrophic areas one sees choroidal blood vessels, retinal vessels and irregularly distributed spots of pigment.

Disseminated choroiditis (Plate 16B)

presents numerous round or irregular yellow spots with fluffy borders scattered over the fundus; later they atrophy and become white with pigmented margins. The choroiditic areas have a tendency to appear in crops. The entire choroid may be studded, and yet vision remains good if the macular region escapes; the retention of good central vision in these cases is quite common. This form of choroiditis runs a *chronic* course. After some time, vitreous opacities may be found; choroiditic atrophy of the optic disk and posterior polar cataract may follow, but not generally.

Circumscribed (nodular) choroiditis (Plate 15 *A* and *B*) is a variety occurring not infrequently in young individuals in whom a *single patch* of yellowish white (occasionally bluish green) color with fading edges is seen near the macula or more peripherally, often accompanied by deposits on the posterior surface of the cornea and by vitreous opacities; there may be but slight damage to vision unless the macular region is invaded. *Relapses* are common, and when they occur the supervening lesion is apt to be contiguous to one of the preceding atrophic spots.

Juxtapapillary choroiditis is a form of circumscribed choroiditis which, as its name implies, is adjacent to the disk; its shape usually is oval.

Anterior choroiditis, presents foci of exudation similar to those found in disseminated choroiditis but limited to the *periphery* of the choroid. The diagnosis usually is made only in the later stage when the exudates have changed to white spots with pigmented margins, and then generally only in the course of an ophthalmoscopic examination made for other reasons. Vision is not affected.

Central choroiditis (Plate 17*B*) is a form of circumscribed choroiditis situated in the *macular region*. There are many variations in the appearance of the macular change. In general there is a gray or white *spot,* usually about half the size of the disk, either mottled or uniform in color, with more or less pigmentation scattered in irregular deposits or forming a border; some choroidal vessels often are seen on its surface. The defect causes a *central scotoma,* usually absolute, and therefore *severe reduction* or loss of *central vision,* but peripheral vision is preserved. This macular lesion may be due to tuberculosis, a septic focus of infection or syphilis. It is found occasionally in children without antecedent history of ocular disease; some of these are toxoplasmic choroiditis (toxoplasmosis) and show cerebral calcification. Central choroiditis must be distinguished from macular degenerative changes of myopia and from senile degeneration at the macula.

SPECIFIC TYPES OF UVEITIS

Syphilitic Uveitis

Syphilis may produce either anterior or posterior uveitis as the result of either congenital or acquired infection.

Syphilitic anterior uveitis is one of the fairly common forms. It occurs in the secondary stage of acquired syphilis, usually during the first year after infection. It usually is acute and generally unilateral but the second eye often is attacked soon after its fellow. In some cases there are no characteristic symptoms distinguishing this from other forms of anterior uveitis though there always are apt to be broad and thick synechiae and pain often is insignificant. In some cases there are yellowish red, highly vascularized nodules the size of a pinhead or larger (Plate 15*C*), usually multiple, situated upon the pupillary or ciliary border (iritis papulosa). There frequently is accompanying disease of the posterior portion of the eyeball (choroid, retina, and optic nerve).

Similar lesions of the iris occur in childhood as a result of congenital syphilis but usually in association with interstitial keratitis, anterior choroiditis and frequently with other ocular lesions of syphilis.

Gumma may occur in the iris in the tertiary stage of syphilis and frequently spreads to involve the ciliary body, cornea and sclera.

An acute serous type of anterior uveitis, which may be quite severe, frequently occurs in the course of a Herxheimer reaction and calls for immediate and intensive ocular treatment.

Posterior uveitis due to syphilis may be diffuse, disseminated or nodular, and usually occurs in secondary syphilis. A particular form of nodular uveitis which is due to syphilis in almost half of the reported cases is chorioretinitis juxtapapillaris.

Treatment for the systemic infection usually results in rapid improvement of the ocular lesions except in those occurring in the course of a Herxheimer reaction. But in all cases general therapeutic measures should be supplemented by intensive ocular measures to prevent sequelae and complications. These include cycloplegia for anterior uveitis and anterior choroiditis.

Gonorrheal Uveitis

Gonorrheal uveitis always occurs as an anterior uveitis or iridocyclitis and may be acute or chronic and recurrent. The acute lesion occurs during the acute urethral infection. It is a severely acute reaction frequently characterized by a fibrin clot in or filling the anterior chamber and occasionally is accompanied by hyphemia. The chronic or recurrent type is associated with recurrent episodes of gonorrheal arthritis and may be plastic in character and as acute as the initial lesion or it may be serous and only moderately severe. However, any or all of the complications

of severe iridocyclitis may result from either type.

Treatment should be directed toward the general infection as well as the ocular inflammation. Penicillin intramuscularly and sulfonamides orally usually accomplish the first aim. Cycloplegia should be obtained and maintained until the ocular inflammation has been completely controlled. Intravenous foreign protein therapy is especially effective in resolving fibrin clots from the anterior chamber as well as stimulating other recovery mechanisms.

Tuberculous Uveitis

Tuberculous iridocyclitis is granulomatous in nature but may be subacute and diffuse or chronic and nodular; the subacute lesion is characterized by a moderately severe inflammation with the exudation into the aqueous humor of cells which appear as fine gray dots circulating in the aqueous humor and fine gray precipitates on the posterior surface of the cornea. Shortly, however, several of these fuse to form typical mutton fat deposits on the posterior surface of the cornea. Some of these also develop as soft gray evanescent deposits near the pupillary margin of the iris (Gilbert-Koeppe nodules) or on the surface of the iris (Busacca nodules).

The nodular lesions are either miliary tubercles or larger tumor-like pale avascular nodules, conglomerate tubercles, which extend into adjacent structures and at times may undergo caseation necrosis (**Fig. 9-7**). These lesions are accompanied by the other usual signs of chronic anterior uveitis. In the miliary variety, the tuberculous deposits may be absorbed completely; in the conglomerate form the process may lead to caseation followed by perforation at the limbus and destruction of the eyeball.

Tuberculous posterior uveitis occurs most frequently in the circumscribed or disseminated form in young patients. Miliary tubercles, yellowish white spots with soft fading edges 1 to 2 mm. in diameter scattered about the posterior pole of the eye occur in acute miliary tuberculosis and in children with tuberculous meningitis. On microscopic examination these are typical miliary tubercles consisting of giant cells and small round cells in which tubercle bacilli are found. Nodular chorioretinitis juxtapapillaris is tuberculous in origin in almost half of the reported cases. Rarely a conglomerate tubercle appears as a single irregular mass resembling a retinoblastoma in infants or malignant melanoma of the choroid in adults. It may involve the sclera and perforate which usually means that the eye must be enucleated.

Tuberculous lesions of the eye require general treatment for tuberculosis. The use of isoniazid, p-aminobenzoic acid and at times streptomycin have improved the prospect for these infections. In addition to the usual ocular treatment for uveitis, bed rest, proper diet and general hygienic measures are important in these patients.

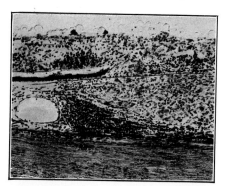

FIG. 9-7. Section of sclera, choroid and retina in tuberculous chorioretinitis, showing nodule of epithelioid cells and lymphocytes with destruction of the choroid and retina.

Sarcoidosis

Anterior uveitis occurs in approximately 45 per cent of patients with Boeck's sarcoid. The lesion is a nodular iridocyclitis. There may be one or more pale slightly vascularized iris nodules accompanied by mutton fat deposits on the posterior surface of the cornea, many floating cells (floaters) in the aqueous humor and a Tyndall's phenomenon. Posterior synechiae develop early or may become extensive. The course is prolonged.

Nodular or circumscribed lesions rarely may occur in the posterior uvea.

Leprosy

Leprotic anterior uveitis usually is insidious in onset and persists as a subclinical infection for months or even years before becoming manifest as chronic serous iridocyclitis, or as nodular uveitis. In the chronic serous iridocyclitis of leprosy there is an occasional fine gray or fine pigment deposit on the posterior surface of the cornea usually the lower portion, an occasional floating cell in the anterior chamber associated with a minimal Tyndall's phenomenon. The iris shows very little change except that posterior synechiae develop slowly and tend to progress slowly unless the inflammation is controlled. However, there is no pathognomonic uveitic sign in this type of inflammation, although there is an absence of photophobia and pain. As in all types of leprotic uveitis these signs are negligible or absent due to anesthesia from early involvement of the sensory nerves of the anterior segment of the eye.

Leprotic nodular iridocyclitis may consist of miliary lepromata or larger nodular lepromatous lesions. Miliary lepromata are small round firm yellowish white round or oval lesions which are seen first as pinpoint spots in the stroma of the pupillary portion of the iris but very slowly increase in size to approximately 1 mm. in diameter. These lesions are called pearls. Some pearls lying close together tend to coalesce to form a small irregular nodule 2 to 3 mm. in diameter. Either single or conglomerate pearls as they increase in size, probably due to movements of the iris, work their way to the surface of the iris and at times break off to float and migrate in the anterior chamber or into the posterior chamber and sometimes even to the internal surface of the retina at the posterior pole of the eye. Miliary lepromata may appear late in the course of a chronic iridocylitis or in the iris which also is involved with large nodular masses. The larger nodular form of iridocyclitis is characterized by the development of masses usually in the ciliary (peripheral) portion of the iris and involving the chamber angle. Other signs of chronic granulomatous uveitis including fine and mutton fat deposits on the posterior surface of the cornea, floaters in the anterior chamber, Tyndall's phenomena, and tendency toward the development of posterior synechiae accompany the various types of iris lesions. The erythema nodosum reaction which simulates the Herxheimer reaction of syphilis frequently is accompanied by an acute serous anterior uveitis.

Lesions of the posterior segment of the eye (choroid, retina, and optic nerve) do not occur due to leprosy, with the exception of the migration of pearls to the internal surface of the retina, probably due to the fact that leprosy bacilli do not seem to localize in these structures.

Treatment. In addition to the general treatment of leprosy with one of the diasone preparations, topical treatment with cycloplegics and steroids are valuable.

Brucellosis

In the acute phase of brucellosis an occasional patient may develop an acute severe uveitis characterized by hypopyon which results in phthisis bulbi. However, more commonly uveitis occurs in the later or chronic stage of the general disease and there may be a simple or nodular iritis, choroiditis or generalized uveitis. These forms of uveitis tend to be recurrent either alone or in association with the periodic exacerbations of febrile, arthritic and neurologic manifestations of the systemic disease. The uveitis occasionally may be accompanied by a nummular keratitis and sometimes may be complicated by cataract formation. Treatment in the acute phase of the disease is most effective with sulfonamides combined with one of the tetracyclines, chloramphenicol or streptomycin. In the chronic phase the use of Foshay vaccine may be more beneficial in addition to palliative, cycloplegic and fever therapy for the uveitis.

Leptospirosis

Uveitis in Weil's disease usually begins some weeks to several months (3 weeks to 5 years, usually 6 months) after the febrile stage of the disease. It may affect only one eye but usually is bilateral. It most frequently occurs as an acute mild iridocyclitis but also typically may produce a severe uveitis with lardacious deposits on the cornea, dense posterior synechiae, and dense opacities of the vitreous humor. Hypopyon may occur at times. In some instances nodular lesions may involve the iris or choroid. Treatment largely is nonspecific and palliative.

Herpes Simplex Uveitis

Herpes simplex virus, presently the most common cause of keratitis in the United States, may cause uveal inflammation in the course of the corneal disease either reflexly from the severity of the keratitis or by extension of the infection into the anterior uvea or by primary infection of the uvea without corneal lesions.

Anterior uveitis always is associated with herpetic keratitis but may be either a mild iridocyclitis or a severe exudative or hemorrhagic type. The mild form consists of a slight ciliary injection, a few fine keratic precipitates, moderate flare and fine cellular floaters in the anterior chamber and subsides with healing of the keratitis. The severe type of anterior uveitis appears with intense circumcorneal injection, numerous keratic precipitates some of which coalesce into mutton fat deposits, heavy flare and numerous floaters in the aqueous humor with a strong tendency to the development of persistent posterior synechiae. Occasionally, hypopyon or hyphema may develop. The lesion produces severe pain. This type of inflammation is persistent, lasting some weeks or months after the corneal lesion has subsided. It may be complicated by secondary glaucoma which serves to accentuate the severe pain.

Primary herpetic iridocyclitis may occur and recur in the absence of other herpetic lesions or in association with herpetic lesions of the skin, the face or elsewhere on the body. The uveitis is acute and severe sometimes showing hyphema as well as many larger keratic precipitates. Pain is severe. Persistent synechiae develop early from the severe iris lesion which frequently results in localized patches of iris atrophy.

Posterior uveitis has not been proved in the adult but may occur in infants in the course of systemic herpetic infection including encephalitis.

There is no specific treatment for herpetic uveitis. The present antiviral agents are ineffective. Therefore, general treatment of uveitis with constant observation for secondary glaucoma so that treatment with one of the carbonic anhydrase inhibitors may be instituted. Steroids are of little value and are contraindicated when the cornea is involved.

Measles

Iritis occurs only secondary to measles keratitis and not as a primary lesion; however metastatic uveitis may occur as a localized patch of choroiditis but usually results in a generalized uveitis, which in young children may be severe and result in the production of a pseudoglioma.

Varicella

Uveitis is rare, occurring in particularly severe cases of chicken pox. Iritis may occur with the fever of the acute infectious stage but more often an iridocyclitis develops in the convalescent period after the eruption has subsided. It usually is mild with fine and fibrinous keratic precipitates and floaters in the anterior chamber. The inflammation may subside or improve but there is a tendency for relapses which are more serious and sometimes repetitive. The exudate becomes more profuse and mutton fat deposits develop on the posterior surface of the cornea. Recovery usually is complete with few sequelae. These may be posterior synechiae or occasionally vitiligo iridis, small round depigmented spots in the iris stroma sometimes referred to as enanthemata of the iris. Very rarely a patch of exudative choroiditis may accompany the anterior uveitis. Complications are rare and include paralytic mydriasis and optic neuritis.

Zoster

A mild transient iritis or anterior uveitis is common in trigeminal nerve zoster but frequently a severe keratic iridocyclitis develops. In some patients the ocular lesion may precede the cutaneous eruption, in others it occurs simultaneously but more commonly it develops later in the course of the disease. Rarely an iridocyclitis may occur without corneal involvement. Hutchinson observed the almost constant relationship between uveitis and involvement of the nasociliary branch of the Vth nerve.

Zoster iridocyclitis is accompanied by severe pain and may be either diffusely exudative or circumscribed eruptive lesions.

The diffuse exudative anterior uveitis may be so mild it is overlooked because of the skin lesions, swelling of the lids and trigeminal nerve pain, but because of its plastic exudative nature may produce extensive posterior synechiae. In other instances it may be severe with profuse exudation into the anterior chamber, keratic precipitates occasionally reaching the proportions of a hypopyon sometimes containing blood. In these patients the uveal inflammation may persist for a long time after the lesions of the cornea and the skin have subsided. Posterior synechiae develop early and extensively. Hypotonia usually accompanies the inflammatory process and persists afterward leading to phthisis bulbi in some cases and may be painful enough to require removal of the globe. Less commonly a very recalcitrant secondary glaucoma may ensue. Ragged patches of stromal atrophy and depigmentation of the iris frequently result and heterochromia occurs occasionally.

Circumscribed eruptive iritis or zoster iridis occurs as localized swollen areas in which the vessels are acutely dilated and often result in repeated and painful hyphema. The iritis is severe and prolonged requiring several months to subside leaving thin atrophic small white scars. Where the ciliary body also is involved there is a more profuse exudation and a haze in the vitreous humor. In rare instances, there is localized focal choroiditis consisting of round cell infiltrations and occasionally small hemorrhages. Even more rarely an exudative retinal detachment may result from a more diffuse choroiditis. These lesions usually resolve.

Ocular complications of zoster include paralytic mydriasis alone or in conjunction with a partial paralysis of the IIIrd nerve or as part of a total ophthalmoplegia. An Argyll-Robertson pupil may be due to a lesion of the ciliary ganglion. These pareses may persist for many months. Glaucoma may occur as an acute hypertensive episode at the onset of the disease at times or secondary to the uveitis at others.

A sympathetic-like involvement of the other eye occurs rarely.

Variola

Primary iritis frequently accompanied by choroiditis was a relatively common complication of smallpox before vaccination was widespread. It developed between the eighth and twelfth days of the disease. It was seroplastic and characterized by localized foci of hemorrhages and necrosis of the iris. The inflammation was moderately severe but was followed by patches of stromal atrophy and pigment dispersion especially in the ciliary portion of the iris (vitiligo iridis).

Vaccinia

Uveal involvement is exceedingly rare except that associated with vaccinial keratitis which frequently is of a disciform type.

Mumps

A rapidly developing unilateral exudative iridocyclitis may occur at the height of mumps or as late as 20 days after the disease has subsided. There is a Tyndall's phenomenon with fine floaters and keratic precipitates, fine posterior synechiae which are easily broken and occasionally there is an increased ocular tension and sometimes endothelial and stromal edema of the cornea. The inflammation may last a few days or as long as a month but usually subsides without serious sequelae. A focal choroiditis occurs rarely.

Cytomegalic Inclusion Disease

In infants, cytomegalic inclusion disease may produce a focal type of peripheral chorioretinitis with patchy perivasculitis which heals leaving slate gray scars and some patches of pigmentation. Occasionally, small lesions may develop in the posterior portion of the choroid. Optic atrophy frequently is associated. The disease also may affect adults since characteristic inclusion bodies have been found in a few enucleated eyes from middle-aged women with chorioretinitis.

Mycotic Uveitis

Although mycotic infection of the uvea has been rare, there has been an increasing incidence in recent years. These infections may occur from a mycotic infection of the external parts of the eye, from intraocular extension of infections from adnexal tissues and from metastatic localizations in the course of systemic disease.

Exogenous fungus infections may arise from penetration of the eye by the fungus responsible for an infectious corneal ulcer, introduction of fungi into the eye with a penetrating injury or introduction of fungi into the eye at or following intraocular surgical procedures. After a latent period varying from 2 weeks to several months a slowly developing infection results in a heavy flare in the anterior chamber with numerous floaters in the aqueous humor followed by haze and floaters in the anterior vitreous humor. There is considerable congestion, visual loss and pain. The vitreous humor progressively becomes filled with exudate until the eye is removed.

The organisms causing this type of infection include the usually pathogenic fungi but in addition many fungi considered nonpathogenic for other areas can establish severe infections when introduced into the eye; these include Cephalosporium, Fusarium, Volutella, Scopulariopsis and many others.

Intraocular fungus infections may extend from the nasopharynx, sinuses and orbit, or rarely from mycotic meningitis or cavernous sinus thrombosis in debilitated or diabetic patients. These usually are terminal events and usually are due to mucor.

Endogenous infection occurs rarely in relatively benign localized fungal infections due to such organisms as Aspergillus, Blastomyces, Candida, Coccidioides, Cryptococcus and Histoplasma. It also occurs rarely as one of the terminal events in severe systemic fungal infections such as blastomycosis or torulosis. The ocular signs vary widely from chronic uveitis, abscess formation associated with disseminated uveal granulomatosis composed of epithelioid and giant cells, to a generalized purulent ophthalmia, all of which are quite painful.

Histoplasmosis

Histoplasmosis, a fungus disease which is endemic in the Mississippi Valley in the United States, also has been found in Canada, Central and South America, India, the Far East and Australia. While not proved it is presumed to be associated with a uveitis which characteristically consists of multiple small white irregular nodules in the peripheral and equatorial choroid which heal leaving discrete depigmented thin choroidal scars and are followed in several months or years later by a central cystic lesion, approximately 1 disk diameter in size in or near the macula, surrounded by a narrow areola of edema and some hemorrhage in approximately half of the patients. The lesion remains active for several months during which the small marginal hemorrhages may recur repeatedly. Central visual acuity is greatly reduced. Healing usually results in a fine chorioretinal scar with little pigment but occasionally results in a thickened and elevated mound of scar resembling a disciform degeneration of the macula (p. 175). Occasionally there may be a mild circumpapillary chorioretinitis. The diagnosis is presumptive for even though the histoplasmin skin test is positive in 67 per cent of the patients with the typical uveitis, 30 per cent of the general population in the endemic area of the United States also show a positive reaction.

Vogt - Koyangi - Harada Syndrome— Uveomeningitic Syndrome

A syndrome consisting of bilateral exudative iridocyclitis associated with alopecia, loss of hair; vitiligo, patchy depigmentation of the skin; poliosis, premature whitening of the hair and eyelashes; and dysacusis was described by Vogt and elaborated by Koyangi early in this century, about the same time Harada described a similar syndrome consisting of bilateral exudative uveitis primarily affecting the posterior uvea resulting in inflammatory detachment of the retina and associated with pleocytosis of the spinal fluid. However, as more examples of the two syndromes have been observed, the distinction between them has decreased as they manifest overlapping or identical involvements and probably should be classified as the uveomeningitic syndrome with a predilection for anterior uveal involvement in some and posterior uveal involvement in others.

The disease occurs in young adults usually in the third decade but may occur between the ages of 10 and 50 years. It has been reported in orientals more often than in other races. It begins as a bilateral chronic exudative anterior and posterior uveitis associated with an edematous retinitis, some retinal hemorrhages and numerous opacities of the vitreous humor. Posterior synechiae develop early and produce seclusion of the pupil and an exudative total detachment of the retina. Visual function is decreased sometimes to loss of light perception. The ocular tension usually is low. When the process subsides, the retina appears yellowish in color with some pigment deposits. The iris may be almost completely depigmentated. The pupil may be secluded or occluded and secondary glaucoma may occur. Cataracts may develop and in some instances, phthisis bulbi may occur. However, the majority of patients recover surprisingly good vision, 30 per cent obtaining normal acuity.

Patchy baldness affects the hair, the lashes and the eyebrows in almost all cases and poliosis occurs in approximately 90 per cent. They begin 3 weeks to 3 months after the ocular signs but may disappear in many patients in 5 to 8 months. Vitiligo and dysacusia begin almost simultaneously with the eye lesion. The hearing impairment may last 4 to 6 weeks. Headache, vertigo, loss of appetite, nausea, vomiting and pleocytosis of the cerebrospinal fluid are almost constant in the predominantly posterior uveal (Harada) type during the first 2 to 3 weeks of the disease, but are infrequent and less severe in the anterior uveal (Vogt-Koyangi) type of involvement.

The cause of the disease is not known. Some indications suggest a virus but bacteria definitely have been excluded. Allergy and immune reactions may be contributing factors.

Pathologically, the lesion is a typical chronic infectious granuloma consisting of inflammatory nodules composed of a core of epithelioid cells surrounded by plasma cells and lymphocytes. There is widespread destruction of pigmented cells of the uvea and retina with phagocytosis of the granules. The retina shows edema, mononuclear cell infiltration and some necrosis.

No specific treatment is known. Steroids appear to be beneficial in the majority, although some are unaffected and others undergo remissions on reduction of dosage.

UVEITIS IN THE RHEUMATOID GROUP OF DISEASES

Uveitis is rare in acute rheumatoid disease, but acute or recurrent anterior uveitis occurs quite typically in chronic arthritic diseases.

Still's disease, a chronic periarticular polyarthritis associated at times with lymphadenopathy and splenomegaly has insidious onset usually in young girls and typically affects the knee, wrist and cervical spine. Band-shaped keratopathy, iridocyclitis and secondary cataract may precede the joint involvement by several months or years but more commonly they follow the arthritic lesions. The iridocyclitis which affects approximately 20 per cent of these patients usually is bilateral with insidious onset and little or no ciliary injection. However, a mild exudation of cells into the aqueous and vitreous humor results in fine keratic precipitates and a faint haze of the vitreous humor which produces a visual disturbance. In older children the onset may be more acute with distinct ciliary injection, photophobia and pain. Posterior synechiae develop progressively in either the acute or chronic form and complicated cataract develops in approximately half of the patients. Occlusion of the pupil, iris bombé and glaucoma or phthisis bulbi may ensue. However, band keratopathy develops in approximately half of the involved eyes and is quite suggestive of Still's disease although it may occur in any prolonged iridocyclitis in children.

Marie-Strümpell Syndrome

Ankylosing spondylitis or poker spine occurs most frequently in young adult males (80 per cent) and usually first affects the lower spine and sacroiliac joints and eventually results in ankylosis of part or all of the spine. Uveitis occurs in approximately half of the patients and most commonly is an acute exudative anterior uveitis with ciliary injection, photophobia and some pain. There are fine keratic precipitates, fine floaters and occasionally fibrinous exudate in the aqueous humor. Posterior synechiae form but are fine and

easily broken by dilating the usually constricted pupil. Occasionally the onset may be more severe and plastic in character resulting in more and larger synechiae and sometimes in cataracts. Generally the uveitis is mild and subsides in several weeks but recurrences are likely to develop over a period of many years.

Chronic Progressive Polyarthritis

In rheumatoid arthritis or chronic progressive polyarthritis of adults, which usually affects women in the fourth or fifth decade of life, uveitis is extremely rare or perhaps coincidental; however, episcleritis, scleritis sclerokeratitis, and scleromalacia perforans with secondary uveitis are more common.

Rheumatic Fever

Uveal involvement is rare in rheumatic fever. An acute iritis, probably coincidental, has been reported occasionally but in severely affected patients small yellow foci of acute choroiditis which do not affect the overlying pigment epithelium or retina have been observed in the periphery of the fundus.

Reiter's Syndrome

Reiter's disease which usually occurs in young men between 19 and 38 years consists of urethritis, polyarthritis, uveitis and mucosal inflammations such as conjunctivitis, stomatitis, balanitis, and frequently carditis. The primary attack usually lasts a few months undergoing some fluctuations in intensity then may disappear or usually a number of recurrences develop after a variable period of remissions but eventually subsides and fails to recur. Rarely repeated recurrences may end in death from cardiac or meningeal complications. The uveal involvement is an acute anterior uveitis which occurs independently of the conjunctivitis. It usually is serous but rarely may be plastic and accompanied by hypopyon or hyphema.

However, it often is recurrent and then synechiae, cataract and secondary glaucoma may occur. No specific treatment is known but cycloplegics and steroids are palliative.

UVEITIS IN OTHER CLINICAL ENTITIES

Psoriatic Arthritis

Psoriatic arthritis which affects the terminal phalangeal joints and is associated with psoriasis and psoriatic changes of the nails frequently also is associated with a mild exudative iridocyclitis and occasionally with conjunctivitis. Cycloplegics and antimetabolites such as methotrexate have been used in treatment.

Behçet's Disease

Recurrent iridocyclitis with hypopyon in association with aphthous sores of the mouth and genitals are the triad of principal symptoms of Behçet's syndrome, a generalized disease, which also involves the skin, joints, blood vessels and nervous system. The disease is chronic with recurrent exacerbations developing up to 4 or 5 times a year over a period of 25 years or more. It affects men more frequently than women and begins most commonly in the third decade. It is rare in children and after 50 years of age. The facial and genital lesions usually precede ocular involvement by several years although occasionally the triad appears simultaneously. In some patients, periodic attacks of fever and malaise may precede the typical manifestations by a year, and in some, recurrent sore throat and joint pains develop some months or years before the typical triad. The cause, although not proved, may be a virus or a combination of virus and autoimmune reactions.

Ocular involvement may begin as a mild iritis or even as an inflammation of the posterior uvea, retina or optic nerve, but the patient usually is seen only after the development of acute anterior uveitis, frequently with hypopyon. At that time there also frequently is macular edema, retinal perivasculitis, thrombosis of some of the vessels and retinal hemorrhages, some of which may extend into the vitreous humor. However, frequently these retinal lesions are obscured by the severity of the anterior uveal reaction and the haze of the vitreous humor. Optic neuritis and subsequent optic atrophy occurs in 15 per cent of patients. One eye usually is involved in the beginning but the other eye becomes affected within a few months as the uveitis undergoes remissions and exacerbations. Conjunctivitis and superficial punctate keratitis, recurrent ulcerations or circumscribed stromal opacities may occur rarely. Severe pain frequently occurs in the acute attacks and may be due to secondary glaucoma. Blindness in one or both eyes usually occurs, but visual loss may progress slowly over a period of years.

The aphthous stomatitis of Behçet's disease consists of 1 to 10 superficial ulcers varying from 2 to 12 mm. in diameter with yellowish necrotic bases surrounded by red areolas. They occur frequently on the lips, gums, cheeks, tongue, palate and pharynx lasting from a few days to a few weeks. They are painful especially during eating.

The genital ulcers (2 to 12) occur usually on the scrotum and less frequently on the shaft or glans penis in males, whereas the labia are more frequently affected than the vaginal wall and cervix in females. They start as vesicles or papules and later ulcerate to form ulcers several millimeters in diameter covered by gray necrotic sloughs which heal by scar formation.

The cutaneous lesions may occur as erythema nodosum, papular rash, pustules, furunculosis, pyoderma, impetigo, cellulitis, or erythema multiforme. The skin, even between exacerbations, is excessively irritable, reacting to a simple puncture by a sterile needle by the production of a papule or pustule.

The central nervous system may become involved within 3 months of onset of the disease or as late as 15 years but usually between the second and fifth years. It varies from a mild cephalgia to severe meningoencephalitis, and may include paralysis of the cervical nerves, hemiparesis, midbrain lesions and involvement of the extrapyramidal tract.

Other systemic involvement includes: arthropathy which is quite common and frequently may be the first sign of the disease; thrombophlebitis which occurs in 12 per cent of patients; epididymitis and orchitis; gastrointestinal lesions; cardiovascular lesions; and bronchopneumonia.

No effective treatment has been developed. Favorable results have been reported from the use of gamma globulin, but this has not been confirmed by all who have tried it. Fever therapy, steroid therapy, anticoagulant therapy, a wide variety of antibiotic therapy, and irradiation therapy have failed to be beneficial.

Serum Sickness

Uveal reactions occur frequently in the course of serum sickness. The majority of patients have a mild bilateral iridocyclitis with a flare and fine floaters in the aqueous humor and fine keratic precipitates. However, a transitory intense bilateral plastic iridocyclitis with much fibrin in the aqueous humor has been reported following autoserum therapy for pneumonia, diphtheria and tetanus. The uveitis usually subsided completely within a week.

Angioneurotic Edema

Repeated episodes or iridocyclitis with hemorrhages in the iris, opacities in the vitreous humor, increased intraocular pressure and corneal edema may occur in patients with angioneurotic edema. A serous choroiditis also may accompany the general attacks. Histamine therapy may be helpful.

Atopic Uveitis

An acute transient fibrinous iridocyclitis similar to that seen in serum sickness but less severe may result from inhaled antigens in patients with severe pollen type hay fever as well as in patients sensitive to animal dandruff, feathers, house dust and orris root. Other allergens which rarely may cause uveitis include foods such as eggs, chicken, beef protein and drugs and chemicals, especially those in cosmetics. The offending agent may be difficult to determine but its elimination gives relief. Desensitization also may be effective therapy in some cases. During the acute episodes cycloplegics and steroids give relief.

Lens-Induced Uveitis

Phacotoxic uveitis occurs following the liberation of lens proteins and their degradation products following a rupture of the lens capsule from trauma or surgery or by the leaking of these products through the lens capsule of a hypermature cataract. An inflammatory uveitis varying from a mild iridocyclitis to a violent endophthalmitis develops in 1 to 14 days following injury or onset of leakage. The reaction consists mainly of mononuclear cells of the lymphocytic and plasma cell type with large mononuclear phagocytes and considerable fibrin resulting in flare and cells in the anterior chamber, fine to large "mashed potato" like precipitates on the posterior surface of the cornea and diffuse or nodular infiltration of the anterior uvea. The inflammation is prolonged unless relieved by removal of the lens or lens remnants.

Endophthalmitis phacoanaphylactica is

a violent uveitis occurring in an individual sensitive to lens proteins following an extracapsular cataract extraction, a discission operation, a traumatic or spontaneous rupture of the lens capsule. The uveitis begins 1 to 14 days after the injury to the lens capsule with severe exudation of cells into the anterior chamber resulting in a heavy flare, many floaters and many fine and large mutton fat keratic precipitates. The cornea may become cloudy along with chemosis of the conjunctiva and edema of the lids. Posterior synechiae develop early and extensively. A cyclitic membrane frequently develops and may occlude the pupil resulting in secondary glaucoma, vascularization of the cornea, and atrophy of the globe may result from the chronic continuous or relapsing course of the disease. Such a course can be prevented by removal of the lens material if the nature of the uveitis is recognized early.

Lens-Induced Uveitis in Second Eye

Lens-induced uveitis may occur in the unoperated second eye provided it also has a cataractous lens. It may be severe and closely resemble sympathetic ophthalmia or it may develop a hypopyon with severe painful glaucoma. Again early recognition of the cause and removal of the cataract is the only method of saving the eye.

Phacolytic Glaucoma

Phacolytic glaucoma results from posterior rupture or leakage of the lens capsule in patients with hypermature cataract. Mononuclear phagocytes overfilled with lens material accumulate in the anterior chamber angle obstructing outflow of aqueous humor producing a subacute or acute glaucoma. Inflammatory reaction is minimal. As in the lens induced uveitides the only effective treatment is early recognition of the situation and removal of the cataract or lens remnants.

SYMPATHETIC UVEITIS

Sympathetic uveitis (sympathetic ophthalmia, sympathetic ophthalmitis) is a plastic type of chronic granulomatous inflammation of the uveal tract in one eye caused by the effects of a similar inflammation in the other. It has an insidious onset almost always following injury of one eye. It runs a progressive course with episodes of exacerbation and unless treated properly may end in blindness of both eyes.

Etiology and Occurrence. Sympathetic inflammation almost always arises out of a traumatic iridocyclitis in the first eye which has been prolonged usually by poor healing of an accidental or operative wound involving the limbus or ciliary body region. Usually there is an incarceration or prolapse of iris, ciliary body or lens capsule in the wound or there may be a retained foreign body in the eyeball. These factors are found in approximately 90 per cent of reported cases. The remaining 10 per cent arise out of the iridocyclitis associated with contusion injury, contusion with subconjunctival rupture of the sclera and poor wound healing, perforation of a corneal ulcer, and very rarely intraocular malignant melanoma and suppurative inflammations of the eyeball.

The prevalent theory is that the disease probably arises as a hypersensitive autoimmune reaction to uveal pigment resulting from absorption and general dissemination of pigment especially in the homologous eye. With continued absorption there is an increase in the allergic intoxication of the second eye which eventually results in sympathetic inflammation. (This shows a very close relationship to lens induced uveitis and these two diseases may occur in the same eye.) However, there probably are additional factors besides pigment involved in the immunizing process; one such could be a simultaneous virus infection.

Formerly more common, sympathetic uveitis now is rare and decreasing in frequency because of greater care and skill in the closure of wounds, either accidental or surgical and perhaps also because of less hesitation in removing an injured eye when its condition or behavior indicates a risk to its fellow. Nevertheless the established disease is most serious because of its tendency to cause blindness. Although sympathetic uveitis occurs at any age it has its highest incidence (20 per cent) in the first decade of life. It affects males twice as often as females and occurs most frequently in winter.

Sympathetic uveitis may begin as early as 5 days or late as 42 years after an injury; however, the usual onset is not until after the ninth day. Approximately 65 per cent develop within 2 months following the injury, 80 per cent within 3 months and 90 per cent within 1 year. The most frequent period appears to be between the fourth and eighth weeks after injury.

The eye originally affected is known as the exciting eye; the one secondarily involved, as the sympathizing eye.

A number of theories have been propounded to explain the occurrence of inflammation in the sympathizing eye; none has been accepted generally as satisfactory. The following have been advanced: (1) *infection* spreading through the sheath of the optic nerve of one side to the chiasm

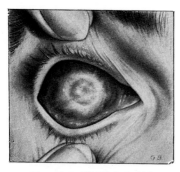

FIG. 9-8. Phthisis bulbi.

and sheath of the optic nerve of the other eye; (2) the action of a *toxin* generated by bacteria which have entered the exciting eye; (3) a focal *allergic* reaction to uveal pigment which is set free in the bloodstream by the injured eye; (4) *metastasis* through the blood of some form of *specific organism* (virus) which is supposed to be pathogenic for the eye only; since such micro-organisms have not been isolated, either they are supposed to be too small to be seen with the microscope, or else the agent is a toxin generated by the specific micro-organisms.

Symptoms. Sympathetic uveitis usually arises out of a persistent angry irritation following an injury but occasionally may begin as the traumatic inflammation seems to be subsiding. The clinical manifestations may begin *acutely* or *insidiously.* When once established the inflammation is *chronic,* and its duration is months or even 1 or 2 years. In many cases *blindness* results, though sometimes, if the inflammation is mild, useful vision may be preserved. The disease is an *iridocyclitis,* most often *plastic,* having the same symptoms and course as when this affection results from other causes. Very rarely sympathetic disease occurs in the form of a neuroretinitis or as a choroiditis.

The symptoms are *photophobia, lacrimation, dimness of vision* and *tenderness* in the ciliary region. There will be circumcorneal *injection,* punctate *deposits* upon the posterior surface of the cornea (keratic precipitates), *increased depth* of the anterior chamber, *contracted pupil* and, at first, increased tension.

In mild cases (*serous type*) the symptoms may not pass beyond those of serous iridocyclitis, but usually they develop into *plastic uveitis* with the following signs: The *iris* is thickened, discolored, its markings obliterated, and it may present new blood vessels upon its surface; it is bound down by extensive posterior *synechiae.*

The *exudation* fills the pupil and more or less of the anterior chamber, which becomes shallow. Later, *tension* is diminished, the choroid and retina participate in the inflammation, the *vitreous* presents many *opacities* and the *lens* becomes opaque. Finally, there is *detachment* of the retina, and the eyeball shrinks and passes into the condition of phthisis bulbi (Fig. 9-8).

Pathology. The changes in the exciting and in the sympathizing eye are identical and begin with a focal infiltration of lymphocytes in and around the large veins of the uveal tract. This expands to a diffuse lymphocytic infiltration of the outer layers of the ciliary body and choroid and the posterior layers of the iris. This is followed by the appearance of large numbers of epithelioid cells some of which tend to coalesce to form giant cells. Nodules develop with the epithelioid cells and giant cells forming a core surrounded by lymphocytes and some eosinophiles which increase diffusely throughout the uveal tract. The posterior layers of the iris are affected most severely resulting in a fibrinous exudate on the lens capsule followed by posterior synechiae and an inflammatory pupillary membrane. The ciliary body is infiltrated early with a resulting decrease in accommodation thus producing blurring of vision. The choroid becomes greatly infiltrated increasing the thickness of the choroid several times, however the choriocapillary layer remains relatively uninvolved. The pigment epithelial layer of the choroid especially peripherally shows isolated small mound-like lesions composed principally of epithelioid cells and some pigment epithelial cells. These are Dalen-Fuch's nodules.

Another characteristic cytologic feature is phagocytosis of pigment by the epithelioid and giant cells as the stroma becomes depigmented and disintegrates. However,

there is little or no caseation or necrosis. The retina and sclera show a lymphoid perivascular infiltration. The optic nerves including the chiasma and the meninges of the optic nerves show perivascular lymphocytic infiltration and at times granulomatous nodules.

Treatment. *Prophylactic treatment* of an injured eye, when there is the possibility of sympathetic inflammation, is of the greatest importance. *The injured eye should be enucleated* if sightless, or if its condition is such (especially when the ciliary region is involved) that useful vision cannot be preserved. This is particularly imperative if it continues to be irritable, has ciliary tenderness and presents persistent signs of iridocyclitis after 2 or 3 weeks, or contains a foreign body which cannot be extracted.

When, however, there is useful vision in the injured eye, or a good chance of obtaining fair sight, the question of enucleation often is a difficult one to decide, since symptoms of irritation may appear and subside and yet sympathetic inflammation may never develop. In such cases, if the injured eye remains quiet and free from inflammation, and the patient is kept under constant observation, enucleation may be postponed until definite indications arise.

Although early enucleation of the injured eye usually will prevent the sympathetic process, removal of the exciting eye will not cure the involvement of the sympathizing eye after sympathetic inflammation has made its appearance; the exciting eye may ultimately possess better vision than its sympathizing fellow. Hence, if sympathetic inflammation is definitely established, the exciting eye should not be removed if it possesses vision; if blind and exhibiting signs of inflammation, it should be enucleated, even with the knowledge that this step will not cure the sympathetic ophthalmia, since its presence may aggravate the condition in the sympathizing eye.

Treatment of sympathetic ophthalmia itself consists in the use of *atropine, hot compresses* and intensive systemic administration of *corticosteroids*. Large doses of *sodium salicylate* often are beneficial.

HETEROCHROMIC CYCLITIS OF FUCHS

Heterochromic cyclitis is an insidious anterior uveitis with little or no external evidence of inflammation and little or no photophobia or discomfort. The cause is not known but there is considerable speculation concerning the role of degenerative, abiotrophic, trophic and genetic factors. It may affect one or both eyes. The structural features of the iris stroma lose their distinctness and character; the surface becomes smoother and more translucent. The pigment epithelium also becomes atrophic especially at the pupillary border and transillumination shows spotty and ragged areas of passage of light. Small, discrete, grayish, round and occasionally fibrin-like precipitates appear on the posterior surface of the cornea. They appear and disappear irregularly. The aqueous humor may be clear or at times show a slight hazy flare with an occasional tiny floating opacity. Frequently cataracts occur, beginning as fine dust-like opacities in the posterior cortex which progress to total opacity. Glaucoma, however, is a more frequent complication and occurs in 15 to 25 per cent of patients. No medical therapy has been found effective against the uveitis. However, the cataracts may be removed where necessary, apparently without the problems usually associated with surgery in other types of uveitis. The associated glaucoma responds to the usual medical therapy and may disappear after cataract extraction.

10

The Retina

Anatomy

The retina is a thin, delicate, transparent membrane which consists, among other parts, of an *expansion of the optic nerve*. It is placed between the hyaloid membrane of the vitreous internally, and the choroid externally. It extends forward to the ciliary body, where, at its termination, the *ora serrata*, it becomes continuous with the epithelium over the inner surface of the ciliary body. The retina is derived from the inner and outer layers of the embryonic optic cup. The outer layer forms the pigment epithelium and is closely attached to the lamina vitrea of the choroid. The inner layer forms the main bulk of the retina and is attached only at the ora serrata and at the optic nervehead. When the retina is detached, the pigment cells, its outermost layer, adhere to the choroid.

The *inner surface* of the retina presents in the axis of the eyeball the yellow spot or *macula lutea*, about 1 to 2 mm. in diameter, and in its center a small depression, the *fovea centralis;* this is the region of most distinct vision. About 3 mm. to the nasal side of the posterior pole of the eye is a pale, round area, the *head of the optic nerve (papilla* or *disk),* corresponding to the point where the optic nerve pierces the sclera (Fig. 2-11). The circumference of the disk is slightly elevated above the surface of the retina, but the center presents a depression, the *physiologic cup* or *excavation;* here the blood vessels of the retina enter the eye. Ophthalmoscopic appearances of the eye grounds and the dis-

tribution of the retinal vessels are given in Chapter 2.

The *central artery* of the retina, accompanied by the corresponding vein, pierces the optic nerve about 12 mm. from the globe, and passes between the bundles of fibers to the inner surface of the retina at or near the middle of the disk. Excepting at the papilla, where communications are sometimes found between retinal and ciliary vessels (cilioretinal artery), the retinal arteries have no anastomoses; they are *terminal* branches; hence in complete obstruction of the central artery, when there is no collateral circulation, blindness results. The retinal vessels lie in the inner layers; the external layers are destitute of blood vessels and are nourished by the adjacent choriocapillaris. The fovea has no blood vessels; in this situation, the choriocapillaris is thickened. The blood vessels are surrounded by sheaths forming the *lymphatics* of the retina.

The *minute anatomy* of the retina is complicated; there are two kinds of tissue: (1) *nervous elements* and (2) *supporting tissue* (Müller's fibers, the internal and external limiting membranes and numerous fibers of glial cells).

Microscopic examination shows the following layers of the retina, from within outward (Fig. 10-1): (1) The *internal limiting* membrane; (2) the layer of *nerve fibers,* consisting of the ganglion cell axons which extend into and form the optic nerve, and containing the main branches of the retinal vessels; (3) the layer of *ganglion cells,* a stratum of large, branching nerve cells; (4) the *inner plexi-*

form layer; (5) the *inner nuclear* layer, made up largely of the bodies and nuclei of the bipolar cells; (6) the *outer plexiform* layer; (7) the *outer nuclear* layer, consisting mainly of the nuclei of the visual cells; (8) the *external limiting* membrane; (9) the layer of *rods and cones,* the light-perceiving layer; (10) the layer of *pigment cells* which bounds the retina externally and consists of a single stratum of hexagonal pigmented cells. The plexiform layers include the synapses between the bipolar cells and the ganglion and visual cells.

The rods are much more numerous than the *cones,* except at the macula, where cones predominate. *At the fovea* there are no rods, and the cones, longer and narrower than elsewhere, are found exclusively. In this spot all other layers of the retina are much *thinner,* there is no nerve fiber layer, and Müller's fibers are arranged obliquely. The *disk* consists mainly of optic nerve fibers and has no power of sight, hence is called the blind spot.

Physiology

The action of light changes the rhodopsin or visual purple contained in the outer segments of the rods in a series of reactions to prelumirhodopsin to lumirhodopsin, to metarhodopsin to retinene to vitamin A and to vitamin A ester. In the dark the process of regeneration of rhodopsin begins with vitamin A ester which is changed to vitamin A then to retinene and to rhodopsin. The pigment epithelial cells function as storage centers for vitamin A and also enter into the esterification of vitamin A.

The *rods and cones,* the terminal visual organs, receive waves of light falling upon the retina and convert these vibrations into nerve impulses which pass through the bipolar cells and are carried by the optic nerves (the fibers of which represent

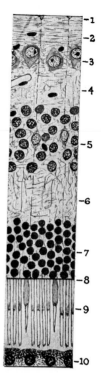

FIG. 10-1. Vertical section of the retina. The *numbers* are explained in the text.

the axis cylinders of the ganglion cells) and the optic tracts to the brain; here they produce the *sensation of light.*

The nerve impulses are propagated by a bioelectric current which can be recorded with the proper equipment, either directly from the receptor cells (rods and cones) in experimental situations, or by electrodes placed on the cornea, clinically. The potentials recorded in this manner are referred to as an electroretinogram (ERG). The clinical electroretinogram is a mass response composed of several waves (Fig. 10-2), some of which come from rods and some from cones. Some differentiation of the source of these several waves in man has been obtained by comparing the response of light adapted and dark adapted eyes (Fig. 10-2). Alterations in the clinical

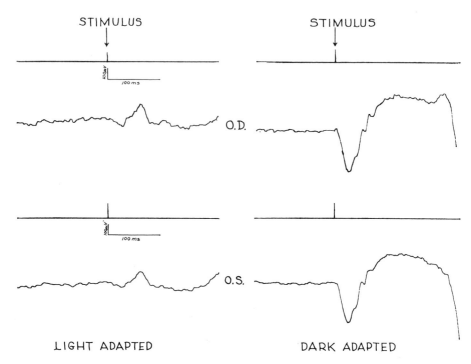

Fig. 10-2. Electroretinograms of the right and left eyes of a normal subject. The light adapted response is shown on the left side and the dark adapted response on the right.

ERG are of limited but definite significance in some patients in whom retinal disease has not developed typical anatomic alterations such as early macular degeneration; early or atypical primary pigmentary degeneration of the retina, early choroideremia, some unusual types of retinal disease such as Oguchi's disease and in some instances the electrical manifestations of retinal integrity can be tested even when the ocular media (lens and vitreous) are cloudy or opaque. Refinements of techniques are slowly extending the usefulness of this method of examination.

Cones are concerned with visual acuity and color discrimination at high intensities of illumination (light adapted or photoptic vision); rods are responsible for vision at low degrees of illumination (dark adapted or scotoptic vision) when sight

is more effective in the periphery of the retina and is colorless. When the image of an object falls upon the macula, there is distinct vision; when it falls upon any other part of the retina, there is indistinct vision. Two points give rise to *separate visual impressions* when their images are at least 0.002 mm. apart, since this represents the diameter of the cones at the fovea. In other words, to be seen distinctly, two objects must subtend a visual angle of 1 minute or more.

Images of an object seen with both eyes give rise to a *single* visual impression when they fall upon *corresponding retinal areas*; otherwise there are double images. In binocular vision certain portions of the retina are *associated*; thus the upper halves of the retinae correspond, as do also the lower halves; but the nasal side of one retina corresponds to the temporal half of the other, and *vice versa*.

Rays of light impinging upon one side of the retina come from the *opposite side of the field*; thus the upper part of the retina is used for seeing objects in the lower part of the field, the temporal portion of the retina for the nasal part of the field, etc. The *image* on the retina always is *inverted*.

Color Vision

Objects have color depending upon the wave lengths of light they reflect and the wave lengths they absorb. The visible portion of light rays is composed of that portion of the spectrum which has wave lengths of 400 to 750 mμ. Where practically all of this portion of the spectrum is reflected from a surface it appears white, when all is absorbed the surface appears black. Objects which reflect light from the 400 end of the spectrum appear blue if they absorb all other wave lengths. Similarly those which reflect light from the 750 end appear red. Those which reflect light of intermediate wave lengths appear to be the color characteristic of the wave length or combination of wave lengths reflected.

Complementary wave lengths are those colors of light which when mixed in the proper proportions produce a white light for example red and blue-green, blue and yellow and orange and blue of the proper wave lengths and mixed in the proper proportions are complementary pairs and produce white light.

The perception of color apparently is dependent upon the presence of three visual pigments (photopsins) in the cones of the retina. Each of the pigments is characterized by a specific sensitivity response with a peak absorption of light rays in a relatively narrow band of the spectrum (Fig. 10-3) thus a surface which reflects light of 540 mμ and absorbs all other wave lengths will stimulate the pigment in the cones which has its maximum sensitivity in this range and the object will appear green. Recent studies tend to show that there are three kinds of cones each with its own pigment and therefore specific spectral absorption curve. These visual pigments each apparently have a degeneration and regeneration cycle similar to the rhodopsin cycle certain phases of which may have excitatory and others have inhibitory effects on the associated ganglion cells. Thus a ganglion cell might receive excitatory stimuli from a group of red sensitive cones and simultaneously be inhibited by a group of green sensitive cones. This suggests that the ganglion cells and intermediate neurons serve a coding function as well as collecting and transmission functions.

Defective Color Vision. Defective color vision then may be explained by the absence of one or more of the cone pigments or by the abnormal presence of a mixture of two of the color sensitive pigments in one cone. Color blindness may be congenital or acquired. The congenital type occurs in 7 to 8 per cent of males and 0.3 to 0.4 per cent of females. It nearly always affects both eyes and usually is hereditary being transmitted as a sex-linked defect. Most often it is a partial achromatopsia a loss of perception of one or two of the fundamental colors; however, rarely there is a loss of appreciation of all colors or total achromatopsia.

Partial achromatopsia may be divided into two main types: (1) dichromasy and (2) anomalous trichromasy. Dichromats perceive all colors as mixtures of two primaries since they lack one of the three receptor pigments. The individual who has lost the red receptor pigment is red-blind. Such a person is called a protanope. A blue-blind is a tritanope and a green-blind individual is a deuteranope. The red-blind and the blue-blind individuals have an absence or great reduction in the specific

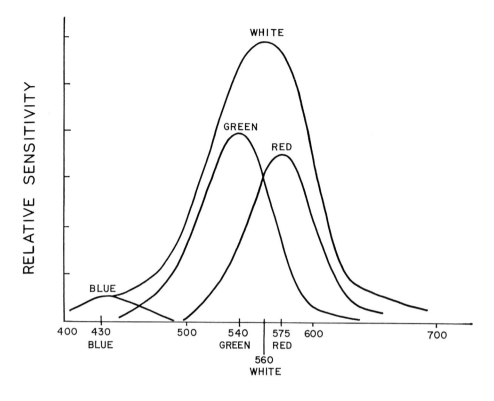

WAVE LENGTH

Fig. 10-3. Relative sensitivity of the human retina to white light and to the blue, green and red portions of the spectrum.

receptor pigment. The green-blind individual may be of this same type or he may have cones in which the red and green receptor pigments are mixed thus producing similar stimuli from either color to both red and green receivers in the brain thus causing confusion and both colors appear yellow. Recent evidence casts doubt on the existence of this mechanism. Anomalous trichomats are individuals with similar but less severe defects than the dichromats. Thus these individuals may have weak perception of red (protanomalous, protans) of green (deuteranomalous) or of blue (tritanomalous). These individuals employ a mixture of the three primaries in anomalous proportions. The more common are the red-weak and the green-weak.

Total achromatopsia or monochromatism prevents all discrimination of color. There are two types, rod monochromatism or cone monochromatism. The rod monochromats have little or no cone function and therefore have greatly decreased visual acuity. The cone monochromat may have either a single color receptor pigment or a mixture of receptor pigments in each cone resulting in a confusion stimulus from all cones.

Acquired Defects in Color Vision. Deficiency in color vision often is found as a symptom of ocular disease. It usually is of the yellow-blue type. It may be due to retinal lesions with changes in the color receptor pigments or due to optic nerve lesions resulting in interference with transmission of color signals. Toxic amblyopia may have a red-green or blue-yellow defect as an initial sign of the disease. Other amblyopias as well as retinal lesions such as macular edema, macular cysts, macular degeneration may produce similar deficiencies in color perception. These usually are mild and may be reversible. Patients with optic nerve lesions such as neuritis may show reversible changes in transmission of color stimuli or permanent defects with optic atrophy.

Affections of the Retina may be divided into (a) *congenital anomalies,* (b) *injury,* (c) *inflammation,* (d) *circulatory disturbances,* (e) *degenerations,* (f) *detachment of the retina,* (g) *tumor:* retinoblastoma (see Chap. 14).

Congenital and Developmental Anomalies of the Retina

Coloboma of the Retina always is associated with coloboma of the choroid, as it represents an imperfect closure of the fetal fissure. Thus it occurs in the lower portion of the eye more or less in a line connecting the 6 o'clock meridian of the iris with the nervehead, and it frequently is associated with coloboma of the iris, ciliary body and nervehead, although occasionally the defect may affect only the choroid and retina, either peripherally or adjacent to the nervehead. It is bilateral in slightly over half of the known examples. The coloboma usually is oval with distinct, frequently pigmented borders and a white background of sclera showing through the thin, transparent, inadequately differentiated retina and choroid. Occasionally tongues of normally developed retina and choroid bridge the defective portions, and retinal vessels may run through either these normal bridges or the defective tissue. At times the sclera of the floor of the coloboma is ectatic in whole or in part. Visual acuity usually is diminished.

Nystagmus and strabismus frequently are associated. However, great variations occur in failure of closure of the fetal fissure, with minimal disturbances producing little effect and perhaps being represented only by alterations in pigmentation in the choroid or retina in this region.

Medullated Nerve Fibers. Normally medullation of the fibers of the optic nerves stops just behind the lamina cribrosa, but at times medullation may continue past this point and develop into the retina as late as the first month postpartum. They produce opaque white patches with fimbriate edges which form a sharp contrast to the orange-red eye grounds. The vessels of the nervehead and retina are obscured as they run through these opaque patches. Commonly the patches cover all or part of the nervehead and extend outward for a short distance into the retina, producing a butterfly wing-like pattern (Fig. 10-4), but occasionally the patch may be separated from the nervehead as an island surrounded by nonmedullated fibers (Fig. 10-5). The opaque patch produces a scotoma corresponding to its outline, but otherwise does not affect visual function.

Congenital Retinal Septum is a recently described but moderately common anomaly characterized by the development of grayish white folds of the retinal layer of the optic cup arising at the nervehead, extending into the vitreous and running out peripherally in any meridian but most commonly in the lower temporal quadrant. In some instances the lesion is hereditary with recessive transmission, but in others it may be developmental and represent an abortive stage of retrolental fibroplasia. Rarely, it may represent an

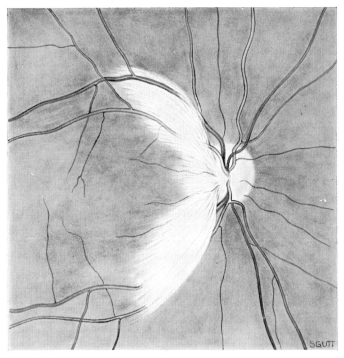

FIG. 10-4. Medullated nerve fibers extending into the retina from the optic nerve, obscuring the inferior temporal vessels completely and the superior temporal vessels partially.

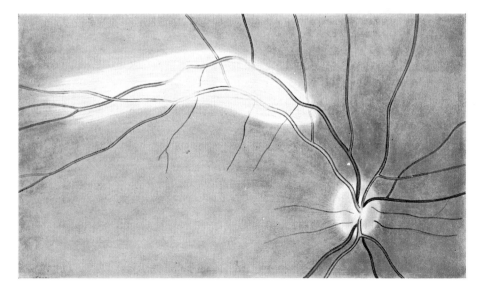

FIG. 10-5. Medullated nerve fibers in the retina. Observe partial obscuration of vessels.

intrauterine or early infantile proliferative retinopathy following a vitreous hemorrhage of undetermined cause.

Retinal Dysplasia, a rare form of disorganized development of the retina, is bilateral, present at birth in eyes that are slightly smaller than normal and appears as a white retrolental mass of fibrous tissue and retinal folds. It may be associated with cataract formation, and secondary glaucoma may develop as a result of malformation of the chamber angle. It may be familial.

Pigmentary Disturbances may be associated with coloboma or may occur as isolated stationary patches of increased pigmentation of the pigment epithelial layer or occasionally as isolated areas in which pigmentation does not develop in this layer (leukosis retinae).

Developmental Anomalies of the Macula. The macula is not developed fully until 16 weeks after full term delivery; however, failure of development is rare but does occur in association with albinism or with familial aniridia. The patient has amblyopia and nystagmus.

Heterotopia of the macula is rare. It usually is displaced temporalward and associated with an abnormal position of the nervehead and with vascular anomalies.

Coloboma of the macula is a misnomer for the scar left by a central chorioretinitis of intrauterine life or which occurred immediately after birth. It frequently is due to infection of the retina by toxoplasma, producing a localized retinitis and choroiditis.

Oguchi's disease is an hereditary, congenital, stationary retardation of dark adaptation in which the eye grounds have a gray color with the retinal vessels in sharp and distinct contrast. On histologic examination of such an eye there is an abnormal increase in number of cones and diminution in number of rods, especially on the temporal side of the nervehead. In addition there is an amorphous layer of tissue containing pigment granules lying between the rod and cone layer and the pigment epithelial layer. Visual acuity is normal in daylight but "night blindness" exists in dim illumination, although dark adaptation may occur after several hours.

Injury of the Retina

Contusion of the Retina (commotio retinae, Berlin's opacity) is a *grayish* or *milky* edema of the retina surrounding the macula, sometimes extending beyond the nervehead, resulting from a contusion of the eyeball. The macula remains relatively bright red in contrast to the surrounding milky retina. Some reduction in vision and changes in the field are present, but generally disappear with the subsidence of the edema in a few days; occasionally degenerative changes are found later at the macula, consisting of a deepening of color and fine pigment stippling; in such cases there is considerable reduction in central vision. Occasionally a *"hole in the macula"* (Plate 27C) results from contusion injury. Treatment consists in rest of the eyes, smoked glasses and atropine. A direct blow on the sclera may be followed by retinal hemorrhages, and rarely by retinal detachment.

Retinal Changes Due to Excessive Light (photoretinitis) are seen after injurious exposure of the eye to the sun (*solar retinopathy*), especially after watching an eclipse with insufficient protection. The subjective symptoms are limited to a central, positive *scotoma*, which may be only temporary or may not disappear entirely. Later there may be pigment changes at the macula with permanent reduction of vision. The conjunctivitis which results from exposure to excessive light is described in Chapter 6.

INFLAMMATIONS (RETINITIS)

Inflammatory disease rarely is limited to the retina, but commonly is associated with disease of the choroid (*chorioretinitis*) and of the optic nerve (*neuroretinitis*). The disease may be confined to one eye, but since it generally is dependent on a constitutional factor it almost always is *bilateral*. It may be acute in course, but as a rule it lasts many *weeks* or even several months.

Signs. There are no external signs; they are all ophthalmoscopic: diffuse *clouding* of retinal details, especially in the region of the papilla; *congestion* of the disk with *indistinctness* of its edges; circumscribed *exudations* appearing as soft, white or slightly yellow spots or patches, discrete or confluent, varying in size and found principally along the retinal vessels and at the macula; *tortuosity and distention of the vessels*, seen principally in the veins, which are darker than normal; the vessels may be obscured in parts by swelling and exudation; *hemorrhages* of various shapes and sizes, rounded when occurring in the deeper layers, and feathery or flame-shaped when superficial; *opacities of the vitreous*.

Symptoms. Diminution in acuteness of *vision* varies with the severity and extent of the retinitis and the situation of the exudates, but generally is considerable. Changes in the *field* of vision may be concentric or irregular contraction, or scotomas. *Alterations* in the *shape* of objects may result in micropsia (objects appearing smaller than normal), macropsia (objects appearing larger than normal) or metamorphopsia (a distortion of the shape of objects, straight lines appearing wavy and bulging). There may be diminution of the light sense, feeling of *discomfort* in the eyes and photophobia may be present, but pain is rare.

Course. The inflammation may *subside* completely and useful vision may return, or, as a result of atrophy and scarring, considerable impairment or complete loss of vision may occur.

The *prognosis* depends upon the severity of the inflammation, the parts of the retina most involved (unfavorable when the macula has suffered and when the deeper layers of the retina have been affected) and the clinical form of the retinitis.

Pathology. The changes consist of congestion, edema, exudation of leukocytes and fibrin, changes in the vessel walls and extravasation of blood; degeneration, scarring and migration of pigment. The white spots seen with the ophthalmoscope in the acute stage are due to exudation of leukocytes and fibrin, swelling of nerve fibers and cells and degeneration of the retinal elements. The walls of the blood vessels become thickened and the lumen is sometimes obliterated. Later, the retina becomes atrophied and scarred and then consists largely of connective tissue containing considerable pigment.

Etiology. Retinitis occurs rarely as a local lesion. Generally it is merely a manifestation of a *constitutional disease* and usually is due to the etiologic agents which produce chorioretinitis (see Chap. 9). It may depend upon neighboring focal infections such as accessory sinus disease, or it may be an extension from an iritis, cyclitis or choroiditis.

Treatment. It is of the greatest importance to treat the *constitutional* condition which is the cause of the retinal lesion. *Local* treatment consists in absolute *rest* for the eyes, *protection from light* by smoked glasses and often the use of *atropine. Diaphoresis* is useful, and sometimes cathartics.

Toxoplasmic Retinitis

One of the most common causes of retinitis and retinochoroiditis at present is localization of *Toxoplasma gondii* in the retina in the course of a general congenital or acquired infection. The organism, presumably a protozoan, is a nonmotile obligate intracellular parasite which divides by longitudinal fission forming round or oval cells which become crescentric with one end rounded and one pointed. The mature parasite measures 2 to 4 by 7 mμ. It is Gram-negative and with Giemsa the nucleus stains red to purple and the cytoplasm blue. It multiplies in the host cell until it bursts the cell wall or if the latter is resistant it becomes stretched to form a pseudocyst wall containing a group of parasites.

The mode of infection of man is not known although infection is widespread only Eskimos apparently not being infected. The organisms are found in many animals of the rodent class (gondi, rabbit, mouse, rat, squirrel, guinea pigs) and others (dogs, monkey, deer) and many types of birds. This infection may occur through breathing dust infected from saliva or excreta of birds or animals, by eating infected meat or contaminated milk, or by inoculation of infectious material by ectoparasites. However, once infected mothers may transmit the disease during pregnancy to the unborn child.

Clinically the acquired general infection is insidious and asymptomatic in the majority of instances. Occasionally, however, the infection becomes overt and may present in either of 4 types: (1) a febrile lymphadenopathy similar to glandular fever (most common); (2) a nonfebrile lymphadenopathy with tender enlarged nodes and without other symptoms; (3) a typhus-like fever with chills, cough, red macular eruption and at times meningoencephalitis; and (4) a cerebrospinal form with fever, delerium convulsions and lymphadenopathy. Only a small proportion of these cases are associated with ocular lesions. On the other hand, 99 per cent of cases of generalized toxoplasmosis of congenital origin have retinal lesions. The exact mechanism of congenital infection is not understood for few women with positive serologic tests transmit the disease and it is exceptional for a woman to infect more than one child. The mother usually is asymptomatic and in good health but does have positive serologic reactions. However, when the infection occurs early in pregnancy abortion or miscarriage almost always follows. Later in pregnancy a severe infection of the fetus produces widespread systemic infection resulting in diverse manifestations such as neonatal jaundice, splenohepatomegaly, interstitial pneumonitis, anemia, leukopenia, hydrocephalus, convulsions, cerebral calcifications of various forms, mental retardation and epileptic fits in addition to retinochoroidal lesions. In less severe infection late in pregnancy a subacute type of systemic infection occurs with few or no signs and symptoms but with ocular lesions developing subacutely or asymptomatically in the first 6 months of life. Years later acute reactivation or relapse of the ocular lesion is common.

The acute ocular lesion of toxoplasmosis whether congenital or acquired begins with localization of the parasites in the retina. This is followed by severe necrosis of the surrounding retina and is accompanied by an intense inflammatory reaction in the underlying choroid. At this stage there is an irregularly round reddish brown or yellowish brown mass involving the retina and choroid with slight hemorrhage and a varying amount of edema and of pigmentation in the surrounding retina. The vitreous humor rapidly becomes hazy with many inflammatory cells some of which find their way into the aqueous humor and may be deposited as fine or lardaceous precipitates on the posterior surface of the cornea. However ciliary flush practically never occurs. After several weeks or months the inflammatory reaction subsides and the chorioretinal lesion heals leaving a heavily pigmented sharply marginated glial scar with erose edges. The lesion may be single or there may be several. In the congenital type several small peripheral lesions are common but frequently in both congenital and acquired toxoplasmosis a single large lesion occurs close to the posterior pole in the macular or juxtapapillary region with the remainder of the fundus apparently normal. In the most severe cases generalized uveitis occurs producing iritis and posterior synechiae, neovascularization of the iris, opacities of the lens, proliferative retinopathy, organization of the vitreous humor into a pseudogliomatous mass, microphthalmos or phthisis bulbi.

Late relapses of congenital toxoplasmosis usually occur in the first 30 years of life. These may result from trauma, general stress or lowered resistance of the host. A fresh satellite lesion occurs in the margin of an old scar. Rarely a distant lesion may develop. In either case it runs a subacute or acute course similar to that of the initial lesion. After several relapses the inflammation may become disseminated. Rarely a generalized exudative reaction, probably a delayed allergic response in a highly sensitized eye, may occur.

Pathology. The acute lesion of toxoplasmosis is characterized by acute necrosis of the retina surrounding the free or encysted parasites. In the adjacent choroid there is a diffuse infiltration of lymphocytes and an ill-defined core of granulomatous reaction consisting of large mononuclear phagocytes, epithelioid cells and giant cells. The retinal necrosis extends into the choroid with increase in the lymphocytic infiltration and exudation into the vitreous humor. The parasites are never found in the uvea although in diffuse lesions the iris and ciliary body may show granulomatous nodules and in some instances the ciliary body also may show some necrosis.

Serologic Tests. A number of tests have been developed and are in use. These include: (1) The Sabin-Feldman dye test which takes advantage of the fact that antibody inhibits the staining of the cytoplasm of parasites with methylene blue by using the patients' serum as an unknown. Inhibition in a dilution of 1:16 or higher is considered significant in patients under 10; 1:32 in patients in the second decade and 1:64 in patients over 20 years of age. (2) The complement fixation test becomes positive in 3 to 4 weeks after the onset of infection and remains positive for years. (3) The hemagglutination test has about the same reliability as the dye absorption test. (4) The direct fluorescent antibody test. (5) The indirect fluorescent antibody test. (6) The direct agglutination test. (7) The serum neutralizing test. (8) The toxoplasmin skin test of Frenkel which is similar to the tuberculin skin test.

Diagnosis. Congenital toxoplasmosis may be diagnosed clinically when the typical ocular lesion in the infant is accompanied by cerebral calcification, hydrocephalus or other signs of encephalitis and positive serologic tests in both the infant and mother. Acquired toxoplasmosis on the other hand, only can be a presumptive diagnosis even if the clinically typical lesion at the posterior pole of the eye is accompanied by a positive serologic test.

Treatment. Both pyramethamine (Daraprim) and the sulfones are effective therapeutic agents *in vitro* but are less satisfactory *in vivo*. Daraprim in combination with sulfonamides may be more effective especially if used for several weeks; for example, Daraprim 25 to 50 mg. daily and 0.5 gm. of one of the triple sulfa preparations 3 or 4 times daily for 5 weeks followed by one-third of that dosage for an additional 3 weeks or longer. To reduce the danger of leukopenia and thrombocytopenia folinic acid also should be given in 10- to 15-mg. doses daily. Spiramycin also may be of some value and the steroids may be of assistance in controlling the excessive inflammatory reaction which develops in the recurrent episodes. Because of the unsatisfactory results of all these methods some ophthalmologists have used photocoagulation or laser therapy on the acute or subsiding lesions in an effort to destroy the parasites. However the healing time seems to be about the same regardless of type of treatment.

Syphilitic Retinitis

This is a *common* form, usually involves both eyes and occurs with *acquired* as well as with *hereditary* syphilis; in the former, it is found in the secondary stage, during the first or second year; in the latter, the lesions accompany but usually are seen after the subsidence of interstitial keratitis. It is associated with choroiditis (hence properly called *syphilitic chorioretinitis*), and often with iritis.

Ophthalmoscopic Signs vary according to whether the affection is due to acquired or hereditary syphilis.

In the acquired form, there is clouding of the fundus caused by *swelling* of the retina and disk, and by fine, *dust-like opacities* of the posterior portion of the *vitreous*; these opacities cause the disk to appear red and hazy; scattered grayish or white *spots* often fringed with *pigment,* especially in the macular region and in the periphery; degenerative changes in the *blood vessels,* causing the edges to present white lines; later, the deposits of pigment may be so diffuse as to resemble somewhat the picture of pigmentary degeneration of the retina. The changes may be more circumscribed and be represented principally by a large, white exudate, macular or peripheral, changing later to an atrophic area with more or less pigmentation.

In the hereditary form there is a leaden or brownish *discoloration* of the fundus upon which there are patches of *pigment* of various shapes and reddish yellow *spots* or gray or white *patches.* All these lesions are most severe in the *periphery.*

Symptoms consist of more or less diminution in the acuteness of *vision*, diminution in the light sense, *night blindness,* annoying flashes of light, *distortion* and changes in size of objects; central, paracentral or ring *scotomas* and concentric contraction of the *field* of vision.

Course and Prognosis. The progress is *slow* and the *prognosis* depends upon the stage during which treatment is begun; if begun early and vigorously, the prognosis is good, though some impairment of vision usually remains. Neglected cases often are followed by atrophy of the retina and optic nerve.

Treatment consists in intensive *antisyphilitic* treatment and cycloplegic drops to keep the eyes at rest.

Metastatic Retinitis

This form of retinitis results from the lodgment of *septic emboli* in the retinal arteries in the course of puerperal and other forms of septicemia. It may develop also as part of a more widespread ocular infection from infected ocular wounds and foreign bodies. In the first stage there are small white *spots* and *hemorrhages* around the disk and in the macular region; very soon the uveal tract is invaded and the signs of *suppurative choroiditis* appear. The inflammation ends in endophthalmitis or panophthalmitis or in degeneration of the eyeball without perforation (pseudoglioma). In rare instances the process does not spread to the uvea and then the patient may recover with some vision. Noninfected embolus gives rise to the characteristic retinal change occurring with obstruction of the central artery or of one of its branches.

Periphlebitis Retinae is an uncommon form of retinitis seen in young adults, of *tuberculous* origin in most cases; areas of exudation are seen along the retinal veins; profuse, recurring hemorrhages into the vitreous may occur. The condition often responds to general treatment of tuberculosis (isoniazid, *p*-aminosalicylic acid and streptomycin), rest and improvement of the *general health*.

Massive Exudative Retinitis (Coats' disease) is a rare condition seen in the young, usually boys, which presents a large, raised, yellowish white mass of cicatricial tissue or several smaller ones, the result of hemorrhages into the deeper layers of the retina; ophthalmoscopically it resembles conglomerate tubercle. Later there may be retinal detachment, cataract or glaucoma.

CIRCULATORY DISTURBANCES

Hyperemia of the Retina, when slight, is recognized by increased *redness of the disk* and by slight *striation* of its margins and, when more intense, is characterized by congestion of the vessels, hemorrhages and edema. Hyperemia is seen as a result of local pressure, in certain general diseases (especially heart disease), emphysema, convulsions, polycythemia and in most severe form in thrombosis of the central vein.

Cyanosis of the Retina is found in patients with congenital heart disease and general cyanosis, presenting great distention of the blood vessels, especially the veins, and a dark color of the blood contained therein.

Anemia of the Retina may be merely the ocular expression of a *general* condition, or it may be *local*; its onset may be sudden or gradual. *Acute* anemia, also known as *ischemia of the retina*, may result from occlusion (embolism), compression (sudden increase in tension), cardiac failure (syncope, cholera), vasomotor spasm and profuse loss of blood from any cause. There are extreme *narrowing* of the retinal arteries, *pallor* of the disk and *blindness*. Examples due to vasomotor spasm are furnished by quinine poisoning, in which some reduction of vision and some contraction of the field are permanent, and migraine, in which the effects are transient. The *chronic* form occurs with general anemia and in blood diseases, and

is seen frequently after *retinal disease*, causing atrophy in which the vessels become narrow, bordered by white lines of connective tissue or even changed into empty threads.

Hemorrhages in the Retina

These often occur without signs of inflammation.

Signs (Plate 21*A*). Retinal hemorrhages *vary in size, shape and position*; they are found most frequently in the neighborhood of the larger blood vessels and also in the macular region. When situated in the nerve fiber layer, they have a *striate* or flame-shaped form; when deep they are *rounded* or irregular in outline Sometimes a large, round extravasation is seen in the region of the macula, between the retina and vitreous; this is known as a *subhyaloid* (or *preretinal*) hemorrhage; it is usually of large size with round outline below and straight edge above. Retinal hemorrhages become *absorbed slowly*; the smaller ones may leave no traces; but frequently white residues, occasionally *pigmented spots*, indicate their previous site; when large they may get into the vitreous and be replaced by connective tissue (*retinitis proliferans*). They may be followed by glaucoma, opacities of the vitreous and occasionally by detachment of the retina.

Symptoms. *Interference with vision* depends upon the amount of damage to the retina, the size and particularly the situation of the hemorrhage; if at the macula, vision is much diminished. A *scotoma* results if the retinal tissue has been permanently injured.

Etiology. The causes of retinal hemorrhages are (1) *injuries*; (2) *local* disease of the vessels of the retina and choroid; (3) *cardiac disease* (hypertrophy and valvular); (4) diseased state of the *blood vessels*, especially arteriosclerosis, frequently associated with heart and kidney disease in old persons, and often a warning of cerebral apoplexy; (5) disturbances in the *circulation* (retinal embolism, thrombosis, hemorrhages in the newborn, menstrual disturbances and after intraocular operations); (6) changes in the *composition of the blood* and in the walls of the blood vessels, seen in anemia, pernicious anemia, leukemia, hemophilia, purpura, scurvy, nephritis, septicemia, diabetes, malaria, jaundice, poisons (phosphorus, etc.); (7) *loss of blood* (hematemesis, menorrhagia, etc.).

Treatment of the etiologic factor is indicated, and, in addition, avoidance of exertion or excitement, rest of the eyes, *cardiac sedatives*, iodides, *calcium* chloride or gluconate and measures to reduce the blood pressure if this is elevated.

Retinitis Proliferans (Plate 22*A*) presents whitish connective tissue membranes of varying density, supplied with blood vessels from the retinal system, projecting from the retina into the vitreous, usually at or near the disk. They result from vitreous hemorrhages when the blood clot becomes organized instead of being absorbed. The condition is found in syphilis, in diabetes, in young persons following the recurrent hemorrhages into the retina and vitreous, which are considered tuberculous, and after traumatism, especially perforating wounds. One form, known as *massive retinal fibrosis*, occurs in children as a result of hemorrhage occurring at birth. There always is great reduction in

vision and sometimes resulting detachment of the retina. No method of treatment is of any value.

Obstruction of the Central Vessels

Obstruction of the Central Artery. Obstruction of the central artery of the retina by a *noninfected embolus or thrombus* is of *infrequent* occurrence; though it causes sudden blindness, this is sometimes unrecognized by the patient, because it is *unilateral* and there is no pain. The *left eye* is the one generally affected by embolus, *either* eye by thrombus. The obstruction usually is at the lamina cribrosa.

Signs. There are no external signs, but the ophthalmoscopic picture is *characteristic* (Plate 22*B*). Within a few hours, the fundus becomes *pale* and edematous, *grayish* or even milky; this is most evident around the macula and fades out toward the periphery. In the situation of the fovea there is a bright *cherry-red spot* which stands out in contrast to the neighboring grayish white retina. The *arteries* are *very thin* and can be followed only a short distance from the disk; beyond this point they may be lost entirely. The veins also contain less than the normal amount of blood, especially on the disk, and may present a beaded appearance. Pressure upon the eyeball gives rise to the appearance of *broken columns of blood* with clear spaces between them, especially in the veins; this intermittent blood column is sometimes observed without pressure. Rarely the obstruction can be seen; often its presence is shown by a swelling in the artery, beyond which the vessel is thin or obliterated.

After a few days, *degeneration* of the retina occurs, and at the end of a few weeks *atrophy* of the nerve fiber and ganglion cell layers. The edema subsides; retina and disk atrophy, the latter becoming white with sharply defined outline; the arteries become shrunken and may be represented by white lines; the larger veins are partially filled with blood; the rest of the fundus retains its normal color. If there have been hemorrhages, these are replaced by spots of degeneration, sometimes marked with cholesterin or pigment deposits.

Symptoms. There is *sudden and complete blindness*; even perception of light is lost. Secondary glaucoma develops rarely. Occasionally a small part of the retina preserves its function when there is a cilioretinal artery (anastomosis between retinal and ciliary systems) or a macular branch given off proximal to the block; this region usually lies between the disk and the macula.

The foregoing description applies to cases in which the main trunk of the central artery is occluded. The embolus or thrombus, however, may lie in one of the *branches* of the central artery. In such cases the interference with sight and the changes will be limited to the *area supplied by the occluded branch*, central vision will be preserved, but there will be a sector-shaped defect in the field.

Occasionally there is the history of short prodromal attacks of blurred vision, probably due to spasm of the central artery.

Etiology. Although the obstruction may result from either embolus or thrombus, the latter is supposed to occur more frequently; differential diagnosis between these two processes is difficult or impossible. *Thrombosis* follows an *endarteritis* in arteriosclerosis or as a complication of various diseases such as nephritis; the lumen of the artery, already narrowed, then suddenly becomes occluded. When *embolism* is the cause, it usually is dependent upon the liberation into the arterial circulation of a thrombus from a diseased heart or aorta. In the rare instances in which the patient has recovered good vision, the blocking probably resulted from a temporary spasm of the walls of the artery.

Treatment usually is not effective. If seen early, paracentesis of the anterior chamber may be beneficial. Inhalations of amyl nitrite, nitrites intravenously, acetylcholine subcutaneously or subconjunctivally and massage of the eyeball often are employed to drive the plug into a smaller branch where it will be less serious. Good results have followed in some cases.

Thrombosis of the Central Vein (Plate 23) may affect the *trunk* (the obstruction is situated at the lamina cribrosa) or merely one of its *branches*. The former is infrequent, the latter more common. The symptoms and prognosis are quite different under the two conditions. Occasionally the occlusion is incomplete.

Signs. There are no external signs. When the *trunk* of the vein is blocked, the ophthalmoscopic signs are striking (Plate 23B): The *retinal veins are enormously distended* and very tortuous; blood escapes from the veins at many points so that the entire fundus is covered with *hemorrhages* and these are constantly being added to by recurrences. The arteries are attenuated. The disk is blurred. Ultimately the whole, or merely the involved portion, of the retina becomes atrophic and somewhat pigmented. When the obstruction is limited to a *branch*, the changes are similar, but they are confined to the area supplied by this branch (Plate 23A).

Symptoms. When the trunk of the vein is blocked, *vision* is impaired immediately, but sight is lost gradually over a period of several hours. Secondary *glaucoma* often develops. When merely a *branch* is occluded, there will be loss of a sector of the field corresponding to the affected area; central vision is reduced when a temporal branch is involved.

Etiology. Thrombosis generally is an

addition to diseased walls and contracted lumen of the veins. The disease occurs in elderly persons suffering from *cardiac disease or arteriosclerosis*, often with nephritis or diabetes and usually with high blood pressure. However it may occur in younger individuals in association with periphlebitis in the course of febrile affections. Sometimes it may be due to local causes such as orbital cellulitis.

Prognosis is *bad* when the vein itself is blocked; it is much more *favorable* when only a *branch* is occluded. The condition should be regarded as a warning of the possibility of a similar cerebral lesion and calls for investigation of the cardiovascular system.

Treatment. When the trunk of the vein is blocked, the use of *miotics* may prevent glaucoma; *atropine is contraindicated*. At times anticoagulants may be beneficial. *Rest* and attention to the general health are advisable. If glaucoma develops, operation is rarely effective; enucleation is indicated if the affected eye is painful.

THE RETINOPATHIES

The Blood Vessels of the Retina

The central retinal artery in the optic nerve just prior to and as it passes through the lamina cribrosa is identical with arteries of similar size in other locations in the body. The thickness of its wall is approximately one-fourth the diameter of its lumen. Both the internal elastic lamina and the muscular coat are well developed and the endothelium lies directly on the internal elastic lamina. As the vessel passes through the cribriform plate, its wall is reduced to less than one-half its former thickness. The adventitiae of the artery and vein fuse to form a common layer between the two vessels. As the artery crosses the disk margin, the elastic lamina thins out and disappears and the muscular coat abruptly becomes thinned but continues as a recognizable layer up to the second bifurcation. However, beyond this point the muscular coat is continued only as isolated muscle fibers separated from one another by increasingly wider gaps. Thus only the central retinal vessel and its first or second branches are true arteries, and the remainder of the visible retinal vascular tree is composed of arterioles and venules.

At the arteriovenous crossings within the retina, the vessels are so intimately joined that the wall between their two lumina is a common structure, and the adventitiae of the arteriole and venule are fused.

Normally the walls of the retinal vessels are transparent and therefore are not visible with the ophthalmoscope. The red line which ordinarily is referred to as the vessel actually is the column of blood cells. In the arterioles, the column of cells occupies the central three-fifths of the lumen, being concentrated there by centrifugal force (Fig. 10-6); the peripheral portion of the lumen contains only serum. In the venules, however, the cells are dispersed throughout the full width of the lumen. This may account in part for the apparent difference in size of corresponding vessels, the arterioles being smaller than venules in a ratio of 2:3.

Arteriolar spasm becomes apparent by the resultant constriction in diameter of the column of cells, even though the wall is not visible; but as the result of inflammation or sclerosis the vessel walls may become opaque and therefore visible as gray or white streaks along the side of the column of cells and, when sufficiently opaque, may obscure the red column. In-

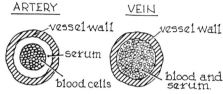

FIG. 10-6. Diagram showing distribution of cells in artery and vein as a result of differences in centrifugal force. The blood cells are concentrated in the central three-fifths of the lumen of the arteriole, with serum only between them and the cell wall. In the veins the cells are more evenly distributed throughout the lumen, but possibly are more concentrated centrally.

creasing density or opacity of the wall first is evident by an increase in the width of the light reflex, producing the "copper wire" reflex.

Arteriosclerosis of only two types affects the arteries of the eye: intimal atherosclerosis and elastic intimal thickening. Although the latter may affect the central retinal artery, it does not produce recognizable ophthalmoscopic manifestations. Arteriolosclerosis and regenerative intimal thickening occur in the arterioles of the retina.

Arteriolosclerosis is believed to be the result of hypertension. Regenerative intimal thickening occurs in primary pigmentary degeneration of the retina, the late stages of glaucoma and optic atrophy. The two most common types producing ophthalmoscopic manifestations, however, are intimal atherosclerosis and arteriolosclerosis.

Arteriolosclerotic Retinopathy

The changes of arteriolosclerosis are organic damage of the retinal blood vessels caused by the functional increase in blood pressure in hypertension. The ophthalmoscopic signs of hypertension, which may be transitory, precede the signs of arteriolosclerosis, which are permanent or progressive.

Evaluation of the degree of retinal arteriolosclerosis is important not only because it reflects similar changes in arterioles elsewhere (brain and kidney) but also because it indicates the duration of the hypertension and therefore has prognostic significance.

Arteriolosclerosis produces changes in the vessel wall which are evident in changes of transparency, changes of the light reflex and changes at the arteriovenous crossings.

Normally the vessel wall is transparent and therefore not visible with the ophthalmoscope, and usually it is possible to see the column of venous blood through the column of arterial blood. With the development of sclerosis this transparency is lost gradually, and usually the changes are most noticeable at the arteriovenous crossings. One of the first indications of sclerosis is loss of visibility of the column of venous blood through the arterial blood, but almost simultaneously there is an increase in width and brightness of the light reflex. As the sclerosis increases, the light reflex becomes broader so it occupies most of the space over the column of blood, giving the appearance of burnished copper to the vessel; thus the descriptive term "copper wire reflex." As the sclerosis increases, the vessel wall becomes increasingly opaque, and light streaks develop alongside the column of blood; with time this spreads and eventually results in opaque white walls which completely hide the red column of blood, giving the appearance of a white cord or silver wire.

Changes in the arteriovenous crossings begin with compression of the vein and banking of the vein or broadening of the column of blood on the side of the arteriole away from the optic disk. This sign may develop during the period of hypertension, but the first sign of sclerosis and loss of transparency of the wall at the crossing is concealment of the vein. The column of venous blood ordinarily seen through the column of arterial blood is no longer visible at the crossing. This is followed by tapering of the vein at the crossing, which results from spread of the sclerosis and loss of transparency from the crossing along the wall of the vein. Later depression of the vein into the retina is followed by deflection of the vein in the direction of the flow of blood in the crossing arteriole. However, the deflection of the vein is a sign of the lengthening of the arterioles, which, in the case of the smaller arterioles, causes them to develop a corkscrew appearance. These phenomena may be grouped according to increasing severity into four grades:

Grade 1 is early compression with concealment of the vein at the crossing.

Grade 2, in addition to the signs of grade 1, shows beginning of the copper wire reflex on the arterioles.

Grade 3 shows an advance of the copper wire reflex with beginning white streaks along the arterioles, depression and deflection of the vein at the crossing.

Grade 4 shows more intense perivascular streaking and silver wire arterioles.

Retinopathy consisting of hemorrhages and edema residues usually is seen by the time the vascular sclerosis has reached grade 2 or grade 3 at the latest, inasmuch as it almost always is preceded by hypertension and the changes coincident to it. Thus most patients, especially those with mild or chronic hypertension, also show arteriosclerosis, and these changes must be added and evaluated with those of hypertension.

Arteriosclerotic Retinopathy

This condition accompanies generalized *arteriosclerosis* (atherosclerosis), and the fundus changes indicate similar lesions in other tissues of the body, especially the brain. The retinal arteries are actually *arterioles*, and degenerative changes in them represent *retinal arteriolosclerosis.* The blood pressure in the patients of this group is normal or moderately elevated. The fundus presents *increased tortuosity* of the vessels, *narrowing* of the lumen of the vessels, especially the arteries, *widening of the light reflex* on the arteries, slight *indentation of the veins at the arteriovenous crossings* and *white lines* along the borders of the arteries. If the vascular disease advances, the above changes become more severe (Plate 21*B*) and may be accompanied by the appearance of *"silver wire"* arteries and *hemorrhages,* scattered or along blood vessels. The hemorrhages may absorb completely, or they may leave pigmented areas or white spots. *Thrombosis* of the central vein of the retina or one of its branches may occur (Plate 23) or obstruction of the central artery (Plate 22*B*).

Hypertensive Retinopathy

The retinal changes in the *mild or benign types of vascular hypertension* are similar to those noted above, although the blood pressure is more elevated.

The changes just described may be so great that the blood supply is lessened and the nutrition of the retina suffers, resulting in atrophy of the retina and optic nerve.

Slight changes in the retinal blood vessels, merely *suggestive* of those described above, are found frequently in *elderly* individuals enjoying good health; they must be regarded as *normal* and can scarcely be considered pathologic.

The retinal lesions in hypertensive retinopathy are dependent upon spasm of the vessels (*angiospasm*) and, later, permanent changes (*angiosclerosis*) of the vessel walls; these changes bear no relation to the presence or degree of renal insufficiency. The most prominent retinal and neuroretinal lesions are *edema* and *vascular changes.* Hypertensive retinopathy may occur in children and in the aged, but is most common between the ages of 35 and 55.

Ophthalmoscopic Signs (Plate 24). The earliest signs in the fundus are slight narrowing of the arteries, slightly increased light reflex of the arteries and occasional areas of transitory irregularity in the lumen of the arteries (due to *spasm*). If the hypertensive disease is controlled at this time, permanent arteriolar damage and its serious sequelae are avoided. *If the vascular disease progresses*, the retinal *arteries* become *sclerosed* and their walls become thickened and irregular, together with severe *indentation of the veins at the arteriovenous crossings, engorgement* of the retinal veins and the development of flame-shaped and rounded retinal *hemorrhages. Edema* of the retina in the form of a grayish haziness and swelling of the nervehead are prominent features. The borders of the disk become indistinct, and whitish deposits (*cotton wool patches*) form in the retina. Edema in the macula results in the development of a partial or complete *star-shaped figure* made up of white dots with the fovea as its center. Occasionally the papilledema is severe; rarely retinal detachment occurs. Hypertensive retinopathy is divided into four grades, depending upon the severity of the ophthalmoscopic changes (see "Course").

Symptoms. The degree of *disturbance of vision* depends upon the severity of the inflammation and especially upon the position of the exudations and hemorrhages. Minute changes in the macular region will cause considerable reduction in acuteness of vision, while extensive involvement of the rest of the fundus may affect the sight comparatively little.

Pathology. The retina presents edema, cotton wool patches, edema residues, hemorrhages and papilledema. As the edema persists or subsides, it may become concentrated, leaving residues which form

hard shiny yellow-white deposits which are prone to occur in the macular region in the fiber layer of Henle. Because of the radial arrangement of the fibers in this layer, the deposits produce radiating striae which have become known as a "star figure." Cotton wool patches are the soft, fluffy, white patches seen with the ophthalmoscope. They are in the nerve fiber layer and may be due to transudate, cellular infiltration, cytoid or granular degeneration of the ganglion cell or the nerve fibers or to edema of these layers. They usually clear without residue. Hemorrhages may be superficial or deep and repeated. They may be transitory, clearing without trace, or they may be followed by the hard yellowish white residues described above. Edema of the disk may be due to local hyperemia in the beginning but later other factors, such as increased intracranial pressure, may contribute.

Course. The *visual disturbance* may be the *first symptom* which brings the patient to a physician. Occasionally the hypertensive disease is discovered first upon ophthalmoscopic examination made in the routine of prescribing glasses. During the course of the disease, there often are *variations* in the degree of disturbance of vision, corresponding to the absorption and reappearance of retinal hemorrhages and deposits. The *blood pressure* of patients with well-defined hypertensive retinopathy always is *high*, with elevated diastolic pressure.

The course of the disease may be divided into the following groups:

Group I consists of patients with mild hypertension who have barely recognizable and usually transitory narrowing or spasm of the arterioles. This stage of the disease often is not discovered.

Group II consists of patients with definite hypertension who have definite generalized spasm or narrowing of the retinal arterioles; the arteriole to venule ratio may be 1:3 or 1.5:3 instead of 2:3, but in addition there are transitory localized constrictions of greater amount (focal spasms) of the arterioles.

Group III consists of patients with moderately severe hypertension and retinopathy in addition to general and focal vasospasm. The retinopathy may consist of hemorrhages, alone or in combination with edema, cotton wool patches and edema residues. The generalized narrowing of the vessels usually is greater, and the arterioles seem to run straighter courses, with branching occurring at more acute angles and with some compression of the venules at the crossings.

Group IV consists of patients with severe hypertension, usually of long standing (or malignant hypertension, see below), and who, in addition to accentuation of all the signs of group III, have papilledema.

Prognosis. Group I has an expected mortality of 30 per cent within 5 years; group II, approximately 45 per cent; group III, approximately 80 per cent; group IV, approximately 95 per cent. However, adequate early control of the hypertension improves the prognosis.

Treatment consists in placing the patient under medical care immediately.

Malignant Hypertension

A malignant type of hypertension has its onset in patients between the ages of 20 and 30 years. The blood pressure in these patients is extremely high, the ocular findings fall into group IV with severe papilledema early in the disease, and progressive renal insufficiency develops rapidly and progresses to uremia and death. Fortunately this is rare.

Nephritic Retinopathy

In general, retinal lesions occur only in those forms of nephritis which are associated with *vascular hypertension* or with severe secondary *anemia*. Retinal changes in *nephrosis* are exceedingly rare. *Acute glomerulonephritis* is rarely accompanied by spasm of the retinal vessels and retinal edema; the retinal lesions disappear unless the nephritis goes into the chronic form, in which case it closely resembles typical nephritic retinopathy.

The retinopathy of *chronic nephritis* begins with retinal edema and an absence of outstanding vascular changes; occasional flame-shaped hemorrhages are seen. As the disease progresses, the retinal vessels become narrow and sclerosed, and the *retinal signs approximate those of hypertensive retinopathy* (Plate 24). In some instances in which renal insufficiency is associated with secondary anemia, the fundus will resemble that seen in pernicious anemia, with the addition of vascular constriction. It usually is impossible to distinguish between the advanced forms of hypertensive and nephritic retinopathies. In the latter, the retinal edema is apt to be more extensive and the disk is likely to be paler.

The fundus changes in the advanced stages of both hypertensive and nephritic retinopathy formerly were known as "*albuminuric retinitis.*" In both hypertensive and nephritic retinopathy the retinal arteriolosclerosis is a part of a generalized arteriolosclerosis; the onset and history of these two varieties of retinopathy may differ, but the end stage is similar.

The course, prognosis and treatment of advanced nephritic retinopathy are the same as in hypertensive retinopathy.

Uremic Amblyopia is the term used for *loss of sight* during an attack of *uremia*, occurring in the course of nephritis and in pregnancy. The fundus presents some of the signs of nephritic retinopathy although rarely these are absent. It appears *suddenly*, affects *both eyes* and is associated with other symptoms of uremia: headache, vomiting, dyspnea, convulsions and coma; the pupils are dilated but usually respond to light. After lasting for a day or two, vision returns to what it was previous to the attack, provided that the patient recovers. The affection is not retinal but *cerebral*, and is caused by the retention of excretory substances in the blood. Treatment is that of uremia.

Toxemia of Pregnancy

Pre-eclampsia and eclampsia are responsible for only approximately half of the cases of hypertension in pregnancy, the remainder being chronic hypertensive disease. However, pre-eclampsia is likely to develop in approximately one-third of the patients with chronic hypertensive disease. Thus it is important to the obstetrician to differentiate between simple toxemia of pregnancy and that superimposed upon chronic hypertensive disease. Fortunately an evaluation of the ophthalmoscopic findings can be helpful.

The retinal changes in pre-eclampsia are those of hypertensive retinopathy without organic changes of arteriolosclerosis. The first signs occur on the nasal side of the disk and consist of general and focal spasm of the arterioles, which are transistory at first but soon affect all the arterioles, become more and more severe and result in the development of cotton wool patches, hemorrhages and retinal edema which may progress to flat detachment of the retina. The detachment frequently is bilateral and usually affects the lower portion of the retina, but is an indication for prompt termination .of the pregnancy, because it indicates severity of the general disease. The retinal detachment usually reattaches spontaneously and the retinopathy clears within 10 to 14 days following delivery. Prolonged toxemia may result in chronic hypertensive disease and eventually arteriolosclerosis, or, when superimposed upon pre-existing chronic hypertensive disease, hastens the advance of arteriolosclerosis and its sequelae.

Pheochromocytoma

Pheochromocytoma may cause an intermittent elevation of blood pressure with evidence of hypertensive changes in the retinal vessels or hypertensive retinopathy during these episodes. However, in other patients there is a sustained elevation of blood pressure between episodes of exacerbation, and in these patients arteriolosclerosis develops in addition to hypertensive retinopathy. After removal of the tumor, hypertensive retinopathy clears but arteriolosclerosis persists in the cases in which it existed prior to surgery.

Diabetic Retinopathy

Diabetic retinopathy (Plate 25A), seen only in elderly patients in the preinsulin era, now is recognized as a complication of the disease which is related to both poor control and duration of the disease. In general, the better the control of the blood sugar the better the chances of avoiding or at least of delaying the complications of diabetes mellitus.

The severe diabetic seldom is able to break his diet or avoid taking insulin for even a short time without developing acute problems. One of these is general lipemia, which occurs in patients who have developed high blood levels of fats and lipoids in association with acidosis and are in or near coma. In these patients, ophthalmoscopic examination reveals *lipemia retinalis* in each eye. The blood vessels appear dilated and almost the same size. Both arterioles and venules are pale pink, pale salmon or creamy white in color throughout the eye in severe lipemia, but in milder states the vessels near the disk may be partially differentiated with the arteries bright red and veins purplish red. The general background of the fundus may appear nearly normal in color or only slightly pale, but this probably is only in contrast with the retinal vessels, for the choroidal vessels are equally affected. The nerveheads usually appear slightly pale but ordinarily there are no other changes. In a few patients, however, a few small hemorrhages have been observed, and they appeared unusually dark. In the preinsulin days, these patients invariably died without recovering from the coma, but with insulin and better methods of control of acidosis they usually recover.

As the result of prolonged poor control or many repeated episodes of vacillating control, more permanent changes are produced and eventually become evident in the retina. These include capillary microaneurysms, pinpoint hemorrhages, transudates and residues, larger retinal hemorrhages, venous dilatations, venous occlusions, vitreous hemorrhages and proliferative retinopathy.

Capillary microaneurysms develop as minute dilatations, outpouchings or buddings on the venous capillaries. Quite a number of these may develop some time before any of them becomes large enough to become visible with the ophthalmoscope. (A microaneurysm must be at least 50 microns to be visible with the 14× magnification of the ophthalmoscope.) They appear as pinpoint, round red spots in the retina and usually are found in the perimacular region within or just outside the superior and inferior temporal vessels as they course around the macula. The microaneurysms appear and remain for many weeks before increasing in size, rupturing or disappearing. They tend to appear intermittently.

Hemorrhages may be the first visible sign of diabetic retinopathy, especially in juvenile diabetics, for tiny pinpoint red spots appear in the macular region and disappear within 8 to 12 days and at times others appear in nearby locations. Some or all of these may result from microaneurysms, and frequently definite microaneurysms occur. However, transitory pinpoint hemorrhages which disappear without trace frequently are the only retinal evidence of periods of poor control in the early stages of adult diabetes and especially in juvenile diabetes. Sooner or later, however, definite microaneurysms become interspersed, and some time thereafter transudates and residues make their appearance (see below), but with continued difficulties and the passage of time larger round hemorrhages, then striate hemorrhages and eventually large hemorrhages, pass into the preretinal position and into the vitreous.

As the result of residues from repeated hemorrhages, or from deposits in the walls and organization of microaneurysms or from localized transudates around or near these retinal changes, hard, yellowish white, glistening deposits become visible in the macular and perimacular region. These may be scatterd diffusely, in which case they sometimes are described as central punctate retinopathy; or they may be deposited in a circular band around the macula on either or both sides of the temporal vessels as they arch around the macula, in which case they are described as circinate retinopathy; or, finally, they may be concentrated in Henle's fiber layer immediately around the macula and in this location they tend to form radiating lines but seldom produce a symmetrical figure as is produced by the star figure at the macula in hypertensive renal retinopathy. In some cases the deposits have a more crystalline character with an iridescent display of colors with slight motion of the light from the ophthalmoscope.

In patients with prolonged retinopathy, the venules may develop varices along their courses, so they come to resemble an irregular string of beads. This condition is found only in a small percentage of advanced examples of diabetic retinopathy; however, many show fullness or generalized dilatation of the veins and venules with some irregularities in their diameters and kinking. Eventually small venules become occluded with increasing hemorrhage in the periphery of the retina, and later larger veins become occluded, producing extensive retinal hemorrhage, preretinal hemorrhage and vitreous hemorrhage.

As a consequence of repeated or extensive hemorrhage, organization with glial proliferation in the retina and into the vitreous occurs with the development of new blood vessels into the proliferating scar tissue. This is proliferative retinopathy. After it has existed for some time the scar tissue contracts and frequently pulls the neural layers of the retina away from the pigment epithelial layer (retinal separation or detachment). In some patients with proliferative retinopathy a heavy meshwork of capillaries and fine vessels invades and sometimes overshadows the development of the glial tissue, producing a rete mirabile. This is most likely to occur at the disk.

Diabetic retinopathy always is bilateral. Although the two eyes may not be exactly identical, there usually is little difference. The end stage usually is either extreme proliferative retinopathy and detachment of the retina or secondary glaucoma following vitreous hemorrhage.

The Blood Diseases

Anemic Retinopathy is seen in any type of anemia and is characterized by pallor of the general background of the fundus. It loses its reddish appearance and becomes of a more yellowish as well as paler hue. The disk is pale and the vessels usually are somewhat dilated and paler; the veins become rose-red and closer to the color of the arteries, hence somewhat more difficult to distinguish from them. With more severe anemia, edema involves both the retina and the nervehead, and in some patients cotton wool patches and occasionally hemorrhages occur. These usually are reversible, but optic atrophy may follow very severe anemia as a consequence of excessive hemorrhage, for example, or after prolonged anemia.

Polycythemia Vera and Secondary Polycythemia both show distention and engorgement of the retinal veins, which is apparent in the smaller as well as the larger vessels. The veins have a darker purplish red color; the arterioles usually are darker and in advanced polycythemia appear to be dilated slightly and indent the veins at the crossings, thus sometimes causing the veins to resemble a string of sausages. Rarely there may be hemorrhages in the retina, but since the vessels in the choroid also are distended the general color of the background is darker than usual. Edema of the nervehead may develop rarely.

Leukemia, of all types, produces changes in the retina. These consist of anemic retinopathy, venous engorgement, retinal hemorrhages, leukemic nodules, papilledema and preretinal hemorrhages.

The anemic retinopathy is similar to that described above: pallor of the fundus and the retinal vessels and at times edema, hemorrhages of the nervehead and cotton wool patches. However, some of these may be merged with or lost in the later developments of leukemia. After the white blood cell count has been elevated quite considerably, the retinal veins and venules become distended and darker than normal. Once developed, these changes persist through remissions in the blood disease even with return of the white blood cell count to normal ranges. With distention of the veins the arteriovenous crossings appear more accentuated, with deep indentations of the venules, which develop the appearance of a chain of sausages. With the distention, the veins also become more tortuous. The arteries and arterioles tend to retain their normal calibers for a long time, but eventually they too may become dilated and tortuous. Hemorrhages occur repeatedly after the engorgement of the veins has developed. They may be round or flame-shaped and moderate to large in size. The most common and most typical hemorrhage is the flame-shaped one, which rapidly develops a large round or oval white center. Infrequently a round hemorrhage will have a white halo around it. These white centers or halos probably represent separation of the large number of white blood cells from the red blood cells but may be due, in part, to other factors. In fact, some of these may be leukemic infiltrations of the retina with some hemorrhage around them. However, leukemic infiltrations generally have been described as being larger, measuring one-third to one-fourth the disk diameter, elevated and with only a slight amount of blood, if any, around them. Actually they are loci of proliferation of leukocytes in the retina. As the disease progresses the venous engorgement of the retina increases, retinal hemorrhages increase in number and size, preretinal hemorrhages occur and retinal edema and neuroretinal edema develop.

Retrolental Fibroplasia (retinopathy of prematurity) occurs as a bilateral disease in premature infants of low birth weight before the age of 3 months. The incidence of the disease is related to exposure of the premature infant to oxygen. Oxygen should be restricted to the minimal amounts required for the survival of the infant. The acute stage, characterized by dilatation and tortuosity of the retinal vessels, hemorrhages, neovascularization and transudation, subsides at the age of about 3 months. The following cicatricial stage of organization and contracture causes retinal folds or detachment. Spontaneous regression may take place in the active phase. The pathologic process is a neovascularization which extends from the peripheral retina toward the vitreous.

Although the incidence was high for a few years it has become negligible, but not entirely eliminated, because of improved methods of control in administration of oxygen to premature infants.

Degenerative Affections of the Retina

Night Blindness (*nyctalopia*, sometimes incorrectly called hemeralopia) is a condition in which the *sight is good by day* or with good illumination, but *deficient at night* or with reduced illumination. It is a symptom of certain forms of secondary atrophy of the optic nerve, especially retinitis pigmentosa.

A form of diminished light sense occurs *without ophthalmoscopic changes* and is due to fatigue of the retina, probably from defective regeneration of the visual purple; this variety is sometimes congenital, or it depends upon *diminished ocular nutrition* for a *debilitated* state in starvation, profound anemia and scurvey, and in cases due to *deficiency in vitamin A;* sometimes there is the history of exposure to bright light; xerosis of the conjunctiva often is present at the same time. The condition often is found in the tropics, among inmates of prisons, workhouses and asylums; it is endemic in some countries, Russia for example; it is found most frequently in adult males. The prognosis is favorable, though there is some tendency to recur, and the defect usually disappears with improvement of the general health by good and sufficient food, vitamin A preparations, tonics (liver, cod liver oil, iron) and the use of dark glasses.

Pigmentary Degeneration of the Retina (retinitis pigmentosa) is a *chronic*, progressive degeneration, consisting of *atrophy* of the retina with characteristic deposits of *pigment*.

Symptoms consist of *night blindness* (nyctalopia), increasing concentric *contraction of the field* of vision and progressive *diminution in sight*.

In early life there is but slight reduction in the extent of the field with good illumination, and central vision often is perfect. But with feeble illumination, the peripheral parts of the retina do not react, and the patient cannot find his way about at night, because the field is small. With increasing years, the field becomes contracted even with good illumination. Finally, in advanced life, central vision becomes poor, but usually does not end in complete blindness.

Ophthalmoscopic examination (Plate 26*A*) shows *black spots* in the *periphery* of the fundus; these have the shape of branching cells, like bone corpuscles with connecting processes, and are found especially along the blood vessels and covering them; they commence at the equator. In the course of years new spots form, and in this way the *pigment circle* gradually approaches the disk and macula as well as increases its width towards the periphery; the process is one of migration from the pigment layer of the retina. The larger *choroidal vessels* become plainly visible on account of absorption and decoloration of the pigment epithelium. The disk and retina are *atrophied*; the disk has a *yellowish, waxy* appearance. The retinal *blood vessels* are much *attenuated* and in the periphery are represented by mere threads. Posterior cortical cataract often develops and may require extraction.

Atypical forms. There are cases of retinitis pigmentosa with all the symptoms of this disease, and the ophthalmoscope shows all changes *except* the presence of *pigment*, and others in which the pigment is distributed in an atypical manner and the spots are rounded or irregular in shape.

Syphilitic chorioretinitis, which also causes night blindness, may present a picture similar to that of retinitis pigmentosa, but may be differentiated by the patches of choroidal atrophy, the absence of characteristic shape of the spots, their more irregular distribution and their position beneath the blood vessels, and by differences in the character of the field.

A rare affection, similar to retinitis pigmentosa, having all of its symptoms except the pigmentation, is called *retinitis punctata albescens*; it presents a great number of small, white spots scattered all over the fundus.

Pathology. This disease is thought to start with degeneration of the choriocapillaris, depriving the outer layers of the retina of their nutrition, or to be primarily a change in the pigment epithelium. There are degenerative and proliferative changes in the pigment epithelium with migration of pigment cells into the retina and around the blood vessels. The rods and cones degenerate and are replaced by neuroglia; with the progress of connective tissue and pigment invasion, the retina becomes atrophic and the ganglion cells are destroyed with degeneration of their axis cylinders and of the optic nerve, so that in the advanced stage there is disappearance of all nervous elements and replacement with glial tissue in which are imbedded masses of pigment; the retina then is adherent to the choroid. The blood vessels of the choroid and of the retina suffer hyaline and endovascular obliterating changes. All these changes begin at or near the equator and then spread anteriorly and posteriorly, the macular region becoming affected only late in the disease.

Occurrence. The disease is fairly common and affects *both* eyes. It is either *con-*

genital or develops in childhood. It is *hereditary*, with or without consanguinity of parents; it occurs often in several members of the same family; frequently other congenital defects, such as deafness, defective color vision and defective intelligence, are present in the patient or in the family. It may be complicated with other ocular anomalies.

Treatment is unsuccessful in arresting the progress.

Choroideremia

Choroideremia is a sex-linked recessive tapetoretinal degeneration producing night blindness which begins in males in childhood (10 to 13 years) with atrophy of the choroid and secondary atrophy of the external layers of the retina. The lesion, like that of primary pigmentary degeneration of the retina, begins in the midperiphery with fine stippled pigmentation followed by atrophy of the choroidal vessels and pigment epithelium. These changes extend both peripherally and centrally until after several years, usually 10, there is only a small remnant of choroid at the macula. The retinal vessels appear normal against the white background of sclera with only an occasional choroidal vessel visible. Eventually the disease ends in blindness. The female carrier is asymptomatic but has a nonprogressive pigmentation and spotty depigmentation in the equatorial region.

Amaurotic Family Idiocy is an uncommon affection which occurs in *infants* in the course of the first year, with general muscular and mental *weakness* and gradual *loss of sight*, ending *fatally* within 2 years. It is *bilateral*. Several children of the same parents sometimes are attacked, and most are of Jewish parentage. Ophthalmoscopically the picture resembles that of embolism of the central artery: a dark red spot at the macula surrounded by a grayish white zone somewhat larger than the size of the disk (Plate 25*B*), followed by optic nerve atrophy. Pathologically, degenerative changes are found in the ganglion cells of the retina and in the entire central nervous system.

Macular Degeneration may be *hereditary* or due to *senile* and *atherosclerotic* disease. The condition is *bilateral* and may occur at *any age* (congenital, juvenile, adult, presenile and senile). The macular region is the seat of *pigmentary changes*, and central vision is reduced. The most frequent variety is found in elderly persons (*senile degeneration of the macula*): The retinal changes often begin with small hemorrhages in the macular area, followed later by pigmentary disturbances in the form of yellowish spots with irregular black stippling (Plate 27*B*). In the course of this progressive process a so-called *"hole in the macula"* may be seen; this is a deep red, round, punched-out patch, with clean-cut grayish edges, situated at the macula (Plate 27*C*); this lesion may also result from contusion. A rare form of macular degeneration is associated with mental deficiency (familial cerebromacular degeneration).

Disciform degeneration of the macula occurs in late middle life, and consists of a slightly raised, irregularly pigmented, round or oval lesion. It is due to organized hemorrhage from the choriocapillaris beneath the macula.

Colloid bodies (drusen) result from hyaline excrescences of the lamina vitrea, and appear as yellowish spots showing through the retina (Plate 18*A*).

Uncommon Forms of Retinal Degeneration include:

Retinitis circinata, in which there is a more or less complete wreath of white spots surrounding the macula, developing slowly, probably is caused by previous deep hemorrhages, occurring in one or both eyes. It occurs frequently in elderly women but may occur in men and in younger members of either sex. It is frequently associated with hypertensive, arteriolosclerotic or diabetic retinopathy.

Angioid streaks are dark brown, pigmented, anastomosing striae, resembling obliterated blood vessels with irregular borders, near the disk, and placed beneath the retinal vessels. They are believed due to choroidal vascular disease with ruptures of the lamina vitrea and often are accompanied by macular hemorrhages and degeneration of the diskiform type. This condition frequently is associated with generalized degeneration of the elastic tissue of the body, pseudoxanthoma elasticum.

DETACHMENT OF THE RETINA

Retinal detachment is a separation of the retina occurring between the layer of pigment epithelium and the layer of rods and cones. The name usually refers to a separation by serum (*serous or simple detachment*), but detachment also may occur as a result of choroidal hemorrhage, exudate or tumor.

Subjective Symptoms. There is *loss of vision* in the field opposite to the detachment, causing the appearance of a dark *cloud* before the eye and a corresponding field defect; early symptoms are *metamorphopsia* and flashes of light (*photopsia*). Central vision is preserved at first, but is lost if the macula is included; with total detachment even perception of light may be abolished.

Ophthalmoscopic Signs depend upon the degree and extent of detachment.

When the detachment is flat, the color appears but slightly changed and the diagnosis is not always easy; however, the retina is somewhat *cloudy* and its *vessels* are darker and more tortuous and show some diminution in light reflex; the variation in level of the affected portion can be recognized by the difference in the refraction of a blood vessel on the separated part as compared with the rest of the fundus.

When the detachment is steep, as is generally the case, it usually is near the *periphery.* It is limited in extent at first and may commence at any part of the retina, but as a result of sinking of the subretinal fluid to a dependent position in the eye, it usually is found *below.* The rest of the fundus appears normal. The detachment tends to become *complete,* then involving the entire retina, which remains attached only at the disk and the ora serrata. It presents a collection of grayish, bluish gray or greenish *folds* (Plate 26*B*) with white tops presenting a bright sheen, *projecting* a variable distance into the vitreous. The *blood vessels* pass over and follow these folds and therefore are very *tortuous,* and *hidden* at places; they appear *prominent* and of a dark red, almost black, color and smaller than normal.

In most cases a *hole or rent,* not infrequently several, can be found in the detached retina; often a *peripheral* tear at the ora can be seen (termed *disinsertion*); through the hole or tear the red choroid is visible (Plate 28*A*). It sometimes is difficult to find the hole, especially if far forward or behind a fold; repeated ophthalmoscopic examinations may be necessary before the tear can be seen, and sometimes it becomes visible only after change of posture or evacuation of the subretinal fluid. Holes are more common in the upper segment, disinsertions in the lower.

In the later stages, retinal degeneration, cataract, uveitis and secondary glaucoma often may be added.

Etiology. Retinal detachment may be due to *disease* or *injury*; occasionally no cause can be found. *Myopia* and *myopic* *degeneration* are causative factors in about one-half of the cases of serous detachment. *Senile* and *chronic inflammatory chorioretinal changes, adhesions* of the vitreous to the retina and *loss of vitreous* during cataract operations may result in retinal tears and lead to separation of the retina. *Ectasia of the sclera* is responsible for some examples. *Uveitis* may lead to retinal separation from the *shrinking* of the organized exudates in the vitreous, which thus pull off the retina. The *organization of vitreous hemorrhage* and the contracture of connective tissue upon the inner surface of the retina (retinitis proliferans) often tear the retina and give rise to detachment. It may occur in the course of nephritis and in the toxemia of pregnancy, and then is preceded by retinal edema. It also may result from choroidal hemorrhage, exudate and tumor, in which instances the retina is *pushed* forward. *Traumatic* detachment usually is the result of a blow, but occurs also after accidental or operative wounds, especially when there has been loss of vitreous. Moderate trauma (stooping, lifting weights) may precipitate retinal detachment in a predisposed eye.

Holes or tears in the retina are considered the main factor in the production and persistence of the detachment, by allowing the fluid part of the vitreous to pass beneath the retina. Such holes tend to occur in parts of the retina previously damaged by disease or injury. The incidence of detachment increases with age.

Diagnosis is made readily by ophthalmoscopic examination, especially with the ophthalmoscope at a distance of 1 foot and an 8.00 or 10.00 D. convex lens in the sight hole. A visual field examination also may be helpful, showing a defect corresponding to the detached portion of the retina. But it is sometimes difficult to decide whether the detachment is *serous* or due to *tumor* of the choroid; if due to

malignant melanoma (Plate 19*A*), there is apt to be an absence of tremulous folds, the detachment often rises abruptly from the surrounding area, it is occasionally nodular, at times vessels belonging to the tumor and not retinal may be seen, and transillumination gives a shadow if the new growth is situated sufficiently forward.

Prognosis, formerly considered practically hopeless, has become much more favorable since the introduction of operations directed to the closure of holes and tears in the retina and to the production of an adhesive inflammation at the seat of the detachment. During the past few years more than one-half of the cases so treated have been reported as cured (Plate 28*B*). *Early operative treatment* is essential, since the separated retina tends to atrophy and the detachment to become complete. The chances of reattachment after operation are best in recent cases, less favorable in high myopia, aphakia, soft eyes and iridocyclitis, and unfavorable in old cases. If the macula has been detached, good central vision is never restored, even if the retina is reattached successfully. Unless the retina can be reattached by operation, the detachment generally *extends* and becomes *complete,* and *blindness* results, though rare cases of spontaneous reattachment as well as stationary cases do occur. The prognosis is much better when detachment is a complication of nephritis or of toxemia of pregnancy; in the latter case spontaneous reattachment generally occurs. Detachment following vitreous hemorrhage and proliferative retinopathy does not respond to treatment.

Treatment. *Operation* is indicated except in cases associated with nephritis and toxemia, in hopeless cases and in certain infrequent examples of stationary detachment.

The operations which are employed

DETACHMENT CHART

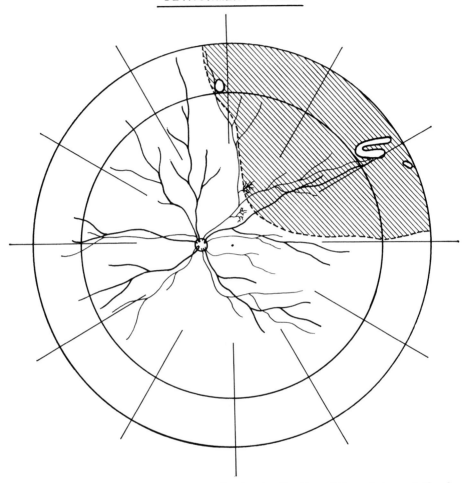

Fig. 10-7. A retinal detachment chart showing localization of three holes and the detached portion of the retina (shaded area) as sketched preliminary to surgical repair.

now with good results aim at *closing the retinal tear by creating a line of adhesive choroiditis around the hole* in the retina or over the entire area of detachment with *release of subretinal fluid*; when the latter is allowed to escape, the retina falls back into position and adheres to the choroid at the sites of reaction induced by the operative procedure. All of these operations begin with dissection of a conjunctival flap and retraction or division of a rectus muscle or two if necessary.

In recent cases of detachment of the retina the patient should be put to bed at once, *atropine* instilled and a careful *search made for holes* and tears. When these are found, their position should be *localized* and recorded (Fig. 10-7). The meridians in which they lie are given by clock-like notation.

The operations now generally favored include diathermy coagulation (penetrating or surface) and scleral buckling procedures. Ancillary use of photocoagulation or cryotherapy may supplement either surgical method. Vitreous implantation also has proved of supplementary value.

Diathermy procedures are dependent upon accurate localization of the tear or tears and careful coagulation all around them so that the subsequent scar will seal the retina and choroid around the tear.

Penetrating diathermy coagulation makes use of weak currents (75 to 125 milliamperes). The sclera is punctured by short needles which extend into but not through the choroid until the tears have been properly surrounded. At the end, a longer needle is inserted within the diathermized rim and after application of current is withdrawn to permit the escape of fluid vitreous from under the retina.

Surface coagulation is applied to the bared sclera over and around the tear by means of various types of electrodes or with the thermophore. This procedure takes in the entire area of detached retina and usually ends with drainage of the subretinal fluid by means of a diathermy perforation of the choroid.

Scleral buckling has the effect of shortening the eye slightly and moving the choroid toward the detached retina. A number of variations of this principle are employed successfully. After careful localization a scleral flap is elevated over the tear or tears, the base is treated by penetrating or surface diathermy and a specially shaped piece of material consisting of cartilage, preserved sclera, or silastic is sutured into place under the flap (Fig. 10-8). In some instances an encircling band of plastic material or fascia lata may be placed under a scleral flap which extends all or most of the way around the globe.

Photocoagulation of the choroid is produced by focusing a powerful beam of light by means of a specially constructed instrument onto the desired area of the choroid for a specific exposure. The light photocoagulator uses white light whereas laser ophthalmoscopes usually use red light. The light passes through transparent media but is absorbed by and destroys or coagulates pigmented tissue. The beam from either type of apparatus may be used through the pupil postoperatively to supplement surgical procedures or in selected instances may be used as the primary method of treatment. However it is essential that the retina is in apposition with the choroid for adhesions to form between them. Therefore these are of little value except in so called flat detachments.

Cryotherapy also is used to produce choroiditis and chorioretinal adhesions. Special cryoprobes have been developed for use in retinal detachment. They do not affect the conjunctiva or sclera but produce a satisfactory focal exudative choroiditis at temperatures between −40 and −90°C. After careful localization of the tear the region is treated by repeated applications of the cryoprobe as is done with diathermy to insure complete sealing of the area. The cryoprobe usually is applied to the bare sclera but it also is used postoperatively and in some instances prophylactically by application to the conjunctiva without exposing the sclera.

Vitreous humor implantation is another supplemental method of treating retinal detachment in cases in which the entire retina is detached and drawn forward in a funnel or morning glory shape because of massive contraction of the vitreous humor; in cases in which there are numerous retinal folds which do not settle out after drainage of the subretinal fluid; in cases in which there are vitreous bands; in cases in which the retina appears to have

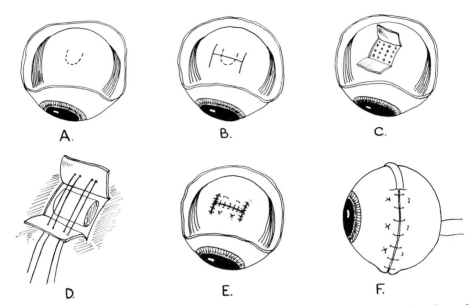

A.　　　　B.　　　　C.

D.　　　　E.　　　　F.

Fig. 10-8. Scleral buckling procedures. *A*, Localization of a tear on external surface of sclera; *B*, incisions made part way through sclera in relation to tear; *C*, lamellar scleral flaps turned back and diathermy coagulation shown in sclera under flaps; *D*, plastic material placed under flaps; *E*, flaps closed by sutures causing inward buckling of inner layers of sclera and choroid; *F*, method of using encircling band for buckling.

shrunken; and as a supplement to some of the buckling procedures.

The *after-care* consists of rest in bed in the supine posture, or semirecumbent if the detachment is inferior, for a few days. During this period the operated eye is atropinized. The patient often is required to wear central aperture goggles (loch-brille) for a month or two, after which he is allowed to resume his usual mode of life gradually, but is cautioned to avoid bumps and blows upon the head, and also jolts.

Failure of reattachment can be seen with the ophthalmoscope during the stay in bed. Redetachments of the retina, if they take place, usually occur after the patient gets up; in such cases one or more subsequent operations may give a satisfactory result. In cases with large detachments, it sometimes is advisable to operate on a part and later upon the rest of the detachment.

Retinoschisis is a condition in which the retina becomes split into two layers and probably arises out of extension or coalescence of peripheral cystoid degeneration of the retina (Illig-Blessig-Iwanoff cysts). Peripheral cystoid degeneration of the retina probably is physiologic for it may occur in childhood but occurs more frequently after the age of 20 and increases in both incidence and extent with increasing age. The microcysts first appear just posterior to the ora serrata as small isolated cysts in the external plexiform layer of the retina. As they increase in size they stretch and condense the surrounding glial fibers (Müllers fibers) to form cyst walls. As the microcysts enlarge and coalesce they extend from the inner to the outer limiting membranes of the retina then along the retina and rupture the cyst wall to split the retina into two layers. Retinoschisis affects the temporal side of the eye most often and frequently is symmetrical in the two eyes. It usually begins in the lower temporal quadrant and slowly spreads circumferentially greater than posteriorly. It may be confused with retinal detachment at times. Lack of a tear may be a significant differential feature. However detachments may follow or develop out of retinoschisis occasionally.

Tumor of the Retina (retinoblastoma). See Chapter 14.

11

The Optic Nerve

Anatomy

The optic nerve may be divided into (1) an *intraocular* portion, the head of the optic nerve, (2) an *orbital* portion extending from the eyeball to the optic foramen and (3) an *intracranial* portion situated between the optic foramen and the chiasm.

The nerve pierces the sclera and choroid a little to the inner side of the posterior pole of the eyeball. At this point the outer layers of the sclera become continuous with the sheaths of the nerve, while the inner layers stretch across the foramen, presenting numerous openings for the passage of the separate bundles of the optic nerve; this sieve-like arrangement is known as the *lamina cribrosa*. Here the *nerve fibers lose their myelin sheath* and become transparent. Spreading apart before reaching the level of the retina, they leave a funnel-shaped depression at the middle of the disk (Fig. 2-11), the *physiologic excavation* or *cup*.

The *lamina cribrosa* represents the weakest portion of the layers of the eyeball, and in increased tension is the first to recede, resulting in pathologic or glaucomatous cupping.

The *orbital portion* of the optic nerve presents a sigmoid curve permitting free movement of the eyeball. The nerve consists of bundles of nerve fibers separated by connective tissue septa. The optic nerve is surrounded by *three sheaths* originating from the three envelopes of the brain, known as the pial, arachnoid and dural sheaths; between the pial and the dural sheaths is a space, the *intervaginal space*, divided into two parts by the arachnoid sheath. The two spaces thus formed are *lymph spaces*, which communicate with the corresponding cerebral spaces. Anteriorly, the intervaginal space ends in a blind extremity and the sheaths unite with the sclera.

A short distance from the eyeball, the *central artery* (a branch of the ophthalmic) enters, and the *central vein* emerges; the latter empties into the superior ophthalmic vein or directly into the cavernous sinus.

The *intracranial portion* of the optic nerve is short and flattened. The *optic foramen and canal* form an unyielding bony ring in the lesser wing of the sphenoidal bone which compresses the nerve in inflammation and injury. The optic canal contains the optic nerve, the ophthalmic artery and sympathetic nerve fibers from the carotid plexus.

The *normal disk (papilla)* varies greatly in appearance; hence it is often very difficult to decide whether it is congested. Its apparent size and shape differ with the state of refraction; in myopia the nervehead appears large or tilted, in high hyperopia it seems small and in astigmatism it seems oval. In the congenital anomaly known as *pseudoneuritis* or *pseudopapilledema,* seen usually but not exclusively in high hyperopia, the disk appears hyperemic with blurring of its margins (Plate 5A); this condition can be distinguished from inflammation or edema of the nervehead by the absence of venous engorgement and the presence of fair or good vision and normal blind spots.

Congenital Anomalies of the Optic Nervehead

Coloboma of the nervehead may occur as a part of a more extensive defect involving the retina, choroid, ciliary body, iris and even the sclera at times; but in the majority of instances the lesion is situated in the choroid adjacent to the nervehead without actually including the nervehead. Although coloboma of the nervehead varies considerably from a large retrobulbar cyst to a slightly enlarged physiologic cup, the usual or average anomaly appears to be a round or vertically oval deep pit, 2 to 4 times the average diameter of the nervehead. The vessels of the nervehead, which are difficult to see in the pit, emerge from the rim individually in the manner of cilioretinal vessels. With extensive defects the vision usually is poor, but with minor variations, which sometimes appear as crater-like holes, pits or simply enlarged physiologic cups, vision may not be disturbed.

Rare anomalies of the optic nerve include congenital absence, hypoplasia and aplasia of the optic nerve.

Heterotopia of the nervehead usually is due to a temporal displacement of the entrance of the optic nerve into the globe. It usually is associated with a temporal displacement of the macula and divergence of the optic axis.

Abnormal shape of the nervehead is common. It may be oval, square, triangular or polygonal, but must be distinguished from the apparent change in shape caused by high astigmatism.

Pseudoneuritis is due to excessive glial tissue in the nervehead, resulting in fullness and elevation of the nervehead which may resemble swelling or inflammatory changes. It is distinguished from papilledema and papillitis in that it is stationary and congenital, does not show hemorrhages or exudates, and the caliber of the arteries or the veins is not altered (Fig. 11-1).

Failure of complete absorption of the glial tissue which surrounds the hyaloid artery may leave remnants on

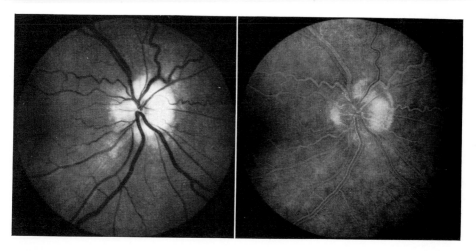

FIG. 11-1. Pseudopapillitis. Photograph before (*left*) and after intravenous injection of fluorescein dye (*right*). The dye appears white or gray in the photograph and is filling the arteries and just beginning to fill the veins. There is no diffusion of the dye into the tissues of the optic nerve and there are no dilated vessels in the nerve head.

the nervehead. A conical projection into the vitreous of this type is known as *Bergmeister's papilla,* whereas a flat membrane-like structure with an angular outline partially covering the nervehead is known as an *epipapillary membrane.* Either with or without these, short or long remnants of the hyaloid artery may project forward into the hyaloid canal of the vitreous, occasionally.

Conus or inferior crescent is a semilunar, white area adjacent to the nervehead, frequently below it although it may occur in any position, and associated with poor vision, which usually cannot be improved to normal even though the usually associated hypermetropic astigmatism is properly corrected. It must be differentiated from *myopic crescent,* which usually is on the temporal side or completely surrounds the optic disk and is associated with other manifestations of myopia.

Diseases of the Optic Nerve

Optic Neuritis is divided into:

(1) *Papillitis* (intraocular optic neuritis), in which the *head* of the optic nerve is involved, and in which there are *visible* changes in the disk.

(2) *Retrobulbar neuritis,* in which disk changes are *slight* or *absent,* and existence of inflammation in the optic nerve *behind the eyeball* is inferred from subjective symptoms.

The above division is anatomic, since the same etiologic agent may affect either the disk or the retrobulbar portion of the nerve. However, certain diseases, such as multiple sclerosis, more frequently produce retrobulbar neuritis, while others, such as syphilis, more often cause papillitis.

Papillitis

This affection must be distinguished from papilledema (see paragraph following description of papilledema); in their early stages, both must be separated from pseudoneuritis.

Symptoms. There usually is great *disturbance of vision,* not always proportionate to the degree of changes as revealed by the ophthalmoscope; there may be complete blindness. There may be *pain* around the eye or on movement of the eyeball, and the globe may be *tender* to palpation. The affection usually is *unilateral*; it may, however, be bilateral, in which case one eye may be affected before the other.

Signs. In the *very early stage* it may be difficult to make the diagnosis of papillitis by the appearance alone. There may be merely congestion of the disk with blurring or striation of its margins; such changes may be present in pseudoneuritis or in early papilledema. If only one eye is affected, a comparison between the two sides is useful. But a careful study of the visual fields almost always will establish the correct diagnosis; a central scotoma without enlargement of the blind spot is characteristic of early papillitis and retrobulbar neuritis.

But when the condition is fairly established, the *disk* is *swollen,* projecting and enlarged, of *whitish* or gray color with reddish center, *striated* and often presenting white spots and *hemorrhages* (Fig. 11-2); its situation often is recognized only by the convergence of the retinal blood vessels, its margins having become indistinguishable. The retinal *vessels* are altered and seem *interrupted* where they are covered by the swelling; the arteries appear thin, the *veins* much distended and very *tortuous.* The adjacent retina is edematous and congested, and presents white patches and hemorrhages. When there is added evidence that the retina is extensively involved, such as hemorrhages along retinal vessels and spots of exudate and degeneration (Plate 24-B), the term *neuroretinitis* is used.

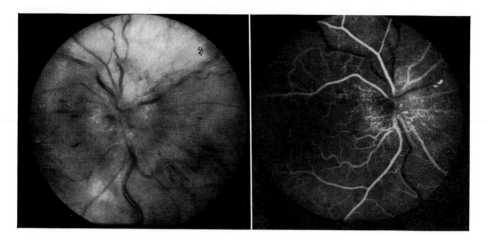

Fig. 11-2. Papillitis. Photograph before (*left*) and after intravenous injection of fluorescein dye (*right*). The dye has filled the arteries and arterioles and is just beginning to enter the veins. Notice the dilated fine arterioles in the nerve head. Also the dye is beginning to diffuse into the tissues of the nerve head. The black elongated spots in each photograph are hemorrhages.

Etiology. A common cause is *syphilis.* Less frequent causes are encephalitis, meningitis, multiple sclerosis, acute febrile diseases, focal infections (teeth, tonsils, nasal accessory sinuses) and occasionally poisoning (especially lead) and vascular disease. It may accompany intraocular disease (uveitis) and injuries, as well as orbital and periorbital inflammation.

Pathology. There are edema, exudation of leukocytes, venous engorgement and hemorrhages.

Course and Prognosis. Though usually *rapid,* the course may be chronic, extending over many months. The changes may subside and the disk may regain its normal appearance with the preservation of good sight (especially in syphilitic cases), and in others in which the cause of the affection is removed before the process has advanced too far or lasted too long. But in most instances intraocular neuritis is followed by *postneuritic atrophy*: The disk becomes white or grayish white, its margins irregular, and

surrounded by changes in the choroid, while the exudation changes into connective tissue which covers the lamina cribrosa; the blood vessels are contracted, the veins preserving some of their tortuosity, and are frequently bordered by white lines (Plate 30*B*). The prognosis, therefore, always is *serious*; when the course is unchecked, vision is finally either much impaired or lost.

Treatment is directed against the *cause.* In syphilis, the appropriate *antisyphilitic* measures are indicated. Removal of foci of infection is important. Orbital and periorbital affections require appropriate surgical treatment. Locally, rest of the eyes and shading from light are indicated.

Retrobulbar Neuritis

Retrobulbar neuritis (*orbital optic neuritis*) involves the *orbital or intracranial portions* of the optic nerve. With few or no visible changes in the disk, at first, the diagnosis is made from the visual dis-

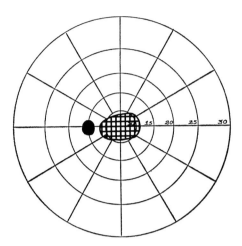

FIG. 11-3. Bjerrum screen visual field, showing an absolute central scotoma.

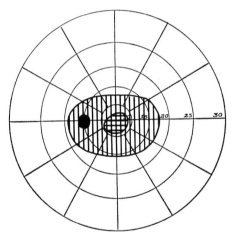

FIG. 11-4. Bjerrum screen visual field, showing a relative (present only with small target) centrocecal scotoma surrounding and including an absolute (present with both small and large targets) central scotoma.

turbance. Usually the *papillomacular* fibers are affected; hence the change in the field of vision is a *central scotoma*. The affection is rather uncommon, generally *unilateral*, occasionally bilateral.

Symptoms and Signs consist of *head-*

ache on affected side, *pain* in the *orbit* aggravated by movements of the eye and upon pressing the eye backward, rapidly progressing *impairment of sight* and *central scotoma*, either relative or absolute (Figs. 11-3 and 11-4). The pupil often reacts sluggishly. Externally the eye appears normal.

Ophthalmoscopic Signs. At first there are no changes; later there may be slight *hyperemia* of the disk and *haziness* of its margins, with slight distention and sometimes diminished caliber of the retinal vessels.

Course. The disease runs an *acute* course, and after a period varying from 2 weeks to 2 months, the sight usually becomes normal; or recovery may be partial and a *central scotoma* be left, in which case there is pallor of the temporal portion of the disk corresponding to degeneration of the papillomacular fibers. Very rarely it terminates in permanent and total blindness. Relapses are observed.

Etiology. The causes may be *general or local. Multiple sclerosis* is the most common cause, the disease occurring as an early symptom in about one-half of the cases; less frequent causes are general diseases (syphilis, so-called rheumatism, diabetes), acute infectious diseases (influenza), septic foci (mouth, intestinal tract) and poisons (alcohol, especially methyl alcohol, lead, thallium used in depilatory creams).

Local causes comprise extension from the orbit (periostitis) and extension from the nasal accessory sinuses, especially the sphenoidal sinus. Sometimes no cause can be found.

Prognosis depends upon the cause and the possibility of its removal. In general the prognosis is *good*; in multiple sclerosis the involvement of the optic nerve rarely leads to complete blindness.

Treatment. Although there is a strong tendency to spontaneous recovery, the responsible *cause* should be attacked. The patient should be placed in the best possible physical condition. Fever therapy may be of service. Large doses of vitamin B complex often are given; also histamine and other vasodilators.

Leber's disease (hereditary optic neuritis). Occasionally *bilateral acute retrobulbar neuritis* occurs as a *hereditary* affection, generally attacking males, often several in the same family, commencing at any time of life but usually about the 20th year; the transmission commonly is through unaffected females. Vision usually fails rapidly at first and then remains stationary or improves, and there may even be complete recovery. Commonly there is a *central scotoma,* either relative or absolute, which is permanent, with little contraction of the peripheral field. The fundus presents little if any change at first; later there is pallor of the temporal segment of the disk, rarely of the whole disk. The cause of the disease is unknown. No form of treatment has been of any value.

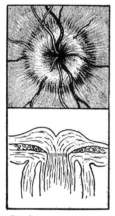

FIG. 11-5. Papilledema. The *upper portion* represents the ophthalmoscopic appearance; the *lower portion,* a longitudinal section.

Papilledema

Papilledema (choked disk) is a *noninflammatory swelling of the optic nervehead* resulting from *increased intracranial pressure* and from obstruction to the orbital venous outflow (Figs. 11-5 and 11-6). The condition usually is *bilateral,* although one eye may be affected before the other. The degree of swelling may dif-

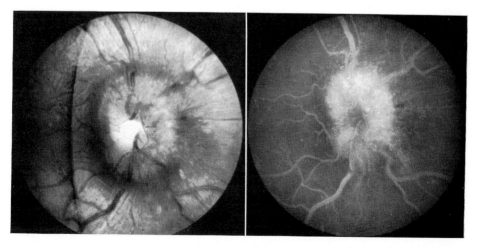

FIG. 11-6. Papilledema. Photograph before *(left)* and after intravenous injection of fluorescein dye *(right).* The dye has filled the arteries, arterioles and veins. It also has diffused out of the vessels into the edematous tissues of the nerve head.

fer considerably in the two eyes. Though numerous hypotheses have been advanced to explain the production of choked disk, the exact mechanism is still unsettled. At present it generally is believed to be due to *increased intracranial pressure* forcing cerebrospinal fluid into the intervaginal space of the optic nerve, causing stasis in the region of the lamina cribrosa and compression of the vessels, resulting in venous engorgement.

Signs and Symptoms. In the early stages there may be only slight edema of the disk; only by observing an increase in this swelling can the ophthalmoscopic appearance of the nervehead be distinguished from pseudopapilledema or a physiologic variation from the normal. Later examination shows *great swelling* and protrusion of the *disk,* distortion and *tortuosity of the retinal veins* and *hemorrhages* upon and near the edematous papilla. The lesions are limited to the disk and immediately adjacent retina (Fig. 11-6). The degree of projection of the disk is estimated by the difference in refraction between the most protruding part of the disk and some unaffected portion of the retina, measured with direct ophthalmoscopy; this often is more than +2.00 D. in papilledema.

In the early stages there is no impairment of vision. The *blind spot is enlarged.* Later, reduction in vision may occur and progress to blindness if the intracranial pressure is not reduced. Oculomotor and field changes may be found when the causative intracranial lesion also affects the nuclei or nerves to the eye muscles and the optic pathways.

Etiology. Brain tumor is the most frequent cause. Choked disk occurs in 80 per cent and may be the first symptom of the intracranial growth. Tumors of the midbrain, parieto-occipital region and the cerebellum furnish the greatest percentage of papilledema; swelling of the disk is apt to be especially well developed with cerebellar tumors. The size of the tumor is not as great a factor in determining the degree of papilledema as its situation; the greater swelling is most often on the same side as the tumor, but there are many exceptions to this: Tumors of the sphenoid ridge may cause ipsilateral optic atrophy and contralateral papilledema (Foster Kennedy syndrome). Occasionally brain tumor gives rise to changes resembling those of nephritic retinopathy with an incomplete star-shaped figure at the macula. Syphilis is a frequent cause, acting generally through intracranial gumma, less often as a basal meningitis. Tuberculous meningitis and abscess of the brain are not uncommon causes. Tumors of the pituitary body usually do not produce choked disk. A considerable degree of papilledema may be present in malignant vascular hypertension; this is accompanied by hypertensive retinopathy; this condition rarely may be mistaken for brain tumor; however, the edema extends outward from the disk and involves much more of the retina, so neuroretinal edema is a preferable term in contrast to papilledema of brain tumor.

Course and Prognosis depend upon the duration and extent of the papilledema and upon the amount of damage to the optic nerve fibers. Vision which has been reduced by swelling of the nerve may be restored if the intracranial pressure is reduced in time. As a rule, long continued choked disk results in more or less permanent loss of vision associated with secondary optic atrophy.

Treatment consists of removal or treatment of the causative lesion if possible. A decompression operation may improve vision temporarily as a palliative measure in otherwise inoperable malignant tumors.

Cerebral decompression (temporal for pretentorial, suboccipital for subtentorial tumors) often is done to relieve the intracranial pressure, thus enabling the optic nerves to resume their functions. The operation causes subsidence of the papillary swelling and improvement in vision within a week or two, if done before much degenerative change in the nerves has taken place; incidentally other symptoms are relieved and life prolonged.

Lumbar puncture may be used not only for diagnosis but also to reduce intracranial pressure and relieve choked disk; however, care must be exercised not to withdraw more than 5 cc. at one time, especially with posterior fossa tumors, since sudden death has followed this procedure. Puncture of the corpus callosum with drainage of the ventricle also has been used for the same purpose.

Differential Diagnosis among papillitis, papilledema and retrobulbar neuritis:

Papillitis. Vision poor; pain around the involved eye, or on movement or palpation of the globe; moderate swelling of the nervehead with inflammatory signs; vitreous opacities frequently; central field defect, but there may be any kind of scotoma or complete loss of the visual field; secondary atrophy may develop later.

Papilledema. Vision not impaired; headache frequently; swelling of disk; enlarged blind spot with other field changes if the visual pathway is involved; loss of vision and secondary atrophy may develop later.

Retrobulbar neuritis. Usually sudden onset of poor vision; pain around eye and tenderness to palpation of globe; normal appearance of disk; central scotoma; temporal atrophy of nervehead may develop later.

Amblyopia

Amblyopia is a reduction in the acuteness of vision which cannot be relieved by glasses and is not dependent upon visible changes in the eye. The term sometimes is used in a less restricted sense to designate *poor sight,* even when changes are found in the eye, as, for instance, toxic amblyopia in which temporal pallor of the disk exists. The name *amaurosis* has been associated with *absolute blindness when* unaccompanied by discoverable ocular changes but now is seldom used.

Toxic Amblyopias

Tobacco alcohol amblyopia is a chronic poisoning of the orbital portion of the optic nerve of fairly *frequent* occurrence, usually attacking *both eyes,* generally in middle-aged or elderly men, and due in many cases to excessive indulgence in *tobacco, alcohol* or both combined, with failure to eat an adequate diet.

Symptoms. There is gradual diminution in acuteness of sight; *foggy vision;* the patient sees better in the evening and the visual disturbance is *worse in bright light.* The field of vision presents the normal peripheral boundary, but there is a *central scotoma* for red and green (Figs. 11-3 and 11-4) corresponding to the distribution of the papillomacular fibers of the optic nerve; bilateral cecocentral (extending from the blind spot toward the area of fixation) scotomas, most easily demonstrated with red test objects, always are present.

Ophthalmoscopic Signs. At first there are no changes in the papilla, or merely some hyperemia and slight blurring of the margin; later, there is *pallor of the temporal side of the disk.*

Course and Prognosis. The progress of the disease is *slow.* If poisoning continues, vision becomes worse and may suffer very much. If the cause is removed, there usually is *gradual improvement* in sight, often to normal, with complete disappearance of the scotoma. In severe cases, there may be some permanent reduction in vision, and the scotoma may be permanent.

Etiology. The condition results most often from overindulgence in *tobacco*, smoking or chewing, occasionally after snuff taking; the stronger tobaccos of cigars and pipes most often are responsible. Some individuals are especially susceptible. Poor general health predisposes; recent investigation has shown that *vitamin deficiency* is an important factor; typical cases are seen in pellagra. *Alcohol* constitutes a frequent cause; in most cases both alcohol and tobacco act together. *Other poisons* which in toxic doses may cause similar amblyopia include chloral, lead, arsenic, male fern, methyl alcohol, carbon disulfide, thallium, nitrobenzol and aniline.

Pathology. The process consists of a degeneration of the ganglion cells in the macular region (these are particularly susceptible and vulnerable), with *interstitial neuritis* of the papillomacular bundle in the optic nerve, and subsequent degeneration of these fibers.

Treatment consists in *abstinence or great reduction* of tobacco and alcohol, an important part of the treatment; if some stimulant or tobacco is required, it must be restricted to a small amount with meals. Attention to *general health*, proper hygiene and especially a *high vitamin diet* with added vitamin B complex are very important. In cases due to poisoning by organic arsenic compounds, such as tryparsamid, British anti-Lewisite (5 per cent in 10 per cent benzyl benzoate in peanut oil, 2 cc. twice daily for 4 days) has proved valuable.

Malarial Amblyopia has been observed, without apparent changes in the fundus or disks. It affects one or both eyes, lasts some hours or days and usually disappears completely as a result of the use of antimalarial drugs.

Quinine Amblyopia occurs after large quantities of quinine have been taken, occasionally with moderate doses in susceptible individuals. Besides other symptoms of cinchonism there may be great reduction in vision or complete *blindness*, often noticed suddenly, *contracted fields*, dilated pupils and intense *pallor of the disk*, with extreme *contraction of the retinal vessels*. The condition is due to *spasm* of the retinal vessels causing anemia of the retina, degeneration of the ganglion cells and nerve fibers of the retina and later atrophy of the optic nerve. After a time, central vision is restored completely or partially, and the field widens but rarely regains its full extent. The disk may regain its normal color, but it may remain pale for a long period; the retinal vessels usually do not resume their full normal caliber. Occasionally pigment deposits occur similar to those seen in pigmentary degeneration of the retina. Treatment consists in discontinuing the drug, inhalations of amyl nitrite and the use of vasodilators, such as sodium nitrite intravenously.

Similar symptoms may follow toxic doses of ethylhydrocupreine (Optochin).

Methyl Alcohol Amblyopia results from the drinking of variable quantities of wood alcohol in the form of cheap whiskeys, cordials, essences and other alcoholic beverages, which often are adulterated with Columbian spirits, the trade name for rectified methyl alcohol; it also has been caused by inhaling the fumes to which the varnishers of the interior of beer casks, for instance, are exposed. The general symptoms consist of *severe gastrointestinal disturbance*, headache, vertigo and sometimes coma, and not infrequently terminate fatally. The ocular symptoms are *great reduction of vision*, peripheral contraction of the *field* and absolute central *scotoma*; *blindness* often follows. The ophthalmoscopic appearances are hyperemia of disk with blurring of edges and, later, atrophy of the optic nerve with small retinal vessels. The prognosis is *unfavorable* both to life and to sight; some cases recover, but very few with useful vision. The anatomic changes are alterations in the ganglion cells of the retina with extension to the optic nerve. Treatment consists in the use of pilocarpine, nitroglycerine and alkalis by mouth and intravenously.

Congenital Amblyopia and Amblyopia ex Anopsia

Congenitally defective vision usually affects *one eye*; it frequently is associated with high degrees of *hyperopia, myopia* and *astigmatism*; some may be due to retinal hemorrhages in the newborn which is a fairly frequent occurrence, all traces of the hemorrhages having disappeared. Probably in many of the so-called congenital cases, the amblyopia is really acquired; a relatively greater error of refraction of one eye may have prevented a perfect image from being focused on the retina, and this has resulted in a lack of development of the retinal function at the macula. The most careful correction of any error of refraction fails to produce normal acuity; in children, the sight frequently can be improved or brought up to normal with the wearing of suitable glasses and occlusion of the sound eye. Unilateral amblyopia may have existed many years, unknown to the individual, and discovered only when, for some reason such as an accident or a functional examination, the good eye is closed or covered.

Amblyopia ex anopsia. Any interference with vision, either congenital or dating from early life, which prevents perfect focusing upon the retina, such as cataract, causes *amblyopia from non-use;* hence the advisability of operating upon congenital cataracts early. An obstacle to vision beginning after the age of 8 years usually does not result in amblyopia from disuse.

Unilateral amblyopia predisposes to *strabismus* by lessening the value of binocular single vision. Very often amblyopia develops in an eye which has squinted from early life on account of its exclusion from the visual act, the retinal image in this eye being suppressed. Exercise of such an eye before the seventh year, by forcing it to work while the sound eye is occluded, frequently will improve its visual power. *Nystagmus,* due to poor development of fixation, often is found in bilateral amblyopia, especially when the latter is of high degree.

Congenital word-blindness occurs occasionally, and is supposed to be due to a defect in the visual memory center for words and groups of letters. With normal fundus and good vision there is inability or difficulty in recognizing printed or written words, although auditory memory is normal. If this condition is detected early in life, much improvement follows training.

Hysterical Amblyopia

This affection usually occurs in *young* girls and women, occasionally in young persons of the male sex; it is most often *bilateral,* but it may be unilateral.

Symptoms. The most constant symptom is *reduction in vision,* frequently amounting to complete blindness. The *field* of vision is *contracted* concentrically, both for white and for colors; it may be tubular; since the retina becomes exhausted rapidly, the contraction often becomes greater with each succeeding test during the same examination (spiral field). The *color fields* have abnormal relative areas; they may be larger than that for white; their order often is *reversed; i.e.,* green the largest, red next, and blue the smallest. There may be central, annular or irregular scotomas or hemianopsia. A *great variety* of other ocular symptoms may be present, such as photophobia, flashes of light, blepharospasm, corneal anesthesia, monocular diplopia, ptosis and metamorphopsia. The pupillary reflexes and ophthalmoscopic appearances are normal.

With these ocular manifestations there usually are *other hysterical symptoms,* especially hemianesthesia of the affected side. It is sometimes difficult to distinguish between this affection and malingering. It sometimes follows injuries (*traumatic neurosis*) even when these do not involve the eye.

Prognosis is *good,* but the affection may last many months.

Treatment is directed to the hysterical condition.

Simulated Amblyopia (Malingering)

Not infrequently persons pretend various degrees of loss of vision in one or both eyes in attempts to recover damages for alleged injury. They may claim blindness in one eye, but rarely blindness in both eyes; more often the claim is for a reduction of vision in one or both eyes.

Tests for Monocular Blindness. In these the person is made to believe that the good eye is being examined while actually the vision of the defective eye is being tested.

(1) With an electric light 15 or 20 feet away, a prism of 6°, base upward or downward, is placed before the sound eye; if the patient sees *double* it is an indication of binocular vision.

(2) With the light in the same position, the supposed blind eye is covered; then *monocular diplopia* is produced by moving a 6° prism, base upward or downward, until the apex corresponds to the center of the pupil. Next the blind eye is uncovered and at the same time the prism is moved until it covers the entire pupil. If now there still is double vision (binocular diplopia) it is evident that both eyes see.

(3) A *strong convex lens* (+6.00 D.) is placed before the good eye and a weak concave lens (0.25 D.) in front of the supposed blind eye; the patient is directed to read distant test types. If he succeeds, it is proof of malingering, since it is impossible to see with the sound eye when covered by the strong lens.

(4) Snellen's test types of alternate *red and green color,* made of glass and *illuminated from behind,* often are used to detect malingering: A red glass is placed before the admittedly sound eye; if the subject reads the green letters, he must do so with the so-called blind eye, since only the red letters can be seen through the red glass.

There is an instrument available in which, by mirrors or prisms attached to binocular tubes, the image of test types at the end of the right tube is seen by the left eye and *vice versa.* The test types, having a relationship to those of the Snellen charts, disclose the real acuteness of vision of the alleged poor eye while the malingerer imagines he is reading with the good eye.

These tests are apt to be unsuccessful if the claimant closes one eye and then the other during the test, in order to ascertain which eye is being examined; this he will do if he has been coached beforehand.

Tests for Reduction of Vision in One or Both Eyes. When the patient claims a mere reduction in vision in one or both eyes it often is difficult to decide whether the claim is justified. Suspicion of malingering is excited when there is an absence of agreement between the functional and objective examinations, or contradictory statements during the different steps in the functional tests upon using different test charts. A method which sometimes succeeds is to record the visual acuity at 20 feet and then, later on, at 10 and at 5 feet; the claimant may be unaware of the relationship between the size of the Snellen letters and the distance from the chart; he may have memorized the letters which he has decided upon when he was placed at 20 feet and declare his inability to read smaller ones at 10 and at 5 feet.

Tests for Blindness in Both Eyes. This is more difficult to detect. Contraction of the pupils to light is presumptive evidence of some sight, but in rare instances the pupils react to light in absolute blindness, the lesion being situated in the visual centers or in the connection between these centers and the corpora quadrigemina (3, Fig. 11-8). In feigned binocular blindness a close watch must be kept on the patient when he thinks he is free from observation, and the following test may be employed: A lighted candle or electric bulb is placed in front of the patient and a 6° prism held base outward before one eye; if both eyes see, the one covered by the prism will move inward in order to avoid diplopia; on removal of the prism it will move outward, the other eye remaining fixed.

Atrophy of the Optic Nerve

Optic atrophy occurs either (1) as *simple* atrophy (primary) or (2) as *secondary* atrophy (postneuritic or secondary inflammatory atrophy). In simple atrophy, there is degeneration of the nerve fibers; in secondary atrophy, resulting from a previous inflammation or edema, this degeneration is accompanied by proliferation of connective tissue upon the nervehead.

Symptoms. There are *reduction* in the acuteness of *vision*, concentric *contraction* (Fig. 11-7) or irregular or sector-shaped peripheral defects *of the field*, first for colors and then for form, rarely scotomas, diminution in the light sense and *color*

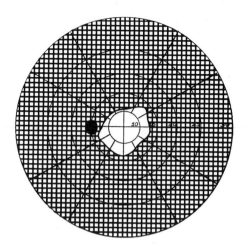

FIG. 11-7. Bjerrum screen visual field, showing severe generalized contraction resulting from optic nerve atrophy.

blindness (first for green, then for red, then for blue). The behavior of the pupils depends upon the degree of atrophy; when the latter is complete, the pupils are dilated and immobile. These symptoms tend to *progress* and end in complete *blindness*.

Ophthalmoscopic Signs depend upon whether the type is simple (primary) or secondary.

Simple atrophy (Plate 30A). The *disk* is *white*, grayish or bluish white, its edges are *sharply defined* and regular, its size is somewhat diminished, and it presents a saucer-shaped excavation (Fig. 15-3, *center*); the *lamina cribrosa* often is seen very *plainly*; the minute vessels of the disk have disappeared; the surrounding retina has its usual appearance; the retinal vessels often appear normal, but the arteries usually are diminished in caliber.

Secondary atrophy (Plate 30B). The *disk* is *dense white* or grayish in color, its margins *irregular* and somewhat *hazy*, its minute vessels lost, and it is *covered by connective tissue* resulting from the preceding inflammation or edema; on this account the lamina cribrosa is hidden; the retinal arteries are narrow, the *veins* normal in size or contracted and generally *tortuous,* and both sets are apt to be enclosed by *white lines.*

Retinitic and choroiditic atrophy.

The disk has a grayish red or yellow, waxy appearance, its outlines are somewhat indistinct, the vessels are exceedingly narrow and many disappear entirely, and the retina presents evidences of the antecedent choroiditis or retinitis.

It should be borne in mind that the *disk varies in color in health* and may appear atrophied as the result of congenital or senile peculiarities, although vision is normal and the field perfect; hence the diagnosis of simple optic nerve atrophy cannot be made, in some cases, from the ophthalmoscopic signs alone, especially when these signs are not definite.

Etiology. *Simple atrophy* frequently is due to cerebrospinal diseases, especially tabes, developing as an early symptom in one-third of the cases of this affection. It is common also in multiple sclerosis and general paralysis of the insane; when it occurs in multiple sclerosis, it follows retrobulbar neuritis and rarely results in complete blindness. It also may be due to systemic syphilis, malaria, diabetes, acromegaly, oxycephaly, excessive hemorrhage, arteriosclerosis and certain poisons (including wood alcohol, lead and arsenic). It is seen with pigmentary degeneration of the retina, and embolism and thrombosis of the central artery; it also may be consecutive to choroiditis, retinitis, glaucoma, pituitary tumor, aneurysm of the internal carotid and orbital inflammations. It may result from injury to the optic nerve caused by fracture of the orbital canal or hemorrhage into the sheath of the nerve, following a blow or other violence; in such cases the atrophy does not show itself for a number of weeks, though reduction of

vision and contraction of the field or even blindness ensue immediately. In some cases *no cause* can be found. Occasionally it is hereditary (Leber's disease).

Secondary atrophy follows papilledema, optic neuritis and tumors of the optic nerve.

Pathology. The process consists of increase in the interstitial connective tissue with atrophy and disappearance of the nerve fibers and the medullary sheaths. In the secondary form there is proliferated glial tissue on the nervehead.

Course and Prognosis. Simple atrophy occurs chiefly in *middle life;* the course is *slow,* extending over many months, and the prognosis is *unfavorable,* the condition usually progressing to absolute blindness. In *secondary* atrophy the prognosis is *better,* and depends upon the extent to which the optic nerve has escaped from the destructive influences of the preceding processes.

Treatment consists in attempting to control the *cause.* For the atrophy itself very little can be done. Atrophy of the optic nerve is considered a contraindication to the use of tryparsamide in central nervous system syphilis. However, the subdural treatment of the early stage of syphilitic optic nerve atrophy with arsphenaminized serum, neoarsphenamine or bichloride of mercury dissolved in salt solution, or spinal fluid or mercurialized serum, injected intraspinally or intracisternally, has been found of some value, and the results of such treatment have been fairly encouraging. Fever therapy, by artificially induced malaria or by mechanical means, has given rather encouraging results in some cases, especially those due to syphilis.

Tumors of the Optic Nerve are rare, being derived from the nerve sheaths (meningioma, "endothelioma") and from the glial framework (glioma). They produce early loss of vision and proptosis.

Treatment consists in removal of the growth by lateral canthal exploration of the orbit or by the Krönlein operation. This condition is unilateral, and must be distinguished from orbital inflammatory processes and other causes of unilateral exophthalmos.

Hemianopsia

Connection between the Retinae, the Fibers of the Optic Nerves and Tracts and the Cerebral Cortex (Figs. 9-1 and 11-8; Plate 32). Familiarity with the course of the optic nerve fibers from the eye to the cortex is of great practical value in the localization of various lesions causing defects in the field of vision.

The *optic nerves* terminate at the *chiasm*, which lies in the optic groove on the body of the sphenoid bone, in front of the infundibulum and above the hypophysis; here they *semidecussate*; from the chiasm they are continued backward as the optic tracts which wind around the crura cerebri to the *primary optic ganglia* —the external geniculate body, the anterior corpus quadrigeminum and the pulvinar of the thalamus opticus (*POG*, Figs. 9-1 and 11-8). Here the fibers divide into two portions: (1) a smaller part passing to the *nuclei of the oculomotorius* and presiding over the reflex action of the pupils and the movement of the ocular muscles and (2) a larger bundle, composed of visual fibers, transferring its impulses (Fig 9-1) to other fibers which carry the *visual impressions* to the cortex; the latter fibers pass through the posterior portion of the internal capsule, then form the *optic radiations* or fibers of Gratiolet, and end in the cortical ganglion cells of the mesial surface of the cuneus and the parts surrounding the *calcarine fissure;* this portion of the occipital lobe is known as the visual *area of the cortex* (*O*, Fig. 11-8).

In the ganglion cells of the visual area, an excitation in the optic nerve fibers is

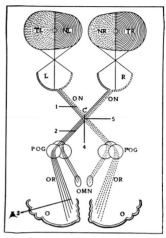

Fig. 11-8. Schematic representation of the visual paths. *L*, left eye; *R*, right eye; *TL*, temporal field of Left eye; *NL*, nasal field of left eye; *NR*, nasal field of right eye; *TR*, temporal field of right eye; *ON*, optic nerve; *C*, chiasm; *POG*, primary optic ganglia; *OMN*, oculomotor nuclei; *O*, occipital lobe; *OR*, optic radiations. Division of fibers at *1* causes complete blindness of the left eye and loss of direct pupillary reaction; at *2*, right homonymous hemianopsia with loss of reaction of the pupil when the left halves of the retinae are illuminated; at *3*, right homonymous hemianopsia with preservation of the reaction of the pupil when the left (and right) halves of the retinae are illuminated; at *4*, bitemporal hemianopsia; at *5*, right nasal field loss.

changed into a sensory perception (sight) or into permanent changes (memories, optical memory pictures). After destruction of this area, excitation of the optic nerve fibers either fails to arouse visual sensation of any kind (*blindness*) or fails to summon forth any recollection of objects or circumstances acquired through previous education; in the latter case, objects are seen but not recognized (*psychical blindness*).

Each retina is supplied by optic nerve fibers passing to *both sides of the brain.* Each *optic nerve* is composed of an *ex-*

ternal set of fibers, derived from the outer or temporal half of the retina, and an *internal* set, derived from the inner or nasal half of the retina. In the axis of the optic nerve is found a special set of fibers which pass to the *macula* and the space between it and the disk. These macular fibers, when they reach the eyeball, are collected into a sector corresponding to the outer third of the disk, the apex directed toward the center and the base toward the margin of the papilla. The *external* or temporal fibers are continued along the lateral part of the chiasm and tract and pass to the primary optic center of the *same side*. The *inner* fibers, derived from the nasal half of the retina, pass into the chiasm and *decussate;* they are continued in the tract of the *opposite side,* thus passing to the side of the brain opposite to the eye which they supply.

The *chiasm* presents laterally the direct or temporal fibers of both eyes, and, in its center, the decussation of the inner or nasal fibers of both retinae. Consequently, the decussation in the chiasm is not complete but partial—a semidecussation.

Each optic tract contains fibers from both eyes. The right optic tract consists of nondecussating fibers from the right (temporal) half of the retina of the right eye, and decussating fibers from the right (nasal) half of the left eye. Hence the *right halves of both retinae* and thus the *left halves of both visual fields* are connected with the *right tract* (Plate 32). It follows, therefore, that the visual impulse excited by objects placed to the left of the median line passes to the cortex of the right hemisphere by means of the right optic tract, and that the perception of all objects placed to the right of the median line is conveyed by the left optic tract to the cortex of the left hemisphere.

Hemianopsia. This arrangement of fibers in the chiasm explains the occurrence of a form of visual disturbance known as hemianopsia (hemianopia, hemiopia), by which is meant the loss of vision for *corresponding halves or sectors of the visual fields.* If a lesion interrupts the continuity of the right optic tract, the right cortical visual area or any portion of the visual path between these parts, there will be blindness of the right halves of both retinae; as a result, the left halves of the fields of vision of both eyes will be lost, and only objects which are placed to the right of the median line will be perceived. This is known as *homonymous* or lateral *hemianopsia,* and in this particular case the condition is called left homonymous hemiopia, because the left halves of the fields of vision are wanting. Homonymous hemianopsia (Fig. 11-9), therefore, always points to a lesion situated in the visual

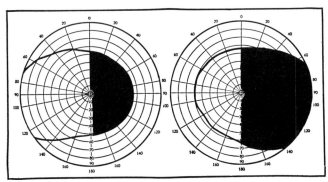

Fɪɢ. 11-9. The fields of vision in right homonymous hemianopsia.

path or cortex on the *central side of the chiasm* and upon the *same side as the blind halves of the retinae*. It is the most common form of hemianopsia.

If a lesion extends anteroposteriorly through the chiasm, or presses upon these fibers, it will destroy the decussating fibers supplying the inner or nasal halves of both retinae; there will be loss of vision in the outer or temporal halves of the field of both eyes; this is *bitemporal hemianopsia* (*4*, Fig. 11-8). It is seen often in pituitary body disease.

If a lesion attacks each side of the chiasm, it will destroy the nondecussating fibers which come from the temporal halves of the retinae, and therefore will cause a loss of the nasal or inner half of the field of vision of each eye; this is known as *binasal hemianopsia*. Bitemporal and binasal hemianopsia are known as *crossed hemianopsia*. Binasal hemianopsia occurs very rarely; another rare form of hemianopsia is altitudinal (inferior or superior), when the upper or the lower half of each field is wanting.

Hemianopsia is said to be *complete* when there is a symmetrical absence of the *entire half* of the field of vision. It is *incomplete* when there is an absence of a *small portion* or *sector* occupying a symmetrical portion in the visual fields of the two eyes; the lesion then involves only a portion of the fibers of a visual tract or cortical visual area.

Even in cases of complete hemianopsia, the line between the absent and the preserved portion of the field seldom extends through the fixation point, the portion of the field corresponding to the *macula* being usually preserved. In the rare instances in which both halves of the fields are lost successively (double homonymous hemianopsia), there will be blindness except at the situation of these macular fibers; this occurrence has been explained by supposing (1) that each macula is represented in both hemispheres and (2) that the cortical center for the macula receives a special and abundant blood supply both from the posterior calcarine and from the middle cerebral artery.

Hemianopsia is known as *absolute* when there is loss of light, form and color sense, and *relative* when only the color sense is destroyed over the symmetrically defective areas. When the hemianopic defect is present for colors alone, the condition is known as *hemiachromatopsia*; it is believed to point to a lesion of less intensity than that which causes absolute hemianopsia.

Complete blindness in one eye only always is due to a lesion situated *in front of the chiasm*. The same applies to *scotomas*, which are defects in the visual field of one eye or nonsymmetrical defects in the fields of both eyes; when central, they indicate an involvement of the papillomacular sector of the optic nerve.

The Hemiopic Pupillary Reaction (Wernicke) is of value in determining whether a lesion causing homonymous hemianopsia is situated *behind* or in *front* of the *primary optic ganglia*. Light is thrown into the eye obliquely so as to illuminate one or the other side of the retina. If the lesion is back of the ganglia, the pupillary light reflex will be preserved whether the blind or the seeing half of the retina is lighted up; if in front of these ganglia (in the optic tract), the pupil will respond when light falls upon the seeing half of the retina, but there will be no contraction or only a feeble reaction when the blind half of the retina is illuminated (Fig. 9-1). This test is difficult to make conclusively.

Scintillating Scotoma (*transient hemianopsia*) is a form of temporary blindness generally associated with *migraine* and probably due to a circulatory disturbance in the occipital lobe. Food allergy may be a cause. The attack begins with a central *dark spot* before both eyes, which spreads by *scintillating* and colored zig-zag lines until there is a considerable *gap in the field*, often assuming the form of homonymous hemianopsia. Accompanying the attack are *headache*, general malaise, vertigo and sometimes nausea and vomiting. The attacks vary in frequency and last about 15 minutes, after which the amblyopia disappears entirely. The attacks may occur after excessive mental or physical exertion or follow severe ocular fatigue. Unless associated with paralysis, aphasia or other symptoms of cerebral trouble, the affection has no importance. Treatment consists in attention to the general health, correction of refractive errors, avoidance of fatigue of any kind, the use of remedies suited to migraine and antiallergic measures.

12

The Lens

Embryology, Anatomy and Physiology

The *crystalline lens* develops in the embryo from an invagination of thickened ectoderm covering each optic vesicle. Originally a hollow sphere of epithelial cells, its posterior cells elongate into lens fibers which soon fill the lens vesicle and form the *embryonic nucleus*. The anterior cells form a layer of cuboidal epithelium. Lens fibers develop from the cells at the equator; they lengthen and are pushed into the interior by later-forming fibers. The lens capsule forms as a secretion from the epithelial cells. The process of formation of lens fibers continues throughout life, at a progressively slower rate. Where the fibers come in contact anteriorly and posteriorly with the fibers from the opposite side, visible *suture lines* are formed. As aging takes place, the central portion of the lens is more and more compressed by the continuous growth of lens fibers surrounding it; in this process, known as *sclerosis* of the lens, there is a loss of water and an increase in density.

The *crystalline lens* is a *transparent* body, *biconvex* in shape, measuring 5 mm. in thickness and 9 mm. in diameter in the adult, suspended in the anterior portion of the eyeball between the aqueous and the vitreous chambers. It presents an anterior and a posterior surface, the latter being the more curved; an anterior pole, a posterior pole; and a rounded circumference, the equator. It is devoid of blood vessels except in fetal life, its nourishment being derived from the intraocular fluids. It is enclosed in a transparent *capsule*, and held in position by its *suspensory ligament*. The adult lens consists of a peripheral portion, the *cortex*, and a central part, the *nucleus*. The cortex is semisolid, softer than the nucleus and colorless; the nucleus is harder and has a yellowish tint; there is, however, no sharp limitation, the transition being gradual. The nucleus increases in size with advancing years, and the cortex diminishes in proportion; in old age the entire lens is of the consistency of the nucleus and is hard and unyielding.

In *structure* the lens consists of concentric *lamellae* formed of long, *hexagonal fibers*, the edges connected by cement substance. The fibers either start or end along *Y-shaped or stellate figures*, the lines of which radiate from the anterior and posterior pole to the equator. These figures can be seen in the adult lens, the Y erect anteriorly and inverted posteriorly, with slit lamp examination.

The *capsule of the lens* is a thin, homogeneous, elastic membrane which covers the lens, being known as the anterior capsule in front and as the posterior capsule behind. The anterior capsule is the thicker, and its posterior surface is lined by a layer of cuboidal epithelium.

The *suspensory ligament of the lens* (zonular fibers) is a delicate bundle of fibers, extending from the ciliary body to the equatorial region of the lens capsule.

The *function* of the lens is to *focus rays* so that they form a perfect image on the retina. To accomplish this, the refractive power of the lens must change with the distance of the object, according to whether the rays are parallel or divergent.

This alteration in the refractive power of the lens is known as *accommodation,* and is produced by a change of shape mainly affecting its anterior curvature.

The lens presents variations in physical characteristics at different periods of life. *In the fetus,* it is nearly spherical and softer than at a later period. *In the adult,* its anterior surface is less convex than the posterior, and its substance is firmer. *Sclerosis* begins in the center of the lens in childhood and advances slowly until adult life, after which its progess is more rapid, increasing the size of the nucleus at the expense of the cortex. *In old age,* the lens increases in size, is flattened and assumes a *yellow* tinge, becoming tougher and less transparent; this process of sclerosis accounts for the *gray reflex* seen in the pupil of the aged, which may be mistaken for cataract (*senile reflex*); it also explains the inability on the part of the lens of advanced years to change its shape for the purposes of accommodation (*presbyopia*).

Congenital and Developmental Anomalies of the Lens

Absence of the lens or congenital aphakia is extremely rare and probably occurs only in association with anomalies that occur quite early in fetal life and therefore involve extensive anomalies of the eye. *Failure of separation of the lens vesicle* from the ectoderm or from the posterior surface of the cornea also is rare but has been observed. *Microphakia,* or small lens, which usually is spherical in shape, *spherophakia,* and frequently is ectopic, occurs as a hereditary defect frequently in association with other anomalies, especially brachydactylia (Marchesani's syndrome).

Ectopia lentis, an asymmetric defect in the zonule resulting in displacement or partial dislocation of the lens, frequently bilateral, is hereditary and familial and frequently associated with other deformities such as dwarfism, other skeletal anomalies and especially arachnodactyly (Marfan's syndrome). *Coloboma* of the lens usually is found inferiorly as a notching defect of the lens border in association with deficient zonule in this location, and frequently is associated with coloboma of the iris, ciliary body and choroid. *Anterior lenticonus* is a rare anomaly in which a conical or spherical projection of the anterior surface occurs; usually it consists of clear cortex but eventually may develop into an anterior polar cataract. *Posterior lenticonus* or, more correctly, posterior lentiglobus is a prominent spherical projection of the posterior surface of the lens and occurs more commonly than anterior lenticonus, producing a refractive type of high myopia. Congenital cataract, which may take any of a variety of types, is the most common congenital anomaly (see below).

CATARACT

A cataract is any *opacity of the lens* which affects the cortex or nucleus. The capsule of the lens never becomes opaque.

Varieties and Classification. Cataracts may be classified under two main divisions:

Developmental cataracts, in which the normal development of the lens fibers and epithelium has been affected during growth by hereditary, nutritional or inflammatory changes, with consequent loss of transparency. This group includes the congenital forms of anterior (Fig. 12-1) and posterior polar cataracts, central cataract, zonular (lamellar) cataract, coronary and punctate cataracts and complete congenital and juvenile cataracts.

Degenerative cataracts, in which normally developed lens substance loses its transparency as a result of degenerative changes from various causes. In this group are placed senile nuclear and cortical cataracts, radiation cataract, lightning, electric and heat ray

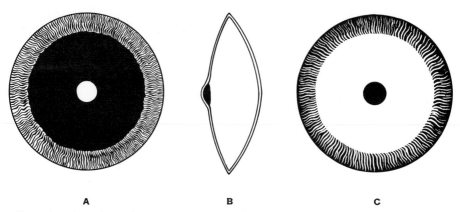

FIG. 12-1. Anterior polar cataract as seen by direct or oblique illumination (*A*), on schematic cross section of the lens (*B*), and by retroillumination with the ophthalmoscope or retinoscope (*C*).

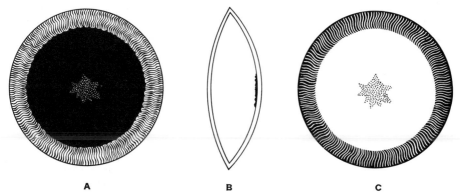

FIG. 12-2. Complicated cataract (posterior subcapsular cataract) as seen by direct illumination (*left*), on cross section of the lens (*center*) and by indirect illumination (*right*).

cataracts, complicated cataract, cataract associated with systemic disease or poisoning and traumatic cataract.

Cataracts also can be grouped *anatomically*, according to the part of the lens involved, into anterior or posterior subcapsular (Fig. 12-2), cortical or nuclear. They also can be divided into progressive and stationary cataracts; or, according to consistency, into hard, soft and fluid cataracts; or into partial or complete cataracts.

Symptoms. There is (1) *diminished acuteness of vision*, depending upon the situation and extent of the cataract, greatest when central or axial and diffuse, least when peripheral. When central, vision is best in dim light—with dilated pupil. Reduction in vision increases with the progress of the cataract, until finally there is mere perception of light. (2) In the incipient stage, the patient may complain of seeing *spots* which occupy a fixed position in the field. (3) Occasionally there is annoying diplopia or polyopia, due to irregular refraction of the lens. (4) Myopia often develops in the early stages because of increased refractive power of the lens;

the patient then may be able to discard his reading glasses and his vision for distance may be improved with concave lenses.

Physical Signs. There are no inflammatory symptoms except with complicated cataracts resulting from intraocular disease. Examination by oblique illumination shows a *grayish* or whitish *opacity* on a black ground, and with a low plus lens in the *ophthalmoscope* held at a distance from the eye, a *black opacity* upon a red field (Plate 2). The pupil should be *dilated*, and the position and extent of the lens opacity studied with the slit lamp and biomicroscope. If the cataract is progressive, the lens opacities increase in size and extent; later, the entire pupil appears *grayish*, and there is an *absence of fundus reflex*. If there is *swelling of the cataract* (intumescent stage) the anterior chamber is reduced in depth, and glaucoma may occur in predisposed eyes.

Treatment. In general, *operation* is the only method for improving the vision of an eye with cataract of the progressive type. The need for operation depends upon the vision of the better-seeing eye, the visual acuity required by the patient for his work or comfort and the presence or absence of intraocular complications.

Vision of an eye with cataract in the early stages often can be made adequate by careful correction with *lenses,* or by the use of *tinted lenses* in patients with central or nuclear cataracts of moderate extent. *Advanced age* is not a contraindication to a needed cataract operation; nor is *diabetes* which is under medical control. In cases of *unilateral* cataract, the question of operation must be carefully considered, since every surgical procedure is attended with a small risk. Removal of a unilateral cataract for cosmetic reasons often is justified, especially in young persons, but the patients must be told that binocular vision is impossible even when

the aphakic eye has normal vision with correcting lenses in ordinary glasses. However, contact lenses, if tolerated by the individual, may restore binocularity.

The type of operation needed for removal of a cataract depends upon the *consistency* of the cataract, the *age* of the patient and the presence of intraocular complications such as posterior synechia.

In patients *under* 25, all cataracts, except those which have become calcified, are of *soft* consistency throughout and of a grayish white color; such cataracts have no hard nucleus and are known as *soft cataracts*. After this period the nucleus becomes hard and of a *yellowish* tint, and the lens opacity is known as *hard cataract*.

It is unwise to operate upon eyes with *active uveitis* or iridocyclitis, or upon eyes which have not been free of inflammation for at least 6 months.

Details of treatment will be discussed under the various types of cataracts.

Prognosis as to the result of operation for cataract depends upon the condition of the macular region and upon the presence or absence of a complicating ocular disease such as glaucoma, detachment of the retina, pigmentary degeneration of the retina or previously existing amblyopia.

Congenital and Developmental Cataracts

Anterior Polar Cataract (pyramidal or anterior capsular cataract). This partial and stationary lenticular opacity occurs in the form of a small, round, white opacity, often pyramidal in shape, situated at the *anterior pole* of the lens, beneath the capsule (Fig. 12-1). It may be *congenital* or *acquired*. The acquired form originates from an ulcer of the cornea in early childhood; such an ulcer perforates and allows contact and pressure between lens and cornea, setting up an irritation which results in a proliferation of the subcapsular

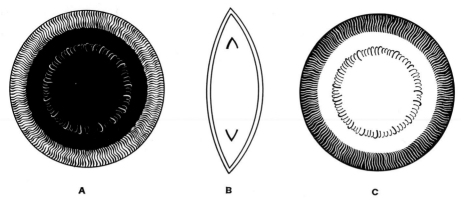

FIG. 12-3. Zonular cataract as seen by direct illumination (*left*), on cross section of the lens (*center*) and by direct illumination (*right*).

epithelium. Afterward the anterior chamber is restored; sometimes there is an accompanying corneal opacity. As a rule this form of cataract causes little if any reduction in vision.

Posterior Polar Cataract is a *congenital* form of *capsular opacity*, consisting of a small, round, white deposit, situated at the posterior pole. It causes but trifling interference with vision and requires no treatment.

Zonular (Lamellar) Cataract (Fig. 12-3). This variety of *partial,* stationary cataract is either *congenital* or forms in *infancy,* and usually affects *both eyes.* It is the most common form of cataract seen in children. It is sometimes hereditary, and often associated with a history of convulsions and with the changes of rickets, especially in the teeth, cranial and other bones. It may occur alone or frequently in combination with a nuclear cataract. It consists of a gray disk-like opacity in a layer of cortex outside the nucleus and separated from the nucleus by a clear layer of cortex and with clear cortex between the opacity and capsule of the lens. When the pupil is dilated, examination by oblique illumination shows a *grayish disk surrounded by clear lens substance;* from the margin of the opacity

short striae (called riders) are seen projecting into the surrounding transparent cortex. The cataract is most dense at the margin of the disk; this distinguishes it from nuclear cataract. A dark disk with radiating short spoke-like striae extending into the center is seen on an orange-red fundus reflex by indirect illumination.

Lamellar cataract usually remains stationary, but occasionally may show several of the diskiform opacities separated by clear layers of cortex and rarely may progress to complete opacification of the cortex and complete cataract. It causes *interference with vision;* the amount may be slight or decided, depending upon the density of the opacity.

Treatment. When sight is considerably affected, as is usually the case, iridectomy may improve visual function. *Iridectomy* (small coloboma downward and inward) is indicated when the vision is materially improved after the use of a mydriatic and correction of any existing error of refraction; this presupposes that the child is old enough to respond to tests of vision. This operation, if applicable, has the advantage of retaining the lens and accommodation, and the avoidance of the wearing of strong convex lenses. As a rule, however, the patient is brought for examination during infancy, and the opacity is found so dense that it is considered unlikely that an optical iridectomy later will answer; then discission is necessary but must be repeated in many cases; the first needling is done as soon as the infant is 6 months old, so that vision will not suffer from disuse.

Central cataract (nuclear cataract, cataracta centralis pulverulenta, Fig. 12-4) is a rare stationary congenital or familial cataract affecting the embryonic nucleus as a granular or uniform opacity. Occasionally the center of the nucleus may remain clear with a diskiform opacity in the outer portion. Any of these varieties may occur in association with zonular cataract. More common and less extensive opacities occur familially and in *anterior axial cataract,* which consists of stationary minute white dots in the neighborhood and posterior to the anterior Y suture; they do not affect visual function and occur in 20 to 30 per cent of children; or in *floriform cataract,* which consists of independent or grouped annular or petal-like opacities in the axial portion of the nucleus near the anterior and posterior Y sutures, some-

times in the neighboring cortex. *Axial fusiform cataract* is a central nuclear opacity which is prolonged anteriorly and posteriorly to the poles subcapsularly, producing a spindle-shaped opacity in the axis of the lens. *Coralliform cataract* is a more complex form of axial opacity of hereditary developmental origin. Round or elongated spokes radiate outward from the axial opacity in the center of the lens but never reach the capsule. A variation of this form has been described as a spear cataract. *Sutural or stellate cataract* is a congential opacity involving the Y-shaped sutures. It may be a dense opacity or feathery, or composed of numerous fine distinct dots.

Coronary cataract of Vogt, a common developmental cataract which affects approximately one-fourth of all individuals to at least a minor degree, is characterized by the occurrence of club-shaped opacities arranged radially in a zone in the outer layers of the adult nucleus and the inner layers of the cortex, mixed with punctiform, ring-shaped and small disklike opacities, leaving the central and peripheral portions of the lens clear. The opacities vary in color from gray to brown, yellow, red or blue. Frequently coronary cataract is associated with other types of congenital, developmental or acquired cataract. Because of its position, coronary cataract usually is covered by the iris, does not interfere with vision and is discovered only after wide dilatation of the pupil. It usually remains stationary but occasionally may become progressive either around puberty or in the third decade of life.

Punctate cataract consists of variable numbers of punctiform opacities scattered irregularly through the nucleus and cortex, and may be either congenital or developmental. They occur so frequently that at least a few may be found on careful biomicroscopic examination of al-

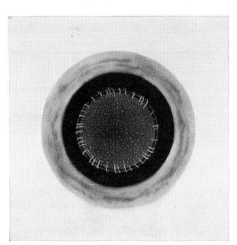

FIG. 12-4. Zonular cataract and congenital nuclear cataract.

most any lens. Occasionally the dots appear to be bright light blue and therefore this type has been called *caerulean cataract* and is frequently found in association with coronary cataract.

Galactosemia Cataract

Bilateral cataracts may develop in infants who have the congenital, hereditary anomaly of lactose metabolism called galactosemia. These infants are normal at birth but develop vomiting, diarrhea and fail to gain weight unless all sources of galactose (milk, etc.) are excluded from the feeding. The lens is clear at birth then the nucleus or central portion of the lens becomes visible as a transparent lens within the lens. At this stage correction of the diet will reverse the process but later an irreversible zonular cataract may develop. Then surgical correction is necessary and is satisfactory.

Down's Syndrome (Mongolism)

Cataract occurs in approximately 50 per cent of patients with mongolism (trisomy 21) in the first or during the second decade of life. The lens changes develop as a layer of punctate powdery or fine flaky opacities which are numerous in the axial portion of the lens and may have a stellate arrangement posteriorly. Other ocular anomalies include nystagmus, high myopia, hypertelorism (widely spaced eyes), narrow downward and inward slanting palpebral fissures and epicanthus.

Cretinism

In cretinism a layer of flaky opacities mixed with iridescent crystals develops in the superficial cortex but seldom progresses to cause interference with visual function.

Lowe's Syndrome

Nuclear, posterior polar or complete cataracts have been observed at birth in males in association with dwarfism due to a congential defect of reabsorption in the renal tubules causing aminoaciduria. In addition there may be nystagmus and glaucoma at times. In addition to physical retardation these children are mentally retarded and frequently die young.

Other Developmental Cataracts

Cataracts of various types, lamellar, nuclear, posterior subcapsular, sutural or peripheral occur as part of the developmental anomalies of a number of syndromes such as: Apert's acrocephalosyndactylism syndrome, Block-Sulzberger's incontinentia pigmenti syndrome, Cockayne's syndrome, Crouzon's dysostosis craniofacialis, oxycephaly syndrome, Marincesco-Sjögren syndrome, and Rothmund's teleangiectasia-pigmentation cataract syndrome.

Rubella Cataract

Cataract is one of the numerous developmental defects which may result from rubella of the pregnant mother especially if the infection occurs during the first trimester of pregnancy. The lens may show a dense white opacity of the embryonal and fetal nuclei or the lens may be completely opaque. Both lenses are affected in 75 per cent of patients. The pupil dilates poorly if at all. Associated ocular anomalies include corneal opacities, strabismus, nystagmus, retinal pigmentation, microphthalmus, and infantile glaucoma. Results of surgical treatment of rubella cataracts have not been satisfactory.

Congenital complete and juvenile complete cataracts are rather infrequent. The lens is uniformly *white*, bluish white or pearly, and always *soft*, sometimes fluid and milky. These cataracts may occur in otherwise perfectly healthy eyes, or they may be complicated cataracts, with changes in the retina, choroid or optic nerve. One or both eyes are affected. The *congenital* complete cataract is due to a disturbance of development or intrauterine ocular inflammation. The complete cataract of young people (*juvenile*) may be hereditary, or arise without known cause; in some cases there is a history of convulsions, and at times it may be the result of uncontrolled diabetes mellitus.

Treatment consists in *discission* (needling) at an early age, so that disuse of sight may not cause amblyopia. Needling sometimes must be repeated. Some surgeons prefer *linear extraction* with injection of air into the anterior chamber as a primary procedure. Semifluid cataracts are removed by linear extraction. Recently an aspiration technique has found increasing favor for infantile and juvenile cataract. After the capsule is opened, the cortex is aspirated through a specially designed 18-gauge needle. Irrigation may be combined with the aspiration.

Senile and Degenerative Cataracts

Senile cataract is the most *frequent* form of cataract. It is quite common after the 50th year; occasionally it is seen as early as 40. Almost always *both eyes* are involved, but generally one in advance of the other. The opacity may begin either in the superficial part of the cortex (*cortical*, Fig. 12-5; Plate 2*E* and *F*) or in the part immediately surrounding the nucleus (*nuclear*, Fig. 12-6; Plate 2*G* and *H*). More often, senile cataracts begin in the *cortex* and the nucleus remains transparent. The time required for *full development varies* from a few months to many years; it may become stationary at any stage. The reaction of the pupil to light is not affected.

The Stages of Sensile Cataract are four in number:

(1) *Incipient stage.* The opacity most frequently begins as *streaks* which extend *from the periphery* of the cortex, where they are wider, to the center of the lens, where they narrow like the spokes of a wheel (Fig. 12-5); the periphery is affected first. These streaks appear grayish by illumination, and black when seen by indirect illumination or light reflected from the interior of the eye. Between these sectors, the lens is transparent. Less frequently, senile cataract begins with dot-like or cloud-like opacities situated in any

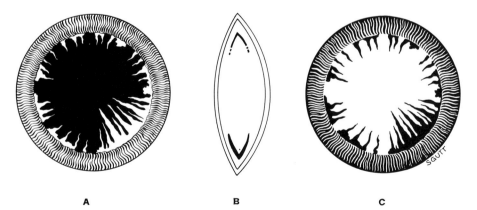

       A   **B**   **C**

Fig. 12-5. Senile cortical cataract, showing large opacities, as are usually found, in inferior nasal quadrant, as seen by direct illumination (*A*), on cross section of the lens (*B*) and by indirect illumination (*C*).

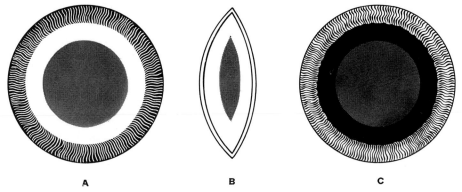

A   **B**   **C**

Fig. 12-6 Senile nuclear cataract as seen by direct illumination (*left*), on cross section of the lens (*center*) and by direct illumination (*right*).

portion of the lens; sometimes the portion immediately surrounding the cortex becomes opaque. The nucleus itself may become denser or opaque (*nuclear cataract,* Fig. 12-6); this form often is spoken of as lenticular or nuclear *sclerosis*; it causes relatively great visual disturbance. Cataracts often remain *stationary* in the incipient stage, with little or no impairment of vision, and the lenticular opacity is discovered when using direct or indirect illumination with the ophthalmoscope in the course of examination of the eyes for glasses. Hence it is a question whether the existence of incipient opacities should be revealed to the patient; it may be better not to alarm him but to wait until, at some future date, the lens changes give evidence of progression and the patient notices some reduction in visual function.

(2) The stage of swelling (intumescent stage). The lens absorbs fluid, swells, pushes the iris forward and *reduces* the *depth of the anterior chamber.* It appears bluish white, shining, and presents distinctly the markings of the stellate figure. During this stage, the *iris casts a shadow upon the lens* when the eye is illuminated from the side, since the superficial portion of the lens is still transparent, and hence the opaque layer is

some distance behind the iris. Some senile cataracts, especially those of the nuclear sclerosis type, do not pass through this stage but directly into the mature stage.

(3) Mature stage. The lens loses its excess fluid, shrinks somewhat and becomes perfectly *opaque* and of a dull *gray or amber color,* the stellate markings still being recognizable. The *anterior chamber* regains its *normal* depth, and there is *no shadow* thrown by the iris on the lens with focal illumination. In the mature stage, the cataract can be separated easily from the capsule of the lens; it is then said to be *"ripe"* for operation, since extracapsular extraction can be made without leaving much if any of the cortex behind, thus diminishing the chances of subsequent opacity (after-cataract).

The mature stage of nuclear sclerosis is a completely opaque dark brown opacity of the lens known as *cataracta brunescens* or later as "black cataract."

(4) Hypermature stage. The cataract may continue in the mature stage for a long time. If changes continue, the surface of the lens loses its radial markings and becomes *homogeneous,* or presents irregular spots. The cataract may continue to lose water, and thus a dry, flattened mass results (*shrunken cataract*), with deepening of the anterior chamber. Or, the cortex may become soft, liquid and milky, and the nucleus sink to the bottom of this fluid (*Morgagnian cataract*), the cataract appearing white with brownish coloring below or when the head is bent forward and the nucleus floats down on the capsule in the pupillary area. Very old hypermature cataracts often present the deposit of *cholesterin* or of *lime* salts; the latter change (*chalky cataract*) is found chiefly in complicated cataracts. The lens (and iris) may become *tremulous* through stretching of the suspensory ligament. For these reasons, operation upon hypermature cataract is less favorable and more difficult than it is with mature cataract.

Pathology. At first there is separation of the lens fibers with formation of drops of fluid in spaces thus created (*Morgagnian spherules*); then the fibers swell, become vacuolated and cloudy, of uneven caliber, and disintegrate. Finally the cortical lens tissue is changed into a soft mass consisting of spheres of Morgagni, remains of lens fibers and albuminous liquid; this mass separates from the capsule. The *nucleus* usually suffers no change except sclerosis.

Treatment. *Extraction* of the cataract by operation is the only means of relief. *Discission* and *linear extraction* are applicable only to cataracts in young persons. There is no evidence that any remedy, local or systemic, is effective in curing cataract or altering its course of development, but it must be remembered that many examples of incipient cataract never advance beyond this stage although nothing is done.

In the incipient stage the eyes should be examined periodically, *errors of refraction* corrected and systemic derangements and *neighboring ocular disease* treated. When the opacity is central, sight may be improved by keeping the pupil dilated with weak solutions of *mydriatics*

(if no tendency to glaucoma exists), thus permitting vision through the peripheral, transparent portion of the lens. *Smoked glasses* accomplish this to a certain extent.

The *favorable time for extraction* of senile cataract is when the vision of the better-seeing eye has failed enough to interfere with the patient's normal daily activities and comfort. It is not necessary to wait until the cataract is mature. *Monocular cataract*, with good vision in the other eye, generally is not removed, since the difference in refraction between the two eyes will not permit them to work together with ordinary correcting lenses in glasses, but some individuals who can tolerate contact lenses may obtain binocular visual function with them after unilateral cataract extraction. Removal of both cataracts should never be performed at one sitting.

Radiation Cataract is a slowly developing form, beginning peripherally and progressing centrally in the *posterior cortex* between 6 months and 2 years after exposure to *radium or roentgen rays*. Some persons appear to be more susceptible to radiation than others. The cataract which develops is characterized by subcapsular proliferation of epithelium into a fibrous plaque; this fact makes intracapsular cataract operation ideal for its removal.

Lightning, Electric and Heat Ray Cataracts. Persons struck by lightning or shocked by a high voltage electric current may develop bilateral lens opacities beginning peripherally and progressing centrally in the posterior and anterior cortex of the lens. These opacities become visible more rapidly than those of radiation cataract. Operation is indicated, by linear extraction in young individuals and combined extraction in persons over 35 years of age. Long-continued exposure to high temperatures in the glass-blowing and iron-puddling industries may give rise to slowly progressing posterior cortical lens opacities which require the same treatment.

Complicated Cataract accompanies or follows *other diseases of the eye.* The most frequent ocular affections which lead to cataract are iridocyclitis, choroiditis, uveitis, high myopia, severe forms of corneal ulcers, glaucoma, retinitis pigmentosa, detachment of the retina and intraocular tumors. Such cataracts usually begin in the center of the *posterior* part of the lens (Fig 12-2) and later spread so as to involve the whole cortex; at a still later period they tend to *degenerate* and shrink; the capsule thickens and often becomes calcified, and there is tremulousness of the iris. Sometimes a complicated cataract begins with scattered opacities, which later coalesce so that the entire lens becomes opaque. It is important to establish that a cataract is complicated when the question of operation presents itself. The *treatment* of complicated cataracts must be directed to the cause of the complication but usually is very unsatisfactory and the prognosis always is much less favorable than in uncomplicated cases. This is because the complicating ocular disease renders the operation difficult and associates it with risk, and the effect on sight may be disappointing; many cases cannot be operated upon; in others extraction may be made merely for the cosmetic gain of a black pupil, if the eye is free from inflammation.

Cataract Associated with Systemic Diseases and Poisoning. *Diabetes* predisposes to the development of senile cataract, but causes either a rapidly developing bilateral complete cataract or a slowly developing punctate or "snowstorm" variety of subcapsular opacity in poorly controlled juvenile diabetes.

The cataracts which sometimes develop suddenly in cholera or after prolonged starvation may be related biochemically in their origins to diabetic cataract.

Parathyroid tetany in childhood produces opacities of the zonular type in the crises which produce convulsive states. As these sometimes are recurrent, several layers of zonular opacities may occur in one patient, the width of the clear zones between the layers of opacities indicating the approximate time between the convulsive episodes. In the adult relatively rapidly developing cataracts may follow the accidental removal of the parathyroids along with the purposeful subtotal removal of the thyroid gland. The opacity may develop quickly to complete cataract in some instances, but usually it consists of punctate white opacities, some of which coalesce into flakes with some interspersed iridescent crystals in the superficial layer of cortex anteriorly and posteriorly. These gradually increase and produce complete opacity of the cortex. This type of cataract is sometimes called *parathyroidea priva cataract.* A similar type of slowly developing cataract occurs in association with idiopathic hypoparathyroidism and in pseudohypoparathyroidism.

Cataract occurs in *myotonic dystrophy* as a subcapsular cortical layer of opacities composed of punctate and small angulated flakes intermingled with small iridescent crystals, which eventually may coalesce to form opaque plaques at the anterior and posterior poles and later, with continued development, form an intumescent and eventually a mature cataract. These opacities as well as the general manifestations of the disease usually begin between the ages of 20 and 30 years and progress slowly, with complete cataracts developing more rapidly in some, but most of the patients usually die of secondary disease before the age of 45. A similar type of cataract is seen rarely in familial hypertrophic muscular dystrophy (myotonia congenita or Thomsen's disease).

Cataract is associated with *atopic dermatitis* associated with other allergic disorders such as hay fever and asthma. The opacity develops rapidly to complete cataract usually in late childhood or early adult life. Discission or linear extraction usually results in good visual function. Cataract occurs in other skin diseases at times (neurodermatitis, Rothmund's disease or poikiloderma atrophicans vasculare and Darier's disease or keratosis follicularis).

A number of toxic agents cause bilateral cataract. *Paradichlorobenzene,* an insecticide used principally as a moth repellant, may produce a similar type of cataract in some individuals by inhalation of the chemical. *Ergot,* when used as a medication or after eating rye products contaminated by the fungus, may result in cataract formation. Naphthalene also may cause the production of cataract. Extraction in all of these usually produces good results. Dinitrophenol produces fine superficial opacities mixed with iridescent crystals which increase rapidly in number and cause the formation of an intumescent cataract. The ingestion of *dinitrophenol,* taken for reducing weight, is responsible for a number of examples of rapidly maturing, bilateral, soft cataracts which, by swelling, produce glaucoma in a fair proportion of cases, and require linear extraction. Triparanol produces a similar cataract.

Corticosteroids administered in large doses over a period of several months to a year or more tend to produce cataract which begins as a posterior subcapsular iridescent opacity and develops peripheral cortical opacities. It affects vision early and usually leads to cataract extraction.

Traumatic Cataract results from a perforating *wound of the lens capsule* and occasionally from contusions of the eyeball without visible perforation but with rupture of the lens capsule (*contusion cataract*). Within a few hours after the perforating injury, the lens becomes *cloudy* at the seat of the wound from absorption of aqueous, *swells,* protrudes through the capsule wound and fragments often fall into the anterior chamber; swelling and clouding continue until, after a few days, the entire lens has become opaque. Then the lens substance becomes *absorbed;* in favorable cases in young persons, spontaneous cure with a clear, black pupil results. More often, part of the lens remains opaque and requires subsequent operation. Occasionally the opacity of the lens remains limited to the injured portion, owing to closure of a small capsule opening. The course may be less favorable; iritis, iridocyclitis or secondary *glaucoma* from swelling of the lens may occur. Most frequently, contusion cataract develops many days or weeks after the injury; rarely, contusion of the eyeball causes rapid swelling and opacification of the lens substance. Contusions of the eye may be followed not only by contusion cataract, but by a brownish ring-shaped opacity (Vossius' ring) on the anterior capsule, corresponding to the margin of the iris and supposed to represent deposits of blood pigment.

Treatment. Immediately after the injury, absolute *rest* and a cycloplegic are employed. If the rapid swelling of the lens causes inflammation and much increase of *tension,* the cataract should be removed by irrigation through a keratome incision or by extraction. But if such complications do not arise, it is wiser to allow absorption to proceed, and to defer operative intervention until there is no irritation or inflammation and spontaneous improvement has come to a standstill.

Operations for Cataract

Combined and Round Pupil Extraction. Extraction may be performed with *complete iridectomy,* in which case it is known as *combined extraction,* or the lens may be extracted with one or more *peripheral iridectomies or iridotomies* and the operation is then called *round pupil extraction.* The removal of a cataractous lens by *simple extraction without iridectomy* or iridotomy so increases the risk of postoperative prolapse of the iris or glaucoma or both complications that it should not be employed. Combined extraction is the operation of choice in many cases; it always is indicated when the iris interferes with easy delivery of the lens or protrudes during the operation and does not stay reduced, when the lens is very large, or with ocular complications. Round pupil extraction with peripheral iridectomy is the operation of choice of many surgeons although it involves a greater danger of postoperative prolapse of the iris than the combined extraction. The retention of the iris diaphragm in the round pupil operation is a safety factor in holding back the vitreous and preventing loss of this substance during the operation. With adequate sedation and anesthesia and the use of corneoscleral sutures to make a watertight closure of the wound, the choice of type of extraction depends upon the surgeon's preference.

Aphakia. After extraction of cataract, the patient is compelled to wear *strong convex glasses,* since the loss of the lens (*aphakia*) causes a high degree of *hyperopia,* amounting to about +10.00 D., and with it there usually is considerable *astigmatism* (+2.00 to +3.00 D.), generally "against the rule" as a result of the corneal incision. In an average case, a convex spherical lens of approximately +10.00 D., combined with a convex cylinder of +2.00 to +3.00 D., must be worn for distant vision; to this spherocylinder an additional convex sphere of +3.00 D. must be added for reading. Any previous error of refraction will, of course, modify this correcting lens. Temporary glasses may be prescribed between 4 and 8 weeks postoperatively, but changes in refraction, usually a change or lessening of the postoperative astigmatism, may continue for several months and permanent glasses usually are not prescribed until about 1 year postoperatively. In some individuals contact lenses may be tolerated and usually produce better visual results than glasses in aphakia. The *aphakic eye* presents, besides hyperopia and loss of accommodation, a *deep anterior chamber* and usually a *tremulous iris.*

Prognosis. A *favorable result* and *useful vision* should follow cataract extraction in almost all uncomplicated cases; there generally is good vision and often this is perfect. The success of the operation is dependent not only upon skillful operation, but upon *exclusion* of those *complicated cases* which cannot be improved by an operation, no matter how successful, and also those in which there is a neighboring source of *infection.* Hence conjunctiva, lid margins and lacrimal sac must be inspected carefully, and if disease is found, this must be cured before operation. Careful operators examine the conjunctiva bacteriologically in every case. Disease of the deeper structures of the eye and especially of the retina must be excluded or taken into consideration in making a prognosis. The condition of the optic nerve and retina is tested with the candle or lighted electric bulb for *light perception* and *light projection.* There should be good perception of light, even with feeble illumination, and also a good field and projection.

Projection is tested by throwing light from the ophthalmoscope upon the upper, lower, inner and outer portions of the pupil; there is good projection if, with the eye steadily directed forward, the patient is able to state correctly the direction from which the light comes; this test also may be applied with the *lighted candle* made to approach the eye from various directions, at a distance of 1 meter and also at 3 or 4 meters.

Cataract Extraction

Besides the division of cataract extraction into combined, round pupil and simple, as explained above, there are two forms of removal: In one, the capsule of the lens is opened by means of the cystotome or the capsule forceps and the nucleus and cortex are removed; this operation, called *extracapsular extraction,* was the more common method of extracting senile cataract. In the other, no opening is made in the lens capsule and the lens is delivered enclosed in its capsule; this type of operation is known as *intracapsular extraction.*

Operation. A sedative is given at the proper time before operation to quiet the patient.

The corneal section. After thorough cleansing of the face, lids, lid margins and conjunctival sac, local anesthetic, rarely a general anesthetic, is administered. Incision is made into the anterior chamber by Graefe knife section (Fig. 12-7, *left*), which is continued to produce a conjunctival flap (Fig. 12-7, *center*), or a conjunctival flap is made and the incision made through the limbus by keratome and scissors.

Iridectomy. The conjunctival flap is reflected upon the cornea, and iridectomy performed, making as narrow a coloboma as possible.

Opening the capsule (capsulotomy). The capsule forceps are introduced, closed, then opened, and as large a piece of the capsule is removed as possible. Some operators prefer division of the capsule with the cystotome; this is introduced and the capsule cut gently and without pressure.

Delivery of the cataract. The lens is expelled by pressing gently upon the lower part of the cornea upward and slightly backward with the back of a Daviel spoon (Fig. 12-7, *right*), following the cataract in its upward course through the corneal wound (Fig. 12-7, *right*), where it passes out and is received upon the wire loop, its exit being facilitated by gentle depression of the posterior lip of the wound with the loop. If the corneal wound is found too small for easy exit of the lens, it is enlarged with Stevens' scissors.

Cleansing ("toilet") of the wound. Lens debris in the anterior chamber and in the wound is liberated by gently stroking the cornea upward with the back of the Daviel spoon. Blood clots in the wound are removed with forceps. If remnants of cortex persist, the anterior chamber is irrigated gently with warm sterilized physiologic saline solution. The iris is smoothed with the repositor and freed from any entanglement in the wound; the repositor also is swept over the edges of the incision,

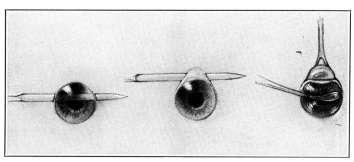

Fɪɢ. 12-7. Cataract extraction. *Left,* corneal section; *center,* conjunctival flap; *right,* delivery of the cataract.

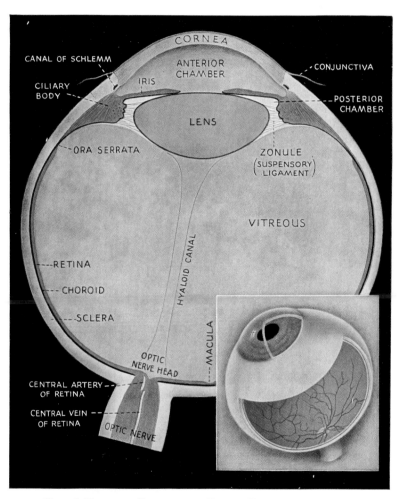

PLATE 1. HORIZONTAL SECTION OF THE EYEBALL MAGNIFIED NEARLY 4 X.

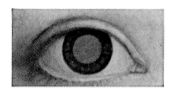

A. Normal Fundus Reflex;
Ophthalmoscope at a Distance.

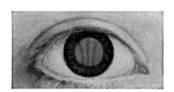

B. Fundus Reflex in Ametropia;
Ophthalmoscope at a Distance.

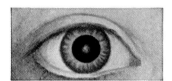

C. Opacity of the Cornea;
Oblique Illumination.

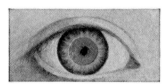

D. Opacity of the Cornea;
Ophthalmoscope at a Distance.

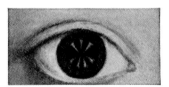

E. Senile Cortical Cataract;
Oblique Illumination.

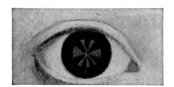

F. Senile Cortical Cataract;
Ophthalmoscope at a Distance.

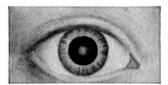

G. Senile Nuclear Cataract;
Oblique Illumination.

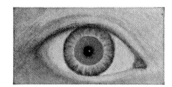

H. Senile Nuclear Cataract;
Ophthalmoscope at a Distance.

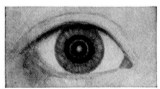

I. Lamellar and Nuclear
Cataract; Oblique Illumination.

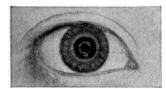

J. Lamellar and Nuclear
Cataract; Ophthalmoscope at
A Distance.

Plate 2. The Media as Seen with Oblique Illumination and the
Ophthalmoscope at a Distance; Pupil Dilated.

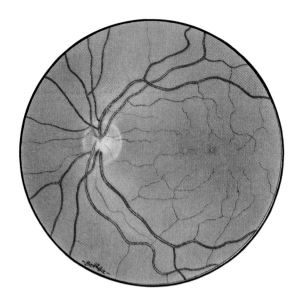

A. NORMAL FUNDUS.

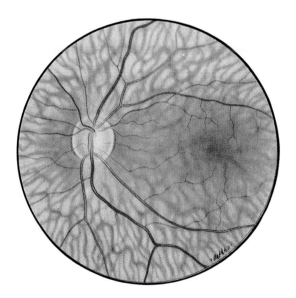

B. ALBINOTIC FUNDUS.

PLATE 3.

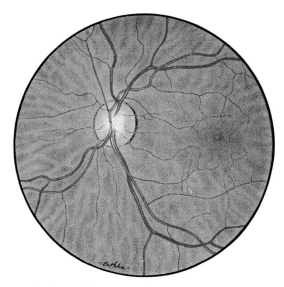

A. Normal Fundus in an Individual of Dark
Complexion (Tessellated Fundus).

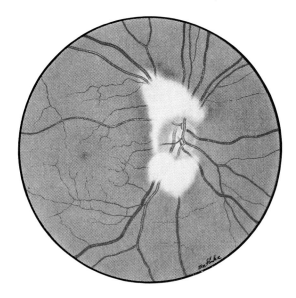

B. Opaque Nerve Fibers.

Plate 4.

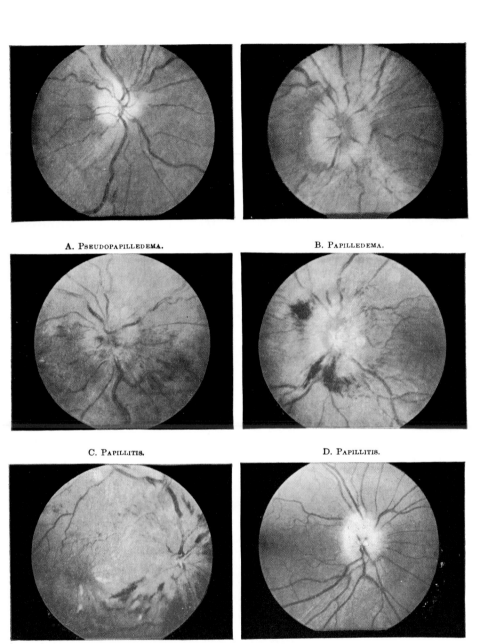

A. Pseudopapilledema.

B. Papilledema.

C. Papillitis.

D. Papillitis.

E. Neuro-retinal Edema, Grade IV
Hypertensive Retinopathy.

F. Drusen of the Nerve Head.

Plate 5.

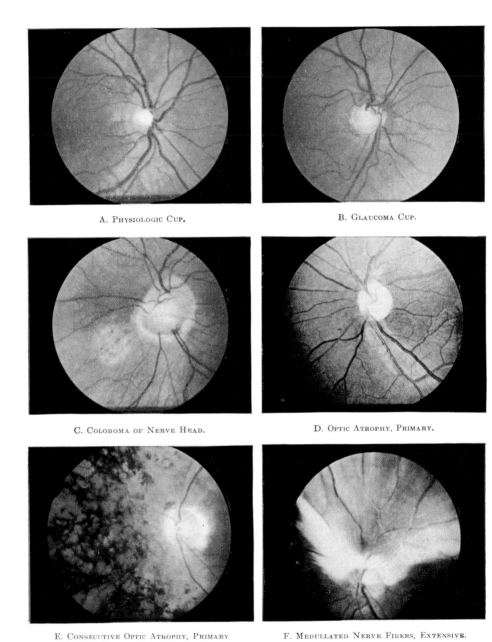

A. Physiologic Cup.

B. Glaucoma Cup.

C. Coloboma of Nerve Head.

D. Optic Atrophy, Primary.

E. Consecutive Optic Atrophy, Primary
Pigmentary Degeneration of the Retina.

F. Medullated Nerve Fibers, Extensive.

Plate 6.

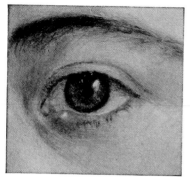

A. Hordeolum.

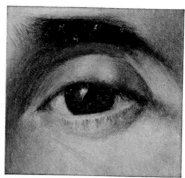

B. Chalazion.

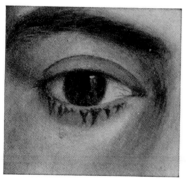

C. Blepharitis.

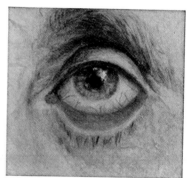

D. Ectropion.

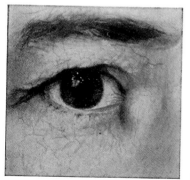

E. Chronic Dacryocystitis with
Distention of the Lacrimal
Sac (Mucocele).

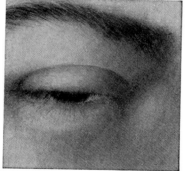

F. Acute Dacryocystitis.

Plate 7.

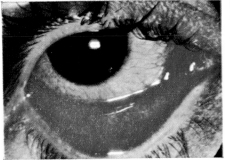

A. CONJUNCTIVAL INJECTION.

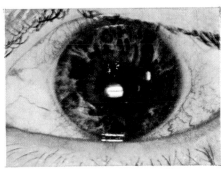

B. CIRCUMCORNEAL INJECTION EARLY.

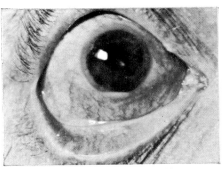

C. CILIARY INJECTION, IRITIS WITH HYPOPYON.

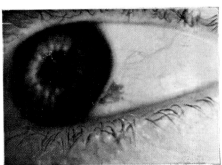

D. SUBCONJUNCTIVAL HEMORRHAGE.

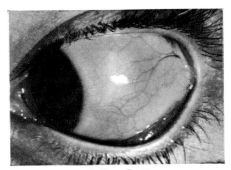

E. BLUE SCLERA.

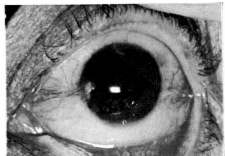

F. PTERYGIUM.

PLATE 8.

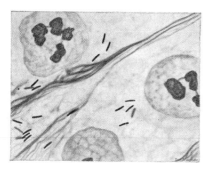

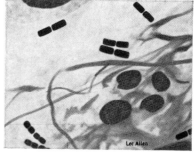

A. Hemophilus Conjunctivitis.

B. Hemophilus Duplex.

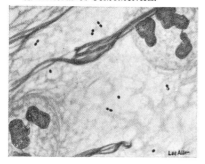

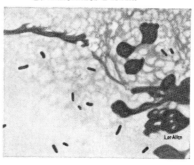

C. Hemophilus Influenzae.

D. Aerobacter Aerogenes.

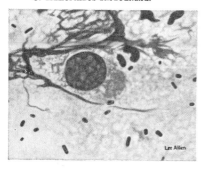

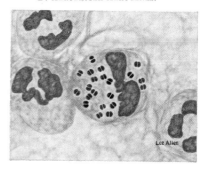

E. Pseudomonas Aeruginosa.

F. Neisseria Gonorrhoeae.

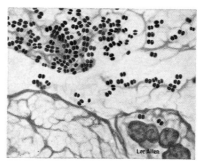

G. Neisseria Catarrhales.

Plate 9.

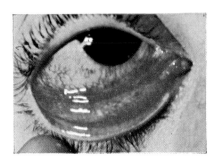

A. Acute Catarrhal Conjunctivitis.

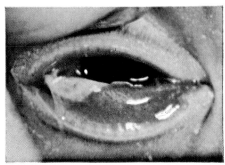

B. Acute Purulent Conjunctivitis of the Newborn.

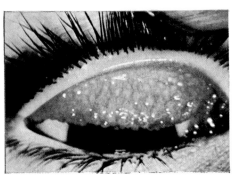

C. Folliculosis of Conjunctiva.

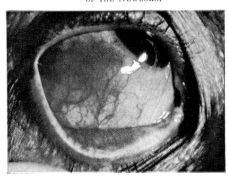

D. Episcleritis.

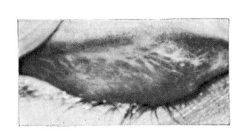

E. Trachoma, Scarring of Palpebral Conjunctiva.

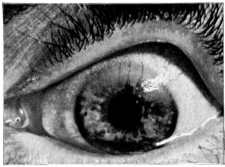

F. Trachoma Pannus.

Plate 10.

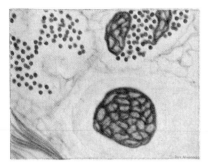

A. Eosinophiles in Conjunctival Smear.

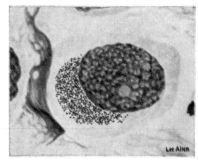

B. Inclusion Body in Epithelial Cell.

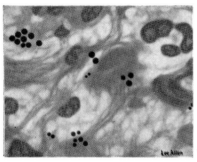

C. Staphylococci—Conjunctival Smear.

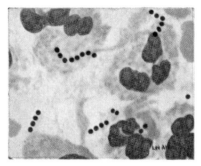

D. Streptococci from
Lacrimal Sac Secretion.

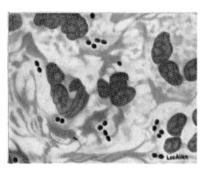

E. Streptococci from
Conjunctival Secretion.

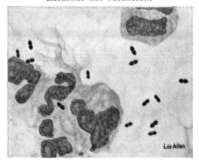

F. Pneumococci from Conjunctival Smear.

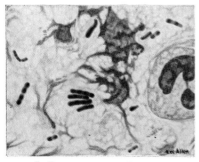

G. Corynebacterium Xerosis—
Conjunctival Scrapping.

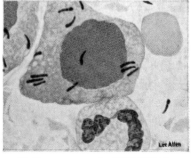

H. Corynebacterium Diphtheriae—
Conjunctival Scrapping.

Plate 11.

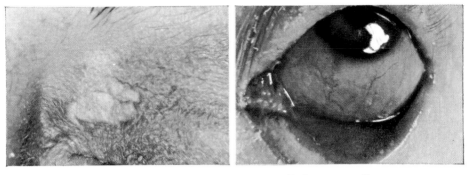

A. Xanthelasma.   B. Argyrosis of Conjunctiva.

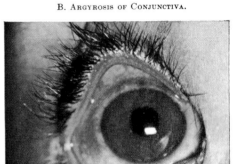

C. Vernal Conjunctivitis, Giant Papillary   D. Limbic Vernal Conjunctivitis.
Hypertrophy of Conjunctiva.

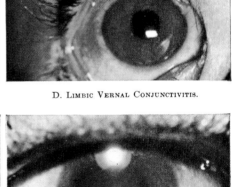

E. Marginal Catarrhal Ulcers.   F. Herpetic Keratitis, Dendritic Figure
Stained with Fluorescein.

PLATE 12.

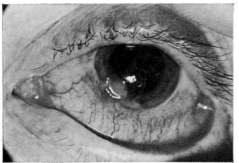

A. Corneal Ulcer with Ciliary Injection.

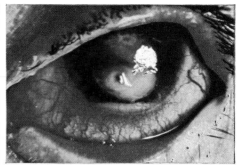

B. Pneumococcic Ulcer with Hypopyon.

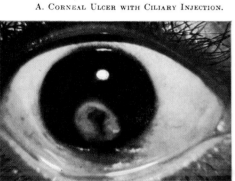

C. Adherent Leukoma.

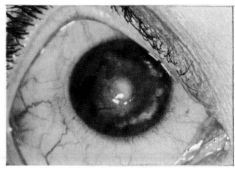

D. Disciform Keratitis.

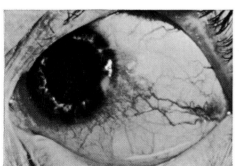

E. Phlyctenular Conjunctivitis.

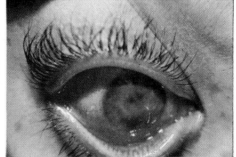

F. Interstitial Keratitis.

Plate 13.

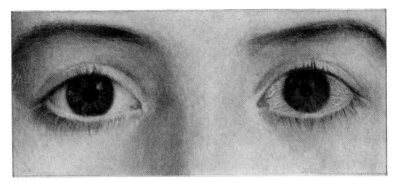

A. Left, Normal Eye (for Comparison); Right, Iritis.

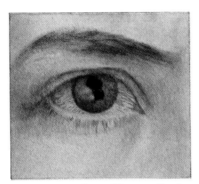

B. Syphilitic Iritis (Nodular Type).

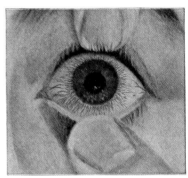

C. Iridocyclitis.

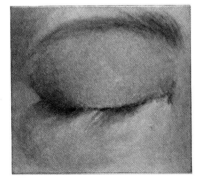

D. Panophthalmitis.

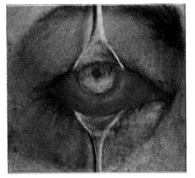

E. Panophthalmitis.

Plate 14.

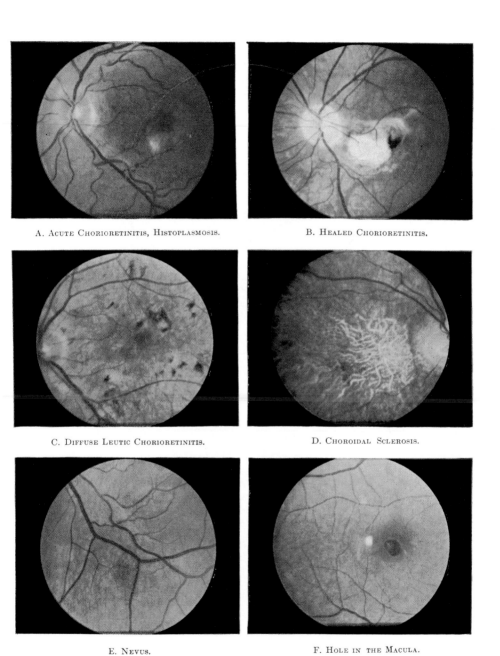

A. Acute Chorioretinitis, Histoplasmosis.

B. Healed Chorioretinitis.

C. Diffuse Leutic Chorioretinitis.

D. Choroidal Sclerosis.

E. Nevus.

F. Hole in the Macula.

Plate 15.

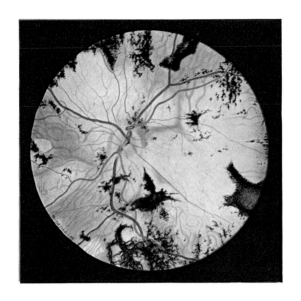

A. Diffuse Exudative Choroiditis.

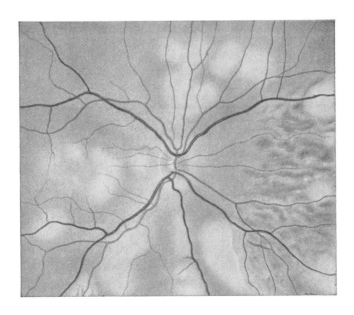

B. Disseminated Choroiditis (Tuberculous).

Plate 16.

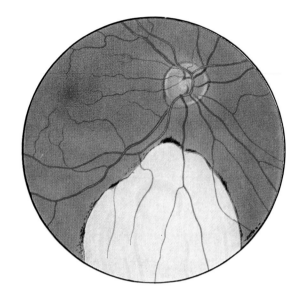

A. Coloboma of Choroid.

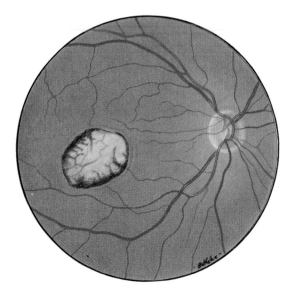

B. Central Choroiditis.

Plate 17.

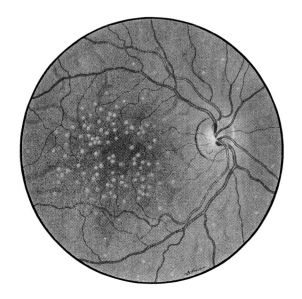

A. Colloid Bodies (Drusen).

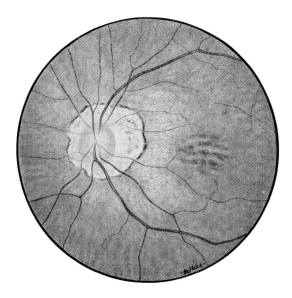

B. Myopic Degeneration.

Plate 18.

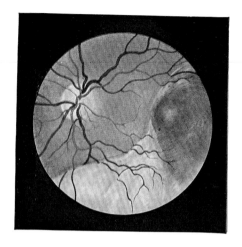

A. Malignant Melanoma of the Choroid.

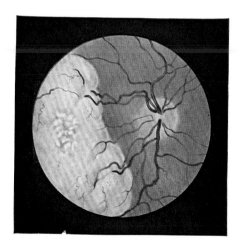

B. Retinoblastoma.

Plate 19.

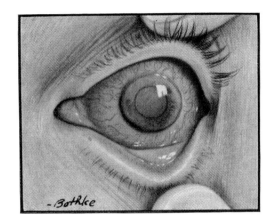

A. Acute Congestive Glaucoma.

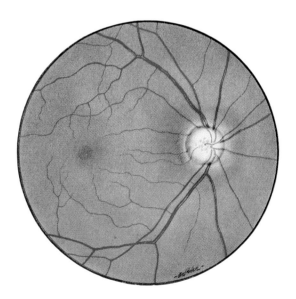

B. Glaucomatous Cupping of the Nervehead.

Plate 20.

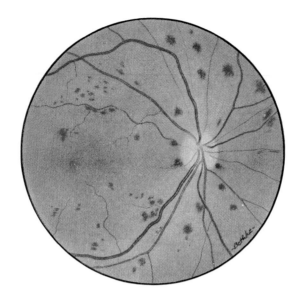

A. Retinal Hemorrhages.

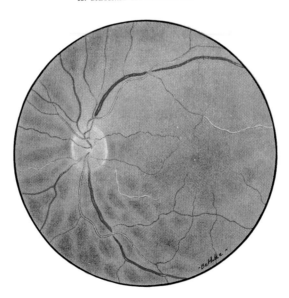

B. Retinal Arteriosclerosis.

Plate 21.

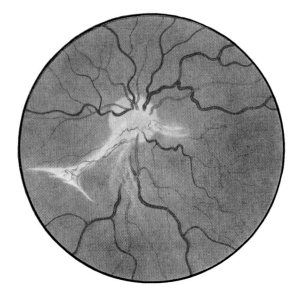

A. Retinitis Proliferans.

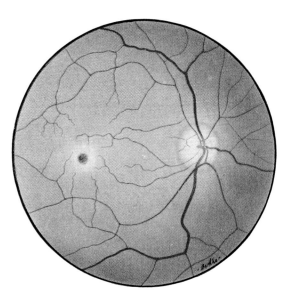

B. Recent Obstruction (Occlusion) of Central Artery of Retina.

Plate 22.

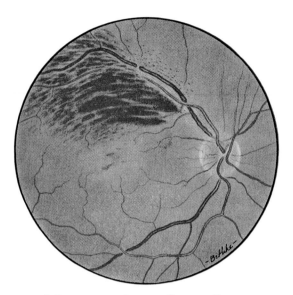

A. Thrombosis of Superior Temporal Branch
of the Central Vein of the Retina.

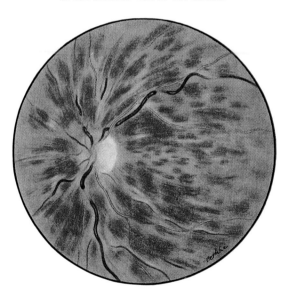

B. Thrombosis of the Trunk of the Central
Vein of the Retina (Early).

PLATE 23.

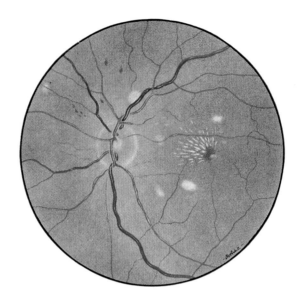

A. Hypertensive and Nephritic Retinopathy.

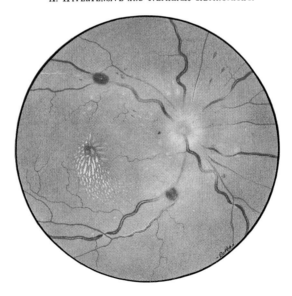

B. Hypertensive and Nephritic Retinopathy;
Advanced Changes, with Neuroretinal Edema
(Grade IV).

Plate 24.

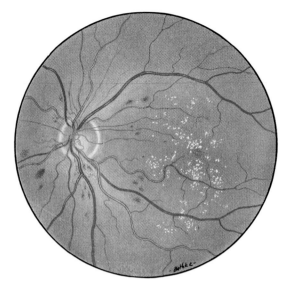

A. Diabetic Retinopathy.

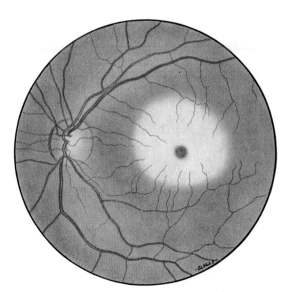

B. The Fundus in Amaurotic Family Idiocy.

Plate 25.

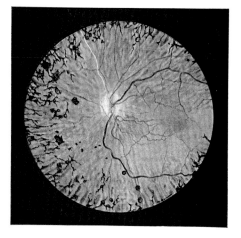

A. Pigmentary Degeneration of the Retina.

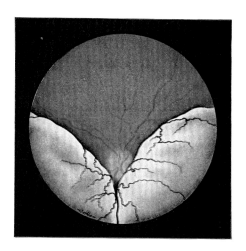

B. Detachment of the Retina.

Plate 26.

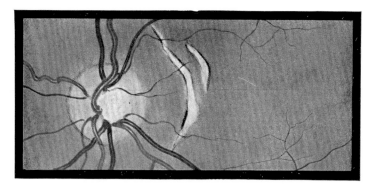

A. Rupture of the Choroid.

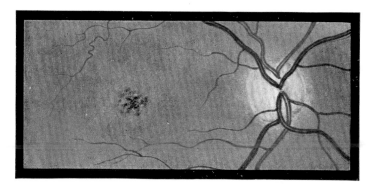

B. Senile Degeneration of the Macula.

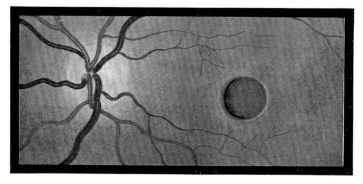

C. Hole in the Macula.

Plate 27.

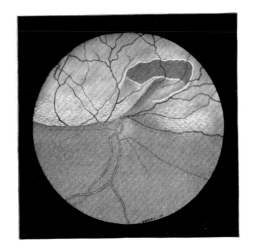

A. Detachment of the Retina, Showing a
Large Tear.

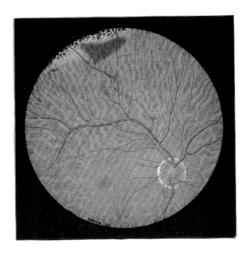

B. The Same Fundus as Shown Above, after
Electrocoagulation Operation.

Plate 28.

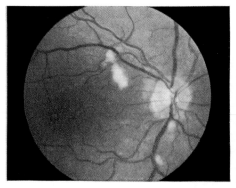

A. Cotton Wool Spots in Retina.

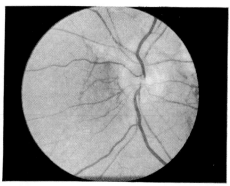

B. Angioid Streaks.

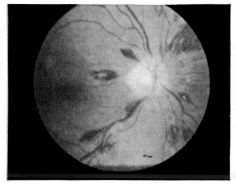

C. Leukemic Hemorrhages.

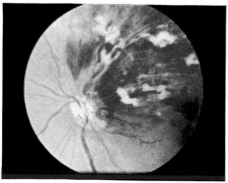

D. Occlusion of the Superior Temporal Vein.

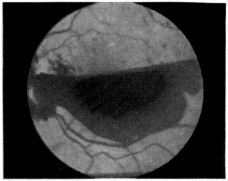

E. Preretinal Hemorrhage.

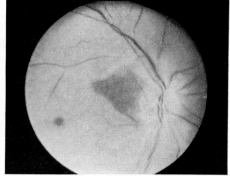

F. Occlusion of Central Retinal Artery.
Cilio-retinal Artery Patent.

Plate 29.

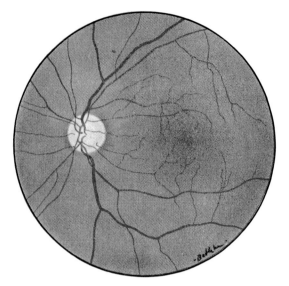

A. Simple (Primary) Atrophy of the Optic Nerve.

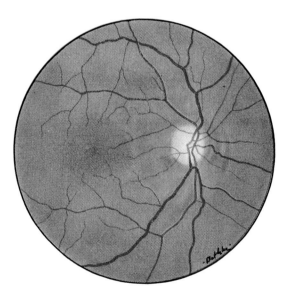

B. Secondary Atrophy of the Optic Nerve.

Plate 30.

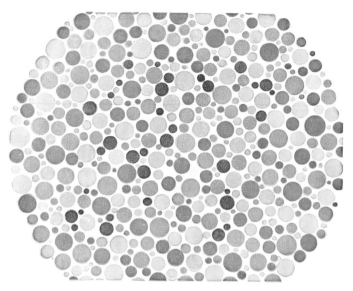

A. One of a Series of Pseudoisochromatic Plates
for Testing Color Perception.

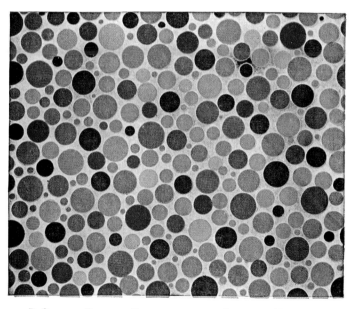

B. One of a Series of Pseudoisochromatic Plates for Testing
Color Perception.

Plate 31.

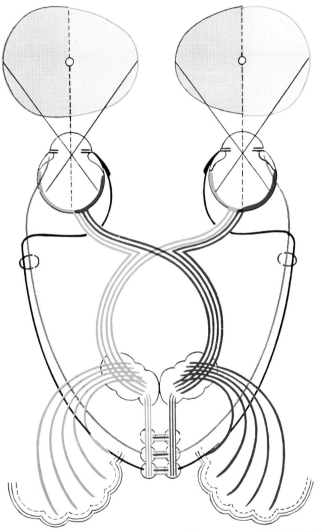

PLATE 32. SCHEMATIC REPRESENTATION OF THE VISUAL AND THE PUPILLARY PATHS.

especially at the ends, to free any tags of capsule. The limbic incision and the conjunctival flap are closed separately, and a drop of cycloplegic instilled onto the cornea.

Dressing. The lids of the operated eye are covered with a round piece of gauze fastened with three strips of adhesive plaster and covered by a perforated metallic protective mask.

After-treatment. The patient must lie quietly upon his back, recumbent or semi-recumbent; after 24 hours he may change to the unoperated side. The patient should be helped to sit up after 24 hours. Food need not be changed from the patient's regular diet, and his bowel habits should be disturbed as little as possible. The dressing is changed daily for 7 days, then removed. A cycloplegic drop is used daily for 1 to 2 months postoperatively.

Round Pupil Extraction. This modification of simple extraction is often used. One or two small pieces of iris are removed from the iris as peripherally as possible, before or after removal of the cataractous lens. This allows the aqueous to circulate freely between the posterior and anterior chambers and thus diminishes the risk of prolapse of the iris. Some surgeons replace peripheral iridectomy by peripheral iridotomy or by a small iridodialysis.

Linear Extraction. In this modification, suitable for *soft* and traumatic cataracts and cataract masses produced by needling, *a small corneal section* (about 5 mm.) is made at the limbus with the keratome, the pupil having been dilated; the capsule is torn widely with a cystotome or opened with the keratome directly after it penetrates the cornea; then the lens masses are evacuated by depressing the posterior lip of the wound with a Daviel spoon and gently pressing upon the cornea. Most of the soft lens matter will escape; sometimes irrigation of the anterior chamber is necessary to wash out additional fragments; the small portion which cannot be removed easily is allowed to remain and is absorbed.

Extraction of Cataract in Its Capsule (*intracapsular extraction*) is being increasingly employed in favorable cases and with cooperative patients. It is a combined extraction in which the lens is dislocated and expressed within its capsule by pressure upon the cornea with a squint hook aided by more or less traction with capsule forceps grasping the lens capsule. Its special indication is found in the extraction of incipient cataracts; but even in other forms, the absence of remnants of cortex, the impossibility of incarceration of tags of capsule in the wound and the avoidance of after-cataract constitute distinct advantages.

Intracapsular Extraction by Suction (phacoerisis), as advocated by Barraquer, occasionally is practiced. After corneal section and peripheral iridectomy, the cup-shaped extremity of a special apparatus is applied to the lens, suction made, the suspensory ligament ruptured and the cataract withdrawn in capsule.

Extraction by Cryoprobe. Recently a number of cryoprobes have been devised especially for use in cataract extraction. The probe must be small and care must be exercised to touch the freezing tip of the probe to the cataract only. Once the tip has frozen onto the cataract, it is extracted in the same manner as with an erisophake (suction apparatus).

The Complications of Cataract Extraction include insufficient opening in the cornea or capsule, wounding the iris, prolapse of the iris, incomplete evacuation of the cataract, loss of vitreous, dislocation of the lens and intraocular hemorrhage.

Postoperative Complications of Cataract Extraction include prolapse of the iris, temporary striate opacity of the cornea (consisting of delicate gray lines running vertically downward from the corneal section, caused by wrinkling of the cornea, and disappearing spontaneously), glaucoma, iritis, iridocyclitis, cyclitis, suppuration of the wound, intraocular hemorrhage and panophthalmitis.

After-cataract (often called *secondary membrane*) is an opacity remaining after extracapsular cataract operation; it consists of remnants of lens cortex, of proliferation of remaining subcapsular epithelium or rarely of inflammatory products (new connective tissue). The *membrane* thus formed may be thin and delicate, or thick and tough, and the degree of impairment of vision following the cataract operation varies accordingly. When due to inflammatory products, the membrane is apt to be thick and the iris adherent.

Treatment consists in *dividing* the membrane (*discission*), after all signs of irritation or inflammation have subsided, usually 2 or 3 months subsequent to the cataract extraction.

Discission or Needling

This operation is indicated in zonular, congenital complete and juvenile complete cataracts (*soft cataracts*), previous to the 20th year, preliminary to extraction in occasional cases of high myopia and for the division or hastening absorption of *after-cataract*.

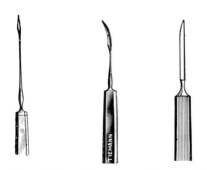

FIG. 12-8. Discission knives. *Left*, Knapp's needle-knife; *center*, Ziegler sickle-shaped knife; *right*, Wheeler's knife.

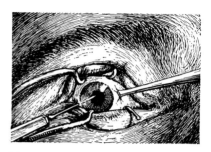

FIG. 12-9. Discission of the cataract.

Discission of Cataract. In very young children a general anesthetic is required; in others, local anesthesia is sufficient. The *pupil* must be *dilated*. A knife-needle, Wheeler or Ziegler knife (Fig. 12-8) is thrust through the conjunctiva 1 to 2 mm. from the limbus and then through the limbus into the capsule of the lens, making three or four cross cuts, each about 6 mm. in length (Fig. 12-9). The cortex may be broken slightly by rotating the needle. The swollen lens matter continues to absorb for several weeks or months. If the pupil is not clear, a second operation may be needed, but the incision should not include the posterior capsule of the lens.

After-treatment. There usually is very little reaction. The pupil must be kept dilated with atropine or scopolamine. The lens substance swells, protrudes through the opening in the capsule and is absorbed. The entire duration of treatment is several months.

Complications. Rapid and extensive swelling of the cortex, especially if the capsule has not been opened widely or the pupil kept dilated at a maximum, may cause a sudden rise of tension requiring removal of the swollen cortical material by *linear extraction* without delay. A bold discission is sometimes made, with a view of extracting the lens a few days afterward, as soon as there is maximal swelling; this is the usual procedure in the occasional extraction of the lens in high degrees of myopia. *Iritis* may occur after discission, occasionally iridocyclitis and, very rarely, loss of the eye.

Discission for after-cataract. If the membrane is *thin* it is divided with a discission knife (Fig. 12-8) introduced through the cornea near the limbus or through the conjunctiva 1 mm. external to the limbus, the pupil having previously been dilated; a linear, T-shaped or cruciate incision is made. The instrument must be sharp, and dragging on the iris or ciliary body avoided for fear of subsequent inflammation. If the membrane is *thick and tough*, it may be divided by two Ziegler knives inserted at each side of the periphery of the cornea, meeting in the center of the pupil and then separating, or with de Wecker's scissors after a limbic incision into the anterior chamber. When the pupil is displaced, it may be necessary to perform iridotomy. Discission of after-cataract is occasionally followed by iridocyclitis and glaucoma, rarely by suppuration.

DISLOCATION OF THE LENS

Dislocation of the lens may be either *congenital* or *acquired*; it may be *partial or complete*. In order that the lens can become dislocated there must be some *defect in the suspensory ligament* (zonula), such as atrophy, rupture, stretching or imperfect development.

The *congenital form* is partial, with the lens usually displaced upward, often becomes complete in after years, generally is bilateral and symmetrical, and often hereditary. It frequently is associated with *arachnodactyly*, a peculiar malformation of the hands and feet, which are exceptionally long.

The *acquired forms* are either *traumatic* or *spontaneous*. Traumatic dislocation generally is the result of a blow upon the eye. The predisposing cause of spontaneous dislocation is degeneration of the suspensory ligament seen in fluid vitreous, choroiditis and myopia of high degree, detachment of the retina and hypermature cataract; in such eyes, the zonula being defective, the exciting cause may be insignificant, such as sneezing or various straining efforts.

Symptoms are disturbance of vision, interference with accommodation, a change in refraction, monocular diplopia and tremulous iris (iridodonesis). They differ according to whether the displacement is partial or complete. In addition there are complications and sequelae which often are serious.

Partial Dislocation (*subluxation*) may consist of a *tilting* of one edge of the lens, or of a lateral displacement upward, downward, inward or outward. In such cases the anterior chamber is of unequal depth, being increased where the lens is absent. The convex edge of the lens usually can be seen (Fig. 12-10) in some part of the pupil, the portion of the latter which is free from lens being particularly black. With the indirect method of ophthalmoscopy, the optic *disk appears double*, one image being seen through the lens and the other through the free pupil. Movements of the eyeball disclose a tremulous condition of the lens and iris. There is considerable *myopia* and astigmatism through the lens, the convexity of the latter being increased through relaxation of the sus-

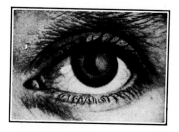

FIG. 12-10. Dislocation of the lens upward and outward.

pensory ligament, with high *hyperopia* in the aphakic portion of the pupil, thus *monocular diplopia* (two images being formed on the retina).

Complete Dislocation (*luxation*) occurs when the lens is displaced *anteriorly* into the aqueous, or *posteriorly* into the vitreous cavity. In traumatic cases in which there is rupture of the sclera, the lens may lie beneath the conjunctiva.

When dislocated *anteriorly*, the lens is recognized easily. If transparent, it looks like a large drop of oil with a curved, golden margin when seen by oblique illumination. The anterior chamber is increased in depth. Blood staining of the cornea may be mistaken for dislocation of the lens into the anterior chamber.

When displaced into the *vitreous*, the lens sinks into the lowest part and either becomes attached by exudation or moves about; when opaque, it can be seen with the ophthalmoscope and sometimes with the unaided eye. The anterior chamber is deep, the iris tremulous and the pupil very black. The eye, for practical purposes, is aphakic, for it is in a condition of extreme hyperopia and has lost its power of accommodation.

Complications and Sequelae. A partial dislocation often changes to a complete one. When subluxated, the lens may remain clear a long time, but completely dislocated lenses soon become opaque. Displacement into the vitreous is tolerated better than anterior luxation. When the lens is dislocated into the anterior chamber, it almost always excites severe inflammation, becomes attached to the cornea and iris by exudates and usually produces an acute secondary glaucoma. Displacement into the vitreous also is followed by the development of secondary glaucoma, but usually slowly and insidiously.

Treatment. In *partial* dislocation, if no symptoms of irritation are produced, treatment consists in prescribing suitable glasses, usually *strong convex lenses*, to correct the refraction of the aphakic portion. When the lens is dislocated into the *anterior chamber* it should be *removed*. If it is dislocated into the *vitreous* and symptoms of irritation arise, extraction is indicated but difficult; strong convex glasses are required subsequently for the aphakia. Operations for removal of a dislocated lens may be complicated by loss of vitreous, since the latter reaches the anterior chamber through the rupture in the suspensory ligament. If inflammatory symptoms occur in a case in which the dislocated lens cannot be removed, an iridectomy may be tried; if, in such cases, the eye is sightless, enucleation is indicated.

13

The Vitreous Humor

Anatomy

The vitreous humor is a *transparent, colorless* mass, of soft *gelatinous* consistency, which fills the posterior cavity of the eyeball behind the lens. Its outer surface presents a thin, structureless condensation, the *hyaloid membrane*. The vitreous humor is traversed from the optic disk to the posterior capsule of the lens by a canal, the *hyaloid canal*, which during fetal life contained the hyaline artery. The vitreous humor is attached to the pars plana of the ciliary body (the "base of the vitreous humor") and to the optic nerve. In structure the vitreous humor consists of a *transparent network*, in the meshes of which are *clear liquid* and a few branching *cells* and an occasional white blood corpuscle. The vitreous humor has no blood vessels, but receives its nourishment from the surrounding tissues: the choroid, ciliary body and retina.

Persistent hyaloid artery. The hyaloid artery usually disappears entirely during the later months of gestation; occasionally a remnant persists. This can be seen with the ophthalmoscope as a *grayish cord or thread*, which arises from the nasal half of the optic disk and stretches into the vitreous humor, with a free extremity or occasionally attached to the anterior face of the vitreous humor; sometimes there is an accompanying opacity of the posterior portion of the lens. Rarely, the hyaloid canal is abnormally dense and is visible as a grayish, tubular cord extending from disk to lens.

Persistent Hyperplastic Primary Vitreous Humor

This condition, known as *tunica vasculosa lentis*, is seen occasionally in infants as a concave opaque mass of tissue, densest in its center, behind the lens. The condition is unilateral; the involved eye is smaller than its fellow. There is gradual absorption of the lens, often with hemorrhages in advanced cases. The ciliary processes are elongated. The retina usually is in place. The anterior chamber is shallow, and glaucoma is a common complication. This process must be distinguished from retrolental fibroplasia, retinoblastoma and pseudoretinoblastoma. Treatment consists in needling the lens, followed by discission of the membrane.

A tiny or insignificant remnant of the hyaloid vascular system occurs quite commonly as a dot-like grayish spot when seen with focal illumination, or black in an orange-colored background with reflected light. This is known as Mittendorf's dot; it is located in the hyaloid membrane just above and just nasal to the posterior pole of the lens and represents the remnant of the anterior end of the hyaloid artery. Occasionally a small corkscrew-like "pig tail" hangs down in the vitreous humor from this dot. This is the remnant of the anterior portion of the hyaloid artery.

Fluidity of the Vitreous Humor

Synchysis is a liquid alteration in consistency occurring as a senile change or due to degeneration from neighboring disease, and found often in high myopia. When opacities are present, these move freely in such fluid vitreous humor. There often is diminished tension of the eyeball, tremulousness of the iris, weakness of the suspensory ligament of the lens and sometimes predisposition to detachment of the retina; these complications increase the risk of loss of vitreous humor in intraocular operations.

Occasionally small glistening white opacities are found in association with synchysis in degenerated eyeballs and in some which are normal in other respects; they fall in a silvery shower when the eyeball is moved. This is known as *synchysis scintillans.*

Opacities of the Vitreous Humor

These are quite common. They may occur as a consequence of changes in the vitreous humor itself, but usually they are the result of disease or of hemorrhages from the *neighboring structures.* They may be fixed or mobile and vary in number, shape, and size. (1) A diffuse cloud or *dust-like* haziness often accompanies cyclitis, choroiditis and retinitis; (2) the opacities may occur in the form of dots, flakes, threads or membranous masses, the result of exudations or hemorrhages; (3) sometimes extensive *membranes (retinitis proliferans)*, attached to the retina, result from organization of exudate and hemorrhages, and often produce detachment of the retina; (4) opacities may accompany or precede retinal separation.

Asteroid hyalosis is an anomaly in which the vitreous humor is studded with dull white globules; the condition is seen most frequently in elderly persons and has little if any effect upon vision.

Etiology. Opacities of the vitreous humor are very common in *myopia* of high degree associated with changes in the choroid; they accompany *diseases of the uvea* and retina; they occur after injuries which have caused *hemorrhage* from the choroid or ciliary body; they may result from certain systemic diseases; and they often exist in patients in whom no cause can be found, especially in the aged.

Symptoms. There may be *disturbance of vision* depending upon the situation, size and density of the opacities. The latter often are movable, indicating a fluid vitreous humor (synchysis); on this account, the visual disturbance may vary according to whether the opacity has gravitated into the line of vision, and the patient may be able to move the eyeball or toss the head so as to throw the opacity out of the line of sight. Occasionally there is the complaint of flashes of light referred to the temporal field.

Diagnosis is made with the *ophthalmoscope*, using a +12.00 or +10.00 diopter lens. The opacities appear as *dark spots* upon a red ground, moving with greater or lesser rapidity, depending upon the consistency of the vitreous humor, when the eye is turned in various directions. When faint, the opacities are seen best with diminished illumination.

Prognosis *varies* with the size, density and nature of the opacity. Uveitic opacities and small hemorrhages often are absorbed. Others become smaller and less dense and give little annoyance. A great many are permanent.

Treatment. The cause must be determined and treatment directed against it when possible. Many empirical measures have been advocated for hastening the absorption of exudates and hemorrhages, but these are of little value if the cause is not corrected.

Muscae Volitantes

This term is employed for the appearance of *spots* (motes) before the eyes, *without appreciable structural change* in the vitreous humor or other media. They are caused by the shadows cast upon the retina by the cells normally found in the vitreous humor or by tiny developmental remnants, and occur in all eyes, being seen in certain conditions such as exposure to a uniform bright surface or in looking through a microscope. They are found more frequently in patients with *errors of refraction* (especially *myopia*), and the symptom may be aggravated temporarily during digestive derangements. They are *annoying* and sometimes alarm the patient, but are of *no importance*, and do not affect the acuteness of vision. The treatment consists in correcting errors of refraction, or in relieving the disturbance of digestion. They persist and annoy the patient until he ceases to look for them and thus forgets their existence.

Hemorrhage into the Vitreous Humor

This produces *interference with vision,* the degree depending upon its size and position. When small, hemorrhages are red as seen with the ophthalmoscope, when larger they appear as dark red masses and when very extensive they fill the vitreous cavity and no red reflex can be obtained. Small hemorrhages often are absorbed; others may be partially absorbed and leave opacities; larger ones may result in permanent membranous masses and bands originating from the retina or ciliary body, and these, by contraction, sometimes cause detachment of the retina.

Hemorrhages into the vitreous humor occur after *injuries* (contusions and wounds), arteriosclerosis, pernicious anemia or other blood dyscrasias, malaria, diabetes, vicarious menstruation and spontaneously from unknown cause. The exciting cause may be a strain of some kind, such as a cough.

One form, usually due to periphlebitis retinae, occurs in *young adults,* usually males, with unknown cause, although tuberculosis and defective blood coagulability are thought to be factors, and presents frequent recurrences in one or both eyes. The blood may be absorbed completely, but sometimes absorption is incomplete with organization of the blood clot into dense opacities or *retinitis proliferans* with some risk of subsequent detachment of the retina.

Treatment consists of absolute *rest*, dressing of both eyes, attention to any predisposing systemic affection, reduction of blood pressure if elevated, and *calcium* chloride or gluconate to increase coagulability of the blood. In the recurrent hemorrhages of young adults, thought to be tuberculous, administration of vitamin C and general treatment for tuberculosis are indicated. Later, to favor absorption, *dionine* and hot compresses may be prescribed.

Abscess of the Vitreous Humor

This term is used to designate those cases of suppurative endophthalmitis (Chap. 17) in which the purulent exudate remains confined to the vitreous humor and internal layers of the eyeball and does not spread to all the structures of the eyeball, causing panophthalmitis (Chap. 17).

Foreign Bodies in the Vitreous Humor are discussed in Chapter 17.

14

Intraocular Tumors

Intraocular tumors are *rather rare.* Their recognition, however, is important, since early enucleation of the eyeball may save life. There are two principal varieties: (1) malignant melanoma and (2) retinoblastoma.

Malignant Melanoma

This malignant growth occurs in *adults,* usually being recognized between the ages of 40 and 60. It is always *primary* and involves *one eye* only. It is composed of round or spindle-shaped cells, usually pigmented, rarely nonpigmented. It begins as a flat disk-shaped mass in the outer layers of the choroid, most commonly near the posterior pole; later it perforates the lamina vitrea, grows more rapidly and forms a *globular* or mushroom-shaped *mass* in the subretinal space, pushing the retina forward at its summit and causing *detachment of the retina* at its sides (Fig. 14-1). This tumor rarely may arise in the ciliary body or iris.

Symptoms. There are four stages.

In the first or insidious stage there are no symptoms and the only sign may be discovered merely by chance; a brown or black, flat or slightly elevated, circumscribed mass in the choroid which slowly increases in size, eventually producing interference with visual function by elevation of the overlying retina. However, the tumor may exist for a long time without causing symptoms. Thus melanomas found in this stage are the result of complete, routine or casual, ophthalmoscopic examinations.

In the second stage (clinical symptoms), a defect in the visual field or diminution in vision is the initial symptom, depending upon the exact location of the tumor. The melanoma which produces the earliest disturbance in vision is the one which originates closest to the macula, but even peripheral tumors produce field defects after a time. At this stage there is definite elevation of the tumor but it still remains circumscribed, yellowish brown, brown or black. Sooner or later the retina immediately around the tumor becomes detached (Plate 19*A*), and as time passes the retina becomes detached more diffusely, thus tending to obscure the underlying tumor. The anterior ciliary veins may be dilated in the vicinity of the intraocular tumor. The ocular tension usually is normal or slightly lower than that of the unaffected eye in this stage.

In the third stage (secondary glaucoma), the tumor continues to increase in size and may produce inflammatory signs as a result of the production of secondary glaucoma and of release of irritating necrotic products. Circumcorneal injection, cloudy cornea or turbid aqueous humor and vitreous humor usually are accompanied by pain, which at times may become intense.

The fourth stage (extraocular extension or metastasis) may follow Stage 3 or at times Stage 2, skipping Stage 3. The tumor grows out of the globe usually through one of the emissaria of the sclera, through which vessels or nerves pass. Once outside the globe, the growth usually increases more rapidly, producing a visible pigmented mass anteriorly, or proptosis when the extraocular extension is posterior. In either case neighboring tissues or structures soon are invaded. Metastasis to the liver frequently occurs before extraocular extension.

Pathology. The tumor is composed of spindle or round cells with more or less pigment. The spindle cells may have nuclei with uniformly delicate, reticulate structure without apparent nucleoli (spindle cell type A) or nuclei with coarse nuclear networks and prominent, usually centrally placed nucleoli (spindle cell type B). The round or sometimes polygonal cells have an abundant amount of cytoplasm with round or oval nuclei, each containing distinct nucleolus (epithelioid type). A large number of malignant melanomas are composed almost entirely of one of these cell types; however, some tumors are composed largely of elongated cells but with some rounded or polygonal cells arranged in columns with their long axes at right angles to the axes of the columns and converging toward a central vessel. This has been called the fascicular type. A fifth or mixed type is composed of mixtures of spindle and epithelioid type cells in varying proportions.

As a rule, the epithelioid type or the mixed type in which the epithelioid variety of cell predominates is most malignant. However, the assessment of relative malignancy on a histologic basis also requires an estimation of the amount of reticulum in and around the tumor. Silverstained sections are used for this evaluation. The more argyrophil fibers in the tumor, the less malignant it is likely to be. This is considered as well as the cell type.

Differential Diagnosis. Malignant melanoma of the choroid may be mistaken for *primary detachment of the retina* or *glaucoma*; it cannot be mistaken for retinoblastoma since this occurs during the first years of life. Ordinary detachment of the retina usually occurs suddenly in a myopic eye or after a blow, tension often

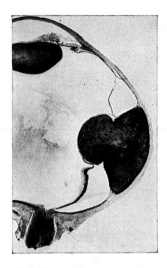

Fig. 14-1. Photomicrograph of an eyeball containing malignant melanoma of the choroid.

is much diminished, a retinal tear most often is found and the retinal folds undulate with motion of the eyeball; while in malignant melanoma, the protruding retina over the summit of the tumor may be rounded and give one the impression of solidity without motion, and there may be some pigment deposit and the addition of blood vessels differing from those of the retina. From primary glaucoma, malignant melanoma of the choroid is distinguished by the fact that sight is involved before the inflammatory symptoms appear, there are no prodromal symptoms such as usually precede glaucoma nor remissions in symptoms, one eye only is involved, the characteristic field of vision in glaucoma (nasal limitation) is not present and the unaffected eye presents no symptoms whatever of glaucoma. However, if the accompanying detachment is extensive, differential diagnosis may be difficult; under such circumstances, the eye usually is blind and enucleation is indicated. Transillumination often is valuable for diagnosis; the pupil

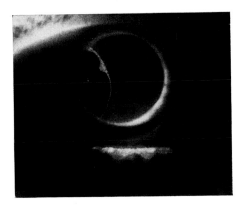

Fig. 14-2. Transillumination of globe, showing the elliptical opacity in the pupil produced by failure of light to pass through a malignant melanoma of the choroid.

or a portion of it remains dark (Fig. 14-2) when the instrument is placed upon the lids or sclera corresponding to the seat of the tumor; it usually will reveal any solid mass situated in the anterior hemisphere; when the tumor is situated near the posterior pole this test is of much less value. A significant uptake of radioactive phosphorus is found in intraocular tumors which are situated anteriorly enough to be accessible to the Geiger counter probe. Counts made 24 hours after injection of P^{32} give best results in differentiating neoplastic from non-neoplastic lesions.

Prognosis. When the eye is enucleated early, cure results in about one-half of the cases. But even after early removal of the eye, death results in many cases from metastases in internal organs, occurring within a few years: rarely there is local recurrence in the orbit. The disease always is fatal, usually within a few years, if the eye is not enucleated.

Treatment. *Enucleation* is indicated as soon as the diagnosis is established, cutting the optic nerve far back, but it is necessary to remove the entire contents of the orbit if the growth has broken through the globe.

Retinoblastoma

This *malignant* growth, formerly known as *glioma of the retina*, probably always congenital, occurs in *children* under 5, usually in *one eye*, at times in both, and occasionally in successive children of the same family.

Symptoms. The clinical manifestations may be divided into four stages, and as in malignant melanoma they are (1) the insidious stage, (2) the stage of signs and symptoms, (3) the stage of inflammation and reaction and (4) the stage of extraocular extension and metastasis.

In the first stage there are no signs or symptoms. Thus, if the tumor is discovered it is only by chance or the result of a complete ocular examination. Small, opaque, white or yellowish white plaques are seen in one or more locations in the retina with the ophthalmoscope. These increase in size, sometimes fusing into a single large whitish mass projecting into the vitreous humor (Plate 19B) or elevating the surrounding retina, causing a white reflex in the pupil producing the so-called amaurotic cat's eye and thus instituting the second clinical stage. The pupil usually becomes dilated and the child begins to bump into things on the side of the affected eye, indicating visual loss.

With continued growth, an acute inflammatory reaction results from extensive necrosis within the tumor (Stage 3). There is increasing circumcorneal congestion and later conjunctival injection and chemosis. The cornea becomes hazy because of numerous fine precipitates on the posterior surface, among which larger grayish white clumps appear. The anterior chamber becomes cloudy because of similar material floating in the aqueous, which at times settles out to form a pseudohypopyon. The vitreous cavity is frequently filled with tumor, producing an appearance resembling a vitreous abscess. The eye becomes painful, and if not enucleated may seem to rupture with extrusion of tumor into the orbit. However, this simply may be the rapid development of extraocular extensions (Stage 4).

The most frequent route of extraocular extension is through the optic nerve and on into the brain; however, others occur through the scleral emissaria, especially along the posterior ciliary nerves. These develop rapidly, producing proptosis and limitation of rotation of the globe.

Metastases usually localize in the skull, long bones and later all organs.

Pathology. The tumor is composed of small, round, densely packed cells arranged around blood vessels or in the shape of tubes, or aggregated in the form of rosettes, in which case the central cells resemble the rods and cones of the retina. The mass usually is permeated with calcium deposits; a short distance from the blood vessels, the cells show a tendency to necrosis. The mass originates either from the outer or the inner surface of the retina; in the former case it causes detachment of the retina (Fig. 14-3); if the growth is inward, the tumor invades the vitreous humor. The tumor always is multiple, there being scattered foci in various parts of the retina. Extension of the growth usually is along the optic nerve and thence into the cranial cavity.

Differential Diagnosis. Retinoblastoma must be distinguished from a number of conditions which have been grouped together under the term *pseudoglioma*. These include (1) vitreous abscess or purulent endophthalmitis, which frequently follows meningitis or pneumonia in children. The pupil usually is irregular, the anterior chamber is deep and a yellowish, avascular mass lies behind the lens; (2) remains of the tunica vasculosa lentis, which may present as a vascularized membrane immediately back of the lens, with

or without a strand of tissue extending back to the optic nerve but through which the retina may be seen somewhat indistinctly but relatively normal in position; (3) retrolental fibroplasia, which is a form of peripheral proliferative retinopathy occurring in premature infants shortly after birth and may be localized to a portion of the peripheral retina or may be extensive and associated with complete detachment of the retina; however, with the pupil widely dilated, pigmented dentation (probably stretched ciliary processes) may be seen in the extreme periphery with the ophthalmoscope.

In x-ray films of eyes containing retinoblastoma, in most cases, there are mottled shadows of calcium density, which are typical of this tumor and are unlike the curvilinear shadow seen in degenerated eyes containing bone. In some instances, however, the differential diagnosis during the first stage may be difficult. When in doubt, such eyes, when sightless, should be enucleated.

Treatment. *Enucleation* is indicated as soon as possible, cutting the optic nerve

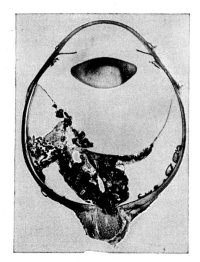

Fig. 14-3. Photomicrograph of an eye containing retinoblastoma.

far back. If microscopic examination of the cut end of the optic nerve shows that the tumor has invaded this part, or if the growth has perforated, exenteration of the orbit is necessary; even then there is danger of recurrence. When enucleation is done early there is a fair chance of cure. Unless this is done death occurs within a few years. In the sad cases in which both eyes are involved, one eye should be enucleated and an attempt made to destroy the tumor without removing the second eye; for this purpose roentgen radiation in divided doses over a protacted period, combined with chemotherapy, is being used, and is now giving encouraging results. There is a high incidence of retinoblastoma in the offspring of cured patients.

Metastatic Tumors

Although metastatic tumors involve the eye only rarely, the choroid at the posterior pole is the most common site of localization by a ratio of approximately 9:1. Carcinoma of the breast is the most common primary lesion to cause metastasis to the choroid, with other metastatic lesions occurring in descending order of frequency: from carcinoma of the lungs and bronchi; the alimentary tract, mostly the stomach; the thyroid gland; prostate; the ovary; the parotid gland; liver; testicle; pancreas; kidney; uterus; and squamous cell carcinoma of the face. On several occasions, metastatic lesions of the choroid have been discovered before the primary lesion was known to exist. Metastases involve both eyes in approximately 25 per cent of cases, but frequently there is some time between involvement of the two eyes. Simultaneous metastases to the brain and eye, however, are quite common.

The patient usually complains of defective vision in one eye, which upon ophthalmoscopic examination shows a pinkish white, solid appearing, indefinitely outlined elevation of the retina at the posterior pole. The surface of the tumor usually has a mottled appearance and may show an occasional hemorrhage. The retina soon becomes detached. The eye becomes painful and frequently inflamed, and glaucoma may develop later.

Treatment should be directed toward control of the primary lesion, and if it is sensitive to irradiation therapy the eye may be treated in an effort to preserve it. If the eye is painful, it may require enucleation.

15

Glaucoma

Anatomy

The anterior chamber is bounded in front by the posterior surface of the cornea, peripherally by the recess of the chamber angle and posteriorly by the anterior surface of the iris and the pupillary aperture. The recess of the chamber angle is bounded by the iris-ciliary body juncture, the ciliary body band and the posterior sulcus of the cornea which is partially filled by the meshwork of the chamber angle overlying the canal of Schlemm (Fig. 15-1). The narrowest part of the anterior chamber is between the last roll of the iris and posterior surface of the cornea and varies considerably between individuals but usually is similar in the two eyes of one person. The deepest part of the anterior chamber is in the pupillary area and also varies considerably between individuals but ranges between 3.0 and 3.6 mm. in general.

The posterior chamber is continuous with the anterior chamber through the pupillary aperture which together with the posterior surface of the iris forms its anterior boundary. The posterior chamber extends between the iris and lens backward along the inner surface of the ciliary body to the ora serrata and between the vitreous humor and lens to the capsulo-hyaloid ligament (Fig. 15-2).

The meshwork of the angle is formed by the breaking up of Descemet's membrane at the margin of the cornea into bundles which connect the sclera with the root of the iris. These elastic laminae are covered by endothelium extended from that covering the posterior surface of the cornea. In this way endothelial-lined spaces are formed which are continuous with the anterior chamber, and are known as the *spaces of Fontana.* To their outer side, in the posterior corneal sulcus, is *Schlemm's canal,* communicating laterally with the anterior ciliary veins.

The aqueous humor which fills the anterior and posterior chambers and permeates the vitreous humor is a crystal clear liquid with a refractive index of 1.336. It contains approximately 0.02 per cent protein in comparison with 7 per cent in the blood plasma. Sugar, urea and bicarbonate also are lower in concentration in the aqueous humor whereas ascorbic acid and chloride are considerably higher than in plasma.

Aqueous humor is produced largely by the ciliary body, partially by diffusion, partially by filtration and partially by active transport from the blood into the posterior chamber by enzymatic activity (carbonic anhydrase and sodium and potassium adenosine triphosphatase) of the cells of the ciliary processes. The composition of the aqueous humor is modified by the diffusion of water from other vascular structures in the eye such as the iris stroma, and the diffusion of metabolites such as lactic acid from the lens and cornea.

In addition to furnishing nutritional support to the avascular lens and the cornea, the aqueous humor contributes to the maintenance of the intraocular pressure. Produced largely by the ciliary body the aqueous humor passes between the iris and lens and leaves the posterior chamber through the pupil, passing into the anterior chamber then a portion passes through

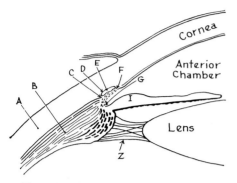

FIG. 15-1. Section of the eye at the sclerocorneal junction showing the angle of the anterior chamber. *A*, Sclera; *B*, ciliary body; *C*, scleral spur; *D*, posterior corneal sulcus; *E*, canal of Schlemm; *F*, meshwork of chamber angle; *G*, ciliary body band; *I*, last roll of iris; *Z*, zonular fibers.

the spaces of Fontana of the meshwork of the chamber angle into the canal of Schlemm and out through the Collector channels or aqueous veins into the anterior ciliary veins. A portion of the aqueous humor is absorbed through the iris vessels, in the stromal spaces of the iris, and some diffuses into the vitreous humor and leaves the eye by posterior drainage routes.

Since the eye does not possess lymphatic vessels some have suggested that aqueous humor also serves a lymph function even though its composition is unlike that of lymph.

When the aqueous humor is drained from the anterior chamber by paracentesis, by other intraocular surgery or by trauma, the composition of the aqueous humor changes to resemble very closely that of plasma. This secondary aqueous humor is referred to as plasmoid aqueous humor. A similar change in aqueous humor composition occurs in the course of intraocular inflammation. This probably is a protective and healing mechanism. The plasmoid aqueous humor persists for several days after wound healing and restoration of normal intraocular pressure. It persists longer after an inflammatory process.

Glaucoma

Glaucoma is a complex of ocular diseases all of which share the characteristic sign of increased intraocular pressure which in time is sufficient to produce visual impairment causing typical defects in the visual field caused by atrophy of retinal ganglion cells and atrophy of the optic

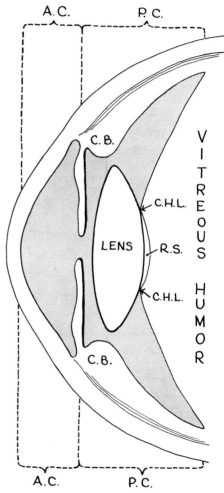

FIG. 15-2. Diagrammatic section of the anterior portion of the eye showing: *AC*, anterior chamber; *PC*, posterior chamber; *CB*, ciliary body; *lens*; *CHL*, capsulohyaloid ligament; *RS*, retrolental space; and *vitreous humor*.

nerve. Specific types of glaucoma have additional characteristic features.

Glaucoma occurs most commonly in adults. Various surveys have shown an incidence varying between 2 per cent and 4 per cent in unselected persons over 40 years of age. This type of glaucoma probably is hereditary and transmitted as a recessive which would mean that approximately 4 per cent of the population should be homozyous and eventually develop the disease, 32 per cent should be heterozygous, and 64 per cent should be normal.

Primary congenital glaucoma which usually appears at birth or shortly thereafter also is inherited as a recessive with only a small pool of phenotypically normal carriers in the general population. Therefore the incidence is quite low (in the region of 0.01 per cent). However it affects males twice as often as females and is bilateral in 75 per cent of patients.

Glaucoma occurs in association with other congential anomalies but frequently is not present at birth and may not become manifest until during the second or third decade.

Secondary glaucoma occurs at any age as a consequence of ocular inflammation, ocular tumor or trauma thus the several varieties of glaucoma may be classified:

A. Adult glaucoma—Primary
  1. Open angle (wide angle, simple, chronic simple, compensated) glaucoma
  2. Angle closure (narrow angle, closed angle, acute congestive, uncompensated) glaucoma
     a. Acute
     b. Chronic
B. Congenital glaucoma
  1. Primary congenital glaucoma (infantile glaucoma, hydrophthalmos)
  2. Glaucoma associated with other congenital anomalies (juvenile glaucoma)
C. Secondary glaucoma

  1. Congenital (buphthalmos)
  2. Juvenile
  3. Adult

Open angle glaucoma occurs in individuals who appear to have normal chamber angles but who have resistance to flow of aqueous humor out of the chamber angle. The resistance may be in the meshwork, in Schlemm's canal, in the aqueous veins or in the ciliary veins.

Angle closure glaucoma results from forward displacement of the last roll and root of the iris against the cornea and obstruction of flow of aqueous humor into the chamber angle and the spaces of Fontana of the meshwork of the chamber angle (Fig. 15-3). In patients in whom the distance between the posterior surface of the cornea and the anterior surface of the iris especially at the last roll of the iris, is slight the entrance to the chamber angle is narrow and more susceptible to closure than in the normal individual. In such a person with a narrow angle, sudden dilatation of the pupil, swelling of the iris from inflammation, swelling of the lens or slight forward movement of the lens and iris may be sufficient to produce a sudden and complete obstruction to outflow of the aqueous humor.

Diagnostic Methods

The diagnosis of glaucoma depends upon the demonstration of increased intraocular pressure, typical visual field defects and glaucomatous cupping and atrophy of the nerve head. However it is important to recognize and treat glaucoma before retinal and optic nerve damage has been produced. Therefore studies of the ocular tension, rate of production and flow of aqueous humor, configuration of the chamber angle, the visual fields and the appearance of the optic nerve head may permit an early presumptive diagnosis.

Tonometry. Ocular tension is measured most commonly by tonometry with the

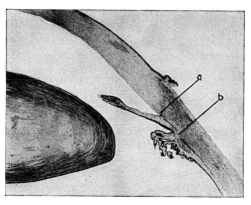

Fig. 15-3. Photomicrograph of anterior portion of the eye in advanced glaucoma, showing iris atrophy and anterior synechia from *a* to *b*.

Schiötz tonometer (p. 7 and 8). However the Goldmann applanation tonometer has become more widely used by ophthalmologists recently. The applanation tonometer is used in conjunction with the slit lamp and biomicroscope after the instillation of a topical anesthetic and measures the force required to flatten a segment of cornea 3.06 mm. in diameter. The mean average intraocular pressure measured in this way is 15.4 mm. Hg. with a standard deviation of ±2.5 mm. The normal eye will tolerate an intraocular pressure of 20 mm. Hg indefinitely without damage; however, those showing pressures of 23 to 25 mm. Hg should be kept under observation and further testing but those showing pressures over 25 mm. Hg should be classed as glaucoma suspects or glaucoma patients.

Ocular tension varies slightly with pulse pressure, respiration and activity but in addition shows a diurnal rhythm usually with a high pressure occurring early in the morning and a low in the evening. In some instances study of the diurnal pressure curve will show a rise above 20 mm. Hg in the morning for a period before there is a gradual elevation of the pressures both in the morning and in the evening. Further aid in arriving at a diagnosis may be ob-

tained by tonographic studies and by provocative tests.

Tonography. Since increased intraocular pressure almost always is due to diminished flow of aqueous humor out of the eye, studies of aqueous flow can aid in arriving at a diagnosis. Pressure applied externally to the eye causes an increase in the outflow of aqueous humor from the anterior chamber. The weight of a tonometer causes an increased outflow of aqueous humor so the plunger gradually indents the cornea further and further with time. The amount of aqueous humor thus expressed from the anterior chamber can be calculated from the tonometer readings at the beginning and at the end of a given period of time. An indentation type of tonometer, similar to the Schiötz tonometer, has been modified electronically so that a record of the pressure is made on a moving drum while the tonometer rests on the eye. This electronic tonometer is allowed to rest on the patient's eye for 4 minutes. From the record made the coefficient of outflow of aqueous humor can be calculated. In normal eyes the average outflow coefficient is 0.28 with a standard deviation of ±0.05. Only 2.5 per cent of normal eyes have a coefficient of outflow as low as 0.18. Therefore a coefficient of outflow below 0.18 would suggest impairment of outflow. Another valuable relationship which can be determined from the tonogram is the Po/C ratio or the intraocular pressure at the beginning of tonography divided by the coefficient of outflow. Normally the ratio will have a value of less than 100. Values of more than 100 occur in only 2.5 per cent of normal eyes. Most glaucoma patients will have a value of 140 or higher without treatment.

Provocative Tests. Tonometry and tonography may separate definite glaucoma subjects from normal individuals but they leave a group of patients in a doubtful or suspect category. In addition some patients may have normal ocular tension at the time of examination, whereas early in the morning their tensions may have been elevated. Thus tests which tend to cause a rise of intraocular pressure in the normal individual usually will show a much more than normal response in a borderline, early or overt glaucoma patient. These tests are not always dependable and in some instances may cause severe or dangerous increases in intraocular pressure; therefore, they should be done only by and under the supervision of an ophthalmologist who from experience and training can handle such problems and immediately institute the necessary therapy to control the pressure.

Provocative tests should be considered on patients who have an intraocular pressure of 22 mm. Hg or higher, a coefficient of outflow value of 0.18 or less, a Po/C ratio of 100 or more, visual field changes suggestive of glaucoma if other confirmatory signs are not present, or optic nerve head changes suggestive of glaucoma if other diagnostic criteria are doubtful.

The water drinking test depends upon the reduction of blood osmolarity and consequent increase in intraocular pressure following the rapid ingestion of a liter of water. Normal eyes may show an increase of 3 to 5 mm. Hg pressure in this test, therefore a rise of 6 mm. Hg pressure or more is considered to indicate glaucoma. The patient is not permitted to use ocular medication for 48 hours preceeding the test. The test is done in the morning and the patient is not permitted breakfast. The intraocular pressure is taken and the patient is given a liter of water to drink within 2 minutes. At the end of 45 minutes the intraocular pressure is recorded again or a tonogram is made. A Po/C value of more than 100 is indicative of glaucoma.

The dark room test depends upon the physiologic dilatation of the pupil in a dark room for 60 minutes. In patients with narrow angles or closure of a considerable portion of the chamber angle, dilatation of the pupil by crowding the iris into the angle may complete the obstruction and cause a rise in intraocular pressure. This test should be performed only after an examination of the chamber angle by gonioscopy to eliminate patients with obvious angle closure for this test could precipitate an acute angle closure glaucoma unless the pupil is promptly constricted following the test. Normal eyes frequently show a rise of 3 to 5 mm. Hg by this test, therefore a rise of 6 mm. Hg or more is required to be significant of glaucoma. Unfortunately some patients with open angle glaucoma also show a significant rise in the intraocular pressure on this test, therefore the eyes should be examined by gonioscopy after the tension is taken at the end of the test to determine whether the angle is open or closed.

Mydriatic dilatation of the pupil may serve the same purpose as a dark room test. However a short acting easily controllable mydriatic should be used because the same dangers and precautions apply to this test as apply to the dark room test.

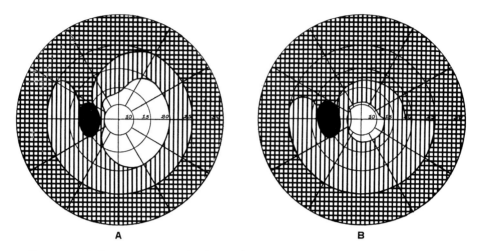

A　　　　　　　　　　　　　　　　　B

Fig. 15-4. *A*, Tangent screen visual field in glaucoma showing upward and downward enlargement of the blind spot, early generalized contraction and baring of the blind spot. Two different size targets were used in making the examination. The clear central portion is visible to both targets. The portion of the field crossed by the vertical "hatch" lines is seen only with the larger target (relative scotoma), but the portion with the double "hatch" lines and the black blind spot are seen with neither target (absolute scotoma). *B*, Tangent screen visual fields in glaucoma at a later stage showing enlargement and baring of the blind spot, generalized contraction of the visual field greater on the nasal side and with a Roenne's nasal step.

The pupil should be constricted at the end of the test.

Corticosteroids when instilled in sufficient concentration (0.1 per cent betametasone) 4 times a day for 3 or 4 weeks will cause a decrease in the coefficient of outflow of aqueous humor in nearly 100 per cent of open angle glaucoma patients, in nearly all of the 32 per cent heterozygous carriers of open angle glaucoma, and in approximately 40 per cent of patients with angle closure and secondary glaucomas. This is not only a valuable test in early glaucoma but also in studying the families of glaucoma patients.

Visual Fields. The visual fields show the effects of increased intraocular pressure upon the optic nerve and retina relatively early. Thus early examination of the visual fields may show defects which may be restored by prompt early control of the intraocular pressure or at least may be prevented from extending into more serious damage.

In uncontrolled glaucoma the visual field defects are progressive. These consist of an upward and downward enlargement of the blind spot (Seidel's sign) with slight general contraction of the field with corresponding changes in the color fields. One of the early changes is baring of the blind spot (Fig. 15-4*A*), then development of arcuate scotomas (island of diminution or loss of vision within the field) which begin in the blind spot and extend in an arching manner around the central portion of the visual field (Fig. 15-5). These are Bjerrum scotomas and may simply represent an extension of Seidel's sign and a variation of the process which produces baring of the blind spot. With progress the general contraction of the visual field continues, especially on the nasal side (Fig. 15-6), often producing a greater contraction in the upper field with a sharp horizontal shelf-like or step-like retention of the lower field (Fig. 15-4*B*), which is known as Roenne's nasal step. The central visual field is not affected by glaucoma until late in the course of the disease. Thus, the visual acuity remains good, unless it is reduced for some reason other than glaucoma; the patient with greatly contracted fields will have difficulty in walking and moving about, continually bumping into or stumbling over things. However, the central fields eventually are lost and the last remnant of vision is a small island in the temporal field (Fig. 15-7) which persists for some time but is of little or no practical value to the patient.

The course of simple glaucoma is very *insidious* and its duration is *years*; if unchecked, it terminates in *blindness*.

Ophthalmoscopy. Ophthalmoscopic evaluation of the optic nerve head is directed toward the condition of the vessels, the color of the tissue and the character of the cup. Increased intraocular pressure tends to effect vessels with lower blood pressure first. Thus the small vessels of the optic nerve head derived from the arterial circle of Zinn which in

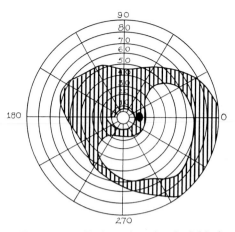

Fig. 15-6. Perimetric visual field in glaucoma showing enlargement and baring of the blind spot, general and nasal contraction of the visual field, Roenne's nasal step, and Bjerrum scotoma.

turn is derived from the short posterior ciliary vessels become decreased in diameter and lost to view as the intraocular pressure increases. At the same time the tissue of the nerve head loses some of its pinkness and begins to appear pale. The physiologic cup, at first normal, is gradually widened and deepened as the result of increased intraocular pressure. The widening begins on the temporal side and progresses to the rim of the disk so there apparently is no tissue left between the margin of the cup and the margin of the nerve head on the temporal side (Fig. 15-8). Along with this the cup enlarges under the nasal rim of the nerve head and the major vessels appear to be pushed nasally disappearing from view at the rim of the cup but become visible again in the depths of the cup (Plate *6B*). As the cup deepens and widens the floor of the cup appears to be stippled, probably the fenestration in the lamina cribrosa. The pallor of the optic nerve head increases to a definite whiteness with the development of optic atrophy. In elderly patients or patients with secondary glaucoma the color changes

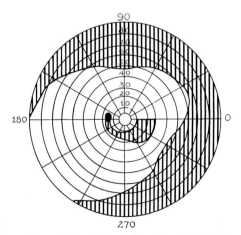

Fig. 15-5. Perimetric visual field in glaucoma showing a Bjerrum scotoma.

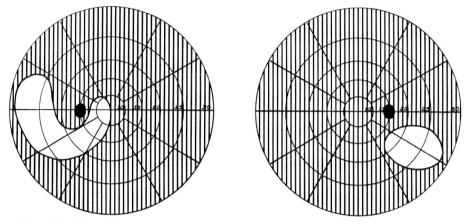

FIG. 15-7. Bjerrum screen visual field in late glaucoma, showing late contraction of fields with temporal field remaining on left but only temporal island remaining on right.

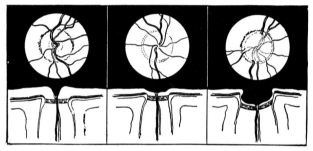

FIG. 15-8. Ophthalmoscopic appearances and longitudinal section of the optic nerve disk. *Left*, normal disk; *center*, disk in optic nerve atrophy; *right*, glaucomatous excavation.

must be evaluated with the fact in mind that opacities of the media (lens and vitreous humor) tend to make the optic nerve head and fundus appear redder than is actually the case.

Gonioscopy. Examination of the angle of the anterior chamber is made possible by the application of a contact prism to the cornea and observing the angle through the biomicroscope with slit lamp illumination. The angle appears to be normal in open angle type of glaucoma. It appears normal but is difficult to see into or to see completely due to proximity of the last roll of the iris to the posterior surface of the cornea in patients with narrow angles.

These people are potential candidates for acute angle closure glaucoma. In patients with angle closure glaucoma the meshwork of the chamber angle is completely obstructed by attachment of the peripheral portion of the iris to the posterior surface of the cornea. Closure of a portion or several portions of the angle may exist before complete closure develops. In some types of congenital glaucoma the angle is obstructed by failure of cleavage and absorption of embryonic tissues which occupy this part of the eye. In secondary glaucoma the chamber angle or the spaces of Fontana of the meshwork of the chamber angle is obstructed by inflammatory cells, red blood cells, pigment granules, crystaline deposits or by scar tissue and synechiae.

PRIMARY GLAUCOMA

Acute Angle Closure Glaucoma (Acute Congestive)

Symptoms. The affection can be divided into three stages: (1) the *prodromal stage*, (2) the stage of *acute glaucoma* and (3) the stage of *absolute glaucoma*.

The Prodromal Stage. This stage is present in most instances in the form of transitory attacks; however, it may be absent. During the attack there is some diminution in the acuteness of *vision;* the sight appears to be obscured by *fog*. A *halo* of *rainbow tints* is seen around lights; the *cornea*, especially at its center, upon careful inspection is slightly *clouded*; this condition is the cause of the preceding symptoms. A feeling of dullness or *slight pain* in the eye and head may occur. The *anterior chamber* is rather *shallow*, and the *pupil* somewhat *dilated* and *sluggish* in reaction. The *tension* of the globe is slightly or moderately increased. There often is slight circumcorneal injection. These symptoms last for a number of hours and then disappear entirely; the eye returns to normal including normal intraocular pressure, except that there often is a *diminution* in the power of *accommodation,* so that the patient requires stronger glasses than are natural at his age. Hence a rapid increase of presbyopia should always excite suspicion of glaucoma. Such prodromal attacks often are excited by insomnia, worry, emotional excitement or some condition which causes venous congestion, and sometimes by overeating, indigestion or the local use of mydriatics. They are relieved by sleep in many cases. At first the attacks are separated by *intervals* of weeks or months, but they soon become more frequent.

This stage, when present, lasts a number

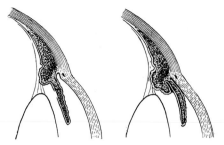

FIG. 15-9. Angle of the anterior chamber: *left*, in the normal eye; *right*, in congestive glaucoma.

of weeks or months, sometimes several years; then the disease passes into the second stage.

The Stage of Acute Glaucoma ("glaucomatous attack"). The *sudden onset* which characterizes this stage usually is due to one of the exciting causes which bring on the prodromal attacks. There are *rapid failure of sight* and *severe pain* in the eye, radiating along the branches of the fifth nerve and causing violent *headache*; this pain sometimes is so severe that it occasions nausea and vomiting, such attacks having been mistaken for "bilious attacks."

Examination reveals a great *increase in intraocular pressure*. The lids are swollen and edematous. The bulbar conjunctiva is intensely congested and chemotic. The *cornea* is clouded or *steamy*, often presents punctate opacities and is insensitive (from pressure upon nerve filaments); there is intense circumcorneal *injection* of a dark red color; the episcleral veins are prominent (Plate 20*A*). The *anterior chamber is shallow* and the aqueous humor sometimes turbid. The *pupil is dilated,* immobile and often presents a greenish reflex. The iris is congested, discolored and dull. The lens and the periphery of the iris are pushed forward (Fig. 15-9). No details of the fundus can be seen with the ophthalmoscope, because of the *clouding of the media.*

In many cases, *decided improvement* takes place within a few hours as a result of treatment. Pain subsides, congestion and edema of lids and conjunctiva disappear, the cornea clears and sight improves. Unless the glaucoma is controlled by medical or surgical means, the eye is left in a condition which resembles chronic congestive glaucoma. Vision is less acute than before the attack, the visual field is contracted, especially on the nasal side, and the light sense reduced. After a more severe attack the pupil remains dilated and sluggish, the iris discolored, the anterior chamber shallow and tension increased, and there is more or less circumcorneal injection; the power of accommodation is diminished.

After a period of quiescence of variable length, *another attack*, similar to the first, occurs, succeeded by others; each attack causes greater reduction in sight.

After a time, the increased tension causes *excavation of the optic nerve disk* (Fig. 15-8, *right*), recognizable with the ophthalmoscope in the intervals between attacks, when the media are clear. The lamina cribrosa, the portion of the sclera which is perforated by the optic nerve fibers, is most yielding and hence bulges backward with the fibers of the nerve as a result of increased intraocular pressure. With the ophthalmoscope a *deep depression* with very steep or *overhanging margins* is seen; this is known as the *glaucomatous cup or excavation* (Plate 20*B*). The *blood vessels bend* sharply over the margins of this excavation and often appear interrupted in this situation, being seen again more or less faintly, at the bottom of the depression. They also are pushed over toward the nasal side. The veins are distended and the arteries contracted. There is *pulsation* in the veins and in the *arteries* at the disk. Pulsation may be seen in the veins in some individuals in

health, but arterial pulsation always is pathologic, and is an important symptom of glaucoma, abnormally elevated pulse pressure, as in aortic regurgitation, or in thyroid disease. The *optic nerve* becomes *atrophied* and the disk appears *pale*, or in late stages white or bluish. The disk often is surrounded by a whitish yellow ring (*glaucomatous ring*), caused by atrophy of the choroid in this situation.

The Stage of Absolute Glaucoma. This is the end stage of all types of primary glaucoma. With each succeeding attack the diminution in vision becomes greater and the tension more difficult to control, until finally, with uncontrollable elevated pressure, pain and *blindness* ensue; the condition then is known as absolute glaucoma. There are no inflammatory or congestive symptoms, except a dark red zone of circumcorneal *injection* and *dilated episcleral veins*. The cornea remains clear or slightly clouded, and often more or less insensitive. The *pupil* is widely *dilated*, immobile, and often presents a *greenish* reflex. The iris is atrophied, narrow and gray, with a border of dark pigment. The anterior chamber is shallow. Ophthalmoscopic examination reveals a *deep excavation* of the disk, the glaucomatous ring, and atrophy of the optic nerve. Pain may disappear entirely, but frequently continues, and the patient suffers from severe attacks at intervals.

After absolute glaucoma has lasted a variable length of time, the eyeball is apt to degenerate. The cornea becomes more or less opaque, and frequently is covered by deposits or vesicles. The sclera bulges, and bluish black staphylomas appear between the cornea and the equator. The lens is apt to become cataractous. The patient may experience subjective sensations of light. The final result is that either the *eyeball* softens, shrinks and *atrophies* or else there are ulceration and perforation of the cornea, followed by iridocyclitis, with subsequent atrophy of the eyeball, or panophthalmitis and phthisis bulbi.

Chronic Congestive Glaucoma

This form of glaucoma is a chronic variety of congestive glaucoma, often complicated by acute or subacute attacks. *Its symptoms resemble those of the acute variety, but are less intense and more gradual in their onset.* Very often the prodromal stage passes uninterruptedly into the subacute or chronic stage of active glaucoma. The bulbar conjunctiva is congested and dusky and the episcleral veins very prominent; there is circumcorneal injection of a dark red color; the cornea is steamy and more or less insensitive; the anterior chamber is shallow, and the lens and iris are pushed forward. The pupil is dilated and rigid, surrounded by the discolored, narrow and atrophic iris, and presents a greenish reflex. There is pain, but this is not so intense as in the acute form. There are gradual loss of sight, progressive limitation of the field, especially on the nasal side, and reduction in the light sense. After these symptoms have lasted a sufficient length of time, the ophthalmoscope reveals the same changes in the fundus that are found in the end stages of acute cases.

The chronic form has the same termination as the acute: absolute glaucoma and finally degeneration of the eyeball. In many cases, no sharp line of differentiation can be drawn between the acute and the chronic forms of congestive glaucoma.

Pathology. The essential histologic features of *acute* congestive glaucoma are *ocular hyperemia and edema.* There may be hemorrhages of the iris. The cornea, iris and ciliary body are edematous, and the anterior chamber is shallow. The angle of the anterior chamber is obliterated by the pushed-forward root of the iris. If the acute attack is not relieved, there often is necrosis and atrophy of the iris and ciliary processes. In *chronic* congestive glaucoma, the *angle* of the anterior chamber is *blocked* by a firm union of the iris to the posterior surface of the cornea over a variable extent (peripheral anterior synechia, Figs. 15-3 and 15-9). In the later stages, *degenerative* changes appear in the ocular tissues.

Treatment. The treatment of congestive glaucoma or angle closure glaucoma, whether acute or chronic, has for its principal aim opening the chamber angle to permit adequate drainage of aqueous. This may be accomplished by medical means, but usually surgery is required eventually if not at once.

The most important medical objective is establishment of miosis, thus pulling the iris out of the chamber angle. The chief medication used for this purpose is pilocarpine. In the prodromal stage or in the interval between acute attacks, instillation of 1 per cent pilocarpine at bedtime or more often may keep the chamber angle open so normal intraocular pressure is maintained.

During acute attacks of angle closure, however, drops should be used as often as every 10 or 15 minutes until the pupil is constricted. The first drop usually is less disturbing if a 1 per cent solution is used, but succeeding drops should be increased in strength up to 4 or occasionally 6 per cent solution during this period of intensive treatment. Miosis should be established in both eyes during an acute attack since this renders treatment of the involved eye more effective as well as tending to prevent overlooking similar but less severe involvement of the fellow eye. Stronger miotics such as eserine and diisopropylfluorophosphate (DFP) should be avoided or used only with great caution in this type of glaucoma, since they may cause swelling of the root of the iris and ciliary body, thus counteracting some of the miotic effect. Supplementation of the topical miotic effect as well as relief of pain is obtained by intramuscular injection of 0.01 to 0.016 gm. of morphine.

Further supplementation of the miotic effect as well as some decongestion, lowering of intraocular pressure and relief of ocular pain is obtained by the retrobulbar injection of 1 cc. of 2 per cent Novocain containing 1:20,000 Adrenalin.

Rapid lowering of the intraocular pressure may be obtained at times by the use of one of the osmotic agents, glycerol or urea, if there are no medical contraindications. Propanetriol (glycerol) is given in a dosage of 1 ml. per pound of body weight in a mixture with equal parts of iced lemon juice. This may be given all at once or divided into two doses one-half hour apart. If this should not be successful or if more rapid action is necessary urea (Urevert) may be given intravenously in a dosage of 1 gm. per kg. of body weight.

Additional lowering of the intraocular pressure is obtained by the oral or intravenous administration of a carbonic anhydrase-inhibiting agent. Diamox may be used for this purpose in an initial dose of 250 or 500 mg. either orally or intravenously, and its effect prolonged by administration of 125 to 250 mg. orally every 6 hours thereafter.

As the acute attack is brought under control, medical therapy is reduced but maintained at a level which controls the intraocular pressure and permits the congestion to subside. Then before the patient leaves the hospital an iridectomy should be made first on the eye involved, then upon the other eye, since similar acute attacks are likely to recur not only in the affected eye but also in the other eye. Should the pressure not be controlled effectively by medical therapy, surgical intervention may be necessary sooner and also may require something in addition to simple iridectomy to insure aqueous drainage (see below).

In the patient in whom such prophylactic surgery is performed acute attacks are prevented, but periodic re-evaluations should be made of the status of the intraocular pressure, the condition of the anterior chamber with special attention to the chamber angle, and the visual field, whereas in the patient in whom such surgery has not been done either for adequate reasons or because of the patient's intransigence, repeated acute attacks are quite likely to occur in either or both eyes. Each attack or any attack is likely to result in increased or permanent closure of the chamber angle and the establishment of severe or absolute glaucoma. In such individuals pilocarpine drops should be used three or four times a day and in addition the patient should be warned that emotional episodes, prolonged periods of visual activity in poor or dim illumination such as prevails in the theatre, or quickly drinking several cups or glasses of any type of fluid are likely to induce acute attacks. He also should be warned that he should waste no time in obtaining ophthalmic care once an acute episode begins.

In absolute glaucoma, with repeated attacks of pain, *enucleation* is indicated.

Prognosis in primary congestive glaucoma is most favorable in acute cases detected and treated early, and especially in those which respond satisfactorily to miotics, for iridectomy can prevent subsequent attacks. Cases of chronic congestive glaucoma do not respond so favorably; retention of ocular function depends upon the extent of damage from the ocular hypertension existing at the time of the operation.

Simple Glaucoma (Open Angle)

In simple glaucoma (chronic noncongestive glaucoma), there are *no congestive attacks and no pain.*

This form develops very *gradually,* and may last some time before the patient becomes aware of the existence of an abnormal condition. The eye may appear perfectly normal externally, or there may be slight circumcorneal *injection* and moderate dilatation of the episcleral veins. The *pupil* is slightly or moderately dilated and is *sluggish.* The *tension is elevated,* often moderately; sometimes the increase is not constant, and the tonometer may disclose a rise in tension only after repeated tests on different days. The instillation of a drop of Adrenalin often causes mydriasis in glaucomatous eyes whereas it has less effect upon the size of the pupil of normal eyes; this may be an aid to diagnosis and also may be the means of permitting a better examination of the fundus. The slit lamp often reveals pigment granules on the posterior surface of the cornea. After the disease has lasted a certain length of time, ophthalmoscopic examination reveals *glaucomatous cupping* of the disk (Fig. 15-8, *right*; Plate 20*B*), atrophy of the optic nerve and the circumpapillary ring of choroidal atrophy, the degree of change depending upon the duration of the process.

There may be periods when the patient complains of *foggy vision, colored halos* around artificial lights and *diminished accommodation.* There are gradual *loss of sight, premature presbyopia* and disturbed dark adaptation.

There are progressive changes in the visual field (p. 230).

Pathology. In the early stages, the iris root, as a rule, is not adherent to the posterior surface of the cornea. There often is thickening or sclerosis of the pectinate ligament. Later, peripheral anterior synechiae usually develop (Fig. 15-3). Atrophy of the iris, ciliary body and choroid appears. The fibers of the optic nerve degenerate, and excavation of the nervehead develops. The nerve fiber

layer and the ganglion cell layer of the retina atrophy. The lens becomes cataractous. Thrombosis of the central vessels of the retina occurs occasionally.

Treatment. This may be *nonoperative* or *operative.* The ideal result is obtained when the disease responds to a weak miotic, pilocarpine (1 to 2 per cent). The patient must be kept under close observation, and the strength and frequency of the miotic regulated to maintain normal tension and arrest visual field changes. Usually, if the disease responds to medical treatment, it will be controlled by the use of pilocarpine hydrochloride or nitrate two to four times a day. Cases which require pilocarpine more often than four times a day or stronger than 4 per cent require operation. Prostigmin bromide in 5 per cent solution or carbamylcholine chloride (carbachol) in 1.5 per cent solution is employed occasionally to enhance or replace pilocarpine. Eserine or DFP may be used at times to supplement the action of pilocarpine or replace it temporarily in this type of glaucoma, but should not be used over prolonged periods without close observation because of the congestion and increased vascular permeability that these drugs induce.

Recently, the use of 1 per cent or 2 per cent epinephrine in the early stages of open angle glaucoma has been just as effective or even more effective than the use of miotics. Later in the course of the disease the miotics may be needed during the day and epinephrine may be used as a supplementary treatment once a day.

General treatment comprises avoidance of physical fatigue and emotional upset. It is best to eliminate coffee, and it is important to maintain the general health at par. Adequate rest is essential; excesses of any kind should be avoided. The possible seriousness of the disease should be explained to the patient. If the glaucoma is unilateral, the patient should be warned that the second eye usually becomes affected and should be watched.

If tension cannot be kept normal, or if there is evidence of advance in the course of the disease, as shown by changes in vision or visual fields, *operative treatment* becomes imperative. Operation also is advisable if the patient is not able to remain under observation. The procedure of choice in these cases is some type of *operation,* having for its object the production of a *filtering scar.*

The operations employed in glaucoma have for their purpose the increased outflow of aqueous humor and are referred to as internal or external "filtering" procedures. The internal "filtering" operations are (1) iridectomy, which increases flow of aqueous humor from the posterior to the anterior chamber and into the chamber angle, and (2) cyclodialysis, which increases the flow of aqueous humor by creation of a passage from the anterior chamber to the suprachoroidal space. The external "filtering" operations are (1) anterior sclerectomy, (2) trephination and (3) iris inclusion operations, all of which have the purpose of creating a passage for aqueous humor from the anterior chamber to Tenon's space.

Iridectomy alone usually is of value only in acute congestive glaucoma in which the intraocular pressure returns to normal after the chamber angle has been opened, but is used in combination with all other filtering procedures. Cyclodialysis is of value in early simple glaucoma in which the intraocular pressure ranges between normal and 40 or 45 mm. Hg, whereas the external filtering operations are valuable when a greater new outflow of aqueous humor is required to keep the intraocular pressure within normal limits. Actually there is little choice between these procedures except the preference of the surgeon; however, iris inclusion operations should not be made when there is associated disease or degeneration of the iris.

In absolute glaucoma enucleation is indicated for the relief of pain. Other surgery, such as a "filtering" procedure, is contraindicated not only because of almost certain failure to accomplish the purposes of lowering intraocular pressure and relieving pain but also because such operations frequently are followed by severe intraocular hemorrhage and occasionally by sympathetic ophthalmia; in addition there is a risk that the glaucoma may have been caused by an intraocular malignant tumor, especially in those in whom previous examinations have not been made. Late infections of the eyeball, made possible by the thin barrier between conjunctival sac and interior of the eye at the scleral opening, occur occasionally after external "filtering" operations, but are rare and do not counterbalance the advantage of this form of operative treatment; cataract also has been attributed to these operations, but it is probable that such lenticular changes occur independently.

Massage of the eyeball, applied gently to the closed lids, may be used with advantage in simple and in chronic forms, and also after operation.

Prognosis is *favorable* in cases which are detected and treated in an *early stage,* even when operation is necessary. When glaucoma has progressed to the extent of producing an extensive contraction in at least one meridian of the visual field, the prognosis is much less favorable. In some of these cases, the ocular changes continue although the tension has been controlled by operation. In general it is safe to say that the disease can be arrested in most cases, so that the patient retains the vision he possesses; however, he always must be told that even the most favorable treatment cannot restore that part of vision or visual field which has been lost as a result of the glaucomatous process.

General Consideration of Primary Glaucoma

Occurrence and Etiology. Glaucoma is a disease of *middle and advanced life,* occurring generally between 40 and 70; infrequently it attacks younger subjects and then is known as *juvenile glaucoma.* The congestive form attacks women more often than men; the simple type occurs equally in both sexes. It usually involves *both eyes,* the second eye generally becoming affected months or years after the first. The exact *cause* of glaucoma is *unknown.* There are a number of *predisposing conditions*: There is a definite hereditary tendency (p. 227). Arteriosclerosis may be a predisposing factor. A disposition toward glaucoma exists in *hyperopic eyes* (myopic eyes are far less liable but not exempt) as well as in small eyeballs with large lenses, and in those in which the cornea is of small size.

Pathogenesis. All the symptoms of glaucoma can be explained by the *increase in intraocular pressure.* But the cause of this increase in tension has not yet been determined; none of the many theories has explained the occurrence of glaucoma adequately in every case. The increased tension must depend upon a disturbed relationship between formation of intraocular fluid and its escape, and although, very rarely, an excessive production of aqueous may play a role, the great majority of cases are due to obstruction of aqueous drainage. As discussed earlier, the site of obstruction in congestive glaucoma is the chamber angle; an anatomically narrow angle may be closed by dilatation of the pupil, crowding the iris into the angle and against the posterior surface of the cornea; a cataract in the stage of swelling (intumescent cataract) may push the root of the iris across the narrow chamber

angle and against the posterior surface of the cornea; a similar mechanism may result from the normal continuous growth of the lens in an anatomically small eye or one with a small cornea and anterior segment (hyperopia, microphthalmia and microcornea); or occasionally vasodilatation and resultant swelling of the ciliary body and root of the iris may occlude the angle. However, in primary simple glaucoma the obstruction to outflow of aqueous humor occurs in the meshwork of the chamber angle, in the canal of Schlemm, in the aqueous veins which pass from the canal of Schlemm through the sclera to the anterior ciliary veins or possibly even in the anterior ciliary veins. Obstruction of the meshwork of the chamber angle may result from thickening of the tissue strands of the meshwork by sclerosis or by swelling or the spaces in the meshwork may be occluded by pigment granules (primary pigmentary glaucoma). Obstruction of the canal of Schlemm or the aqueous veins may result from sclerosis or swelling of the surrounding sclera. Occasionally the obstruction to aqueous humor drainage may be due to excessive hydrostatic pressure in the anterior ciliary veins.

Differential Diagnosis. The *congestive form* of glaucoma has been mistaken for *iritis* and *conjunctivitis*; the use of atropine in such cases has caused great mischief. The dilated pupil, increase in tension, shallow anterior chamber, steamy cornea, altered vision and visual field, as well as the subjective symptoms, ought to be sufficient to differentiate (see Table 9-1). In acute cases, the violent headache and general constitutional symptoms have misled the medical practitioner, and have been responsible for the diagnosis of some *general febrile disease* or of a "bilious attack," at a time when active ocular treatment was urgent.

Simple glaucoma sometimes is mistaken for *simple optic nerve atrophy.* In the

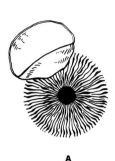
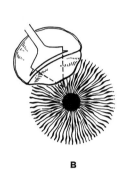
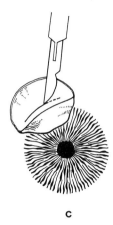

A   B   C

FIG. 15-10. *A*, Conjunctival flap turned downward in preparation for scleral incision. *B*, Keratome incision through limbus and into anterior chamber. *C*, Scratch incision.

latter case, there is no increased tension; the excavation of the disk is shallow and gradual (Fig. 15-8, *center*; Plate 30*A*); there is apt to be greater diminution in central vision; the form fields present more uniform contraction; the color fields show greater peripheral loss, and there is an absence of scotoma directly continuous with the blind spot. There are, however, instances in which the differential diagnosis between these two affections is not easy, particularly when the increase of tension is very slight or happens to be temporarily absent.

Operations for Glaucoma

Iridectomy (Complete or Radial). Iridectomy for glaucoma usually is made in the upper temporal portion of the iris so the defect is covered by the upper lid, thus limiting troublesome optical effects of the coloboma. The conjunctiva and Tennon's capsule are incised 5 or 6 mm. away from the limbus in the superior temporal quadrant and undermined to the limbus, producing a conjunctival flap (Fig. 15-10, *left*) which is turned down over the cornea. An incision is made through the limbus into the anterior chamber with a keratome in patients with a deep anterior chamber (Fig. 15-10, *center*) or by a scratch technique (Fig. 15-10, *right*) in patients with a shallow anterior chamber or narrow chamber angle. The incision is completed and the aqueous allowed to drain slowly. Closed iris forceps are passed through the limbic incision, and the iris is grasped near the pupillary border and withdrawn. The iris is cut with scissors (Fig. 15-11), producing a keyhole-shaped pupil (Fig. 15-12, *left*) when the iris is replaced in the anterior chamber. The limbic incision and the conjunctival wound are closed separately by interrupted fine catgut sutures. A drop of cycloplegic is instilled onto the cornea and the eye dressed for 24 hours. Recovery is uneventful in most instances; in some cases the anterior chamber is not re-formed for several days. Cystoid cicatrix sometimes results—a condition which is not objectionable and is thought to facilitate filtration.

The indications for iridectomy. Besides (1) glaucoma, the operation may be indicated in (2) some cases of chronic and recurrent iritis and iridocyclitis, (3) complete circular synechia, (4) partial corneal staphyloma, (5) tumors and foreign bodies in the iris, (6) recent prolapse of the iris, (7) as a part of the operation of

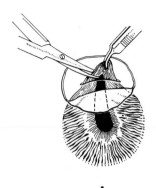 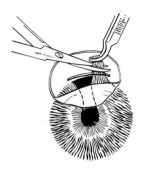

A   **B**

FIG. 15-11. *A*, Complete iridectomy, 1st cut. *B*, Complete iridectomy, 2nd cut.

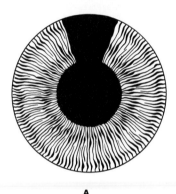 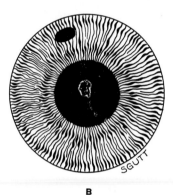

A   **B**

FIG. 15-12. *A*, Complete iridectomy, resulting in a keyhole type of pupillary aperture. *B*, Peripheral iridectomy, leaving the pupil and its reactions intact.

extraction of cataract—here the coloboma should be smaller than in glaucoma—and (8) as a means of improving sight (artificial pupil, optical iridectomy) in central opacities of the cornea and lens, occlusion of the pupil and keratoconus.

Optical iridectomy is made in the manner described above, except that the location usually is different. The best position for the artificial pupil is *downward and inward*; but when there is a corneal opacity, the site must correspond to the most transparent portion of the cornea. The effects of optical iridectomy often are disappointing; hence, before operating, it is well to dilate the pupil and, by applying a stenopeic slit held in different positions, to ascertain whether and where there is an improvement in sight.

Peripheral iridectomy may be adequate to insure passage of aqueous from the posterior to the anterior chamber in many cases, and with this technique there is less trouble from light and glare. The operation is different from complete, radial or optical iridectomy described above, in that the iris is grasped in the ciliary or peripheral portion and gently withdrawn through the limbic incision, and a small piece cut out of the iris around the tip of the forceps. Thus when the iris is reposited a small peripheral "buttonhole" results (Fig. 15-12, *right*).

Cyclodialysis. A conjunctival flap is

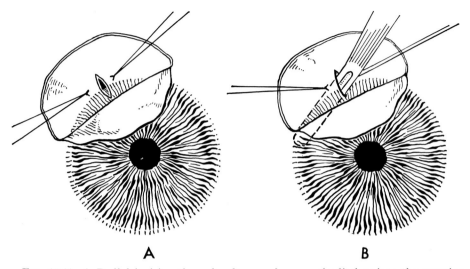

A **B**

FIG. 15-13. *A*, Radial incision through sclera, and across the limbus into the anterior chamber. *B*, Cyclodialysis operation; spatula introduced through radial incision and passed downward separating attachment of the ciliary body to the scleral spur.

made and turned downward over the cornea, as described above. Then an incision 4 to 6 mm. long is made through the sclera parallel with the limbus, taking especial care to open into the suprachoroidal space without injuring the ciliary body. A special thin but grooved spatula is passed forward through the suprachoroidal space into the anterior chamber, separating the attachment of the ciliary body to the scleral spur and thus creating an opening from the anterior chamber into the suprachoroidal space. The spatula is withdrawn slightly and reinserted, repeatedly, gently increasing the extent of detachment of the ciliary body from the scleral spur on either side of the wound until one-third to one-half of this attachment has been severed.

A simplification of this technique has been employed successfully in recent years. After the conjunctival flap has been made it is extended by separating the superficial layers of the cornea for approximately 2 mm. into the cornea. Then a radial incision 3 to 4 mm. long is made

through sclera and limbus (Fig. 15-13, *left*) into the suprachoroidal space and extended into the anterior chamber across the line of attachment of the ciliary body to the scleral spur. The grooved spatula is passed along this line, separating the attachment for approximately one-fourth the distance around the margin of the cornea (Fig. 15-13, *right*) on each side of the incision.

In both methods, after the separation procedure has been completed, an iridectomy usually is made. It may be either of the peripheral or the complete radial variety but is accomplished with more ease following the radial scleral incision method.

The conjunctiva is closed and a light dressing is applied to the eye for 24 hours.

Elliot's Operation (sclerocorneal trephining). A large conjunctival *flap* is dissected from above the cornea to the corneal margin (Fig. 15-14) without detaching the lateral ends. The flap is turned over the cornea and the *cornea* is *split* for a distance of 1.5 mm. with a knife, by means of a number of short lateral strokes; as the dissection proceeds, the deep layers of the split cornea are seen as a dark crescentic area. Care must be taken not to buttonhole the flap. A *trephine*, 1.5 to 2 mm. in diameter, is applied with its center over the corneoscleral junction and with a few semirotary movements with slight pressure the trephine goes through and aqueous escapes. Usually the disk remains attached by a hinge on the scleral side and a knuckle of iris presents in the opening. Disk and bead of iris are grasped together with iris forceps and cut off with a single snip of the iris scissors, thus producing a small peripheral *iridectomy*. If any part of the iris remains in the wound, it must be replaced either by a stream of saline solution or by an iris repositor. The conjunctival flap is replaced and secured with fine silk sutures. A cycloplegic is instilled upon completion of the operation and repeated daily until the iris irritation from the manipulation has passed. A small conjunctiva-covered *bleb* (Fig. 15-15) or a region of conjunctival edema will remain permanently at the seat of the trephine opening in most cases. The operated eye is covered by a dressing for 1 or more days.

Lagrange's Operation (sclerectomy combined with iridectomy). With a Graefe knife the sclera is punctured 1 mm. from the limbus and counterpunctured at a corresponding point 7 mm. removed. The *incision* is made in the iris angle, and at its termination the edge of the knife is directed backward so as to bevel the sclera,

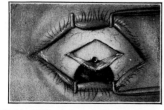

Fig. 15-14. Elliot's operation for glaucoma.

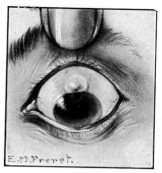

Fig. 15-15. Conjunctival bleb after sclerocorneal trephining.

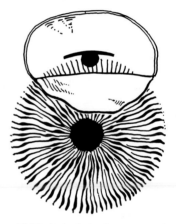

Fig. 15-16. Anterior sclerectomy. A small piece of sclera has been removed from anterior or corneal side of the scleral incision, producing an opening from the anterior chamber into Tenon's space.

then continuing so as to make a 5-mm. conjunctival flap; the latter is grasped and turned back over the cornea, thus tilting the edge of the scleral flap upward, and a piece of the *sclera is excised* (Fig. 15-16). *Iridectomy* is performed, conjunctival flap is closed with sutures and a monocular dressing applied. As a result of the operation, a small dark opening in the sclera is visible through a little cystlike elevation of the conjunctiva or an area of edema, indicating that the aqueous is filtering through the opening.

Holth's punch operation. After a conjunctival flap and a scleral incision into the anterior chamber have been made, a small piece of sclera is removed from the anterior lip by a punch forceps; this is followed by a peripheral iridectomy and replacement of conjunctiva.

Iridotasis. A transverse conjunctival incision, 8 mm. long, is made 10 mm. from the limbus, and the conjunctiva is separated from the sclera by knife or fine scissors down to the limbus; a 4-mm. *keratome incision* is made into the anterior chamber at the limbus; the iris is grasped at its pupillary margin with forceps, drawn into the scleral opening with its posterior surface turned to the front and left there; the conjunctival flap is replaced, covering the *scleral wound*.

Iridencleisis resembles iridotasis except that a radial cut is made in the iris at one side and the iris pillar on this side is replaced in the anterior chamber. This maneuver leaves the other pillar incarcerated in the wound and beneath the conjunctival flap. Both iris pillars may be left incarcerated.

Results of Operations in Glaucoma. The most favorable results of operation are seen in the effect of an iridectomy in *acute congestive glaucoma*; in such instances pain and congestive symptoms subside rapidly and sight returns to the degree possessed before the onset of the attack. Furthermore, the results are generally lasting. If the acute attack has been preceded by chronic glaucoma, the effects of iridectomy may be only temporary; a filtering cicatrix operation then should be done. Exceptionally the effects of an iridectomy are disappointing or temporary, and the operation must be repeated or, better, a filtering cicatrix operation made. Occasionally operation has no effect upon the course of acute congestive glaucoma, and the disease progresses until blindness

ensues. The best time for operation is during the prodromal stage. During the glaucomatous attack iridectomy is very difficult because of congestion and the shallow anterior chamber.

In *chronic congestive glaucoma*, the results of iridectomy often are disappointing. Here, with permanent adhesive blocking of the iris angle, removal of a piece of the iris does not relieve the obstruction of the angle and restore filtration. Therefore iridectomy has been abandoned in chronic congestive glaucoma, and one of the operations which aim at producing a *filtering scar* is used. Although operations very often check the progress of the disease, even in favorable cases existing impairment of function remains. With all operations, but less with trephining and anterior sclerectomy than with iridectomy, tension sometimes increases after a variable period and a second operation must be performed; with trephining this return of increased tension follows blocking of the scleral opening with either iris or dense scar tissue. In occasional cases there will be progressive diminution of vision despite all operations.

In *simple glaucoma* most ophthalmologists commence treatment with miotics and advise *operation* as soon as the field of vision shows any progressive sign of defect. The younger the patient, the more certain it is that operation eventually will be necessary. The results of operation are less permanent than in the acute congestive form. Although in many instances there is arrest in the progress of the disease, there are less fortunate patients in whom operation results in a mere temporary halt and the procedure has to be repeated; and in some of these the disease continues until blindness results. The unfavorable cases are apt to be those in which an associated *optic nerve atrophy* is a prominent feature.

CONGENITAL GLAUCOMA

Primary Congenital Glaucoma

This form of primary glaucoma (hydrophthalmos) is an uncommon hereditary disease of infancy or early childhood. It usually appears at birth with more than 80 per cent of cases occurring before the end of the first year of life. It usually is bilateral and is due to an interference with the outflow of aqueous humor from the eye as a result of a congenital defect in the development of the angle of the anterior chamber.

The typical manifestations consist of photophobia, tearing, blepharospasm, hazy cornea and increased size of the cornea. Photophobia is the most common symptom of congenital glaucoma and may persist through adolescence. When present in an infant it always should call for consideration of a diagnosis of glaucoma. Blepharospasm usually is related to the severity and duration of the photophobia. Tearing varies considerably and at times is insignificant. Clouding of the cornea may be present at birth or develop during the first few months of life. It is due to edema and begins as a slight haze of the epithelium but becomes quite opaque with the development of stromal edema. In the beginning the cornea may show transitory haziness after crying but in neglected cases the cornea may remain opaque even after control of the ocular tension. Increase in size of the cornea is the result of the increased tension on the relatively elastic cornea and sclera of the infant and is an indication of generalized enlargement of the eyeball. This may occur as the first sign of glaucoma in some children. The diameter of the infant cornea is in the range of 10 to 11 mm. at birth increasing to 12 mm. at 1 year of age. Thus an infant having a cornea 12 mm. or more in diameter should be studied for possible glaucoma. With increase in size of the cornea and increase in intraocular tension breaks in Descemet's membrane appear peripherally in the cornea and parallel with the limbus. Later they involve the central portion of the cornea.

The optic disk remains remarkably normal in appearance even though the intraocular pressure may be high. Perhaps this may be due to the yielding character of the sclera and the enlargement of the eyeball in general; however, if left untreated or if the pressure is not adequately controlled typically glaucomatous changes eventually develop in the optic nerve head.

Ocular tension studies are essential whenever congenital glaucoma is suspected. Therefore it is necessary to examine the child under general anesthesia. Unfortunately anesthesia lowers the intraocular pressure, and some anesthetic agents such as the barbiturates (thiopental, thiamylal) and halothane (Fluothane) may lower the pressure by as much as 50 per cent or more. However the most satisfactory anesthesia is obtained with ethyl ether after induction with nitrous oxide or vinyl ether. Deep surgical anesthesia must be obtained to avoid false results. Advantage should be taken to make ophthalmoscopic and gonioscopic examinations while the child is under anesthesia. These examinations should be made in the operating room so that surgery can be done, when indicated, immediately and without subjecting the infant to another episode of general anesthesia.

Differential Diagnosis. Bilateral enlargement of the corneas in otherwise healthy eyes occurs in congenital megalocornea. There is no photophobia, corneal edema, breaks in Descemet's membrane, no abnormality of the chamber angle, no glaucomatous cupping and no increased intraocular pressure. Corneal opacification may occur as the result of ophthalmia neonatorum, birth trauma, congenital hereditary corneal dystrophy, rubella keratitis, Hurler's disease and corneal cystinosis.

Course. Without treatment the disease progresses slowly and the eye enlarges. The cornea becomes enlarged, thin and bulging and usually becomes cloudy and frequently opaque. The anterior chamber becomes very deep, the pupil dilated and the iris atrophic and tremulous. The sclera becomes thinned and bluish due to the uveal pigment showing through. The disk develops pallor, glaucomatous cupping and atrophy. In some cases the disease comes to a spontaneous stop with the preservation of moderately good vision. However, it often progresses to blindness. Therefore the prognosis in general is unfavorable.

Treatment frequently is disappointing. Temporary control sometimes may be obtained medically by use of Diamox in a dosage of 62.5 mg. every 6 hours. However since the cause is an abnormality in the tissues of the chamber angle the best therapeutic results have been obtained from surgical procedures designed to open the chamber angle. Cyclodialysis (p. 241) or goniotomy have been successful in accomplishing this purpose in a number of cases, eliminating some disfigurement and preserving fair vision. Goniotomy is accomplished by making an incision into the canal of Schlemm through the abnormal tissues of the chamber angle, a special goniotomy knife is introduced into the anterior chamber through the margin of the cornea or the limbus and passed across the chamber to incise the tissues of the angle of the opposite side.

GLAUCOMA ASSOCIATED WITH OTHER CONGENITAL ANOMALIES

There are a number of congenital anomalies in which glaucoma occurs in relatively high frequency. However the glaucoma frequently is not present at birth and at times may not develop until during the teens or early twenties.

Aniridia is a dominant hereditary anomaly usually associated with nystagmus. The name implies total absence of the iris but it practically never is complete for rudimentary tags or a small stump of iris tissue usually is present. This rudimentary iris tissue becomes adherent to the meshwork of the chamber angle and reduces the outflow of aqueous humor from the anterior chamber causing a moderately elevated intraocular pressure but without the usual signs of congenital glaucoma, *i.e.*, enlargement and edema of the cornea, and breaks in Descemet's membrane. However the prognosis is poor for the glaucoma usually is refractory to medical and surgical treatment.

Hemangioma of the face (nevus flammeus, encephalofacial hemangioma, Sturge-Weber syndrome) usually is a unilateral hemangioma involving all or any part of the distribution of the Vth cranial nerve. Glaucoma arises because of hemangiomatous involvement of the choroid which is thought to have an associated anomaly of the chamber angle. Often there also is hemangiomatous involvement of the brain resulting in mental deficiency and at times convulsions. Calcification may be demonstrable in the involved areas by roentgenograms. Rarely the anomaly may be bilateral (Fig. 15-17). Any child with nevus flammeus should be examined regularly for glaucoma which usually develops in the latter part of the first or in the second decade. Some cases may be controlled medically but frequently surgery may be necessary.

Mesodermal dysgenesis (posterior embryotoxon, Axenfeld's syndrome) is characterized as a ring-like opacity of the deep corneal layers continuous with the scleral opacity but extending 2 mm. or more into the posterior surface of the cornea from the limbus. This is due to large ropy strands of iris which bridge the chamber angle and attach to the posterior surface of the cornea at the end of Descemet's membrane. There may be associated anomalies including ectopia of the pupil, polycoria, hypoplasia of the iris stroma and cataracts. The glaucoma apparently is due to reduction of outflow of aqueous humor by the anomaly of the meshwork of the chamber angle.

Neurofibromatosis (von Recklinghausen's disease) which involves the upper eyelid may be associated with glaucoma of the eye on that side. Neurofibromatosis nodules often are visible on the iris and probably account for the angle anomaly. The glaucoma resembles infantile glaucoma.

Marfan's syndrome is characterized by arachnodactyly, cardiac anomalies, subluxation of the lenses and glaucoma occasionally. The lenses usually are small, spherical in shape and displaced upward to one side or the other. At times the lenses may become dislocated and displaced into the pupil, obstructing flow of aqueous humor, and producing acute angle closure

glaucoma of the iris bombé type, with the acute signs and symptoms of that syndrome. Rarely dilatation of the pupil will control the acute attack. Usually however surgical treatment is necessary. In such a case, prophylactic surgery should be done on the other eye. In addition to these factors it appears that there also is an anomaly of the meshwork of the chamber angle in these patients.

Marchesani's syndrome (spherophakia brachydactyly syndrome) a recessive hereditary anomaly is characterized by short stubby fingers and toes, short stocky body brachycephaly and spherical lenses. As in Marfan's syndrome the lenses tend to obstruct the pupil causing angle closure glaucoma. The use of a miotic drop may precipitate an attack in these patients or increase the severity of the pupillary obstruction.

Other rare congenital anomalies in which glaucoma is associated at times include the Fanconi syndrome, Ehlers Danlos syndrome, Lowe syndrome, Pierre Robin syndrome, Klippel-Trenaunay syndrome and the von Hippel-Lindau syndrome.

SECONDARY GLAUCOMA

This form comprises examples of increased tension and other symptoms of glaucoma developing as a result of some other *ocular disease* or after *injury or operation*. The clinical picture varies with the disease which it complicates, and the consequences, if the condition is not relieved, are often the same as in primary glaucoma. In infants secondary glaucoma produces enlargement of the globe (buphthalmos). This also may occur in young children as a result of prolonged secondary glaucoma with moderately high intraocular pressure.

The *cause* is *obstruction* in the path of flow of aqueous from the posterior chamber through the pupil to the canal of Schlemm. This is produced by obstruction

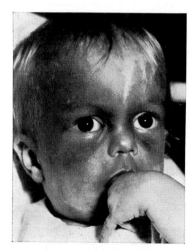

Fig. 15-17. Bilateral glaucoma with bilateral nevus flammeus.

or obliteration of the angle of the anterior chamber from hemorrhage or products of inflammation, by the crowding of a swollen and congested iris and ciliary body against the meshwork of the chamber angle and the posterior surface of the cornea, anterior synechia, swelling or dislocation of the lens or tumor of the iris or ciliary body, by complete adhesion of the pupillary margin of the iris to the anterior lens capsule (iris bombé) or by complete posterior synechia.

The ocular affections which most frequently are followed by secondary glaucoma are ulcers or wounds of the cornea with prolapse of iris, contusions of the eyeball, corneal cicatrices and staphylomas with incarceration of the iris, iridocyclitis, uveitis, annular posterior synechia, dislocation of the lens, swollen stage of traumatic cataract, swelling following discission or extracapsular extraction cataract, intraocular tumors and foreign bodies in the eye.

A form of secondary glaucoma occurs with retinal hemorrhages following thrombosis of the central vein or in diabetic retinopathy or sometimes in old persons suffering from arteriosclerosis; these cases rapidly end in blindness; they are known as *hemorrhagic glaucoma* and usually require enucleation for severe pain.

Treatment consists in removal of the cause. In cases occurring in iridocyclitis in which mydriatics do not give relief, systemic administration of a carbonic anhydrase inhibitor such as *acetazolamide (Diamox)* is helpful. If due to anterior or posterior synechia, *iridectomy* is indicated. When following traumatic rupture of the lens capsule and due to swollen cataractous material irrigation of the anterior chamber through a keratome incision is necessary. When resulting from dislocation of the lens into the anterior chamber, removal of the lens is required. In cases following cataract extraction or discission of a secondary membrane without closure of the chamber angle, cyclodialysis may afford relief if miotics fail. In examples of glaucoma which result from hemorrhage into the anterior chamber following contusion of the globe, irrigation of the anterior chamber and evacuation of the clot are indicated if the intraocular pressure remains elevated. Enucleation is indicated in secondary glaucoma from intraocular tumors.

16

The Orbit

Anatomy

The orbit is formed of bony walls having the shape of a quadrilateral pyramid; the apex corresponds to the optic foramen; the base is directed forward and corresponds to the strong, thick, projecting anterior margin. The nasal wall, the thinnest, is formed largely by the lacrimal bone and the os planum of the ethmoid, also by the frontal and sphenoidal bones; it presents in front the groove for the lacrimal sac. The inner walls of the orbits are almost parallel, but the outer diverge considerably from each other from behind forward.

The posterior portion of the orbit presents three *openings* leading to adjacent cavities: (1) the optic foramen, transmitting the optic nerve and the ophthalmic artery, (2) the superior orbital fissure (sphenoidal), transmitting the ophthalmic vein, the nerves for the ocular muscles and the first branch of the trigeminus, (3) the inferior orbital fissure (sphenomaxillary), transmitting the maxillary nerve and the infraorbital artery.

Besides communicating with the cavity of the skull by means of the openings at the apex, the orbit is *surrounded by a number of other cavities*. These are the nasal fossae and accessory cavities—the ethmoidal and sphenoidal sinuses, the frontal sinus and the maxillary sinus; these relations are important (Fig. 16-1).

The *contents* of the orbit consist of the eyeball and optic nerve, the ocular muscles, the lacrimal gland, blood vessels and nerves; the spaces between these are filled with fat and fasciae.

The *eyeball* is composed of the segments of two spheres: the anterior (cornea), about 12 mm. in diameter, is the smaller and more prominent; the larger, posterior, corresponds to the sclera. The eyeball measures about 1 inch in diameter (24.5 mm. from side to side, 24 mm. from before backward, and 23.5 mm. from above downward).

The orbital fascia is extensive and presents numerous subdivisions. It serves as *periosteum* to the walls of the orbit (*periorbita*). A portion closes in the opening of the orbit, forming an anterior wall, and extends from the margin of the orbit to both tarsi and to the external and internal tarsal ligaments, thus constituting the *septum orbitale*. Prolongations of the orbital fasciae surround the muscles and connect them with one another, the lids and the margins of the orbit.

In addition, a layer of fascia, Tenon's capsule, surrounds the globe from the cornea to the posterior part, separating the organ from the orbital fat and attached to the sclera by fine trabeculae. Anteriorly it merges into the subconjunctival connective tissue; posteriorly it disappears around the optic nerve and is pierced by all the structures which are attached to the globe. In wide movements of the eyeball, both the globe and its capsule move together as a whole upon the surrounding fat. Where the tendons of the ocular muscles pierce Tenon's capsule, the latter is reflected upon them, becoming continuous with their fasciae.

The arteries of the orbit are derived from the ophthalmic. The *veins* empty

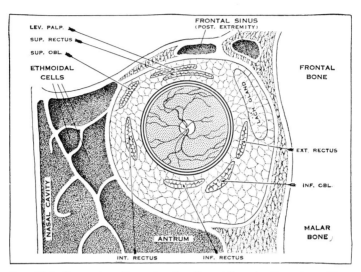

Fig. 16-1. Coronal section, showing the orbit and adjacent cavities.

into the ophthalmic veins, which pass through the superior orbital (sphenoidal) fissure to the cavernous sinus. The *nerves* of the orbit are motor and sensory; the motor nerves, the third, fourth and sixth, supply the ocular muscles; the sensory nerves are the first and second branches of the trigeminus. The *ciliary ganglion* lies to the outer side of the optic nerve; it receives motor fibers from the third, sensory fibers from the fifth, and sympathetic filaments from the carotid plexus; it gives off the short ciliary nerves which enter the eye at its posterior part. The orbit contains no lymph vessels or lymphatic glands.

Affections of the Orbit include congenital and developmental anomalies, displacement of the eyeball (exophthalmos, proptosis and enophthalmos), diseases of the orbital contents and orbital bones, orbital manifestations of diseases of the cranial cavity and of diseases of the nasal accessory sinuses, tumors and injuries.

Congenital and Developmental Anomalies

Congenital anomalies of the eyeball are rare. They may be bilateral. In *anoph-* *thalmos* the eyeball apparently is absent, but careful dissection usually reveals a rudimentary, small, solid or cystic mass. In *microphthalmos*, the eyeball is diminished in size in all diameters.

Anomalies of the orbit may occur as a part of more extensive anomalies of the head, some of which are incompatible with life. *Anencephalia* includes congenital absence of vault of the skull, roof of the orbits, brain above the medulla and sometimes the eyes. *Arhinencephalia* consists of fusion of the two orbits with a single median proboscis. *Cebocephalia* also has a medial single proboscis but has two distinct and closely placed orbits. *Craniofacial dysostosis* (*Crouzon's dysostosis*) is characterized by proptosis, exotropia and nystagmus associated with a small receding maxilla, prognathism, a prominent frontal boss and hooked nose. Papilledema, optic atrophy, blindness and mental retardation are common. *Cyclopia* usually signifies a single eye in a single, median, diamond-shaped orbit, but in some the orbit may contain two distinct or fused eyes.

Dysostosis multiplex (Hurler's disease, gargoylism, lipochondrodystrophy) combines widely spaced orbits with a large head, grotesque facial features, sunken nose, short neck, dwarfism, protuberant abdomen and short limbs with limited movement. The corneas have a ground glass appearance. *Encephalocele* is a herniation of the meninges or the brain and the meninges through the skull. It may affect the orbit anteriorly or posteriorly. Anteriorly, a visible fluctuant mass which increases in size or firmness when the infant cries usually occurs in the frontal region. *Posterior orbital cephalocele* produces a slowly progressive downward and forward pulsating proptosis commonly associated with edema of the upper lid. *Hypertelorism*, due to an abnormal development of the lesser wing of the sphenoid, is characterized by wide-set eyes, exotropia and occasionally optic atrophy. *Mandibular dysostosis*, a hypoplasia of the facial bones, produces downward slanting palpebral fissures temporally, absence of the frontonasal angle, sunken cheek bones, receding chin, abnormal dentition, high palate and various combinations of other deformities. *Oxycephalia* (*tower skull*) is characterized by shallow orbits of reduced volume, proptosis and exotropia in a vertical elongated skull with short anterior posterior and transverse diameters. Papilledema and optic atrophy may follow. Syndactylia may be associated. *Osteochondrodystrophy* (*Morquio's disease*) results in widely spaced orbits in a large head with a sunken nose in association with short neck, thoracolumbar kyphosis, flexion deformities of the knees and hips and dwarfism. *Osteopetrosis* (*Albers-Schönberg disease*), an osteogenetic anomaly, is characterized by a slowly progressive proptosis and optic atrophy.

Displacement of the Eye

Displacement of the eyeball is a common sign in affections of the orbit; however, determination of displacement at times may be difficult, for variations in the size of the globes, in the width of the palpebral fissures and in the development of the orbits may cause considerable difference in the apparent position of the eyes. Because of this, measurements must be made of the distance of the apex of the cornea anterior to the lateral rim of the orbit. This can be done by setting the 0 of a transparent millimeter rule at the palpable lateral rim of the orbit, and, with the rule parallel to the sagittal plane and looking at right angles through the rule at the apex of the cornea, reading the distance. A more accurate measurement can be made with a special instrument, an Hertel exophthalmometer, which permits visualization of the apex of the cornea from in front of the patient by reflection in a mirror placed above a millimeter scale (p. 3). The instrument is made for use on both eyes, with the mirrors adjustable for different distances between the two orbital margins, and a scale for determining the separation so that subsequent measurement may be repeated at the same separation of the mirrors. Thus measurements should be recorded: O.D. = 17 mm., O.S. = 21 mm. at 104 mm. In this example, it would appear that the left eye was displaced anteriorly 4 mm., but since the normal position of the apex of the cornea may vary from 12 to 21 mm. anterior to the lateral orbital rim, the reading might be interpreted to show that the right eye was retracted 4 mm. Thus repeated examinations and additional criteria may be necessary for a proper interpretation. In any case a difference of 5 mm. or more is considered abnormal.

Exophthalmos is active or dynamic forward displacement of the eye and occurs (1) in sympathetic stimulation as in Claude Bernard's syndrome, (2) in endocrine diseases such as thyrotoxicosis (Fig. 16-2), exophthalmic ophthalmoplegia and, rarely, in pituitary adenoma and acromegaly, and (3) in voluntarily induced protusion by muscular contraction, by

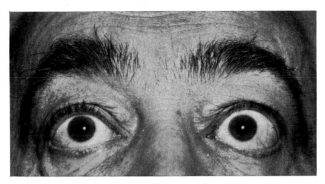

Fig. 16-2. Bilateral exophthalmos in thyroid disease.

increasing intranasal pressure and forcing air into the orbit through a dehiscence in the bony orbital wall and by increasing orbital congestion in orbital varices.

Proptosis is passive or mechanical protrusion of the eyeball. *Acute proptosis*, which may develop quite rapidly, usually is the result of orbital emphysema following a fracture of the medial orbital wall, but also may result from hemorrhage or rupture of an ethmoid mucocele into the orbit. *Intermittent proptosis* may be due to varices of the orbit, highly vascular tumors, recurrent orbital hemorrhages, periodic edema or venous congestion of the orbit, recurrent emphysema, recurrent sinus infection, especially of the ethmoids, and intermittent otitis.

Pulsating proptosis usually is due to carotid cavernous sinus fistula, vascular tumors or aneurysms or cerebral pulsation due to a defect in the orbital roof.

Unilateral proptosis most commonly is due to inflammatory lesions of the orbit, such as cellulitis, pseudotumor of the orbit, abscess, tenonitis, inflammation of the lacrimal gland, or panophthalmitis. Other causes include vascular lesions of the orbit, trauma to the face or orbit, tumors arising in the orbit or eye, and cysts.

Bilateral proptosis most commonly is caused by endocrine disorders (thyrotoxic, ophthalmoplegic) but also may be due to cavernous sinus thrombosis which usually begins unilaterally and a number of rare congenital anomalies such as oxycephaly, craniofacial dysostosis, gargoylism and allied disorders.

Pseudoproptosis, or the appearance of proptosis, occurs in situations in which the eyeball is enlarged or in which the eyelids are retracted or opened widely.

Enophthalmos is a recession or retraction of the eyeball into the orbit as a result of surgical decompression of the orbit, fracture of the orbit especially involving the floor of the orbit, or atrophy of the orbital fat from trauma or senile changes.

Diagnosis. In assessing the position of the eyes it is important to determine whether the change affects one or both eyes; whether it is constant, intermittent or pulsating; whether the change in position is axial or combined with an upward, downward, inward or outward component; whether there is limitation of movement of the globe in one or more directions; and whether there are associated signs of inflammation. In addition, the duration and speed of development of the displacement should be determined; the difficulty of pushing the globe backward into the orbit should be ascertained; and exploration of the orbital contents should be made by palpating with a finger between the globe and the orbital rim. If a mass should be encountered, its position, consistency and fixation should be determined. The visual acuity and visual fields should be tested and an ophthalmoscopic examination made. Finally, x-ray examinations of the orbit and skull should be made and at times planograms will be necessary to complete the local examination, but a general physical examination which includes blood studies and urinalysis should be a part of the complete evaluation of displacement of the eyes.

DISEASES OF THE ORBITAL CONTENTS

Orbital Edema is characterized by variable amounts of axial proptosis and restricted movements of the globe, edema of the lids and chemosis of the conjunctiva with little evidence of inflammation or venous congestion. Orbital edema may occur in the course of an acute febrile illness such as malaria or typhus, in renal disease, in lacrimal sac infections and as a precursor to more serious signs in cavernous sinus thrombosis, intraocular infection, orbital abscess and tumors. Recurrent episodes of orbital edema are likely in angioneurotic edema, drug reactions and recurrent inflammation of the paranasal sinuses.

Orbital Hemorrhage produces axial proptosis with limitation of movement or fixation of the globe, ecchymosis and swelling of the lids and conjunctiva. Dilatation of the pupil, loss of vision, pain in the orbit, nausea and vomiting may occur. At times corneal necrosis and ulceration may occur. Trauma perhaps is the most frequent cause, but general diseases such as hemophilia, leukemia, scurvy and rickets, as well as vascular diseases such as aneurysm and arteriosclerosis, also may cause orbital hemorrhages.

INFLAMMATORY DISEASES

Orbital Cellulitis

Orbital cellulitis is an inflammation of the *cellular tissue* of the orbit. It may run an acute course, terminating in *suppuration*, in which case it is also known as *orbital phlegmon* or *retrobulbar abscess*, or it may run a chronic course.

Symptoms. Great *swelling* of the lids, chemosis, *exophthalmos, impairment of mobility* of eyeball and violent *pain* in the orbit increased by pressure upon the eyeball are accompanied by *constitutional symptoms*, with high fever, nausea, vomiting and prostration. Cerebral symptoms may be added. Vision may not be affected, but usually it is reduced and it may be abolished owing to the occurrence of optic neuritis followed by atrophy. After these symptoms have lasted about a week, *pus* appears at a certain part of the skin of the lids (usually below the supraorbital margin) and perforates or, less frequently, it may empty into the fornix. After the evacuation of pus, the symptoms subside and the opening heals, often leaving the eye with some permanent damage.

Complications include optic neuritis; less frequently, thrombosis of the retinal veins and of the cavernous sinus, and occasionally panophthalmitis. The process may extend to the brain and be fatal.

Etiology. Acute orbital cellulitis may be caused by extension of disease of the *nasal accessory sinuses*, especially ethmoid, or from neighboring foci such as orbital periostitis or the teeth, injuries and operations involving the orbit followed by *infection*, foreign bodies in the orbit, facial erysipelas, septicemia and bacteremia and acute infective diseases, especially influenza.

Treatment. The patient should be placed at bed rest on a force fluid regimen with local application of heat. The cause and source of the infection should be determined and treated. Sulfonamides may be given orally until more specific treatment can be determined, such as penicillin for anthrax and streptococcic infections. Wounds or injuries should be examined and foreign bodies removed. Incision and drainage of abscess formations should be done with care to avoid further injury to orbital contents.

Chronic Orbital Cellulitis. Symptoms of chronic orbital cellulitis are characterized by slowly progressive proptosis, limitation of movements of the globe, edema of the lids, chemosis and chronic injection of the conjunctiva. General symptoms are much less evident than in the acute type.

Etiology. As in the acute type, chronic orbital cellulitis may follow penetrating injuries of the orbit, result from spread of infection from adjacent structures or from metastatic localization, but in addition may follow an acute orbital cellulitis. Among the specific lesions are chronic typhoid abscess, tuberculoma, syphilitic cellulitis, periostitis and osteitis, sarcoid, actinomycosis, aspergillosis, filariasis, hydatid cyst (*Taenia echinococcus*) and cysticercus cyst (*Taenia solium*).

Pseudotumor of the Orbit. A special form of chronic orbital cellulitis is diagnosed pseudotumor of the orbit, for its manifestations often resemble the signs and symptoms of an orbital tumor more than an inflammation. However, it usually occurs in patients of middle age or older with an abrupt onset in one orbit, but sooner or later the other orbit undergoes similar involvement. The lesion runs a chronic course occasionally characterized by pain, tenderness and moderate redness, which usually subside spontaneously but with some optic atrophy and visual loss. No specific causative factor has been found but steroid therapy frequently controls the reaction; however, it may have to be maintained for many weeks to avoid reactivation.

Tenonitis as a primary disease is rare and consists of a *serous* inflammation with effusion into Tenon's space. The symptoms are moderate swelling and redness of the upper lid, vesicular swelling over the insertion of one of the rectus muscles or diffuse chemosis, moderate forward exophthalmos, limitation of movements of the globe and some pain on motion of the eyeball. It may follow an injury or a tenotomy in which the wound has become infected; it also has been ascribed to influenza, gout and rheumatism. It may be difficult to differentiate between this affection and a mild case of orbital cellulitis. It runs its course in a few weeks, leaving no permanent disability, but there are apt to be adhesions between Tenon's capsule and the eyeball. As a secondary affection, it is found to accompany severe forms of iridocyclitis and also panophthalmitis. Treatment consists of hot compresses and attention to the etiologic factor.

Orbital Periostitis

Orbital periostitis is an inflammation of the orbital periosteum, either *acute* or *chronic* in its course, and either *limited* to a portion of the margin of the orbit or *spreading* more deeply. The products of inflammation often consist merely of a *thickening* of the membrane. Sometimes there is a *deposit* of bone or an *abscess* may be formed, with or without subsequent *caries* or *necrosis* of a part of the wall of the orbit.

Symptoms. These depend upon whether the affection runs an acute or a chronic course, the part of the orbit involved, and whether a subperiosteal abscess results.

The most common variety is that attacking the *margin* of the orbit. In such a case there may be no other symptoms than pain, tenderness on pressure at the orbital margin, hard immovable *swelling* in this situation and some swelling of the lids and conjunctiva; the amount of constitutional disturbance will depend upon the acuteness of the process. Such a case frequently results in complete *absorption* of the products of inflammation; less commonly, periosteal *thickening* or bony deposit remains. If, on the other hand, there is pus, a subperiosteal *abscess* is developed at the margin of the orbit which perforates the skin, leaving a *fistula* through which the probe detects either bare or necrosed bone. Such a fistula remains open for months until all the dead bone has been extruded, and after it heals there is a depressed *scar* and sometimes ectropion and lagophthalmos.

If the periostitis is situated more *posteriorly*, there will be more pain, and this will be of a deep-seated character and accompanied by tenderness on pressure upon the globe; there will be considerable swelling and redness of the lids and conjunctiva, exophthalmos and constitutional symptoms. Such cases may result in *absorption* of the products of inflammation, or in periosteal *thickening* or bony deposit; the diagnosis of this type is often difficult. But if such a deep-seated process goes on to the formation of an *abscess,* it becomes much more serious and presents the *symptoms of orbital cellulitis,* from which it frequently cannot be differentiated; the pus finds its way to the surface, but this may take some time. Cases of this sort, especially if they involve the roof, may be dangerous to life through extension to the cranial cavity and the occurrence of meningitis or cerebral abscess.

Etiology. Causes include *tuberculosis* (in children), *syphilis* (tertiary stage, in adults) and extension from affections of nasal accessory sinuses, but trauma often is the exciting factor. Syphilitic cases usually run a chronic course and produce periosteal thickening without any tendency to suppuration.

Treatment is directed against the cause, for example, syphilis or tuberculosis when these are present. In acute cases general treatment by antibiotics or sulfonamides often leads to dramatic improvement. Locally, moist *warm compresses* and *incision* and *drainage* along the wall of the orbit are helpful in suppurative cases. Caries and necrosis may require subsequent operative intervention.

Osteomyelitis

Osteomyelitis of the orbital bones may cause an orbital cellulitis or produce a localized, painful, red swelling which may break down and form a chronic draining fistula. Involvement of the roof of the orbit can lead to meningitis or more serious cranial involvement. It is due to a bacterial infection of the bone which may follow trauma or be metastatic from a primary infection elsewhere in the body. Intense treatment with antibiotics should be started after the causative agent has been isolated and sensitivity tests made. Surgical drainage and removal of necrotic bone frequently are necessary.

LESIONS OF ORBITAL BONES

Hyperostosis

Hyperostosis of the orbit usually is localized in the frontal bone, producing a poorly defined, hard, subcutaneous mass with no inflammation. Slow and progressive enlargement of the mass causes forward and downward proptosis of the globe. Should the lesion occur posteriorly, there is danger of blindness from pressure on the optic nerve, producing atrophy. The growth may follow trauma or result from a meningioma. Treatment is surgical removal or decompression of the orbit.

Morgagni's Syndrome consists of hyperostosis of the frontal bone, obesity and hirsuties of unknown cause; it affects women in the seventh decade almost exclusively.

Leontiasis Ossea

Leontiasis ossea, a chronic hypertrophic disease of the bones of the skull, may take the form of a creeping periostitis or a diffuse osteitis of the bones of the face and skull. The periostitic type usually affects the bones of the lower jaw but can start in the orbit from chronic suppuration of the lacrimal sac. The osteitic type usually affects all the bones of the skull but it may remain localized to the frontal, for example. In either type considerable displacement of the globe may occur without visual symptoms.

Osteitis Deformans

Osteitis deformans (Paget's disease) is an insidious, slowly progressive, chronic disease of unknown cause which affects adults of both sexes with a rarefying osteitis and secondary bone formation, eventually reducing the size of the foramina. Ocular signs and symptoms result from reduction in capacity of the orbit, from compression of the nerves entering the orbit and from the associated arterial disease. They include proptosis, edema of the conjunctiva and lids, optic atrophy, paresis of lateral rectus muscle and others; later, retinal hemorrhages, angioid streaks, macular and choroidal degeneration and cataract. Treatment is unsatisfactory.

Osteitis fibrosis cystica is a rare bone disease in which absorption and replacement by fibro-osteoid tissue which may contain cysts sometimes affect the frontal bone, resulting in proptosis occasionally followed by optic atrophy.

Rickets occasionally involves the skull and produces proptosis with extreme changes resembling oxycephaly at times.

Acromegaly causes prominence of the orbital margins.

Hydrocephalus may cause proptosis as the expansion of the cranial cavity causes encroachment on the orbits.

ORBITAL MANIFESTATIONS OF INTRACRANIAL DISEASE

Arteriovenous Aneurysm with Fistula between the cavernous sinus and internal carotid artery is the most common cause of pulsating proptosis. The clinical manifestations usually are typical, consisting of sudden onset of a rapidly developing unilateral proptosis accompanied by a swishing noise in the head, diminished vision, swelling of the lids, venous congestion and pain in the head. Palpation of the globe may disclose the venous pulsation or a thrill synchronous with the pulse beat and the swishing sound heard by the patient. On auscultation, especially over the inner aspect of the lid, a bruit may be heard which is synchronous with the pulse. In some cases the bruit may be heard all over the head. The pulsation, proptosis, bruit and thrill are increased on stooping and exertion, but they disappear on compression of the homolateral or both common carotid arteries. In many cases papilledema, retinal hemorrhages and vitreous opacities occur, with glaucoma and involvement of the third, fourth, fifth and sixth cranial nerves occurring in some.

Etiology. Trauma is responsible for 80 per cent of cases, the majority being the result of a fracture of the base of the skull involving the sphenoid bone, but some are due to contrecoup rupture from a contusion of the occiput, forehead or temple. In some instances the trauma does not cause an immediate rupture but weakens the arterial wall, producing an aneurysm which subsequently breaks. The remainder result from the spontaneous formation of a fistula, probably from rupture of a pre-existing aneurysm. The majority of this type occur in women.

Treatment. The treatment usually is ligation of the carotid artery on the affected side; however, it should be preceded by intermittent compression of the vessel for increasing periods up to 45 minutes several times a day. A few may respond to the compression alone.

Thrombosis of the Cavernous Sinus (almost always infective and usually fatal) may be due to extension of a thrombus in the orbital veins occurring in orbital abscess; it may be caused by neighboring purulent foci situated in the nose, pharynx, tonsils, teeth and the nasal accessory sinuses; or it may follow erysipelas, caries of the petrous bone and metastasis in pyemia and the infective diseases. The signs and symptoms are similar to those of orbital abscess, from which it can be differentiated by the existence of severe cerebral symptoms, edema over the mastoid region (through venous stasis in the emissary veins), extension to the opposite side, distention of the retinal veins and the more constant existence of papilledema. Early treatment with large doses of sulfonamides and penicillin has given some successful results.

Ocular Manifestations of Disease of the Nasal Accessory Sinuses

These comprise not only affections of the orbit and its contents due to *extension*, but include disease of these parts from an *infective focus* in a sinus. The accessory sinuses of the nose (frontal sinus, anterior and posterior ethmoidal cells, sphenoidal sinus and maxillary antrum) surround the orbit, being separated by bony walls which are very thin in spots. They are lined by an extension of the nasal mucous membrane and as a result of such relationship often become *infected*. When the sinus outlet is blocked, secretion will accumulate; in chronic cases, this may lead to distention of the sinus (mucocele) with encroachment upon the orbit, producing exophthalmos and other signs of an orbital tumor. Such a sinusitis may run an acute or a chronic course.

Frontal Sinusitis may be accompanied by a *bulging* at the upper and inner angle of the orbit with tenderness on pressure over this area and sometimes redness of the overlying skin, severe frontal head-

ache and dizziness on stooping. There may be protrusion of the eyeball downward and outward, diplopia, *edema of the lids*, conjunctival and episcleral congestion and lacrimation. Orbital periostitis and cellulitis may result.

Ethmoiditis may present a *tumefaction* at the upper and inner part of the orbit with *swelling* of the integument of the adjacent lids, *displacement of the globe* downward and outward, diplopia, severe pain, conjunctival and episcleral congestion and lacrimation. The process may involve the orbit, causing periostitis or cellulitis.

The ethmoids may harbor the infective focus responsible for certain cases of uveitis and iritis.

Disease of the Sphenoidal Sinus usually is associated with ethmoiditis. The walls of this cavity and the *optic nerve* are contiguous, and this close relationship explains the occurrence of optic neuritis and of retrobulbar neuritis in affections of the sphenoidal sinus. Examples of disease of this sinus (including ethmoiditis) may present no external evidences of inflammation and yet cause definite ocular complications, among which are *optic neuritis*, neuroretinitis and *retrobulbar neuritis*, leading to optic nerve atrophy if the cause is not removed. With sinusitis there may be a central, paracentral or annular *color scotoma*, which later may become absolute, usually with but little contraction of the visual field. Another fairly frequent symptom is *enlargement of the blind spot*. There also may be asthenopia, deep-seated pain and tenderness when the eyeball is pressed backwards.

Antrum Disease is not often accompanied by ocular symptoms, although infrequently there may be pain, swelling of the lids, conjunctival congestion and lacrimation, but involvement of the orbit is rare.

Tumors of the Orbit are infrequent; they may arise from the walls or contents of the orbit, from neighboring structures involving the orbit by extension or from distant sites involving the orbit by metastatic localization. The symptoms depend upon the size, position and nature of the tumor. The cardinal signs are *unilateral exophthalmos, visual disturbances* and roentgenographic evidence of *bone changes.* The direction of the proptosis and the impairment of motion of the eyeball will be determined by the exact situation of the tumor. Pressure upon the optic nerve may cause papilledema or retrobulbar neuritis and, later, atrophy. When located forward or after it has reached a certain size, the tumor may be felt by the tip of the finger passed between the margin of the orbit and the eyeball. Benign tumors usually grow slowly and frequently give rise to but few symptoms; malignant tumors are apt to increase in size very rapidly.

Primary Benign Tumors of the Orbit

Hemangioma is the most common tumor of the orbit. It may be of any type, but the majority are cavernous, forming a soft mass which, depending upon its position, may produce proptosis in any direction. The proptosis, usually variable in amount, often is compressible by pressure on the globe and increases with crying or straining, and on bending the head forward. Rarely the proptosis is pulsating in type. Ocular motility is not affected unless fibrosis has occurred after the tumor has existed for a long time. Pressure in the orbit and on the eye may cause visual loss.

Dermoid Tumor, composed of abnormal cystic or solid masses of skin and its appendages, usually occurs in the upper temporal and anterior portion of the orbit, producing a firm smooth mass palpable beneath the skin of the lid; frequently it is attached to the periosteum, but not to the skin. Rarely extension pos-

teriorly into the orbit may produce a downward and nasalward proptosis and occasionally cause pressure absorption of part of the lateral wall of the orbit. An oil granuloma may follow degenerative changes in the tumor.

Neurofibroma, a mass of entwined cord-like thickened nerves, is the most common neurogenic tumor of the orbit and frequently is associated with similar lesions of the lids, face, scalp and skin in general, pigmented nevi of the skin producing *café au lait* spots, occasionally so-called multiple drusen of the nervehead or retina and glioma of the optic nerve as part of von Recklinghausen's disease. Neurofibromas of the orbit may cause erosion of the bones of the orbit, producing a pulsating proptosis when the roof is affected.

Glioma of the Optic Nerve, usually occurring before the twelfth year of life, produces a painless, slowly progressive unilateral visual loss and proptosis. Although ophthalmoscopic examination usually discloses a simple optic atrophy, occasionally there is a papilledema-like elevation of the disk. Extension of the tumor backward produces enlargement of the bony optic canal and involvement of the optic chiasm with disturbance of the visual field of the fellow eye.

Meningioma of the Optic Nerve Sheath occurs in older patients, producing unilateral visual loss, interference with movement of the eyes because of involvement of the extraocular muscles, and proptosis, but does not cause enlargement of the optic canal. The tumor is locally malignant but quite slow in growth.

Xanthomatous Disease (see Chap. 23) produces tumor-like lesions either as the benign eosinophilic granuloma of the frontal bone or as the more malignant Hand-Schüller-Christian and Letterer-Siwe disease.

Primary Malignant Tumors of the Orbit

Sarcomas of the Orbit may arise from any of the mesodermal structures of the orbit, usually in children or young adults. They are highly malignant and rapidly fatal. Because they frequently are anaplastic, their cellular origin may be obscure; however, many may be classified as rhabdomyosarcoma, liposarcomas, myxosarcoma and embryonal sarcomas.

Rhabdomyosarcoma, the most common malignant tumor of the orbit in childhood, arises from the extraocular or lid muscles at an average age of 6 to 7 years. It affects males twice as frequently as females.

Lymphosarcoma and related blood cell tumors affecting the orbit, on the other hand, usually occur in older patients, the average age being 55 years. These lesions include lymphocytic cell and reticulum cell lymphosarcomas, lymphomas, giant follicle lymphosarcoma, Hodgkin's disease and, rarely, myeloma and chloroma.

Carcinoma of the Orbit, as a primary lesion, usually arises from the lacrimal gland in the form of an adenocarcinoma, carcinoma or mixed tumor.

Tumors Extending into the Orbit

The more common tumors which involve the orbit by extension from neighboring structures are meningocele or cephalocele, meningioma and mucocele, nasopharyngeal fibroma and carcinoma of the sinus mucous membrane.

Meningocele and cephalocele were described under developmental anomalies.

Meningioma arising from the sphenoid ridge involves the orbit by extension through the superior orbital fissure, producing proptosis with hyperostosis, or by extension through the optic canal, resulting in pressure on the optic nerve causing papilledema, optic atrophy and visual loss

with proptosis developing later. Growth of the tumor usually is very slow.

Mucocele, a closed mucus-filled cyst of the mucous membrane of a sinus, usually the frontal or an ethmoid cell, expands slowly, fills the sinus and continues to expand slowly, encroaching upon the orbital space.

Nasopharyngeal fibroma or angiofibroma extends into the orbit, producing proptosis, and at times paralysis of the third, fourth and sixth nerves and atrophy of the optic nerve.

Carcinoma invading the orbit from a paranasal sinus usually originates in the antrum, but at times may arise in the ethmoid cells or, rarely, in the frontal sinus.

Metastatic Tumors of the Orbit

Neuroblastoma or sympathicoblastoma, the most common metastatic tumor of the orbit, usually arises in the suprarenal medulla or the retroperitoneal ganglia, almost exclusively in infants or young children. The tumor is very malignant, and often produces proptosis before the primary lesion manifests itself. The tumor frequently becomes necrotic, producing inflammatory signs, ecchymosis and at times hematoma. The metastases occasionally may involve both orbits.

Metastatic carcinoma of the orbit may develop from primary lesions of the breast, uterus and cervix, kidney, thyroid gland, prostate gland and pancreas. Proptosis is a common finding.

Malignant melanoma and sarcoma rarely metastasize to the orbit from distant sources.

Benign tumors demanding excision should be removed with preservation of the eyeball, if possible, especially if sight is good. Such tumors, even when situated far posteriorly, often can be removed by a free external canthotomy to the bone, with an incision at right angles to the canthotomy, opening above and below into the upper and lower fornix; additional approach may be provided by temporary tenotomy of the external rectus muscle; this exposure is useful in exploration of the orbit and for obtaining biopsy material. If this would not procure sufficient space, Krönlein's operation (temporary loosening and displacement of the external orbital wall) may be used.

Malignant tumors call for exenteration of the orbit with sacrifice of the eyeball, even though it possesses useful vision.

Krönlein's Operation is a temporary resection of the external orbital wall employed for the removal of deep-seated tumors of the orbit without sacrifice of the eye, and for exploration of the orbit. The operation is performed by extending a lateral canthotomy incision (see p. 50),

cutting the lateral canthal ligament and retracting the upper and lower margins of the skin incision. Identifying sutures are placed in the lateral canthal ligament and in the tendon of the lateral rectus muscle. The exposed outer wall of the orbit with attached periosteum is temporarily resected, by the use of a motor-driven saw, and bent outward. After the operation has been completed, the parts are replaced and sutured in position. The skin incision is closed, the eyelids are sewed together and a pressure dressing is applied.

Exenteration of the Orbit is a radical operation resorted to in certain cases of malignant disease. The periosteum and all the contents of the orbit, including the eyeball, are excised. Skin grafts are used to cover the defect.

17

Trauma

Injuries of the lids and eyes always are serious even though they may seem trivial when compared to injuries elsewhere in the body. However minor injuries to the lids and conjunctiva may cause great disfigurement as well as disturbance in protection of the cornea which in turn could lead to damage and visual loss, while injuries to the globe always are potentially dangerous to vision and frequently may result in loss of the eye or rarely loss of both eyes through sympathetic ophthalmia. For these reasons as well as because of the high emotional concern of the patient for his eyes and his appearance, injuries of and about the eye require particular care.

INJURIES OF THE LIDS

These are quite common, and include contusions, wounds, burns and insect bites. Ecchymosis and edema often produce exaggerated signs in relation to the severity of the trauma because of the looseness of the subcutaneous connective tissue.

Ecchymosis ("black eye") usually is of little importance, merely causing disfigurement, which lasts 1 or 2 weeks; however, a thorough examination of the eyeball and adjacent structures should be made in those which develop immediately after trauma, and x-ray examination of the skull in those which are delayed. In fracture of the base of the skull, blood may travel along the floor of the orbit, and after a day or two appear in the lower lid and bulbar conjunctiva. If the injury is seen immediately, *cold* compresses are of service. After 48 hours, *hot*

compresses are indicated to promote absorption of the extravasated blood. The disfigurement may be concealed by the use of flesh-colored powders or paints. Occasionally in debilitated individuals, especially in association with abrasion, abscess of the lid results, and may require horizontal incision.

Insect Bites give rise to extensive *swelling*, which is controlled best by *cold compresses*.

Wounds of the eyelids are common, especially in automobile accidents, and because of their functional importance require careful consideration and management. Early proper management may prevent serious deformity and numerous reconstructive procedures. A detailed examination must be made prior to any definitive treatment. This includes determination of additional (head or general) injury, whether the patient is in shock and whether treatment for shock is necessary or has been started, and, finally, a detailed examination of the ocular injury. Even small wounds, on the surface of the lid, may extend deep into the orbit or into the eyeball itself. Thus the extent and depth of the wound should be determined with reference to the structures involved, especially observing for damage to the lid margin, the puncta, the canaliculi and the lacrimal sac. Foreign material such as pieces of glass, wood or metal must be removed with as little damage to the tissue as possible. Dirt and finer debris may be removed by irrigation, but all pieces of tissue must be saved, even those attached only by threadlike strands, for repair at times may be likened to the fitting of a piece of a jigsaw puzzle. Bleeding must be controlled before the wound is closed; this often may be accomplished by pressure or hot compresses, though occasionally ligation of a bleeding point with fine white silk suture material may be necessary.

Incised wounds cause considerable gaping, if vertical, on account of division of the orbicularis, and the scar is apt to be noticeable; if horizontal, the lips of the wound do not tend to separate, and usually heal without deformity. Incised wounds should be *cleansed* and *united* at once, with fine silk and delicate needles. A vertical wound of the margin must be sutured carefully so that no indentation will remain.

Lacerated and contused wounds, if extensive and accompanied by much swelling, should not be closed at once. The wound should be thoroughly *cleansed* and a *wet dressing* applied, and after the swelling has subsided the edges of the wound may be brought together. Care must be taken not to produce deformity or shortening. It may be advisable to use skin grafts or sliding flaps.

Thermal Burns of the external surfaces of the lids should have a bland oil or ointment applied, then be covered by a thin rubber membrane, and a pressure dressing should be placed so as to keep the lids closed. In some instances removal of superficially burned tissue and replacement with a split thickness skin graft may be indicated. In all cases the conjunctiva and cornea should be examined before treatment is instituted (see Chap. 6 and 7).

In Chemical Injury of the lids, immediate irrigation with a large amount of water to remove the chemical should be followed quickly by an effort to determine whether the injury also involves the conjunctiva and cornea (see Chap. 6 and 7). If only the skin of the lid is involved,

further irrigation with water or saline solution for 10 to 15 minutes should be followed by the application of a bland ointment and a pressure dressing as in thermal burns of the lids.

In both thermal and chemical injuries, the general condition of the patient should be assessed, sedatives administered, or treatment for shock instituted if indicated.

Emphysema associated with injury to the lids denotes a fracture of the walls of the orbit, permitting communication with the neighboring nasal or nasal accessory cavities. The lids present a soft *swelling* of considerable size, often closing the palpebral aperture; bubbles of air, becoming displaced in palpation, give rise to the sensation of *crepitation.* A firm *dressing* will hasten the disappearance of the air. The patient must be instructed to avoid blowing the nose, which will increase the emphysema and may bring infection from the nasal cavity.

INJURIES OF THE CONJUNCTIVA

These are very common, and include:

(1) *Foreign bodies* in the conjunctival sac, consisting of dust, iron, coal or ashes. They usually adhere to the inner surface of the upper lid, causing severe pain and irritation, and are readily removed after eversion of the lid.

(2) *Wounds;* extensive wounds of the conjunctiva should be closed with one or more fine sutures.

(3) *Burns;* these are quite common, being due to hot liquids, steam, tear gas, lime, powder, molten metal and chemicals. Following the accident a grayish eschar forms, separates and leaves a granulating surface, which heals by cicatrization; thus symblepharon often results. Burns of the conjunctiva are frequently accompanied by injury to the cornea; the results then are more serious. Treatment begins with

complete *removal* of the caustic substance as soon as possible.

The conjunctival sac should be *washed out* with *great quantities of water immediately*, whether the foreign material is acid or alkaline; it is important to remove the destructive material *without delay*, since the extent of injury depends upon the length of time the agent has been allowed to act. Then a topical anesthetic (Pontocaine or Nupercaine, etc.) should be instilled. Solid particles are removed with absorbent cotton or forceps.

Subsequently *cold* compresses and *atropine* are used. Unless the burn is very superficial, there will be eschars; when these loosen and come away, raw and granulating surfaces will be exposed. These have a great tendency to form *adhesions*, which must be separated frequently with a glass rod or smooth probe. Symblepharon, however, is very apt to occur notwithstanding the greatest care in separating these adhesions.

INJURIES OF THE CORNEA

These comprise foreign bodies, contusions, burns and wounds.

Foreign Bodies, consisting of iron, coal, ashes, dust, etc., frequently adhere or become imbedded in the cornea, causing much pain (usually referred to the under surface of the upper lid), lacrimation and photophobia. When the foreign body is small, it may be difficult to detect, unless oblique illumination is used with magnification (loupe or corneal biomicroscope). When minute, its location may be revealed more easily following the instillation of a drop of fluorescein solution. The mischief which a foreign body provokes depends upon the *depth* to which it penetrates and whether it is *infected*. If present for a number of days, a surrounding area of *infiltration* appears, resulting in a small ulcer, and in this manner the foreign body may become dislodged;

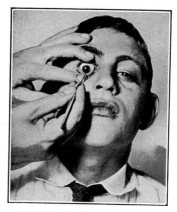

FIG. 17-1. Method of removing a foreign body from the cornea (surgeon standing in front of the patient).

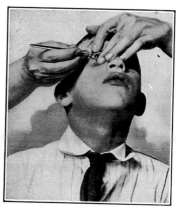

FIG. 17-2. Method of removing a foreign body from the cornea (surgeon standing behind the patient).

if it consists of iron or steel, this ring will become stained by *rust*. Foreign bodies frequently are the cause of ulcers of the cornea.

To remove a foreign body. With the patient seated in a chair with headrest, the surgeon stands in front and to the left; after surface anesthesia, the index finger of the left hand is applied to the margin of the lower lid and the middle finger to the border of the upper lid, separating the lids with gentle backward

FIG. 17-3. Foreign body spud.

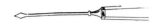

FIG. 17-4. Foreign body needle.

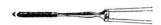

FIG. 17-5. Foreign body gouge.

pressure (Fig. 17-1). Or, lacking a head-rest, the surgeon may support the head of the patient from behind or place the patient on a treatment table, separating the lids by applying the index finger of the left hand to the margin of the upper lid and the middle finger to the border of the lower lid (Fig. 17-2). When the foreign body is quite small the patient is seated at the slit lamp and biomicroscope.

The *instruments* used are either the blunt spud, the gouge or the foreign body needle (Figs. 17-3 to 17-5) *sterilized* before use.

When the foreign body is superficial, the *blunt spud* (Fig. 17-3) will serve. When it is firmly attached or has penetrated into the corneal substance, it must be *lifted or dug out* with spud, gouge or needle (Figs. 17-3 to 17-5); in such a case the instrument is passed *behind* the foreign body. If a ring of *rust* is present, this must be removed (best accomplished with a dental burr). Care must be taken to inflict *as little injury as possible* and, when the foreign body is deep, *not to perforate the cornea*.

After the foreign body is removed a drop of scopolamine or homatropine is instilled onto the cornea and the eye left open or dressed, depending upon the size of the epithelial defect. In either case the eye should be examined in 24 hours.

Contusions of the cornea with some blunt object may give rise to a deep-seated opacity; this usually clears completely. Occasionally there is blood staining of the cornea complicating hemorrhage into the anterior chamber; this disappears very slowly; it may give one the impression of dislocation of the lens into the anterior chamber. Contusions may be accompanied by injury to deeper parts, including hyphema, iridodialysis, rupture of the choroid, traumatic cataract, hemorrhage into the vitreous and edema of the retina.

Burns of the cornea are treated like burns of the conjunctiva.

Wounds may be nonpenetrating or penetrating. *Nonpenetrating* wounds are due to scratches with the fingernail, the twig of a tree or the like. Such injuries, though *painful*, heal readily unless infected; the pupil should be *dilated* with homatropine or scopolamine, sulfonamide drops instilled several times a day and a protective dressing applied if the injury is extensive. Occasionally such superficial abrasions recur after a week or two or after a longer period (*recurrent erosion of the cornea*) and sometimes there are several recurrences, each accompanied by irritative symptoms similar to those originally present; gentle curetting of the abraded area may be necessary to effect a cure and then precautions to prevent infection are important.

INJURIES OF THE SCLERA

The important injuries include *perforating wounds* and *rupture*; these are *serious* because of the danger of injury to the inner layers (uvea and retina), escape of the contents of the globe and infection of the interior of the eye.

Ruptures of the Sclera are produced by blows and blunt instruments; they usually occur a short distance from and concentric with the corneal margin, generally above and internally. The conjunctiva may not be broken (*subconjunctival rupture of the sclera*). The prognosis is unfavorable and most of such eyes are lost, since, with force sufficient to rupture the sclera, there usually are serious lesions in the interior of the eye, such as iridodialysis or tear of the iris, dislocation of the lens, separation of the retina and hemorrhage into the vitreous. If there is good light projection, an attempt should be made to preserve the eye by suturing the scleral and conjunctival wounds after excision of the prolapsed uveal tissue and vitreous.

Perforating Wounds of the sclera are discussed on page 266.

INJURIES OF THE IRIS

Injuries to the iris may be (1) nonperforating or (2) perforating.

Nonperforating injuries (concussion) may cause (a) *traumatic mydriasis* from paresis or paralysis of the motor nerve fibers supplying the sphincter and the ciliary muscle. The pupil will be dilated (*iridoplegia*) and usually there is paralysis of accommodation; there always are accompanying minute ruptures of the pupillary border. This injury is not uncommon. More or less mydriasis *persists* permanently; (b) rarely, a visible tear in the pupillary margin; with both of these injuries, rest, pilocarpine and a dressing are indicated; (c) *iridodialysis*, a separation of the ciliary border of the iris (Fig. 17-6) presenting a black crescentic area at the detachment with some inward displacement of the corresponding pupillary edge; the condition is permanent. Rest, atropine and a dressing are indicated; the iris can be reattached by operation. Whenever the iris is torn there will be blood in the anterior chamber (hyphema).

RUPTURE OF THE CHOROID

Rupture of the choroid sometimes results from *contusions* of the eyeball. The

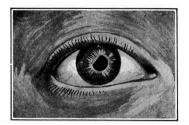

FIG. 17-6. Iridodialysis.

immediate effect of such an injury is an extravasation of blood into the vitreous. After this is absorbed a long, *yellowish white streak* with pigmented edges, curved with its concavity toward the disk, is seen, usually in the neighborhood of the disk and to its outer side (Plate 27*A*). The white color is due to the exposed sclera; the rupture is crossed by retinal vessels. Sometimes a second or even a third rupture occurs, concentric with the first. If the rupture is limited to the choroid and does not approach the macula, there will be little reduction in vision; if the rupture includes the retina, a large scotoma will result; if the rupture is in the macular region, there will be loss of central vision. Treatment consists of rest, both ocular and bodily, atropine and smoked glasses.

INJURIES OF THE OPTIC NERVE

Injuries of the optic nerve result most frequently from fractures of the skull with involvement of the bony optic canal. There is immediate, usually permanent, loss of vision in the affected eye, optic atrophy being observed after 4 or 6 weeks. The injury consists of laceration of the nerve in the optic canal or hemorrhage into the nerve sheath; sometimes roentgenograms of the optic canal will reveal a fracture, and give evidence of the nature of the injury. Surgical decompression of the involved optic canal has been employed rarely. Bullet wounds of the orbit may involve the optic nerves, with immediate loss of vision and with optic atrophy and pigmentary changes in the course of time.

INJURIES OF THE ORBIT

Injuries of the orbit include contusions, incised and penetrating wounds, foreign bodies and fracture of the orbital wall. A prominent sign is *hemorrhage* into the orbit, causing *exophthalmos* and sometimes ecchymosis of the lids and conjunctiva. A blow or stab with a blunt object may rupture the globe or occasionally dislocate the eyeball in front of the lids; such displacement is sometimes produced through gouging with the thumb. *Fracture* may involve the orbital rim, detected as an unevenness by the finger; the inner wall, causing emphysema; the floor, with resulting enophthalmos; or the apex, involving the optic canal and injuring the optic nerve. The last may result from direct injury or indirectly (contrecoup) and produce blindness without immediate ophthalmoscopic evidence, but followed in a few weeks by atrophy of the optic nerve.

Treatment consists in cleansing wounds and extracting foreign bodies. A dressing aids in the absorption of blood and air in the case of hemorrhage or emphysema.

PERFORATING WOUNDS OF THE GLOBE

In all perforating wounds of the globe (as well as in injuries in general) it is advisable to instill a *local anesthetic*; this makes the examination easier for both patient and surgeon, and in extensive wounds tends to prevent squeezing which would expel contents of the globe. If the wound seems dirty, an injection of antitetanus serum (1500 units) is indicated.

Perforating Wounds of the Cornea are subject to a complicating laceration of the iris, prolapse of the iris and injury to deeper parts. If the perforating wound is limited to the cornea, the treatment consists of cleansing, bichloride solution 1:3000, atropine, suturing the corneal wound or covering it with a conjunctival flap slid over from adjacent parts and a firm dressing. Unless there is evidence that no foreign body has entered the globe, an x-ray examination is indicated. With very extensive wounds of the cornea and considerable involvement of deeper parts, enucleation must be considered.

Prolapse of the Iris requires irrigation with a mild cleansing lotion and excision of the prolapse with careful separation of the cut edges from the wound, following which a drop of a cycloplegic solution is instilled and the eye is dressed. A foreign body may pass through the cornea and lodge upon the iris; in such a case, the particle should be removed by forceps after a preliminary incision with the keratome at the limbus; if composed of iron or steel it may be drawn out with a magnet; if these efforts are unsuccessful, the piece of the iris upon which the foreign body lies should be drawn through a keratome incision and excised.

Perforating Wounds Involving the Ciliary Body. The *ciliary region*, represented by a pericorneal band about 6 mm. wide, is known as the *"dangerous zone,"* because penetrating wounds in this situation are apt to initiate *sympathetic uveitis*. After thorough cleansing, extensive ciliary wounds are closed by one or more sutures passed through the superficial layers of the sclera; such wounds are generally covered by a conjunctival flap; if there is prolapse of the iris or ciliary body this should be excised. The presence of a foreign body in the globe must be excluded. Atropine is instilled and the eye dressed. If the wound is very extensive and sight is lost, enucleation is indicated.

Perforating Wounds of the Sclera are serious because of accompanying injury to the inner layers, escape of the contents of the eyeball and possible infection of the interior. *Small, clean, perforating wounds* often heal without reaction if there is no infection at the time of the injury, and merely require cleansing, conjunctival suture and dressing. *Large, gaping wounds* frequently allow escape of the vitreous or hemorrhage in the vitreous, and some of the underlying tissues (choroid or ciliary body, varying with the position) will be found in the wound; if there is a chance for useful vision, such wounds should be cleansed, the prolapsed parts excised, if not too extensive, the opening closed by superficial sutures in the sclera (being careful to avoid the choroid), the patient kept absolutely quiet, atropine instilled and the eye dressed. Sometimes, when there is no infection, such wounds fail to excite much inflammatory reaction and may heal readily, even though there has been extensive prolapse through the wound and remnants of prolapsed parts remain in the cicatrix; but frequently they give rise to inflammation leading to panophthalmitis or to plastic iridocyclitis, in either case with loss of sight. When the wound includes the ciliary body, the injury becomes more dangerous because of the liability of such wounds to excite sympathetic ophthalmitis. When injuries of the sclera are very extensive and there is considerable loss of contents of the eyeball, and when useful sight cannot be expected, the eyeball should be removed at once; this becomes still more urgent when the wound involves the ciliary region. In every case an x-ray examination is indicated; a foreign body in the eye always is a serious complication; if other conditions are such that it seems likely that the eye can be saved, an attempt should be made to extract the foreign body, as described later.

Penetrating Wounds Involving the Orbit. Penetrating wounds of the orbit may destroy the eyeball, injure the optic nerve, causing blindness, or sever some of the muscles, resulting in paralysis and diplopia; if infected, such wounds are followed by orbital abscess. A blow or stab with a blunt object may rupture the globe. Foreign bodes in the orbit may be tolerated if aseptic; if infected, suppuration ensues. Treatment consists in cleansing and endeavoring to extract foreign bodies after an x-ray examination has shown the location; if the situation is such that extensive manipulation is necessary for its removal, and if there is reason to believe that the substance is aseptic (such as shot), it often is better to allow the foreign body to remain; if suppuration follows, the foreign body must be removed and free exit for secretions maintained.

FOREIGN BODIES IN THE GLOBE

The entrance and lodgment of a foreign body (metal, glass, wood, stone, etc.) within the globe usually causes *severe inflammation* and *destruction* of the eyeball as a result of iridocyclitis or panophthalmitis unless the substance is extracted promptly; the gravity of the accident depends upon the nature and size of the foreign body and the presence or absence of *infection.* Particles of iron which penetrate the eye during machinist's work, riveting or stonebreaking usually are so heated as to be sterile; occasionally these substances, when small and free from infection, remain quiescent and become encysted; but even in such cases there is danger of subsequent inflammation.

The presence of a particle of iron for any length of time causes a rusty brown or greenish discoloration of the iris and lens, occasionally in the cornea, known as *siderosis bulbi;* in the lens there is a characteristic rusty deposit just beneath the anterior capsule; in addition, such eyes are apt to suffer from degenerative changes in the retina.

A fragment of *copper* remaining within

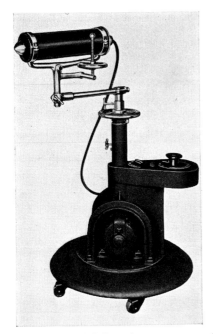

FIG. 17-7. The Müller giant eye magnet.

the globe almost invariably leads to destruction of the eye.

Lead, gold, silver, porcelain or glass, unless septic, may become *encapsulated*, and for a long time may cause little or no trouble; but eventually an eye containing a foreign body posterior to the lens usually becomes inflamed and *disorganized*; and prior to this there are apt to be degenerative changes at the macula as the result of the initial concussion.

Diagnosis. The foreign body may have dropped to the *bottom* of the vitreous cavity, become imbedded in the uvea or sclera or have passed through the eyeball and be located in the *orbit*. If the patient comes under observation soon after the injury, before the media have become hazy, the particle may be seen with the *ophthalmoscope*. A careful examination of the field of vision, disclosing a *scotoma*, also may be an aid in locating its position; this information will be corroborated by a study

of the site of the wound of entrance and the probable *direction* which the foreign body took. In most instances, an *x-ray* examination will reveal its presence and position; to be conclusive the x-ray examination must be made with a *special localizing apparatus*, and above all must be made by an *expert* in this field. If the foreign body is of iron or steel, the giant magnet (Fig. 17-7) frequently will indicate its presence by the production of pain when the point is brought near the eyeball, or by the bulging of the iris or the forward movement of the lens when the particle is within these structures.

Treatment. If the substance is a piece of *iron or steel*, an attempt to extract it with a *magnet* should be made at once. Attempts to remove other foreign bodies (glass, wood, copper, lead) should be made as soon as possible after they have been located, by means of delicate *forceps* introduced through the original wound or through an opening into the vitreous cavity made at the point at which the foreign body has been located. But if this is not accomplished promptly, and very often it is unsuccessful, the foreign body should be allowed to remain rather than stir up the vitreous, especially if there are no symptoms of infection or irritation, and the patient can be kept under constant observation; in such cases, however, the question of enucleation must be considered.

Magnet Extraction. Magnets used for the extraction of particles of iron or steel are small, *portable* electromagnets (Fig. 17-8) or *large*, stationary electromagnets (Fig. 17-7).

A piece of iron or steel imbedded in the *iris* is removed best by keratome incision near the limbus and the introduction of the pole of a small magnet; if this fails, a small iridectomy embracing the foreign body should be performed. If the particle of steel is free in the anterior chamber, a keratome incision is made and the foreign body drawn toward the incision by the portable magnet; as the magnet passes over the incision the posterior lip of the incision is depressed slightly and the foreign body drawn out of the wound. If a magnetizable particle is in the *lens,* an attempt should be made to draw it into the anterior chamber by means of the giant magnet; if this succeeds the foreign body is removed with the small magnet as described above; if it fails, and if the foreign body is nonmagnetizable, the lens should be removed by linear extraction in young subjects and by extracapsular extraction in an older person.

It seldom is possible to remove a nonmagnetizable foreign body from the vitreous. If it is of iron or steel an attempt should be made to extract it with the portable or the giant magnet at the *earliest possible* moment, since the delay of even a few hours may permit the particle to become so firmly fixed by inflammatory exudate that removal is impossible.

When using the *portable magnet,* the point is held at the entrance wound or at an opening made through the sclera, but not through the choroid, corresponding to the location of the foreign body, and then the current is turned on.

For use of the *giant magnet* the patient is seated before the apparatus and the pole of the magnet is brought in contact with the cornea; as the current is turned on and increased gradually, the patient usually feels some pain. In a successful case the foreign body comes forward to the back of the lens or behind the iris, dragging the latter forward; by a little manipulation and adjustment of the eye it may be *worked into the anterior chamber,* whence it may be extracted as already described.

Even after successful extraction the *prognosis* always is *serious;* a small number of patients recover permanently useful vision; in some the form of the eyeball

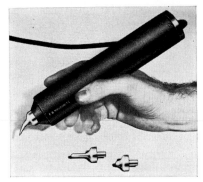

Fig. 17-8. Portable electromagnet.

is preserved, although frequently a detachment of the retina ultimately follows; in many cases destructive inflammation supervenes. If the attempt at extraction fails and the eye remains quiet with no evidence of other injury and with likely preservation of some sight, and if the patient can be kept under observation, the particle may be allowed to remain in the hope that it will become encapsulated and not excite inflammation; but, as a rule, *enucleation* is required to prevent the possibility of *sympathetic inflammation* in the fellow eye.

If the eye presents evidence of *infection* when first seen or after the foreign body has been extracted, *enucleation* is necessary.

SUPPURATIVE OCULAR INFECTIONS

Endophthalmitis and panophthalmitis also are known as purulent uveitis and frequently follow trauma involving the globe.

Etiology. Suppurative infection of the interior of the eye occurs either from without or from within the body. Exogenous infection occurs with penetrating wounds such as operations, injuries and perforating ulcers of the cornea, and by penetration of infectious agents through thin corneal or scleral scars. Endogenous infection results from hematogenous metastasis or septic embolism or general infectious diseases, from direct extension from orbital cellulitis or meningococcic meningitis and occasionally from necrosis of tissues especially a rapidly growing tumor within the eye. The organisms most frequently involved are *Staphylococcus aureus, Pseudomonas aeruginosa,* and Streptococcus. Rarely Pneumococci, *Bacillus subtilis,* various fungi or the gas forming bacilli may be involved.

Endophthalmitis

(1) Infrequently, the process is limited to the choroid (*suppurative choroiditis*); the purulent exudate fills the vitreous humor (*vitreous abscess*) with no external evidences of inflammation, but always with loss of vision. A *yellowish* or grayish yellow *reflex* is obtained from the interior of the eye; the purulent mass degenerates, shrinks and forms a membrane, the retina becomes detached, the eyeball softens and the process ends with *atrophy of the eyeball.* Since the reflex from the pupil resembles in color that in retinoblastoma, the condition is known as *pseudoretinoblastoma* or *pseudoglioma.*

(2) More commonly, the purulent exudate fills the *whole interior* and involves the *entire uveal tract,* constituting septic *endophthalmitis.* Then the symptoms are those of acute iridocyclitis and are severe: much pain, conjunctival congestion, chemosis, swelling of lids, cloudy cornea, pus in the aqueous humor as well as in the vitreous humor, constitutional disturbance and loss of sight; finally, a blind, degenerated, shrunken globe remains (*atrophy of the eyeball*).

Panophthalmitis

An intense *suppurative inflammation of the entire uveal tract,* which fills the eyeball with *pus,* extends to all the structures of the eye and ends in *complete destruction* of this organ. It is due to *infection.* It differs from suppurative endophthalmitis in spreading beyond the uveal tract and involving *all the structures* of the eye.

Symptoms, described in connection with suppurative endophthalmitis, are *acute* and *severe.* The disease usually is ushered in by a rise of temperature, headache and sometimes vomiting. There are severe *pain* in the eyeball, rapid *loss of sight,* intense ciliary and conjunctival *congestion,* severe *chemosis* and *swelling* and redness of the *lids* (Plate 14*D*). The iris soon becomes involved, the anterior chamber and vitreous become filled with *pus,* the cornea is *clouded and yellow* (Plate 14*E*) and tension increased. There is infiltration of Tenon's capsule, followed by *exophthalmos* and limitation of the movements of the eyeball. *Pus* usually *breaks through* the anterior portion of the sclera, after which the pain and other symptoms subside; in the course of several weeks the process has run its course, leaving a shrunken, *sightless eyeball* (*phthisis bulbi,* Fig. 9-8).

Prognosis always is *hopeless;* sight invariably is lost. The condition does not cause sympathetic ophthalmia.

Treatment. It is almost impossible to save sight once either endophthalmitis or panophthalmitis has become established, therefore every precaution should be taken to prevent such infection. Active and intensive treatment of pneumococcic pneumonia and meningococcic meningitis in recent years has reduced the incidence of these two types of endophthalmitis almost to the point of elimination. However once the infection is established, its cause should be determined and specific therapy instituted as quickly as possible. In the interval, general administration of sulfonamides should be accompanied by the use of cycloplegic drops and other pain relieving measures. With persistent pain and progressive suppuration, drainage of the exudate, evisceration or enucleation may be indicated in endophthalmitis. In panophthalmitis drainage or evisceration may be necessary in the acute phase but enucleation should be delayed until after the infection has run its course and the inflammation has subsided.

OPERATIONS UPON THE EYEBALL

Enucleation of the Eyeball

Anesthesia. In enucleation of the eyeball and in substitutes for this operation a *general anesthetic* is necessary in children and in nervous persons. In others either general or local anesthesia can be used.

Operation. The conjunctiva is incised around the cornea as close to its border as possible. Together with Tenon's capsule, it is elevated away from the globe back to the insertion of the rectus muscles. The tendons of these muscles are isolated and divided close to the globe. The eyeball then is dislocated forward to put the optic nerve on stretch (Fig. 17-9), which is then located and cut 0.5 to 1 cm. posterior to the globe. The eyeball then is lifted forward and all unsevered attachments divided as close to the globe as possible. Hemorrhage is arrested by packing the orbit with gauze and applying pressure for several minutes. The conjunctiva and Tenon's capsule then are closed in a horizontal line by use of several interrupted fine catgut sutures, and a firm pressure dressing is applied for 48 to 72 hours.

Care should be taken to avoid rupturing the eyeball, since a collapsed globe makes the operation more difficult. Troublesome hemorrhage may occur; it can be controlled by pressure. When an eyeball containing a malignant growth is enucleated, as much of the optic nerve as possible should be removed. Very rarely, infection of the wound has led to abscess, thrombosis and even fatal meningitis. The tendency to meningitis is increased in enucleation of an actively suppurating eyeball; hence panophthalmitis is a con-

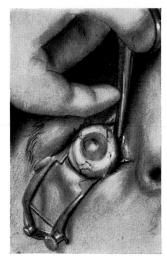

FIG. 17-9. Enucleation of the eyeball.

traindication to enucleation and usually requires evisceration of the eyeball.

The Indications for Enucleation are (1) injuries of the eyeball, especially those involving the ciliary region, when the eye is blind, or the traumatism so extensive that the form of the eyeball cannot be preserved; (2) traumatic iridocyclitis, to prevent sympathetic ophthalmitis; (3) severe pain in a blind eye which cannot be relieved by less radical means; (4) iridocyclitis, phthisis bulbi and glaucoma, when accompanied by severe pain or inflammatory symptoms, and when the eye is blind or is certain to become so; (5) malignant tumors, either intraocular or epiocular (except small tumors of the iris, which can be removed entirely by iridectomy); (6) anterior staphyloma, if the eye is blind, troublesome and disfiguring; (7) panophthalmitis after the suppurative process has ceased; (8) foreign bodies in the eye when they cannot be removed and cause irritation; (9) cosmetic improvement in blind and disfiguring eyes.

Enucleation with Insertion of an Artificial Globe or Implant into

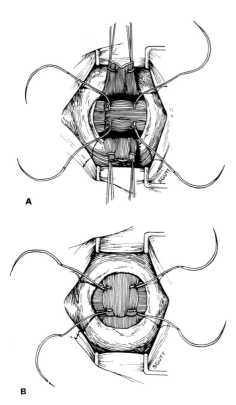

A

B

FIG. 17-10. Insertion of implant. *A*, Cut ends of lateral and medial rectus muscles are overlapped and sutured around implant (redrawn after Lee Allen). *B*, Cut ends of superior and inferior rectus muscles are overlapped and sutured over horizontal muscles (redrawn after Lee Allen).

Tenon's Capsule. Unless there is some contraindication, this operation is preferred to simple enucleation since it provides a less sunken stump and results in an improvement in appearance and motion when the artificial eye subsequently is worn.

During the enucleation procedure as described above, the sutures are placed through the edges of the tendons of the four recti before they are detached from the globe. The muscles then are sutured to each other around the artificial globe

or after they have been passed through special tunnels in the implant being inserted (Fig. 17-10). The conjunctiva and Tenon's capsule are closed in a horizontal line by interrupted fine catgut sutures. This operation is contraindicated when the eyeball is the seat of panophthalmitis, in some cases of suppurative endophthalmitis or when there is an intraocular growth and postoperative radiation is to be used.

Evisceration of the Eyeball

In this operation the cornea and entire contents of the eyeball are removed, the sclera alone remaining.

Operation. The cornea is removed and the contents of the eyeball are removed thoroughly with a sharp spoon, care being taken to leave nothing but sclera. The cavity is wiped out with gauze and hemorrhage is controlled. The sclera and conjunctiva usually are not closed, so as to permit drainage, but a moderate pressure dressing is applied.

Recovery is less rapid than after enucleation, and pain and reaction are greater; however, the support for an artificial eye is better than is obtained with simple enucleation. The operation may be substituted for enucleation after panophthalmitis, but is contraindicated in malignant tumors, foreign bodies, shrunken eyeballs and sympathetic ophthalmitis.

Artificial Eyes (Fig. 17-11), made of glass or plastic, are worn after enucleation and evisceration for cosmetic purposes and to fill out the cavity left between the lids. They can be worn as soon as the socket is free from swelling, usually after several weeks. Plastic artificial eyes are more expensive than those of glass, but need less frequent replacement and are unbreakable.

Either type should be made to conform to the cavity in order to obtain the best

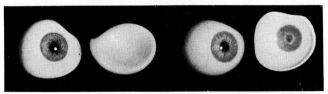

Fig. 17-11. Artificial eyes. Shell prosthesis is seen at *right*.

movement. Thus many artificial eye makers make an impression mold of the socket in beginning the construction of the prosthesis.

The artificial eye (*prosthesis*) may be removed at night.

A shell-shaped prosthesis is occasionally worn over a shrunken globe or over such a globe which has had its cornea denuded and covered by a conjunctival flap.

Contracted Socket may result from cicatricial bands or scar tissue due to injuries, so that after enucleation the capacity of the socket is lessened; or in consequence of the continued wearing of a roughened prosthesis the lower fornix may become shallowed; in either case an artificial eye will no longer stay in place. Operations designed to restore the socket or the lower fornix begin with thorough division and excision of all cicatricial tissue; then the conjunctival sac is relined with a mucous membrane graft, which is kept in place by being wound around an insert of gutta percha, dental wax or a prosthesis, the lid being stitched together until the graft has taken.

COMPENSATION FOR EYE INJURIES

The examination of eyes injured by accident or occupational disease is important; such examinations are necessary not only after industrial injuries and diseases of workmen who seek compensation awards, but also in connection with persons who have met with accidents and who have claims for loss of visual efficiency against insurance carriers. The estimation

of permanent visual disability, after all possible benefits of medical and surgical treatment, forms the basis for compensation.

Such examination must be thorough and complete; it must include not only the injured eye, if only one has been involved, but also its fellow. It is important that all findings be recorded, even if not related to the injury; claims often are made for visual defects that depend upon lesions which were not caused by the accident and which antedated the injury; such claims sometimes lead to legal action at which the examiner may be called to testify, and his written record then will serve as evidence.

After the accident, the individual sometimes claims a greater loss of vision than really exists; this is suspected when the objective examination fails to disclose a cause for the reduction in vision claimed. In such cases it becomes necessary to examine for malingering as explained in Chapter 11.

When determining the loss of visual efficiency, the estimation of which is to form the basis of a compensation award, it is important to distinguish between "central visual acuity" and "visual efficiency." There are three principal factors connected with vision, each of which has an interdependent relation to full visual efficiency; these are (1) central visual acuity, (2) the field of vision and (3) muscle function; accommodation also must be considered.

In determining the amount of industrial visual disability when one eye has been injured and the other has escaped or has suffered less injury, the visual efficiency of the better eye must be taken into account; if one eye is lost through injury and the other eye is normal, visual efficiency of the individual is not one-half, but is considerably more than one-half.

The evaluation of the visual efficiency loss is the basis of compensation awards to workmen who have suffered injury from accidents or disease acquired in industrial pursuits.

There are laws governing compensation for eye injuries in every state. Unfortunately these are not uniform and not always equitable, since they sometimes are framed upon consideration of faulty premises. One source of error is the assumption that the Snellen fraction used in recording central vision for distance represents the fraction of normal vision which is present; the fraction merely indicates that letters of a certain size are seen at a recorded distance; 20/40 for instance, does not denote one-half of normal vision, but merely indicates that the individual's vision is limited to the ability to read at 20 feet the letters which should be read at 40 feet. A second error, which is very obvious, is the provision in the laws of some states that central vision for distance be recorded without glasses, and that this estimation be used as a basis for compensation awards.

The meaning of the term "industrial blindness" varies somewhat in different states. The American Medical Association recommendation regards visual acuity less than 20/200 to be equivalent to industrial blindness.

Since there are variations in the compensation laws of different states, it is necessary to become acquainted with the statutes on this subject in force in the state in which the examiner pratices. In 1955, a committee appointed by the *Council on Industrial Health, American Medical Association,* submitted a revised report on computing visual efficiency loss. This report was approved by the *Section of Ophthalmology,* and has been adopted as a basis for computing compensation for industrial eye injuries in some states. The report follows.

Estimation of Loss of Visual Efficiency

Section I: Essential Factors in Determination of Visual Efficiency. Visual efficiency is defined as that degree or percentage of the competence of the eyes to accomplish their physiologic functions, including (1) corrected visual acuity, for distance and near, (2) visual fields, (3) ocular motility with absence of diplopia, and (4) binocular vision. Although these factors do not possess an equal degree of importance, vision is imperfect without the coordinated action of all. Other functions, such as color perception, adaptation to light or dark, and accommodation, although secondary and dependent, are recognized as important. Because these functions are inherently dependent on the status of the previously mentioned four coordinating functions of vision, they are not included in the basic method of calculation of the percentage of loss of visual efficiency.

Section II: Central Visual Acuity. For purposes of standardization, the Snellen test chart utilizing block letters or numbers without serifs, the illiterate E chart, or Landolt's broken-ring chart is desirable. Illumination of the test chart should be at least 5 foot-candles (f-c.), and the chart or reflecting surface should not be dirty or discolored from age. The test distances should be at 20 ft. (6 meters) and at 14 in. (36 cm.). In line with the recommendations of the American Committee on Optics and Visual Physiology, Subcommittee on the Problem of an International Nomenclature for Designating Visual Acuity, the sizes of letters in the test lines form a geometric progression, as proposed by Green in 1867. With this scale, the size of letters of each successive line is 26% larger than that of the following line, or 20% smaller than that of the preceding line. Visual acuity is most commonly recorded in the form of a fraction in which the test distance, in feet or meters, is expressed as the numerator. The denominator represents the distance at which the smallest letters discriminated by the patient would subtend 5 minutes of arc (Table 17-1). Although this method of

TABLE 17-1

Percentage of Central Visual Efficiency Corresponding to Central Visual Acuity Notations for Distance

Snellen		Visual Angle in Minutes*	Per Cent Central Visual Efficiency	Per Cent Loss Central Vision
English	Metric			
20/16	6/5	0.80	100	0
20/20	6/6	1.00	100−†	0
20/25	6/7.5	1.25	95	5
20/32	6/10	1.6	90	10
20/40	6/12	2.0	85	15
20/50	6/15	2.5	75	25
20/64	6/20	3.2	65	35
20/80	6/24	4.0	60	40
20/100	6/30	5.0	50	50
20/125	6/38	6.3	40	60
20/160	6/48	8.0	30	70
20/200	6/60	10.0	20	80
20/300	6/90	15.0	15	85
20/400	6/120	20.0	10	90
20/800	6/240	40.0	5	95

* Denoting each constituent part of test character. When the visual angle of each constituent part is multiplied by 5, the product is the visual angle of entire test character.

† For purposes of calculation of the per cent of central visual efficiency, 100% is used. This does not consider the fact that the average normal person usually has a visual acuity of 20/16 corrected by ophthalmic lenses.

TABLE 17-2

Percentage of Central Visual Efficiency Corresponding to Central Visual Acuity Notations for Near

Snellen	Jaeger	Point	Visual Angle in Minutes	Visual Efficiency	Per Cent Loss of Central Vision
14/14	1−	3	1.0	100	0
14/18	2−	4	1.25	100	0
14/22	...	5	1.6	95	5
14/28	3	6	2.0	90	10
14/35	6	8	2.5	50	50
14/45	7−	9+	3.2	40	60
14/56	8	12	4.0	20	80
14/70	11	14	5.0	15	85
14/87	...	...	6.3	10	90
14/112	14−	22	8.0	5	95
14/140	...	...	10.0	2	98

designation appears to be a mathematical fraction, it is purely a convenient form of notation by ophthalmologists and does not represent a true percentage of normal visual acuity. For designation of visual acuity for near, a similar Snellen ratio can be utilized using inches, or a comparable Jaeger or a point type system may be used, according to Table 17-2. The visual acuity may also be designated as visual angle, in accordance with the recommendation of the previously mentioned Subcommittee on Nomenclature. A visual angle of 1.0 minute of arc of each constituent part of the test character (or 5 minutes for the entire character) can be discriminated by a "normal" subject.

The best vision obtainable with opthalmic lenses should be used in determining the degree of central visual acuity. It is realized that the use of contact lenses might further improve vision reduced by irregular astigmatism from corneal disease or injury. However, the practical difficulties of fitting, expense, and tolerance of contact lenses are sufficiently important at the present time to favor recommendation that only regular ophthalmic lenses be used to determine the best corrected vision.

The visual disability due to monocular aphakia (with normal corrected vision in the other eye) varies considerably among different persons because of several factors, including age and accommodative power, ability to tolerate a contact lens for adequate periods of time, ability to obtain single binocular vision comfortably when wearing a contact lens, and the importance of binocular vision in the patient's work. If the vision in the aphakic eye can be corrected to 20/20, the disability may be slight in a presbyopic patient who can wear a contact lens comfortably for period of eight hours or more. However, a young person doing close precision work may be incapacitated for this task even when wearing a contact lens. Other persons may not be able to obtain and wear a contact lens comfortably for long periods of time, for one reason or another. However, even an uncorrected aphakia is not equivalent to a blind eye because of the usefulness of side vision, and the possibility of correction if the normal eye should be injured subsequently. The practice of considering monocular aphakia as the full loss of visual efficiency in one eye does not recognize the value of an eye with no abnormality except the loss of the lens. With these considerations in mind, it is recommended that monocular aphakia be considered as a partial visual disability, *viz.*, 50% of the central visual efficiency of that eye when corrected by lenses (Table 17-1). For example, if corrected vision in the aphakic eye is 20/40, the allowable central visual efficiency of that eye would be $0.50 \times 0.85 = 43\%$ or a loss of central vision of 57%.

The visual handicap resulting from aphakia corrected by regular ophthalmic lenses can only be estimated. This factor would be of importance in cases of binocular aphakia, or in monocular aphakia where the corrected vision in the aphakic eye is greatly superior (perhaps 50%) to that of the opposite eye. In such cases where the corrected aphakic vision is used for the patient's activities, it is recommended that this *per se* be considered an additional partial visual handicap of 25% of the best corrected binocular visual efficiency, as calculated under Section VI. For example, if the binocular visual efficiency of the corrected aphakic patient is 75%, the final estimation of the visual efficiency of that patient would be $0.75 \times 0.75 = 56\%$.

A visual acuity of 20/20 or better (6/6 or better, or visual angle of 0.1 minute or less) is considered 100% acuity for distance vision, and Snellen 14/14, Jaeger 1, or 3-point type (with presbyopic correction if necessary) is considered 100% acuity for near vision (14 in., or 36 cm.). A revision of the estimations of percentage loss of visual acuity corresponding to the Snellen and visual-angle notations for distance and near is given in Tables 17-1 and 17-2. This has been done in the light of statistical reports of average "normal" vision, and experience in the disabilities caused by reduced visual acuity. It should be remarked that no scientific studies are available relating central visual acuity, visual field, and motility deficiencies to the actual performance of various duties. This Committee feels that the table set up by the 1925 and 1940 American Medical Association Committees overestimates the loss of visual efficiency for distance acuities poorer than 20/200 and underestimates the loss for near acuities poorer than 14/28, Jaeger 3, or 6-point type. Although the visual angles may be the same, it should not be concluded that the Snellen notation for distance is the exact equivalent of the Snellen notation for near in respect to visual efficiency because of other influences, such as accommodation, size of retinal image, etc. Also, the visual disability in reading with acuity for near of 14/35 (Jaeger 6 or 8-point type) is far greater than the visual disability for distance with 20/50 vision, which has the same visual angle. The revised Tables 17-1 and 17-2 represent an effort to relate more closely visual acuity and visual disability in the light of experience. Because of the importance of good near vision in the performance of work, the revised Table 17-2 weights this disability more heavily than the 1940 American Medical Association table. Calculation of the percentage of central visual efficiency for both distance and near vision would therefore be the average of the two percentages.

Section III: Visual Field. The extent of the visual field is determined by the use of the usual perimetric methods, utilizing a white target which subtends a 0.5-degree angle (that is, a 3 mm. white disc at a distance of 330 mm.) under illumination of not less than 7 f-c. A 6 mm. white disc is recommended for uncorrected aphakia. The test object is brought from the peripheral to the seeing area. At least two peripheral visual fields should be obtained which agree within 15 degrees in each meridian. The reliability of the patient's responses should be noted. The result is plotted on an ordinary visual field chart on each of the eight 41-degree principal meridians.

The minimum normal extent of the visual field from the point of fixation can be defined as follows: temporally, 85 degrees; down and temporally, 85 degrees; down, 65 degrees; down and nasally, 50 degrees; nasally, 60 degrees; up and nasally, 55 degrees; up, 45 degrees, and up and temporally, 55 degrees. These figures are about 10 to 15 degrees less than the average normal, thus allowing for poor or delayed subjective responses or undue prominence of the brow or nose.

The visual field efficiency of one eye in percentage is obtained by adding the number of degrees of the eight principal radii given above for the 3/330 white isopter, which normally is 500 degrees, and dividing by 5. For example, if the field is contracted down to 25 degrees, in all eight meridians, there would be a remaining visual field efficiency of $25 \times 8 \div 5 = 40\%$, or loss of 60%. If the field is contracted down to 5 degrees in every meridian, the remaining efficiency would be $5 \times 8 \div 5 = 8\%$, or loss of 92%. If the entire temporal field is lost, the loss would amount to:

Up and temporally...... 55
Temporally 85
Down and temporally... 85
Average of up and down
   ($\frac{1}{2}[45 + 65]$) 55
                 ——
      $280 \div 5 = 56\%$,

or a remaining efficiency of 44%. If the upper nasal quadrant is lost, the loss of field efficiency would amount to $55 + 52$ (average of up and nasal meridians = $45 + 60 \div 2) \div 5 = 21\%$, or a remaining efficiency of 79%. Loss of visual field efficiency can be calculated for other field defects in a similar manner. Although the extent of loss of visual field efficiency cannot be determined accurately for a ring scotoma, an approximation can be obtained by considering the width of the ring scotoma to be equivalent to loss of peripheral visual field. A similar estimation of visual field loss can be applied to enlargement of the blind spot using a 2 mm. white test object at a distance of 1 meter from a tangent screen with the subject wearing his corrective lenses; for example, a general enlargement of the blind spot of 5 degrees would result in a visual loss of $8 \times 5 \div 5 = 8\%$ loss, or 92% visual field efficiency. Because a central scotoma directly affects the central visual acuity, such loss of visual field is not used in the final calculation of the visual efficiency.

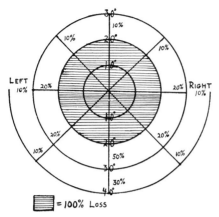

= 100% Loss

Fig. 17-12. Percentage loss of ocular motility of one eye in diplopia fields.

Section IV: Ocular Motility. Visual efficiency is related to the function of extraocular muscles in two major ways: (1) the absence of diplopia, and (2) binocular vision. Except on looking downward, it is doubtful whether diplopia causes significant visual disability unless it is present within 30 degrees of the center of fixation. The extent of the diplopia in the various directions of gaze is determined on the perimeter at 33 cm., or on the ordinary tangent screen at 1 or 2 meters' distance from the patient in each of the 45-degree meridians, utilizing a small test light and without the addition of colored lenses or correcting prisms. The degree of separation of the two lights is plotted along each of the three meridians above for 10, 20, and 30 degrees away from the straight-ahead position and for 10, 20, 30, and 40 degrees away from the straight-ahead position horizontally and below (down and right, down and left). The results of the separation of the two images are plotted on a visual field chart.

The percentage loss of ocular motility efficiency of one eye caused by diplopia in various positions of gaze is given in chart above. Diplopia within the central 20 degrees represents a 100% loss of motility

efficiency in one eye. If diplopia is not present in the central 20 degrees of ocular rotation from the straight-ahead position, diplopia present on more peripheral gaze should be considered as a loss in motility efficiency of one eye, according to the chart. For example, if there is diplopia only on looking straight down between 20 and 40 degrees, the loss of ocular motility efficiency of one eye is 50 + 30 = 80%. Again, if diplopia is present only on looking between 20 and 40 degrees to the right, due to a residual paresis of the right lateral rectus muscle, the loss of ocular motility efficiency of one eye is 20 + 10 = 30%.

If the patient has lost binocular vision as a result of disease or injury and, because of suppression, diplopia is not present, the degree of visual disability will depend on how important good depth perception would be for the performance of the patient's work. However, loss of binocular vision without other ocular abnormalities probably does not represent more than a 50% loss of ocular motility efficiency of one eye in the average case. Tests for binocular vision can be made with any of the well-recognized instruments, such as the major amblyoscope and various forms of stereoscopes.

Strabismus following disease or injury as discussed here is considered only on the basis of the loss of motility efficiency. The cosmetic defect of a strabismus is considered to be a separate factor (see Section VII).

Section V. Calculation of Visual Efficiency of One Eye. Determination of the visual efficiency of one eye considers the average percentage of central visual efficiency for distance and near, percentage of visual field efficiency, and percentage of ocular motility efficiency, including absence of diplopia and binocular vision. For example, with average central visual efficiency for distance and near of 30%, visual field efficiency of 40%, and motor field efficiency of 70%, the total visual efficiency of this eye would be 0.30 × 0.40 × 0.70 = 0.084, or 8.4% of total visual efficiency of this eye. Should the visual efficiency of one eye be reduced to less than 10%, the visual loss is considered to be total from a practical standpoint.

Section VI: Calculation of Binocular Visual Efficiency. If the vision in one eye is completely lost and the fellow eye is normal, it has been found by common experience that the total visual efficiency of such a person is actually more than 50%. In agreement with the opinion of the previous committee of the American Medical Association in 1940, a more nearly correct estimation of visual efficiency can be obtained by weighting the visual efficiency of the better eye three times according to the following method:

$$\frac{(\% \text{ efficiency better eye} \times 3) + (\% \text{ efficiency worst eye})}{4}$$

$$= \text{binocular visual efficiency.}$$

For example, the binocular visual efficiency of a patient with one blind and one normal eye would be

$$\frac{100\% \times 3 + 0\%}{4} = 75\%,$$

or binocular visual loss of 25%.

When disease or injury has involved both eyes, a loss of efficiency in ocular motility is used only in computing the efficiency of the less efficient of the two eyes.

The estimation of the visual efficiency of the better eye is therefore based only on the central visual acuity and the visual field of this eye.

Should the total binocular visual efficiency of the patient be less than 10%, for all practical purposes the patient can be considered blind.

Section VII: Types of Ocular Abnormalities Not Included in the Visual Efficiency Factors. Certain types of ocular disturbances are not included in the previously mentioned computations, and these may result in disabilities the value of which cannot be calculated by any scale as yet scientifically determined. Such are disturbances of accommodation, color vision, light and dark adaptation, metamorphopsia, entropion, ectropion, lagophthalmos, epiphora, strabismus, deformities of the orbit, and cosmetic defects.

Section VIII: Some Considerations in the Final Estimation of Loss of Visual Efficiency. It is recommended that final estimation of visual efficiency be deferred following certain conditions, for example, at least 3 months after all visible evidences of inflammation have disappeared, at least 6 months following surgery, and at least 12, and preferably not more than 16, months in cases of disturbance of the extraocular muscles, sympathetic ophthalmia, traumatic cataract, or optic nerve atrophy.

EDMUND B. SPAETH, *Chairman*
F. BRUCE FRALICK
WILLIAM F. HUGHES, JR.

18

General Optical Principles

Light arising from a point source travels through the medium in straight lines in every direction; the lines of direction are called rays. The speed of light is decreased as the density of the medium is increased. The amount of divergence of the rays of light falling on a given area is inversely proportionate to the distance of the luminous source; the nearer this point, the more divergence. When the distance from a light source becomes *20 feet or more*, the divergence of rays is so slight that for practical purposes we assume them to be *parallel*.

When a ray of light meets an *opaque* body, it is either *absorbed* or *reflected*. When it meets a *transparent* medium, some of it is absorbed and some reflected, but the greater part traverses the medium being *deflected* in its course; this bending is called *refraction*.

Reflection occurs from any polished surface (mirror)—plane, concave or convex. The ray striking the mirror is called the *incident ray* (*IB*, Fig. 18-1); that returning from the mirror, the *reflected ray* (*BR*, Fig. 18-1).

Laws of reflection. (1) The angle of reflection is equal to the angle of incidence. (2) The reflected and incident rays are both in a plane perpendicular to the reflecting surface. In Figure 18-1, *IB* is the incident ray on the reflecting surface *AC*, *BR* the reflected ray and *PB* the perpendicular. The angle of incidence, *IBP*, is equal to the angle of reflection, *PBR*. *IB*, *PB* and *BR* lie in the same plane.

Reflection by a Plane Mirror. The image is formed at a distance behind the mirror equal to the distance of the object in front of it. The image is *virtual, erect* and the *same size* as the object. In Figure 18-2, *O* is the object, *I* the image and *E* the eye of the observer. The image of the candle *O* is found behind the plane mirror *MM*; the observer's eye *S* receives the rays from *O* as if they came from *I*.

Reflection from a Concave Mirror. A concave surface may be considered as made up of a number of plane surfaces inclined toward one another. *Parallel rays falling on a concave mirror are reflected as convergent* rays which meet at a point on the perpendicular axis of the mirror called the *principal focus* (*Pf*, Fig. 18-3); this point is midway between the mirror and its optical center *C*. The distance of the principal focus from the mirror is called the *focal length* of the mirror.

The position of an image formed by a concave mirror varies with the distance of the object from the mirror. If the object is placed at the principal focus, *Pf*, the reflected rays are parallel to each other and to the axis of the mirror. If the object is placed at the center of concavity *C*, the reflected rays return along the same lines. If the object is beyond the center, at *CF*, the reflected rays focus between the center and the principal focus at *cf*; and conversely, if the object is moved between the principal focus and the center, at *cf*, its focus will be beyond the center, at *CF*; these two points, *CF* and *cf*, bear a reciprocal relation to each other and are known as *conjugate foci*; the nearer the object approaches the principal focus, the greater the distance at which the reflected rays meet. If the object is placed nearer the mirror than the principal focus, at *X*, reflected rays will be divergent and never meet; if, however, these divergent rays are continued backward, they will unite at a point, *Vf*, behind the mirror; this point is called the *virtual focus*, and an observer placed in the path of the reflected rays will receive them as though they came from this point.

It follows, therefore, that concave mirrors produce an enlarged, erect and virtual image if the object is placed nearer than the principal focus; no image if an object is placed at the principal focus; an enlarged, inverted, real image if the object is placed between the principal focus and the center; an inverted image of the same size when placed at the center; and a smaller, inverted, real image if the object is placed beyond the center.

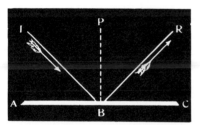

FIG. 18-1. Reflection by a plane surface.

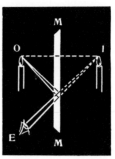

FIG. 18-2. Formation of image by a plane mirror.

Reflection by a Convex Mirror. Parallel rays falling on a convex surface are reflected *divergent* and hence never meet; but if the rays are prolonged backward a *negative image* is formed at a point called the *principal focus* (*F*, Fig. 18-4). The image is always *virtual, erect* and *smaller* than the object, independent of the position of the object before the mirror.

Refraction is the *deviation* in the course of rays of light in passing from one transparent (dioptric) medium into another of different density (refracting medium). The ray which falls *perpendicular* to the surface separating the two media is *not refracted* but continues in a straight course (*PP*, Fig. 18-5).

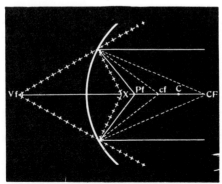

FIG. 18-3. Reflection by a concave mirror.

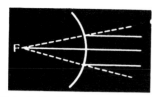

FIG. 18-4. Reflection by a convex mirror.

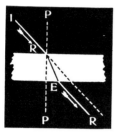

FIG. 18-5. Refraction by a transparent medium with parallel surfaces.

In passing from a *rarer to a denser* medium, a ray is refracted *toward the perpendicular* to the refracting surface; in passing from a *denser to a rarer* medium, the ray is refracted *away from the perpendicular*. In Figure 18-5, the incident ray *IR*, in passing from a rarer medium (air) into a denser medium (glass), is refracted toward the perpendicular *PP*; in passing from a denser to a rarer medium, the emergent ray *ER* is refracted from the perpendicular *PP*. The ray continues in a line parallel to its original course, but has suffered lateral deviation. The angle formed by the incident ray with the perpendicular, *IRP*, is known as the *angle of incidence*; the angle formed by the emergent or refracted ray with the perpendicular, *PER*, is known as the *angle of refraction*.

Index of refraction. The *relative density*, or the comparative length of time occupied by light in traveling a definite distance in different transparent media, is known as the index of refraction. Air being taken as 1.00, the index of refraction of water is 1.33, of the cornea 1.33, of the

lens 1.40, of crown glass 1.5, of flint glass 1.6, and of diamond 2.50.

Prisms

A prism is a piece of glass or other refracting substance bounded by *plane surfaces inclined toward each other* (Fig. 18-6). The angle formed by the two surfaces is called the *refracting angle* of the prism (*BAC*), the thin edge where the intersecting surfaces meet is known as the *apex* (*A*), and the opposite thick portion as the *base* (*BC*).

Refraction by a Prism. Rays of light passing through a prism are *bent toward the base*. In Figure 18-6, the incident ray *IR* is refracted toward the perpendicular *PR*, at *R*, and assumes the direction *RR* in the prism; on emerging, it is refracted away from the perpendicular and continues as *RE* toward the base of the prism. To the eye placed at *E*, the ray *RE* seems to come from *X*; hence *an object seen through a prism appears displaced toward the apex*. A prism has neither converging nor diverging power, and therefore has no focus and cannot form an image; rays that are parallel before entering the prism are parallel on emerging (Fig. 18-7).

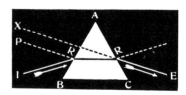

FIG. 18-6. Refraction by a prism.

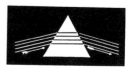

FIG. 18-7. Passage of parallel rays through a prism.

The Numbering of Prisms. The strength of a prism usually is expressed in prism diopters, less frequently in degrees; a third method (the centrad) is not used much. The *prism diopter* is a deviation, the tangent of which is 1/100 of the radius, and is expressed: 1Δ, or 2Δ, etc. In the second method (degrees), which is still used fairly often despite certain faults, the value of the prism corresponds to the refracting angle (geometrical angle) and is expressed: Prism 1°, 2°, 10°, etc. A centrad corresponds to a deviation, the arc of which is 1/100 of the radius, and is expressed 1∇, 2∇, 10∇, etc. Within the limits of common use, the three scales can practically be considered alike.

The Position of a Prism when placed in front of an eye is indicated by the *direction of its base*; "base out" means that the thick part of the prism is toward the temple; the base may be up, down, in or out.

The Uses of Prisms. (1) As a test for heterophoria, (2) to test the extent to which the eyes can be deviated from parallelism, (3) for detecting simulated blindness, (4) to counteract the effects of muscular paralysis or insufficiency, (5) for the exercise of weak muscles.

Lenses

A lens is a transparent *refracting medium*, usually made of glass, in which one or both surfaces are *curved*. There are two kinds: *spherical* and *cylindrical* lenses.

Spherical Lenses are so called because the curved surfaces are segments of spheres (Fig. 18-8); such lenses refract rays of light equally in *all meridians* or planes. There are two kinds of spherical lenses, *convex* and *concave*.

Convex spherical lenses are formed of *prisms* with their *bases together* and toward the center (Fig. 18-9); they are therefore *thick at the center* and thin at the edge. They are known as *converging*,

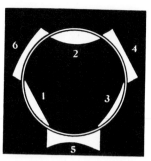

FIG. 18-8. The relation of the surfaces of lenses to spheres. *1*, Planoconvex; *2*, biconvex; *3*, convex meniscus; *4*, planoconcave; *5*, biconcave; *6*, concave meniscus.

FIG. 18-9. The formation of lenses by prisms.

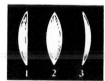

FIG. 18-10. Convex lenses. *1*, Planoconvex; *2*, biconvex; *3*, convex meniscus.

magnifying, positive and plus lenses, and are denoted by the sign +. They have the power of *converging* parallel rays and of bringing them to a *focus* (Fig. 18-12). There are three different forms: (1) *planoconvex*, one surface plane, the other convex (*1*, Fig. 18-10); (2) *biconvex* or double convex, both surfaces convex (*2*, Fig. 18-10); (3) *concavoconvex* (*convex periscopic*, convex or converging *meniscus*), one surface convex, the other concave; the former having the shorter radius of curvature (*3*, Fig. 18-10). The *periscopic* lens (whether + or −) diminishes spherical aberration and enlarges the field of vision.

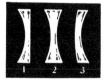

FIG. 18-11. Concave lenses. *1*, Plano-concave; *2*, biconcave; *3*, concave meniscus.

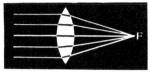

FIG. 18-12. The action of a convex lens on parallel rays.

Concave spherical lenses are formed of *prisms* with their *apices together* and toward the center (Fig. 18-9); they are therefore *thin at the center* and thick at the edge. They are known as *diverging*, reducing, negative or *minus* lenses, and denoted by the sign —. Parallel rays of light after passing through a concave lens are rendered *divergent*. These rays, if projected backward, form an image on the same side as the object (Fig. 18-13). There are three different forms: (1) *planocon-cave*, one surface plane, the other concave (*1*, Fig. 18-11); (2) *biconcave* or double concave, both surfaces concave (*2*, Fig. 18-11); (3) *convexoconcave* (*concave periscopic*, concave or diverging *meniscus*), one surface convex and the other concave; the latter having the shorter radius of curvature (*3*, Fig. 18-11).

The Action of Spherical Lenses. Since spherical lenses are formed of prisms with their bases (convex) or apices (concave) in apposition, and since rays in passing through a prism are refracted toward its base, it follows that *convex lenses cause convergence* (Fig. 18-12) and *concave lenses produce divergence* of rays (Fig. 18-13).

A line passing through the center of the lens (optical center or nodal point, *O*,

Fig. 18-14) at right angles to the surfaces of the lens is called the *principal axis* (*AB*, Fig. 18-14). A ray passing through this axis (*axial ray*) is *not refracted*; all other rays suffer more or less refraction. Rays passing through the optical center of a lens, but not through the principal axis (*secondary rays*), are slightly deviated, but emerge in the same direction as they entered (*CD* and *EF*, Fig. 18-14); the deviation in thin lenses is so slight that practically they may be considered as straight lines and are called *secondary axes*.

Foci of a Convex Lens. The point to which rays converge after refraction by a convex lens is called its *focus*. The *principal focus* is the *focus for parallel rays* (*F*, Fig. 18-15); the distance of this point from the optical center is called the *focal*

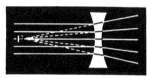

FIG. 18-13. The action of a concave lens on parallel rays.

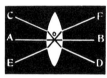

FIG. 18-14. Principal and secondary axes of a convex lens.

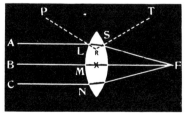

FIG. 18-15. The principal focus of a convex lens.

distance of the lens (*XF*, Fig. 18-15). Since the course of a ray passing from one point to another is the same, independent of the direction, it follows that rays from a luminous point placed at the principal focus will emerge as parallel after passing through the lens.

In Figure 18-15, the rays *ABC* strike the surface of the lens at *LMN*; the axial ray *B* strikes the lens at *M* perpendicular to its surface and consequently continues in a straight line to *F*. The ray *A* strikes the lens obliquely at *L* and is bent toward the perpendicular of the surface of the lens at that point, shown by the dotted line *PR*; on leaving the lens obliquely at *S* it is deflected away from the perpendicular *RT*, being directed to *F* where it meets the axial ray *BF*. The ray *C* is refracted in a similar manner; it is bent upon entering the lens at *N* and rendered additionally convergent when emerging from the lens, and finally it meets the other rays at *F*. If, in this same illustration, the rays proceed from *F*, the principal focus, they emerge parallel (*LA, MB, NC*) after passing through the lens.

Conjugate foci of a convex lens. Conjugate foci are *interchangeable foci* in which the image can be replaced by the object and the object by the image. When divergent rays (*i.e.*, rays coming from a point nearer than 20 feet) proceed from a point beyond the principal focus, they will meet at a point beyond the principal focus on the other side of the lens. The more distant the luminous point, the nearer the principal focus (on the other side of the lens) will the rays be focused. If the luminous point is situated at a dis-

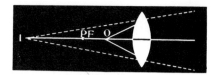

Fig. 18-17. Virtual focus of a convex lens.

tance equal to twice the focal length of the lens, the rays will focus at the same distance on the opposite side. These are conjugate foci.

In Figure 18-16, the rays diverging from *O* and passing through the lens converge at *I*; if they diverge from *I*, they would return in the same path and meet at *O*; the points *O* and *I* are conjugate foci. In the preceding example the conjugate focus is *positive or real*.

Virtual or negative focus of a convex lens. When rays diverge from some point between the lens and its principal focus (Fig. 18-17, *O*), they will continue divergent after refraction, but less so than before entering the lens; if prolonged backward they will meet at a point (*I*, Fig. 18-17) on the same side of the lens from which they diverged; this point is a *negative* or *virtual focus*.

Foci of a Concave Lens. After passing through a concave lens, rays of light, whether originally parallel or divergent, are always *divergent* and the *focus* is, therefore, always *negative* or *virtual*; it is found by continuing these divergent rays backward until they meet at a point (Fig. 18-13).

Formation of Images. The *image* of an object formed by a lens is a *collection of foci*, each corresponding to a point in

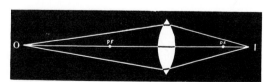

Fig. 18-16. Conjugate foci of a convex lens.

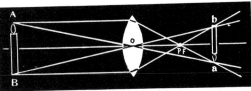

Fig. 18-18. Real, inverted and reduced image formed by a convex lens.

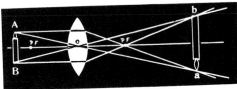

FIG. 18-19. Real, inverted and enlarged image formed by a concave lens.

the object. Such images are either *real* or *virtual*. A *real image* is formed by the *meeting of rays*; it can be projected on a screen. A *virtual image* is formed by the *prolongation backward of diverging rays* until they meet at a point; it can be seen only by looking through the lens.

To find the position and size of an image formed by a lens, it is necessary to obtain the conjugate focus of each extremity of the object: Two lines are drawn from each of these points, one parallel to the axis of the lens and then through the principal focus, and the other through the the point where these rays intersect (Figs. 18-18 to 18-20).

In Figure 18-18, *AB* is the object, *O* is the optical center of the lens and *PF* its principal focus. From *A*, two rays are drawn, one parallel to the axis of the lens and then through the principal focus *PF*, and a secondary ray through *O*; the image of the point *A* is formed at *a*, where these two lines intersect. The conjugate focus of *B* is found in the same manner.

The relation in size between image and object depends upon their respective distances from the optical center of the lens. In Figure 18-18, the object is placed at a distance greater than twice the prin-

cipal focus; hence the image is real, inverted and smaller. If the object is situated at exactly twice the distance of the principal focus, the image will be real, of the same size and inverted. If the object is situated just beyond the principal focus, the image will be real, enlarged and inverted (Fig. 18-19). If the object is placed at the principal focus, the rays will be parallel after refraction and no image will be obtained. If the object is nearer than the principal focus, the rays will be divergent after passing through the lens (Fig. 18-20), and no real image will be formed; but by projecting these rays backward they would meet, and an eye placed at *PF*, Figure 18-20, will receive the rays from *AB* as if they came from *ab*; the image will be enlarged, erect and virtual; it is on the same side of the lens as the object, and is seen only by looking through the lens, which acts as a *magnifying glass*.

Images formed by concave lenses are always virtual, erect and smaller than the object; they are seen only by looking through the lens, which acts as a *reducing glass* (Fig. 18-21).

Cylindrical Lenses. A cylindrical lens or *cylinder* is a *segment of a cylinder parallel to its axis* (Fig. 18-22). Cylinders are divided into *convex* and *concave*. Light passing through a cylinder *in the plane of its axis is not refracted* and behaves exactly as if passing through a plate of glass with parallel sides; in this direction, the surface of the lens is straight. But when light passes through in a *plane opposite* or perpendicular *to the axis* of a cylinder, the rays are rendered *convergent* or *divergent,* according to whether the cylinder is convex or concave; in this direction the surface of the lens is curved. Parallel rays of light after refraction by a cylinder are focused in a straight line which corresponds to the axis of the cylinders (Figs. 18-23 and 18-24). A spherical lens refracts equally in all planes; a cylindrical lens does not refract in the axial plane, but all other rays are refracted, those the most which pass at right angles to its axis. It is necessary to *indicate the direction of the axis of a cylinder;* in the lenses of the trial case, used for the estimation of the refraction of the eye, this is done by a short linear scratch on the lens at its margins or by having a portion of the surface on each side ground parallel to its axis.

The Numeration of Lenses. The *strength* of a lens refers to its power of bringing parallel rays to a focus, *i.e.,* its

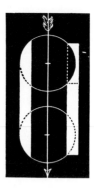

FIG. 18-22. The construction of a convex and a concave cylindrical lens from a cylinder.

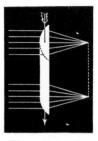

FIG. 18-23. The action of a convex cylindrical lens on parallel rays.

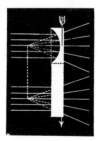

FIG. 18-24. The action of a cylindrical concave lens on parallel rays.

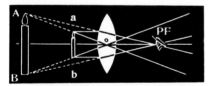

FIG. 18-20. Virtual image formed by a convex lens.

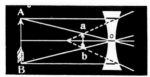

FIG. 18-21. Virtual image formed by a concave lens.

refractive power; this is indicated by its *principal focal distance,* the interval between the optical center of the lens and the principal focus. The shorter this distance, the stronger the lens; the greater the principal focal distance, the weaker

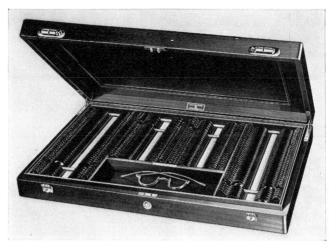

FIG. 18-25. The trial case of lenses.

the lens. *The strength of a lens is the inverse of its focal distance.*

The metric or dioptric system is used to indicate the strength or refractive power of lenses. The *unit* is a lens which has its principal focus at *1 meter* (about 40 inches); this lens is known as 1.00 *diopter* (abbreviated D.). Every lens is numbered by its strength in *whole numbers* and in *decimal fractions.* A lens which has twice the strength of the unit is known as 2.00 D.; its focal distance is 0.5 meter. If the lens has a strength four times that of the unit, it is called 4.00 D., and its focal distance is 0.25 meter. If one-quarter, one-half or three-quarters as strong as the unit, it is known as 0.25 D., 0.50 D. or 0.75 D., respectively; intermediate subdivisions (0.12 D., 0.37 D., 0.62 D., 0.87 D.) also are used. The number of the lens does not express its focal distance; but the focal distance in centimeters is obtained by dividing 100 cm. by the number of the lens; for example a 2.00 D. lens has a focal distance of 100/2 = 50 cm.

The Trial Case (Fig. 18-25) is a box containing + and − spherical, and + and − cylindrical lenses, arranged in pairs. The spherical lenses (30 pairs or more)

run from 0.12 D. to 20.00 D., the weaker ones separated by intervals of 0.12 D. or 0.25 D., those of moderate strength by 0.50 D., and the strongest ones by 1.00 D. The cylindrical lenses usually run from 0.12 D. to 6.00 D. Besides these lenses, the case contains a set of prisms, various metal disks, one of which is opaque, a pinhole disk, a stenopeic disk, red and green glass and a trial spectacle frame (Fig. 20-13).

Recognition of the Kind of Lens and Estimation of Its Strength. By moving a *spherical lens* before the eye and looking at an object, the latter will appear to move, rapidly if the lens is a strong one, slowly if a weak one. If the object seems to move in the *opposite* direction and appears *enlarged*, the lens is *convex* or +. If the object appears to move in the *same* direction and seems *smaller*, the lens is *concave* or −.

When a cylinder is rotated before the eye an object will appear to rotate in the opposite direction when the cylinder is convex, in the same direction when concave.

Having recognized the character of the lens, the *strength* can be determined by *neutralizing.* Lenses of opposite kind and

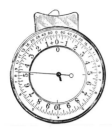

FIG. 18-26. Lens measure.

known strength are placed in front of the one to be tested, and the two lenses moved in front of the eye. The neutralizing lens is the one which *stops all apparent movement* of an object looked at, when the combined lenses are moved in front of the eye. The lens measure (Fig. 18-26) furnishes a quick method of determining the character and strength of any lens; the lensometer, electrically lighted, is a more elaborate instrument for rapidly and accurately estimating the character, strength and axis of any lens or combination of lenses.

Finding the Center of the Lens. Unless especially desired otherwise (for prismatic effect), the optical center of the lens should coincide with the geometric center. To find the optical center we look through the lens held a few inches above two lines at right angles to each other. The portion of the vertical and of the horizontal line seen through the lens is made continuous with the portion seen beyond the lens; then the two lines should cross at the geometrical center of the lens.

Varieties of Lenses Used to Correct Errors of Refraction are (1) simple spherical lens, convex (+) or concave (−), (2) simple cylindrical lens, convex or concave, (3) spherocylinder, a combination of spherical with a cylindrical lens, (4) spherical or cylindrical lens or a spherocylinder combined with a prism.

Abbreviations and Signs Used in Ophthalmology

A. or Acc.	Accommodation
Am.	Ametropia
As.	Astigmatism, astigmatic
As. H.	Hyperopic astigmatism
As. M.	Myopic astigmatism
Ax. or x.	Axis (of cylindrical lens)
B.	Base (of prism)
c.	With (cum)
C. or Cyl.	Cylindrical lens or cylinder
C.F.	Counting fingers
D.	Diopter
E.	Emmetropia or emmetropic
F.	Field of vision
H.	Hyperopia, hyperopic, horizontal
Hl.	Hyperopia latent
Hm.	Hyperopia manifest
H.M.	Hand movements
Ht.	Hyperopia total
M.	Myopia or myopic
M.A.	Meter angle
n.	Nasal
O.D. (R. or R.E.)	Oculus dexter (right eye)
O.S. (L. or L.E.)	Oculus sinister (left eye)
O.U.	Oculus uterque (both eyes)
Oph.	Ophthalmoscope or ophthalmoscopic
P.D.	Interpupillary distance
P.L.	Perception of light
p.p.	Punctum proximum (near point)
p.r.	Punctum remotum (far point)
Pr.	Presbyopia
s.	Without (sine)
S. or Sph.	Spherical lens
t.	Temporal
T.	Tension
V.	Vertical
V.A.	Visual acuity
w.	With
+	Plus or convex
−	Minus or concave
=	Equal to
◯	Combined with
∞	Infinity (20 feet or more distance)
′	Foot, minute
″	Inch, second
‴	Line
°	Degree (prism)
▽	Centrad (prism)
△	Prism diopter

19

Optical Consideration of the Eye

The eye may be considered as an optical instrument, often compared to the photographic camera, in which by means of a refracting (dioptric) system a *small and inverted image* of external objects is formed *on the retina*. It is well adapted for its function of refraction; the outermost portion of the retina consists of a layer of pigment cells which absorbs the excess of light and prevents dazzling. The impression received by the rods and cones is conveyed through the optic nerve to the cortical area where the visual act is completed and results in the sense of sight.

Dioptric Apparatus of the Eye. In passing through the eyeball, rays of light transverse the cornea, aqueous humor, lens and vitreous humor. The *refracting surfaces* of the eye are the cornea, the anterior surface and the posterior surface of the lens; the *refracting media* are the aqueous humor, the substance of the lens and the vitreous humor. These surfaces and media constitute the *dioptric or refractive apparatus of the eye*, a system which is represented by a convex lens of 23-mm. focus; hence in an emmetropic eye, in a condition of rest, parallel rays are brought to a focus on the retina. The greatest deflection of rays takes place at the anterior surface of the cornea; additional deviations occur at the anterior and posterior surfaces of the lens. In each case the effect is one of *convergence. Refraction of the eye* signifies changes which the ocular media exert upon rays of light when the eye is in a *state of rest*.

Cardinal Points of the Eye. It is necessary to know the cardinal points of the eye (Fig. 19-1) in order to understand the course of rays of light through this organ; they are the two principal points, the two nodal points and the two principal foci, all situated on the optical axis.

The principal points (*P*, Fig. 19-1) are two points so related that when an incident ray passes through the first principal point, the corresponding emergent ray passes through the second principal point. These two points are placed so close together in the anterior chamber that they may be considered as one point, situated about 2 mm. behind the cornea.

The nodal points (*N*, Fig. 19-1) correspond practically to the optical center of the dioptric system. They are so close together that they may be considered as one point situated near the posterior pole of the lens about 7 mm. behind the cornea. Rays passing through this point are not refracted and form either the axial or secondary rays.

The first principal focus (*A*, Fig. 19-1) is that point on the axis at which parallel rays in the vitreous meet; it is situated about 14 mm. in front of the cornea.

The second principal focus (*F*, Fig. 19-1) is that point on the axis at which parallel rays meet after being refracted by the dioptric system of the eye; it is situated to the inner side of the macula, between it and the optic disk, about 23 mm. behind the cornea.

The center of rotation of the eyeball (*R*, Fig. 19-1) is situated in the vitreous, about 10 mm. in front of the retina.

The optical axis (*AF*, Fig. 19-1) is

the line connecting the center of the cornea, the nodal point and the posterior principal focus.

The visual line (*OM*, Fig. 19-1) is the line passing from the object looked at, through the nodal point, to the macula.

The line of fixation is the line joining the object looked at with the center of rotation; practically it corresponds to the visual line.

The angle gamma (γ, Fig. 19-1) is the angle formed by the optical axis with the line of fixation (practically with the visual line); it varies with the refraction of the eye, being about 5° in emmetropia, larger in hyperopia and smaller in myopia.

The angle alpha is the angle formed by the visual line with the major axis of the corneal ellipse.

Refraction of the Eye

Emmetropia. When parallel rays are focused exactly on the retina with the eye in a condition of rest, the refraction of the eye is normal or *emmetropic* (Fig. 19-2, *top*) and the condition is known as emmetropia.

Ametropia. The eye, at rest, is ametropic when parallel rays are *not focused on the retina*. The focal point may be behind or in front of it. The condition is known as ametropia. The forms of ame-

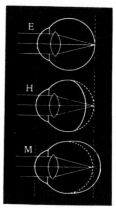

FIG. 19-2. *Top*, emmetropia; *center*, hyperopia; *bottom*, myopia.

tropia (*errors of refraction*) are hyperopia, myopia and astigmatism.

Hyperopia is that form of ametropia in which the axis of the eyeball is too short or the refractive power of the eye too weak, so that *parallel rays* are brought to a *focus behind the retina* (Fig. 19-2, *center*).

Myopia is that form of ametropia in which the axis of the eyeball is too long or the refractive power too strong, so that *parallel rays* are *focused in front of the retina* (Fig. 19-2, *bottom*).

Astigmatism is that form of ametropia in which the *refraction of the several meridians* of the eyeball is *different* (Figs. 20-6 to 20-9).

Accommodation

Accommodation is the *power of altering the focus of the eye* so that divergent rays (those coming from an object nearer than 20 feet) are brought together on the retina; this is accomplished by means of an *increase in the convexity of the lens* and thus in its refractive power. The degree of accommodation must *vary for every distance* of the object; the eye cannot be adapted for two different distances at the same time.

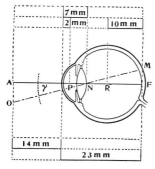

FIG. 19-1. Cardinal points of the eye.

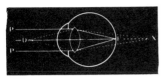

FIG. 19-3. The emmetropic eye in a state of rest.

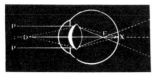

FIG. 19-4. The emmetropic eye during accommodation.

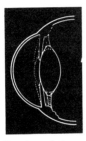

FIG. 19-5. Section of the anterior portion of the eyeball. The *dotted lines* illustrate the changes during accommodation.

In the emmetropic eye *at rest, parallel* rays are brought to a focus on the *retina* (*PF,* Fig. 19-3), but rays coming from a near object (*divergent* rays) are focused *behind* the retina (*DX,* Fig. 19-3); hence distant objects appear distinct and near objects blurred. If the refractive power of the eye is increased by *accommodation, parallel* rays will be brought to a focus in *front* of the *retina* (*PF,* Fig. 19-4), while *divergent* rays will be focused *on the retina* (*DX,* Fig. 19-4); consequently near objects appear distinct and distant objects appear blurred during accommodation.

Mechanism of Accommodation. The *lens* is an elastic structure and, when released from the flattening influence of its suspensory ligament, tends to assume a spherical shape. During accommodation, the *ciliary muscle* (especially the circular fibers) *contracts,* drawing forward the choroid and *relaxing the suspensory ligament;* this diminishes the tension of the lens capsule and allows the inherent elasticity of the lens to *increase its convexity.* The change in curvature affects chiefly the anterior surface of the lens (Fig. 19-5). This is *Helmholtz's theory* and the one usually accepted. Tscherning has advanced a different theory: He maintains that the ciliary muscle increases the tension of the suspensory ligament during contraction, and that this causes peripheral flattening of the lens with bulging anteriorly at its center.

The act of accommodation is accompanied by *contraction of the pupil* and by *convergence* of the visual lines.

The Far Point. When the eye is in a state of rest, with accommodation completely relaxed, it is adapted for its far point (*punctum remotum*). This is the *farthest* point of *distinct* vision, and in the emmetropic eye it is situated at *infinity.*

The Near Point (*punctum proximum*) is the *nearest* point at which the eye can see *distinctly* when employing its maximum amount of accommodation. It *varies* with the amount of accommodation possessed by the eye. The usual plan of determining the near point is to find the shortest distance at which the patient can read the smallest test type (Jaeger, *No. 1,* Fig. 3-4) with each eye separately.

The Range of Accommodation is the *distance* between the far point and the near point.

The Amplitude of Accommodation is the *difference* between the refractive power of the eye when at *rest* and when the *accommodation* is exerted to the utmost. It is *expressed in diopters* representing that convex lens which it would be necessary to place before the eye to take the place of accommodation for the near point.

The amplitude of accommodation in diopters is found by dividing 40 by the distance of the near point in inches, or 100 by the near point in centimeters; for example, if the near point of an emmetropic eye is 8 inches or 20 cm., 40/8 or 100/20 = 5.00 D. = amplitude of accommodation; this rule applies to *emmetropia*.

In *hyperopia* some of the accommodation is required for distant vision; hence we find the apparent amplitude of accommodation and then add that lens which enables the patient to see distant objects without his accommodation; for example, if the near point of a hyperopic eye is 8 inches or 20 cm., and the patient is compelled to use 2.00 D. of accommodation for distant objects, his amplitude of accommodation would be 40/8 (or 100/20) = 5 + 2 = 7.00 D. With the same amplitude of accommodation the near point is farther away than in emmetropia, since some of the power of accommodation is expended in adapting the eye for distant objects; and if the near point were the same, the amplitude of accommodation would be greater in hyperopia than in emmetropia.

In *myopia*, since a concave lens is necessary to enable the patient to see distant objects clearly, we must deduct the strength of this glass from that glass the focal length of which equals the distance of the near point from the eye; for example, if the myopia equals 2.00 D. and the near point is 4 inches or 10 cm., the amplitude of accommodation will be 40/4 or 100/10 = 10.00 D. − 2.00 D. = 8.00 D. With the same amplitude of accommodation, the near point is closer to the eye in myopia than in emmetropia; and if the near point were the same, the amplitude of accommodation would be less in myopia than in emmetropia.

The power of accommodation gradually

TABLE 19-1

Amplitude of Accommodation and Near Point at Various Periods of Life

Year	Amplitude of Accommodation (D.)	Near Point	
		Centimeters	Inches
10	14.0	7.0	2.8
15	12.0	8.5	3.3
20	10.0	10.0	4.0
25	8.5	12.0	4.7
30	7.0	14.0	5.6
35	5.5	18.0	7.0
40	4.5	22.0	9.0
45	3.5	28.0	11
50	2.5	40.0	16
55	1.75	55.0	22
60	1.0	100	40
65	0.75	133	53
70	0.25	400	160
75	0.0	∞	∞

diminishes and the near point recedes as age advances, owing chiefly to loss of elasticity of the lens. In the emmetrope at 10 years, the p.p. is at 7 cm.; at 40 years it has receded to 22 cm.; at 60 years to 100 cm., and at 75 years to infinity, the accommodation being suspended and the p.p. coinciding with the p.r. Table 19-1 gives the amplitude of accommodation and the near point at various periods of life. The near point applies only to emmetropic eyes, but the amplitude of accommodation applies to all eyes, whether emmetropic or ametropic. There is a tendency toward increased amplitude of accommodation in hyperopia, and diminished amplitude in uncorrected myopia.

Presbyopia. When the near point of the emmetropic eye has receded to a distance at which the finer kinds of work become difficult, the condition is known as presbyopia (Chap. 20). This state is the result of a *physiologic process* which affects *every eye* and must not be considered

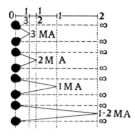

FIG. 19-6. Diagram illustrating the unit of convergence, the meter angle.

a disease. It usually is said to be present when the near point recedes to a distance of more than 22 cm. (9 inches) from the eye, an event which generally happens *between the 43rd and 45th years.*

The Association between Accommodation and Convergence. The preceding considerations of the subject of accommodation referred to monocular vision or sight with one eye. With *binocular vision* it is necessary to consider *convergence* as well as accommodation, for these two actions (together with the contraction of the pupil) normally are *associated.*

Convergence is the power of directing the visual lines of the two eyes to a near point, and results from the action of the medial rectus muscles. When we look at a distant object, accommodation is at rest and the visual lines are parallel. When we look at a near object, we are compelled both to accommodate and to converge for that distance; a certain amount of accommodation is *associated with* a corresponding effort of convergence of the visual lines.

The *angle* which the two visual axes form with the median line in looking at a near object is called the *angle of convergence.* The unit of convergence is the *meter angle* (M.A.), which is the angle formed by the visual line with the median line at a distance of 1 meter (Fig. 19-6). If the eyes look at an object ½ meter distant, the convergence is twice that of the unit, and convergence $c = 2$ M.A.; if directed toward a point ⅓ meter distant, $c = 3$ M.A.; if toward an object 2 meters distant, $c = ½$ M.A.

The *emmetropic* eye requires, for each distance of binocular vision, as many *meter angles* of convergence as it needs *diopters of accommodation.* To see an object at 1 meter distance, 1 meter angle of convergence is required and also 1 diopter of accommodation; at 10 cm., 10 meter angles of convergence and 10.00 D. of accommodation would be required.

This harmonious relationship between accommodation and convergence is not, however, unchangeable. Within certain limits either of these actions may take place independently of the other.

The Range or Amplitude of Convergence. The *far point of convergence* is the point to which the visual lines are directed when convergence is at rest; the *near point of convergence* is the point to which the visual lines are directed with the maximum amount of convergence. The distance between the far point and the near point of convergence is the *amplitude of convergence;* it is expressed by the greatest number of meter angles of convergence of which the eyes are capable. In a state of rest the far point of convergence is at infinity and the visual lines are either parallel or, more commonly, somewhat divergent, in which case convergence is spoken of as *negative.* In cases of convergent squint, the visual lines deviate inward even when convergence is relaxed; convergence then is said to be *positive.* In a case of divergent squint convergence is a negative quantity. Normally, the eyes diverge during sleep.

20

Errors of Refraction

In *emmetropia* (E.) the eye in a state of rest, without accommodation, focuses the image of distant objects exactly upon the retina (Fig. 19-2, *top*); such an eye enjoys distinct vision for distant objects without effort or fatigue. Any variation from this standard constitutes *ametropia*, a condition in which the eye, in a state of rest, is unable to focus the image of distant objects (parallel rays) upon the retina. Ametropia includes *hyperopia, myopia, astigmatism* and *presbyopia*. The effects of ametropia are not only *indistinctness* of vision but various pains and other symptoms comprised under the term *asthenopia* (weak sight, eye strain). *Presbyopia* is a *physiologic* change which affects every eye, commencing between the 42nd and 45th years, caused by a gradual lessening of *accommodation*.

Hyperopia

Hyperopia (*hypermetropia, farsightedness,* H.) is an error of refraction in which, with accommodation completely relaxed, *parallel rays* (rays from distant objects) are brought to a *focus behind the retina* (Figs. 19-2, *center,* and 20-1, *top*); divergent rays (from near objects) are focused still farther back.

Etiology. It is due most commonly to *shortening* of the anteroposterior diameter of the eyeball (*axial H.*), less frequently to diminished convexity of the refracting surfaces of the eye (*H. of curvature*), changes in the media or absence of the lens (*aphakia*). It is by far the *most frequent* error of refraction and is *congenital;* in a certain sense it may be considered to be due to imperfect development of the eye. It is often *hereditary*. Children usually are hyperopic at birth and subsequently become less hyperopic, emmetropic or even myopic.

The Course of Rays. The hyperopic eye cannot, without accommodation, see either distant or near objects distinctly (Fig. 20-1, *top*). To focus parallel rays on the retina either it must *accommodate, i.e.,* increase the convexity of its lens as shown in Figure 20-1, *center,* or a *convex lens* of sufficient strength to focus rays on the retina must be placed before the eye (Fig. 20-1, *bottom*).

To focus divergent rays, *i.e.,* rays from *near* objects, the hyperope must *accommodate* not only the amount required of an emmetropic eye (Fig. 20-2, *top*) but an *additional amount* to compensate for his error. In other words, the hyperope requires some accommodation constantly in order to see distant objects distinctly, and in addition the amount equal to that required by the emmetrope for near vision (Fig. 20-2, *bottom*). Such an eye (when the error is uncorrected) is *never in a condition of rest* as long as it enjoys distinct vision.

Changes in the Eye. As a result of the constant overaction of the *ciliary muscle,* the latter becomes *hypertrophied,* especially its circular fibers (Fig. 20-3, *center*); it remains in a greater or lesser condition of spasm. In high degrees of H. the eyeball may be diminished in size, the anterior chamber shallow, the sclera flat with a sharp curve at the equator, and there may be an apparent divergent squint, owing to the high angle gamma.

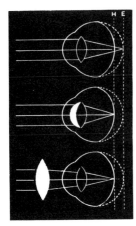

FIG. 20-1. The hyperopic eye: *top*, in a state of rest; *center*, during accommodation; *bottom*, corrected by a convex lens.

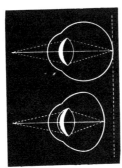

FIG. 20-2. Accommodation for near vision: *top*, in the emmetropic eye; *bottom*, in the hyperopic eye.

Varieties. Hyperopia is divided into (1) manifest, (2) latent and (3) total.

(1) The *manifest* hyperopia (Hm.) is that which is detected *without paralyzing accommodation* and is represented by the strongest convex glass with which the patient sees most distinctly; it corresponds to the amount of accommodation which he relaxes when a convex lens is placed before the eye. Manifest hyperopia may be either *facultative*, when it can be overcome by an effort of accommodation, or

absolute, when it cannot be overcome in this manner.

(2) The *total* hyperopia (Ht.) is the *entire* amount of hyperopia detected after the *accommodation* has been *paralyzed* or during complete relaxation of the ciliary muscle.

(3) The *latent* hyperopia (Hl.) is the difference between the Hm. and the Ht., and is the amount which is *habitually concealed* and is discovered only after the use of a cycloplegic.

The application of these terms can be illustrated by considering an example of H. of 2.5 D. in a young person. If in such a case V.A. = 20/40, and, without the use of a cycloplegic, a + 1.00 D. spherical lens brings the acuity to 20/20, we say Hm. = 1.00 D.; if now we paralyze the accommodation with a cycloplegic and find V.A. = 20/100, and that a + 2.50 D. spherical lens increases this to 20/20, the Ht. = 2.50 D.; the difference between 2.50 D. and 1.00 D. = 1.50 D. = Hl.

The *ratio* between the manifest and the latent hyperopia is not constant; it depends more or less upon the age and vigor of the individual. In *youth*, the amount of Hl. is apt to be considerable, and consequently a cycloplegic is essential in estimating the amount of hyperopia. The *older* a person grows, the less accommodative effort he is able to make; hence the Hl. becomes less, and the Hm. greater. In *old* persons there is no Hl., the total hyperopia becoming manifest.

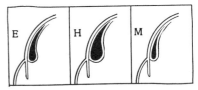

FIG. 20-3. Section of the ciliray muscle: *left*, in an emmetropic eye (*E*); center, in a hyperopic eye (*H*); right, in a myopic eye (*M*).

Symptoms. Unless the error is considerable or the patient advanced in years, there usually is *good vision for distance*. A great many patients with hyperopia present *no symptoms* whatever; this is apt to be the case when the hyperope is young and in good health. In other cases, the accommodative effort will be unequal to the task imposed in near work, and as a result the hyperopia will give rise to *accommodative asthenopia* (eye strain).

The *symptoms of asthenopia* show themselves particularly after reading, writing, sewing and other forms of *near* application, especially in the evening and with artificial illumination. They comprise *pain* referred to the eyes or above the eyes; *headaches*, usually frontal, but also occurring in the occiput and other parts of the cranium; various neuralgias; *congestion* of the conjunctiva and margins of the lids; lacrimation, blinking and slight photophobia; *burning* sensation and heavy, *sleepy* feeling referred to the lids, and *blurring* of near vision. These symptoms are worse whenever the general health is unsatisfactory.

With advancing years, there will be greater difficulty in reading without correcting glasses.

In *early childhood*, hyperopia often favors *convergent squint* in a patient whose fusion sense is deficient.

In *children*, H. shows a physiologic tendency to *diminish* with growth; they may become emmetropic. In the adult it remains stationary; after 50 there is a tendency to a slight increase.

Hyperopic eyes are *predisposed* to convergent squint and glaucoma.

Occasionally hyperopia in children and in young adults is accompanied by *spasm of accommodation*, which not only neutralizes the latent hyperopia but may produce apparent myopia. This condition may result from excessive close work, especially with poor illumination. The diagnosis is made after instilling a cycloplegic; homatropine may be insufficient and atropine may be necessary for this purpose. Treatment calls for the use of a cycloplegic for a few days, thus preventing near use, and the correction of any existing ametropia.

Diagnosis. The tests for hyperopia are given in the division on technique in determining the state of refraction.

Treatment consists in prescribing such *convex spherical lenses* as will make *vision distinct* and enable the patient to do near work *without fatigue*. The mere existence of hyperopia is no indication for the use of correcting glasses unless these are worn in childhood for the cure of convergent squint. It is only when there is a diminution in the acuteness of vision or when symptoms arise indicating eye strain that convex lenses should be used.

Though theoretically it would seem proper to prescribe the full correction (for Ht.), practically there are many objections and exceptions to this. When both the manifest and the total hyperopia have been estimated, the *symptoms* of the individual will give reliable indications as to the *proportion* of the Ht. which ought to be corrected, and the *constancy* with which the glasses should be worn. In cases of squint, and when glasses are prescribed for the relief of headaches which are continuous, or which occur independently of near use of the eyes, they must be worn constantly. In other cases, glasses should be worn either continuously or only for near, according to whether the symptoms are always present or follow only after using the eyes for reading and the like. When distant vision is perfect and comfortable, and when the patient does not suffer from any symptoms except when engaged in near work, glasses need be prescribed only for such use; this is often the case in young adults who enjoy good health. Under such circumstances, the cor-

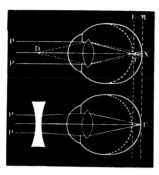

Fig. 20-4. *Top*, the focusing of parallel and divergent rays in myopia; *bottom*, the correction of myopia by means of a concave lens.

rection of the Hm. may be sufficient; or the Hm. and a part of Hl. may be needed; occasionally full correction of Ht. is required. In cases in which the correction is only partial, the glasses may require changing from time to time. In hyperopes after 45, convex lenses should be worn to improve distant vision, and a stronger pair for near; the weaker set is for the H., the stronger pair to correct both the hyperopia and the presbyopia. Under such circumstances, *bifocal lenses* (Figs. 20-22, and 20-23) are very convenient, the upper segment corresponding to the weaker glass, the lower to the stronger.

Myopia

Myopia (*nearsightedness, shortsightedness*, M.) is that refractive condition in which, with accommodation completely relaxed, *parallel rays* are brought to a *focus in front of the retina*. These rays cross in the vitreous; when they reach the retina they have become divergent, forming a circle of diffusion and consequently a blurred image (Fig. 20-4 (*top*), *PPF*). Certain divergent rays, coming from the myopic far point, are focused on the retina (Fig. 20-4 (*top*), *DX*) without accommodation.

The greatest distance at which the pa-

tient can read fine print is the *far point*. This is always at a definite distance *corresponding to the amount of M.*; the higher the M., the closer to the eye is the far point; the distance of the latter is the *measure of the M.* For example, if the far point is at 20 inches (0.5 meter) the M. = 2.00 D. (40/20 or 100/50) = 2; if at 10 inches (0.25 meter), the M. = 4.00 D. In these two instances concave lenses of 2.00 and 4.00 D., respectively, would render parallel rays as divergent as if they came from a distance of 20 and 10 inches (0.5 and 0.25 meter), respectively; and with these lenses, the myope would be able to see distant objects distinctly (Fig. 20-4, *bottom*).

Etiology. Myopia almost always depends upon a *lengthening* of the anteroposterior diameter of the eyeball (*axial myopia*); in M. of 3.00 D., for example, the eyeball measures 24 mm. in its anteroposterior diameter, and in M. of 10.00 D., 27 mm. from before backward, instead of 23 mm., the normal diameter. Much less frequently M. is due to an increase in the refraction of the lens from swelling in incipient cataract, to spasm of accommodation or to increased curvature of the cornea (anterior staphyloma and keratoconus).

Myopia rarely is congenital; there is, however, a *strong hereditary tendency*. It commences at an *early* age and often *progresses*, and is definitely related to a *developmental* factor. There is evidence of a constitutional factor, and endocrine disturbances and various dietary deficiencies are said to play a role. Myopia is a frequent result of prematurity.

The *cause of the lengthening of the eyeball* is attributed (1) to pressure of the extraocular muscles during excessive convergence, causing the posterior pole, which is the least resistant part of the eyeball, to bulge; (2) to congestion, inflammation and softening of the layers of the eyeball, together with increased tension, produced by fullness of the veins of the head as a result of stooping postures and other predisposing causes, and (3) to the shape of the orbit in broad faces, causing excessive convergence.

Clinical Forms. In many instances, myopia of moderate degree develops during youth, and comes to a standstill or increases very little at or soon after puberty, or there is a very limited increase up to the 20th year; this is known as *stationary* or *simple myopia*.

In other cases, the error reaches a considerable height in youth, and *increases* steadily up to the 25th year or even later, resulting in a *high degree* of myopia; this is known as *progressive myopia*. These are the cases which may be accompanied by destructive *changes* in the choroid and other parts of the eye, leading to considerable impairment of vision, and in which myopia may properly be considered *a disease*. Extreme cases of progressive myopia are known as *malignant myopia*.

Thus myopia may be divided into primary or *physiologic* myopia (a biologic variation of refraction) and *secondary* myopia (the result of disease of the coats of the eye).

Symptoms. Many myopes present no symptoms except *indistinct vision for distance*. Near work can be accomplished with comfort; since the myope requires less accommodation than the emmetrope, he often has an advantage in close application. It is on this account that the circular fibers of the ciliary muscle are less developed than in the emmetropic eye (Fig. 20-3, *right*).

In other cases of myopia, especially if astigmatism also is present, not only is there great reduction of vision for distance, but there may be discomfort upon near use and inability to continue at work for any length of time on account of excessive convergence; such eyes may *tire*

easily, and become sensitive to light; often *black spots* before the eyes are complained of, and sometimes bright flashes of light.

In *high myopia*, there often are prominence of the eyes, deep anterior chambers and dilated pupils; the patient is apt to screw the eyelids together since this adds somewhat to his acuteness of vision. The strain of excessive convergence is so great and painful in some cases that the effort is given up and divergent squint results.

Ophthalmoscopic Signs. In myopia the disk appears large. In *low* (less than 3.00 D.) or *moderate* (3.00 to 6.00 D.) degrees, there frequently are no changes; in other cases often there is found a crescent-shaped patch of atrophy of the choroid of whitish or grayish color, embracing the outer side of the disk; this is called a *myopic crescent* (Plate 18B); more or less superficial atrophy of the choroid is often seen, allowing the larger choroidal vessels to become plainly visible.

In *high myopia* (more than 6.00 D.), a well-defined *crescent* is usually found; there will be *posterior staphyloma* (bulging of the sclera), and there may be patches of *choroidal atrophy* with pigmented margins, exposing the sclera. In *progressive cases*, frequently there are added to these lesions atrophic and pigment changes in the *macular region* (Plate 18B), *hemorrhages*, especially at the macula, *fluid vitreous* (sometimes causing tremulous iris) and *opacities of the vitreous* and the posterior pole of the lens. There is a predisposition to detachment of the retina. Thus *vision* often is *reduced* in progressive myopia.

Diagnosis. The tests for myopia are given in the division on technique in determining the state of refraction.

Prognosis. In low and moderate degrees of *stationary myopia*, the prognosis is *good* when suitable glasses are worn and hygienic directions (described under treatment) are followed. *Progressive myopia* always is a *serious* condition especially when the choroidal and vitreous changes are severe, sometimes requiring cessation of all near work. In *malignant myopia* the prognosis is poor.

Treatment consists in prescribing suitable *glasses*, avoiding excessive near work and attempting to *prevent the progress* of the disease as indicated below.

In general terms, it is proper to give a *full correction for low and moderate myopia in young persons*, to be worn for *both distance and near*; this places the eyes under normal conditions of vision and accommodation. Full correction corresponds to the *weakest* concave spherical lens which, with accommodation paralyzed, gives the best vision. In low degrees of M. an adult may be allowed to read without glasses if he finds this convenient.

In *high myopia*, a slight reduction from full correction is prescribed for distance, and about two-thirds correction for near work; the reading glasses should be such as to enable the patient to read at a comfortable distance.

After the age of 45, while no change is necessary in the distance glasses, those used for close work must be reduced by an amount equal to the presbyopic correction, and often even more.

In prescribing glasses in M. every case must be considered on its merits. Many myopes wear strong lenses, representing the full correction, constantly and with absolute comfort; others require two sets of lenses, one for distance and a weaker pair for reading.

In order to check any tendency to increase of M., *rigid hygienic rules*, both local and general, should be obeyed. These are of special importance in the young. The patient's *habits* should be *regulated* to insure good health. He should have an abundance of *outdoor exercise* and plenty of *sleep*.

Near work should be restricted and the patient not be allowed to read too long at a time. The book should be held no closer than 13 inches (33 cm.). In most cases the *full correcting lenses* should be worn for near work. The *illumination* should be good, and should come *from behind or above*, never from a source directly in front so as to shine into the eyes; the myope should avoid reading at dusk or with feeble illumination. The *print* should be large and clear, with ample spacing. *Desks* should be constructed so that the sitting posture is comfortable, and so that the child is not encouraged to stoop over his books; the myope must be taught not to bend over his work, but to lift the latter to the required distance from the eyes.

Even in patients exhibiting a continuous increase in the myopia and the development of pathologic changes in the backgrounds of the eyes, there is little evidence that complete abstinence from close work has any value. There seems to be no valid reason to take the myopic child out of school.

Keeping in mind the predisposition to retinal detachment, it is important to caution myopes against taking the risks involved in falls or injury incident to violent sports, such as football, boxing, etc.

The *operation* of removal of the lens in young adults with uncomplicated myopia of 15.00 D. or more is performed occasionally. After a successful extraction, the aphakic eye will have gained a decided advantage by becoming almost emmetropic. The operation is not used often, since it is considered too hazardous.

Telescopic spectacles occasionally are prescribed for improving vision of myopes of very high degree and of others with very poor vision which cannot be improved with glasses. They act like opera glasses, improving vision by magnifying about 2 diameters. But very few individuals can be aided with these. Such spectacles limit the field of vision and cause distortion and apparent movement of objects upon rotating the head, besides being heavy, clumsy and expensive. Separate combinations are required for distance and for near vision.

Astigmatism

Astigmatism (astigmia; As.) is that refractive condition of the eye in which there is a *difference in degree of refraction in different meridians*, so that each will focus parallel rays at a different point (Figs. 20-6 to 20-11).

In E., H. and M., rays coming from a luminous point are brought to a single focus at a certain distance behind the cornea. In astigmatism, since the refractive surfaces are not spherical, rays from a luminous point are brought to a focus at different points; the shape of the image may be a line, an oval, or a circle, but never a point.

Astigmatism may be (1) *regular*, which is very common, or (2) *irregular*, comparatively infrequent.

Regular astigmatism is that form in which, though the refraction in a meridian is the same throughout, there is a *difference in the degree of refraction in every meridian*; the curvature of the cornea is different in different meridians. One meridian exhibits the *maximum* and the other the *minimum* refraction; these are called the *principal meridians* and are *always at right angles* to each other. The refractive power of all other planes will be regularly intermediate according to their position with regard to the principal meridians.

Irregular astigmatism, on the other hand, is that variety in which there is a difference in refraction not only in different meridians, but also in *different parts of the same meridian.*

When the term astigmatism is used without qualification, it refers to regular astigmatism.

Etiology. Astigmatism usually is due to a change in the *curvature of the cornea*, with or without some shortening or lengthening of the anteroposterior diameter of the eyeball. It also is caused, in part at least, by defects in the curvature of the lens; this *lenticular* astigmatism may partly neutralize that of the cornea. Astigmatism usually is *congenital* and there often is an hereditary tendency; it may, however, be *acquired*, and then is caused by corneal changes from inflammation, injury or operation.

Even the normal eye has a slight amount of regular astigmatism, because of the fact that the cornea is the segment, not of a sphere, but of an ellipsoid; consequently there is a slight difference in the refraction of the two principal meridians, the curvature of the vertical meridian being greater than that of the horizontal; hence the focus of the former is somewhat shorter than that of the latter.

Refraction of Rays in Regular Astigmatism. Parallel rays refracted by a spherical surface form a circular cone and focus at a point. In astigmatism, those rays which pass through the meridian of greater curvature come to a focus sooner than those which pass through the meridian of lesser curvature; the resulting cone will not be circular, but more or less oval; hence the vision of astigmatic subjects is not simply indistinct, but the diffusion images are more or less elongated.

Straight lines (which are made up of a succession of points) appear distinct or indistinct to astigmatic persons according to their direction. If the vertical meridian of an astigmatic eye is out of focus and the horizontal normal, a vertical line will be slightly elongated; but the sides will be distinct since each point of light will be seen as a small vertical line, and these overlap. But if such an eye looks at a horizontal line, each point of light will again be seen as a small vertical line, and consequently the line will appear blurred (Fig.

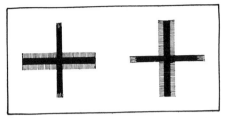

FIG. 20-5. Vertical and horizontal lines as seen by an astigmatic eye: *left,* in which the horizontal meridian is emmetropic; *right,* in which the vertical meridian is emmetropic.

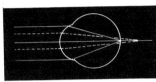

FIG. 20-6. Simple hyperopic astigmatism.

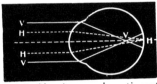

FIG. 20-7. Simple myopic astigmatism.

20-5). There is, therefore, one direction in which straight lines appear most distinct, and another at right angles to it, in which they appear most indistinct; this forms the basis for the construction of the astigmatic dial or fan (Fig. 20-11) commonly used as a test for this error. *The lines parallel with the ametropic meridian are seen most clearly and those parallel with the emmetropic meridian are seen most indistinctly* (in simple As.).

Varieties of Regular Astigmatism. According to the refraction of the principal meridians, astigmatism is divided into:

(1) Simple, in which one meridian is emmetropic and the other hyperopic or myopic; it comprises simple hyperopic astigmatism (As. H., Fig. 20-6) and simple myopic astigmatism (As. M., Fig. 20-7).

(2) Compound, in which both meridians are either hyperopic or myopic, but unequal in degree; it comprises compound hyperopic astigmatism (H. + As. H., Fig. 20-8) and compound myopic astigmatism (M. + As. M., Fig. 20-9).

(3) Mixed, in which one meridian is hyperopic and the other myopic (As. H. + As. M., Fig. 20-10).

In most cases of astigmatism, the cornea presents its *maximum curvature* in or near the *vertical meridian* and the least curvature in or near the horizontal meridian, corresponding to the slight astigmatism of the normal eye; when this is the case, it is said to be *astigmatism with the rule;* when the relative curvatures are reversed, it is *astigmatism against the rule.* In astigmatism with the rule the axis of the cylinder is vertical or nearly so in hyperopic astigmatism, and horizontal or nearly so in myopic astigmatism. The chief meridians, though *vertical* and *horizontal* in the majority of cases, may oc-

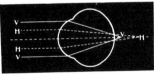

FIG. 20-8. Compound hyperopic astigmatism.

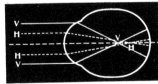

FIG. 20-9. Compound myopic astigmatism.

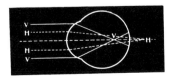

FIG. 20-10. Mixed astigmatism.

cupy an *oblique* position; in such cases they are most frequently *symmetrical, i.e.,* inclined an equal number of degrees from the vertical or horizontal on each side; but this is not always the case.

Symptoms. With small amounts of astigmatism there may be no reduction in sight; but with greater degrees there always is a *diminution in the acuteness of vision,* both distant and near, varying with the degree and variety of astigmatism. There commonly is considerable *asthenopia,* especially upon use of the eyes for near work, but also present with distant vision, such as at theater and movies, during which performances the individual makes an instinctive effort of accommodation in order to neutralize or reduce the effects of his astigmatism. These asthenopic symptoms are similar to those occurring in hyperopia, but are apt to be more severe and continuous. They vary with the degree and variety of astigmatism, the amount of near work indulged in and especially the state of the patient's health; a small amount (0.50 D. or even 0.25 D.) will, for instance, often give rise to severe asthenopic and nervous symptoms in a young, delicate, neurasthenic individual. The involuntary accommodative efforts of the ciliary muscle, instinctively made to diminish the effects of the error, cause continuous *eye strain* and explain the frequency of asthenopia. While there is no fixed rule, a low degree of astigmatism may cause more asthenopia than a high degree; in the latter case, the patient accepts a constant reduction in vision, since he cannot overcome this by any straining effort.

Diagnosis. Astigmatism should be suspected when vision cannot be brought up to 20/20 with spherical lenses, notwithstanding a normal fundus and clear media. In testing for astigmatism in children and in young adults, sometimes even in adults of 40 and occasionally after this age, it is

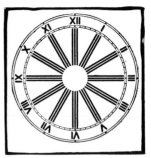

FIG. 20-11. Astigmatic dial.

necessary to have the eye under the influence of a *cycloplegic;* otherwise the results are apt to be unsatisfactory.

The astigmatic dial. The diagnosis of astigmatism is made if the patient, when placed before the astigmatic dial or fan, formed of radiating lines numbered like the face of a clock, (Fig. 20-11), is unable to see all the lines with equal distinctness. The line seen most distinctly and the line seen least distinctly indicate the axes of the two principal meridians; the axis of the former corresponds to the ametropic meridian, that of the latter to the emmetropic meridian (in simple astigmatism).

Suppose, in an example of simple astigmatism, that the patient sees lines XII and VI most distinctly and those at right angles, IX and III, least clearly; then the ametropic meridian is vertical. If a weak convex lens placed in front of the eye makes lines XII and VI indistinct, we know that the horizontal meridian is emmetropic. Next we find which spherical lens clears up lines IX and III; this glass is the measure of the refractive error of the vertical (ametropic) meridian.

The metal disk with stenopeic slit (about 1 mm. in diameter) is another method of discovering the *two principal meridians* (and the amount of astigmatism). It is placed in front of one eye, the other being excluded, and is rotated slowly so that the slit occupies each meridian successively. The patient is placed at 20 feet before the distant test types and the position of the slit in which the best acuity is obtained is noted. Then convex or concave lenses are placed in front of the slit, and the strongest convex or the weakest concave lens which gives the most improvement is the measure of the refraction in this meridian. The slit then is turned 90° and convex and concave lenses again applied until one is found which produces most improvement. In this way the refractive error of the two principal meridians is determined. If, for instance, with slit vertical, the patient reads 20/20, and convex lenses in front of the slit make the types indistinct, the vertical meridian is emmetropic; if, when the slit is horizontal, the patient reads 20/50, but this increases to 20/20 when + 3.00 D. Sph. is placed in front, the horizontal meridian is hyperopic 3.00 D.; this case would be one of simple hyperopic astigmatism corrected by a + 3.00 D. cylinder, axis vertical.

Other means of determining the existence and the amount of astigmatism comprise the subjective method with *test types and lenses, astigmatic dial, cross cylinder, retinoscopy* and the *ophthalmometer.* These methods are described later.

The Correction of Astigmatism. Astigmatism is corrected by cylinders and spherocylinders. The curve of the correcting cylinder corresponds to the ametropic meridian; consequently its axis is at right angles to this meridian.

Notation of Cylinders. *The direction of the axis of a cylinder* generally is indicated by the angle which the axis makes with the horizontal, this angle being numbered from 0° on our right (as we stand before the patient) to 180° on our left (Fig. 20-12); *i.e.,* 0° is placed at the end of the horizontal meridian to the patient's left, and the degrees are counted on the

upper semicircle to 180° at his right (either eye).

Treatment consists in prescribing *glasses* which correct the error. In some cases of high degree it is impossible to obtain V.A. 20/20 even with full correction; we often have to be satisfied with 20/30 or 20/40; but the acuity often improves after the lenses have been worn for a time. The glasses should be *worn constantly.* When the correction has been estimated with the eye under the effects of a cycloplegic, a slight reduction may be necessary in high degrees of astigmatism; after a while, the full correction will be tolerated. The relief which cylinders give, usually, is very good.

Irregular Astigmatism is that variety in which there is not only a difference of refraction in different meridians, but also in *different parts of the same meridian.* It generally is due to changes in the *cornea,* such as opacities and cicatrices following ulceration, interstitial keratitis, injuries or surgical operations, and keratoconus. It also may result from partial dislocation of the *lens,* or from a congenital or acquired change in the refractive power of different sectors of the lens. Visual acuity is diminished considerably and *cannot be improved materially by ordinary glasses,* but may be increased by contact lenses. Fundus details seen with the ophthalmoscope appear *distorted,* and there is distortion of the rings of corneal reflection with Placido's disk (Figs. 1-8 and 20-14, *right*). Insignificant normal irregular astigmatism accounts for seeing stars as stellate points instead of round dots.

Anisometropia

This term is applied to cases of *great inequality* in the state of refraction of the two eyes; slight differences are present in most cases of errors of refraction. Every combination may occur: (1) One eye may be emmetropic and the other ametropic;

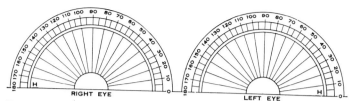

Fig. 20-12. Standard method of designating the axis of cylinders.

(2) both eyes may have the same variety of ametropia, but of unequal degree; (3) less frequently, one eye may be myopic and the other hyperopic, either simple or combined with astigmatism. Notwithstanding the unequal refraction, binocular vision is present unless the variation in the two eyes is very great; sometimes the eyes are used alternately; in other cases one eye is habitually excluded from vision.

In prescribing glasses no arbitrary rules can be followed; each case must be considered by itself. When one eye is emmetropic and the other ametropic, probably no glass will be required, unless to prevent the ametropic eye from suffering from disuse, or for the relief of asthenopic symptoms. When the difference in the refraction is not great (1.00 to 2.00 D.) and there is good binocular vision, each eye may be given its correction. Even when the difference is greater, correcting lenses often will give satisfaction; but when full correction causes discomfort it may be necessary to give only a partial correction in the eye having the greater error of refraction. When there is no binocular vision, a correcting glass is given for the better eye; in such cases, when discovered in a child, there may be some gain in vision if the poor eye, provided with a suitable lens, is forced into use for at least several hours each day, the good eye being occluded. When there is an absence of single binocular vision there is liability to strabismus; this is apt to be convergent in hyperopes and divergent in myopes.

Aniseikonia

Aniseikonia is the name applied to a condition in which the retinal images are unequal in either size or shape. The knowledge of the existence of this anomaly is founded upon research in the physiologic optics laboratory. It has been assumed that such unequal images result in an effort to fuse two disparate images into one coordinated whole upon reaching the brain, and that this accounts for occasional instances in which asthenopia is not relieved by glasses or attention to heterophoria, however perfect such correcting lenses may be. The defect is estimated by examination with an instrument of elaborate construction called the ophthalmo-iconometer. Anisometropia may cause aniseikonia. Aniseikonic lenses consist either of an increase in thickness or curve of ordinary lenses or of double lenses cemented together at the edges with a central air space between them; these are designed to equalize the size and shape of the two retinal images. Although the need of aniseikonic corrections is not frequent, there are some cases in which relief from asthenopia results from the wearing of such lenses after other means of correcting ametropia have failed.

Asthenopia

Asthenopia (*eye strain*) is a convenient term which embraces the group of symptoms dependent upon *fatigue* of the ciliary muscle or of the extraocular muscles.

Symptoms. The condition is of very frequent occurrence and causes a great variety of symptoms. The most common manifestations of asthenopia are: (1) *pain* in or around the eyes or *headache*, usually aggravated by use of the eyes for close work, and in some cases present only after near use; (2) *fatigue and discomfort* upon use of the eyes for near; this shows itself by inability to indulge in such work for more than a short period without dimness of vision and confusion of the lines of print, pain in and about the eyes, headache, drowsiness, lacrimation, photophobia and congestion, and an irritable condition of the lids with itching and burning sensations. These symptoms regularly are worse at night, when the patient is tired, or when artificial illumination is employed; (3) *vertigo* and a tendency to diplopia; (4) *reflex symptoms*, such as neurasthenia, nausea, twitching of the facial muscles, exceptionally migraine, and neuroses.

The term asthenopia refers to the above-mentioned symptoms when produced by fatigue of the ciliary muscle or by muscle imbalance. However, some of these symptoms can be present with chronic catarrhal conjunctivitis in which the conjunctiva is hypertrophied and roughened, without any error of refraction or heterophoria, or after successful correction of such errors.

The amount of asthenopia depends not only upon the kind and degree of defect but also upon the *state of the patient's health*, and therefore is worse in delicate, anemic and neurasthenic individuals.

Varieties are (1) accommodative, (2) muscular, (3) neurasthenic. Two of these varieties may be associated.

Accommodative Asthenopia is the most common variety. It is due to strain and *fatigue of the ciliary muscle* when used too constantly or excessively, in *ametropia*. It is especially frequent in astigmatism and hyperopia, but is common enough in myopia and in presbyopia. Treatment consists in the use of *glasses* that correct the error of refraction as advised in preceding pages. In delicate and neurasthenic individuals attention to the *general health* is very important.

Muscular Asthenopia is due to a want of balance of the motor apparatus of the eye (*heterophoria*), necessitating an abnormal effort to preserve single binocular vision. Its existence may be associated with and depend on ametropia, or it may occur in emmetropia. Heterophoria is described in Chapter 21.

Neurasthenic Asthenopia is a variety which occurs occasionally in emmetropes or in ametropes in whom proper correcting lenses and treatment of any existing heterophoria give no relief. The condition is a neurosis dependent upon an asthenic condition of the nervous system; consequently it is found most frequently in neurasthenic individuals, anemic persons and convalescents from debilitating diseases; it may be a manifestation of reflex irritation from some neighboring infective or inflamed focus, such as a diseased tooth. It often is very *troublesome* and *obstinate*. *The more carefully one investigates the state of refraction and the motor balance of the eye, the fewer cases one finds necessary to classify as neurasthenic.* Treatment consists in improving the general health, rest of the eyes, attention to proper hygiene and elimination of any existing source of neighboring irritation.

Presbyopia

Presbyopia (Pr.) is a *physiologic* change which affects every eye, commencing between the 42nd and 45th years, as a result of which the *near point recedes* beyond the distance at which ordinary print is read; this distance has been fixed somewhat arbitrarily at 22 cm. (about 9 inches). The change is due chiefly to *loss of elasticity of the lens* and, to a much lesser extent, to a weakening of the ciliary muscle; consequently the power of *accommodation is lessened*. As explained previously, this diminution in the power of accommodation begins early, about the 10th year; when approaching the 45th year it becomes sufficient to interfere with the comfortable exercise of near vision; then presbyopia is said to be present.

At the age of 40, there are 4.50 D. of accommodation, and the near point is at 22 cm., or 9 inches. To read at 9 inches, such an individual would require all of his accommodation and the effort would soon become fatiguing, since only one-half or two-thirds of this power can be used for any length of time without causing asthenopia. If this person were to hold print at about 13 inches (33 cm.), he would require 3.00 D. of accommodation, leaving a reserve of 1.50 D., which usually suffices for comfort. At 45 his accommodation would diminish to 3.50 D.; all or nearly all of this would be required to read comfortably at 13 inches, leaving little or no reserve. If he kept one-third of his accommodation in reserve, he would have about 2.25 D. available for near work; with this, his reading distance would be 45 cm., or 18 inches—too great for comfortable and continuous near work. Hence the defect in accommodation must be corrected by a convex lens sufficient to bring the near point to a convenient distance. In the example made use of, the reading distance for the adult is given as 13 inches (33 cm.); as a matter of fact, most adults prefer to read at 15 or 16 inches.

Symptoms. The presbyope is compelled to hold reading, sewing and other forms of near work *farther* away than the usual distance, making reading unsatisfactory. With recession of the near point beyond the usual situation, the *print becomes pale and indistinct,* and fine type can be read only with great difficulty. The patient is apt to use strong illumination; this produces contraction of the pupil, and thus improves the definition by diminishing the circles of diffusion. If the condition is uncorrected, he suffers from *asthenopic symptoms*, especially pain, fatigue, lacrimation and dimness of vision, all of these symptoms being intensified with poor light or at night with *artificial illumination*. Presbyopia has *no effect upon distant vision*.

Treatment consists in prescribing *convex spherical lenses* for near work so as to compensate for the lack of power of accommodation, and to bring the near point back to a comfortable working distance, about 15 inches.

We generally can prescribe approximately correct glasses *according to age*. We usually find that the lens required is as follows: At 45, +0.75 or +1.00 D.; at 50, +1.75 D. or +2.00 D.; at 55, +2.25 D. or +2.50 D.; at 60, +2.50 D.; at 65 and over, +2.50 D. or +2.75 D. These numbers are generally correct; but a *slightly weaker lens* is sometimes preferred by the patient, who usually prefers to hold print at 15 or 16 inches. The *age* at which patients are obliged to wear glasses *varies* within a few years, and is influenced, to a certain extent, by the vigor of the individual; a delicate or neurasthenic person will require glasses for reading earlier than a robust individual.

The glasses also must be selected with reference to the *occupation* or the *special use* for which the patient wishes them. Thus in reading, writing and sewing, 15 inches (38 cm.) is a comfortable working distance for most persons; but a musician will prefer a distance of 20 inches or more (50 cm. or more) for reading his notes, and for this he will need a weaker glass; the same applies to typing and cards; for these longer range purposes, it usually is satisfactory to give one-half of that presbyopic correction which has been selected for ordinary reading.

The existence of *ametropia* will modify the strength of glasses required for presbyopia. Hence the visual function for distance, and the state of refraction, must be determined before estimating the glasses required for near work. In ametropia the *lenses required for distance must be added* to those which would be selected for presbyopia in the emmetrope. This would have the effect of increasing the strength of the convex lens required for presbyopia in hyperopes, and of diminishing its power in myopes. If the lens correcting myopia equals that required for presbyopia, the patient will be able to read without glasses. In astigmatism, the cylinders must be added to the convex lenses required for the correction of presbyopia.

Since presbyopia increases with age, glasses will require *changing* for stronger ones *every 2 years*. When glasses have to be changed for stronger lenses very frequently, *glaucoma* must be suspected.

In prescribing glasses for presbyopia, the patient's *muscle balance* also must be considered. Convergence and accommodation being associated, a patient who has a *weakness of convergence* may suffer discomfort as a result of strain upon his converging power, if glasses are prescribed for the usual reading distance. In such cases, it may be advisable to prescribe a *weaker* presbyopic correction than is usual, so as to lessen convergence. Sometimes such a muscle defect will require the addition of a *weak prism* (base in) to the reading glasses, or the decentering of the lenses to produce the same effect.

On the other hand, when vision is reduced by some condition such as incipient cataract or a fundus lesion, there may be an advantage in prescribing a stronger convex lens than is usually required; this forces the patient to hold reading matter closer than usual, but produces a larger image and in this way may assist near vision.

TECHNIQUE EMPLOYED IN DETERMINING STATE OF REFRACTION

There are two principal methods of testing the refraction of the eye: (1) subjective and (2) objective.

The Subjective Method

This method depends upon an estimation of the acuteness of vision by *test types and trial lenses*. It can be employed only with patients who are old enough and sufficiently intelligent to cooperate; but even in children it has some value; and in illiterates the E chart test (Fig. 3-3) will serve to check results obtained by objective methods. *The objective method* gives information derived from the use of the ophthalmoscope, retinoscope and the keratometer (ophthalmometer).

The subjective method may be divided into (a) *dynamic or manifest* refraction, in which the eyes are examined in their natural condition, (b) *static or cycloplegic* refraction, in which accommodation is eliminated by a cycloplegic, and (c) *postcycloplegic* refraction, in which discrepancies between manifest and cycloplegic refractions are corrected. It is customary to estimate both manifest and static refraction in patients under 40; during this period the patient involuntarily uses his accommodation and this hides or changes the results. On this account accommodation must be abolished so that the true or total error of refraction can be ascertained; this is especially necessary in hyperopia and hyperopic astigmatism, but even in myopia and myopic astigmatism the results are more accurate if accommodation is eliminated. Occasionally a cycloplegic is indicated after the age of 45 if the manifest examination has proven unsatisfactory or inconclusive; such patients must be kept under observation until the pupils have contracted.

Manifest (Dynamic) Tests. External examination and darkroom examination,

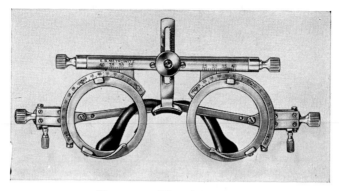

Fig. 20-13. The trial frame.

as described in Chapters 1 and 2, should always precede the examination of refraction. The darkroom examination will not only disclose the condition of the media and fundus and any changes or lesions which would limit improvement with glasses, but also will give information as to the nature of any considerable error of refraction; although this will be only of a qualitative value, the knowledge will be of some assistance in the subsequent examination. At this time retinoscopy will disclose the kind and amount of any error of refraction—not as accurately as when used in the subsequent static examination with the dilated pupil, but sufficiently closely to be of real value in the manifest examination.

The subsequent steps in a complete examination of refraction are, in the order of their sequence: (1) subjective examination (manifest), (2) preparation of the eyes with a cycloplegic, (3) objective methods (ophthalmoscope, retinoscope and ophthalmometer), (4) subjective examination (static) and (5) the prescription for glasses.

The Manifest (Dynamic) Examination. The patient is seated 20 feet (preferably) in front of the test types, which should receive proper daylight or electric illumination; the trial frame (Fig. 20-13) is adjusted to the face of the patient. A manifest retinoscopy having been done, as described briefly above and in more detail later, the examiner will start with some idea of the nature and amount of the refractive error. The examination will proceed by one of three or more methods depending upon the refractionist: (1) the trial and error method, (2) the "fogging" method, (3) the cyclodamic method. All of these methods are in common use.

In the trial and error method, each eye is examined separately. The lenses which correct the error of refraction and bring vision up to the best possible acuity are ascertained.

If the patient reads 20/20, we may assume the absence of myopia; either the patient is emmetropic or he has hyperopia or astigmatism. A weak convex spherical lens is placed in the trial frame; if he still reads 20/20 he has hyperopia, and the strongest spherical lens with which he can read 20/20 is the measure of his manifest hyperopia. If the patient accepts plus spheres, but these fail to bring vision up to normal, plus cylinders are added and rotated in different axes to obtain the axis and the strength of cylinder which gives the best results.

If the patient's vision is below normal, either he has considerable manifest hyperopia or he is myopic or astigmatic. In this instance much information will have been obtained by the manifest retinoscopy. If the patient is myopic, weak concave spherical lenses are placed in the trial frame to give him the best possible vision with the weakest minus lens. If we still are unable to improve the vision to normal we assume the existence of astigmatism, and cylinders either alone or in combination with spheres are added. In determining the amount of astigmatism the astigmatic dial, the cross cylinder, the retinoscope and the ophthalmometer are invaluable aids. The degree of astigmatism can be determined by the trial and error method, but it requires considerable cooperation on the part of the patient.

In the fogging method each eye is examined separately. A convex lens of sufficient strength to blur distant vision is placed in the trial frame and gradually reduced in strength until the best possible vision is obtained. Cylinders then are added if necessary, by one of the various methods described below. The procedure then is repeated for the other eye.

In the cyclodamic method both eyes are examined simultaneously. The strongest spherical lenses which will enable the patient to see 20/200 are placed in the trial frame. The strength of the lenses then is reduced by 0.50 D. and the acuity determined; these lenses should increase the acuity to 20/70. The lenses thereafter are reduced by 0.25 D. steps until 20/20 acuity is obtained; cylinders then are added if necessary by one of the methods described below. The cyclodamic method of refraction is said to be more reliable than the fogging method, since more of the latent hyperopia can be determined.

Each of the methods has its advantages and disadvantages and frequently all three must be used to determine the state of the refractive error. With the trial and error method the tendency is to undercorrect the hyperope and overcorrect the myope. With the fogging method and the cyclodamic method there is a strong tendency to overcorrect the hyperope and undercorrect the myope. When all three are used these tendencies neutralize themselves.

The astigmatic dial. There are two principal methods of determining the amount and axis of astigmatism with the astigmatic dial (Fig. 20-11). With the trial and error method, after the best possible correction with spherical lenses has been obtained, the astigmatic dial, placed at 20 feet, is used and then convex plus cylinders or concave minus cylinders are added to the previous subnormal correction with spheres. The lines of the astigmatic dial which correspond to the axis of the astigmatism will appear blurred, while the distinct lines will correspond to the axis at right angles to that of the correcting cylindrical lens. In general, the blurred axis may be corrected with a minus cylinder placed in this axis; however, a plus cylinder may be placed at right angles to the blurred axis; with the trial and error method it is necessary to try both plus and minus cylinders to see which will correct the blurred axis.

With the fogging method, a strong spherical lens is placed in front of the eye and gradually reduced in strength until one of the axes of the astigmatic dial becomes clear; concave cylindrical lenses then are placed with their axis in the axis of the blurred lines on the astigmatic dial; the strength of the minus cylinder is adjusted until all the lines are equally clear.

The pinhole disk. If little improvement is obtained, trial with a pinhole disk often will give useful information; if there is astigmatism, this will be eliminated, and in consequence there will be considerable improvement in vision. In irregular astigmatism in which vision cannot be improved by glasses, for example opacities of the cornea, the pinhole disk often effects

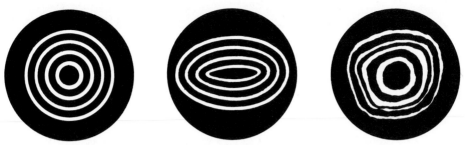

FIG. 20-14. Corneal reflection of Placido's disk: *left*, in emmetropia; *center*, in regular astigmatism; *right*, in irregular astigmatism.

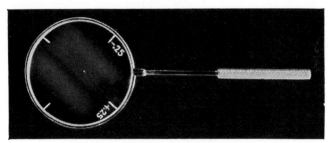

FIG. 20-15. The cross cylinder.

considerable gain through elimination of the irregular refraction of light.

Placido's disk or keratoscope (Fig. 1-7) consists of a circular disk upon which are painted alternate rings of black and white. The patient is placed with his back to the light and fixes the center of the disk, while the examiner looks through an opening in the center and sees an image of the concentric circles reflected upon the patient's cornea. If no astigmatism is present the rings are circular (Figs. 1-8*A* and 20-14, *left*). If regular astigmatism exists, the rings will appear elliptical with the long axis corresponding to the meridian of least curvature (Fig. 20-14, *center*). If the cornea is the seat of irregular astigmatism the rings will be distorted (Fig. 20-14, *right*). This forms a very useful test for irregular astigmatism.

The cross cylinder (Fig. 20-15). Cross cylinders are widely used by ophthalmologists because the test is a more objective

one than the astigmatic dial. Cross cylinders can be of any strength, but the most widely used are the 0.25 D. and 0.50 D. The lens, in effect, consists of a plus cylinder and a minus cylinder at right angles to each other, mounted in a ring attached to a round handle, which permits easy rolling between the thumb and index finger; the handle is attached at 45 degrees from the axis of either cylinder. Actually the 0.25 D. cross cylinder is made by the combination of a plus 0.25 D. sphere with a minus 0.50 D. cylinder.

The cross cylinder may be used to determine both the strength and the axis of the astigmatism. After the best possible spherical correction has been obtained, the cross cylinder is held in front of the eye with the axis of the plus cylinder at 90 degrees and the axis of the minus cylinder at 180 degrees; the cylinders are quickly reversed to place the plus axis at 180 degrees and the minus axis at 90 degrees.

The difference in the degree of vision and clarity of the letters will indicate which is the approximate axis of the astigmatism. A cylinder then is placed before the eye in the axis and of the same sign as the cross cylinder; if, for instance, vision is best when the plus axis of the cross cylinder is placed at 90 degrees, then a plus cylinder is placed in the trial frame at 90 degrees or a minus cylinder is placed at 180 degrees.

The axis of the trial cylinder is checked by holding the handle of the cross cylinder in the axis of the trial cylinder and quickly turning it to determine the position of best vision. The cylinder in the trial frame then is turned toward the side of the same sign on the cross cylinder; for example, the plus trial cylinder is placed at 90 degrees, the handle of the cross cylinder is held in front of the lens at 90 degrees and rotated, best vision is obtained with the cross cylinder held so that its plus axis is at 135 degrees and the minus axis at 45 degrees, then the trial cylinder is turned toward the 135 axis and placed at 105 degrees; the handle of the cross cylinder now is held at the new axis of 105 degrees and rotated about its axis to determine again the position of best vision. The axis of the trial cylinder is the correct axis when the two sides of the cross cylinder blur the test letters equally.

To check the strength of the cylinder selected, the cross cylinder is held so that the axis of the cylinder is in the same axis as the axes of the cylinders of the cross cylinder. The cross cylinder then is rotated, and the patient reports whether blurring or clearing results. If one has a plus cylinder at 90 degrees and if the plus side of the cross cylinder held in the same axis results in better vision, then the plus cylinder in the trial frame is too weak and should be increased in strength; if the minus side of the cross cylinder gives better vision when held in the axis of the trial cylinder, then the cylinder is too strong and should be decreased in strength. The converse is true when one is dealing with minus cylinders. It is essential, when checking the strength of cylinders with the cross cylinder, that the vision of the patient be corrected as completely as possible with spheres.

When the cross cylinder renders the types equally indistinct in both positions, the strength and axis of the trial cylinder will have been proved correct.

The cross cylinder also may be of use in arriving at the estimation of the amount and axis of astigmatism where the usual means fail, such as cases of immature cataract, opacities of the vitreous humor, etc., in which retinoscopy is unsuccessful, thus enabling improvement of poor vision to a certain degree, even though limited; in such cases higher cross cylinders (0.50 D. or 1.00 D.) are used.

At this stage of the manifest examination *vision for near* and the *muscle balance* are investigated, and in the case of adults who have reached the age of 45 and over, the *presbyopic correction* is determined.

The vision for near. A page of Jaeger's test types (Fig. 3-4) is given to the patient, and the smallest type which he is able to read with each eye separately, the distance which he selects, and the nearest and farthest distances at which he is able to read are recorded. In myopia, the patient will hold the print closer than normal. In presbyopia he will hold it at a greater distance than normal.

The Static (Cycloplegic) Examination. After completing the manifest examination, patients up to 45 are re-examined under the influence of a cycloplegic; this examination employs *objective tests* and is *followed by the subjective method.*

Cycloplegics. A description of these agents and of mydriatics is given in Chapter 22.

A cycloplegic is indicated in estimating refraction in *children and in young adults* up to 45, and occasionally in older individuals if the previous examination has been unsatisfactory. Before these agents are used, any suspicion of *glaucoma* must be excluded.

Homatropine (2 per cent), or homatropine (2 per cent) combined with cocaine (1 per cent), is the agent most frequently employed. A drop is instilled every 3 minutes for four instillations, and the examination is begun 1½ hours after the last instillation, when satisfactory cycloplegia will have been produced; if a drop of Paredrine is instilled after 2 successive drops of the homatropine-cocaine mixture, the waiting period is reduced to 1 hour. The effects last from 24 to 48 hours.

In children under 7 years, accommodation is very active and homatropine cycloplegia is incomplete; 0.5 per cent atropine sulfate solution is used, 1 drop instilled three times a day for 3 days preceding the examination, the last drop being instilled 1 hour before the examination. Children may be susceptible to the toxic effects of atropine, and on this account it is well to use the precaution of pressing upon the lacrimal sac for a few minutes after each instillation in order to prevent the solution from passing through the nasolacrimal duct into the nasopharynx. The effects of atropine used in this manner last for a week or 10 days.

Objective Methods

Objective methods of estimating errors of refraction include *ophthalmoscopy, retinoscopy* and the *ophthalmometer*.

The Ophthalmoscope in Relation to Refraction. As has been stated, the ophthalmoscope is not used for the detection and estimation of errors of refraction; but the view of the fundus may be so modified or interfered with by ametropia, if this is of considerable degree, that it is well to know the effects of such errors of refraction upon the appearance of the fundus when this instrument is used.

The ophthalmoscope at a distance gives *qualitative* information. In *emmetropia,* no details of the fundus will be seen; if some part of the disk or vessels is seen, the patient is *ametropic.* If the examiner moves his head from side to side and the *vessels* seem to move in the *same* direction, the case is one of *hyperopia,* if in the *opposite* direction, there is *myopia.* If the vessels of one meridian only are seen, *astigmatism* is present.

The direct method of ophthalmoscopy. If errors of refraction are large, they will interfere with a satisfactory view of the fundus unless a correcting lens is rotated into the sight hole of the ophthalmoscope; this lens then will represent a rough estimate of the error of refraction, provided that the examiner, if ametropic, has corrected his own error of refraction by wearing suitable glasses. In *emmetropia* a distinct view of the fundus is obtained; in *hyperopia* the image of the disk appears small and if the fundus appears blurred it will become distinct upon rotating convex lenses into the sight hole. In *myopia* the image of the disk appears large and it will be blurred to the emmetropic observer, but will be rendered distinct when concave lenses are rotated into the sight hole. In *astigmatism,* if moderate, there is little if any apparent change in the fundus; in greater degrees the disk will appear oval with its long axis corresponding with the axis required in the correcting cylinder.

The indirect method of ophthalmoscopy will give some information regarding the variety of *ametropia* by disclosing changes in the size and shape of the inverted image of the disk and its behavior upon withdrawing or approaching the lens before the patient's eye. If no change takes place in the shape and size of the image when the lens is withdrawn, the

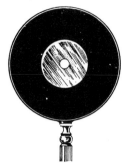

FIG. 20-16. Retinoscopic mirror.

eye is *emmetropic*; if the shape remains
the same but the image becomes smaller,
it indicates hyperopia; if the shape remains the same but the image becomes
larger on withdrawal of the lens, there is
myopia. In *astigmatism* the disk appears
oval and the shape of its image changes in
withdrawing the lens; one diameter decreases or increases and the other remains
stationary in simple astigmatism; both in-
rease or decrease unequally in compound
astigmatism; one increases and the other
decreases in mixed astigmatism.

Retinoscopy (*the shadow test, skias-
copy*) is a very accurate, objective method
of determining the refraction by illumi-
nating the eye with a plane or concave
mirror (Fig. 20-16), and observing the *direction of the movement* of the retinal
illumination and its bordering shadows
when the mirror is rotated. Its *advantages*
are that it can be used in *children, illiterates* and in severely *defective sight*; it is
entirely *objective,* and hence requires no
cooperation on the part of the patient; it
is *quick* and *accurate,* and it requires no
expensive apparatus. While approximate
results may be obtained with the pupil of
normal size, more accurate findings are secured after cycloplegia. The examination
is made in the darkroom.

The principle of retinoscopy is the
finding of the *point of reversal or the
myopic far point.* In myopia an inverted

image is formed in the air in front of the
eye at the far point—the distance from
which rays would be focused on the
retina; this point is known as the point
of reversal. If the eye is hyperopic or emmetropic, a convex lens is placed before
it so as to give it an *artificial far point.*

When light is thrown into the eye by
means of a plane or concave mirror at a
distance of 1 meter, the fundus is illuminated. By looking through the sight hole
of the mirror an observer will see the *illuminated* portion (red fundus reflex) and
also the *shadow* bounding this bright area.
When the mirror is rotated, the illuminated area and the shadow will *move
across the pupil.*

The electric retinoscope (Fig. 20-17),
in which the illumination is produced by
dry cells in the handle or by cords connected with the house current through a
rheostat, now is used almost exclusively.

The patient is directed to *look at the
forehead* of the examiner, who is at a 1-
meter distance (Fig. 20-18) and who
should *wear correcting lenses* if ametropic.
Each eye is tested separately, one eye being covered.

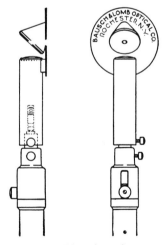

FIG. 20-17. Electric retinoscope.

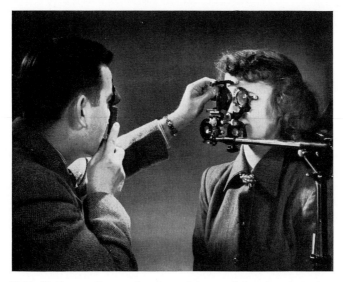

FIG. 20-18. Retinoscopic examination, with use of the electric retinoscope.

If now the mirror is rotated slowly from side to side on its vertical axis, so that the light moves across the pupil horizontally, the observer will see an *illuminated area and a shadow* coming from behind the pupil; if the mirror is rotated on its horizontal axis the light will move across the pupil vertically. The *direction of movement* of this light and shadow as compared with that of the mirror *depends upon the state of refraction* of the eye. The shadow moves either in the same direction (*with*) or in the opposite direction (*against*) to that of the mirror; if the mirror is turned toward the right and the shadow moves toward the right, we say that it moves *with* the mirror; if the mirror is turned toward the right and the shadow moves toward the left, it moves *against* the mirror. *With the plane mirror at 1 meter, the shadow moves with the mirror in hyperopia, emmetropia and myopia of less than 1.00 D., and against the mirror, in myopia of more than 1.00 D.* The illuminated area and the shadow appear to move with the mirror when the ob-

server is within the point of reversal, and against the mirror when he is beyond this point.

Besides the direction of the movement, information is obtained from the *brightness,* the *form* and the *rate of movement* of the light and shadow: If the reflex is bright, its edge sharp and the light and shadow move rapidly, the error of refraction is a low one; if the illumination is dull, its edge indistinct and the movement of light and shadow slow, the error is a high one. If the shadow has a *straight* edge it is an indication of astigmatism (Fig. 20-19, *left*); in hyperopia, myopia or emmetropia the shadow has a *crescentic* edge (Fig. 20-19, *right*).

Next the *correcting lens, i.e.,* the lens which causes a *reversal* of the direction of movement of the shadow, is determined. This lens will be correct for the distance separating the observer from the patient, 1 meter. For infinity, −1.00 D. must be added to all results; this increases the myopia 1.00 D. and diminishes hyperopia 1.00 D.

FIG. 20-19. Retinoscopic illumination and shadow: *left*, in astigmatism; *right*, in hyperopia, myopia or emmetropia.

To be absolutely accurate, the lens which abolishes all shadow should be ascertained; such a lens produces the point of reversal; but practically it is easier to determine the lens which causes a reversal of the shadow and then make a slight reduction from this.

If with the plane retinoscope the *shadow moves against the mirror, concave* spherical lenses are placed before the eye until a reversal of the movement of the shadow occurs, *i.e.*, it moves with the mirror; this lens, to which −1.00 D. is added, is the measure of the patient's *myopia*. Suppose that, when −1.00 D. is added before the eye, the shadow still moves against the mirror, and the same with −2.00 D., but that with −2.50 D. the movement of the shadow is reversed; then −2.50 + (−1.00) D. = −3.50 D. is the correction.

If with the plane retinoscope the *shadow moves with the mirror*, the eye may be hyperopic, emmetropic or myopic less than 1.00 D. In such a case, if adding a convex lens of +0.50 D. causes a reversal of the shadow, the eye is *myopic* 0.50 D., since +0.50 ◌ −1.00 = −0.50 D.

If the +0.50 D. lens does not alter the direction of the movement of the shadow, but the next lens (+1.00 D.) causes the shadow to disappear so that the pupil appears either completely illuminated or totally dark, the eye is *emmetropic*, since +1.00 ◌ −1.00 = 0 = E.

If the +1.00 D. lens has no effect upon the direction of the movement of the shadow, the eye is *hyperopic*, so stronger + spheri-

cal lenses are placed before the eye until the one which causes a reversal of the movement of the shadow is found. Say that this is +4.00 D.; then the hyperopia amounts to +4.00 ◌ −1.00 = +3.00 D.

In the previous examples, the results were the same whether the mirror was rotated upon its vertical or its horizontal axis. In *astigmatism*, upon correcting each of the two principal meridians separately, one meridian will require a different lens to cause a reversal than the other. The most common positions of the two meridians in astigmatism are *vertical* and *horizontal*. But frequently the edges of the shadows lie more or less *obliquely*. In such cases the mirror must be rotated so that the light moves obliquely and parallel with the movement of the shadow.

For example, if *the shadow moves with the mirror* in both meridians, but one shadow is more distinct and moves more quickly than the other, astigmatism is likely. Then if the vertical meridian requires +1.00 D. for the reversal of the shadow and the horizontal meridian +2.00 D., −1.00 D. is added to each of these results, giving +1.00 ◌ −1.00 = 0 or E. in the vertical, and +2.00 ◌ −1.00 = +1.00 in the horizontal meridian. The case is one of *simple hyperopic astigmatism* and requires for its correction +1.00 D. cylinder, axis vertical.

If in the horizontal meridian −2.00 D. are required for reversal, and in the vertical meridian −4.00 D., by adding −1.00 D. to each, the error of refraction is seen to be *compound myopic astigmatism*, and the correcting spherocylinder will be −3.00 D. ◌ −2.00 D. cylinder, axis horizontal.

Finally, an example of *mixed astigmatism*: The shadow will move *with* the mirror in one meridian and *against* the mirror in the other. If in the vertical meridian the shadow moves with the mirror and +2.00 D. are required to cause a reversal, and if in the horizontal meridian the shadow moves against the mirror and −2.00 D. effect a reversal, the correcting lens will be +1.00 D. Sph. ◯ −4.00 D. Cyl. axis vertical.

The results of the retinoscopic examination usually are recorded by two lines at right angles to each other, showing the direction of the axes, and by numbers indicating the kind and strength of the lenses which caused reversal of the shadows; these numbers are then modified by the addition of −1.00, if the distance between examiner and patient was 1 meter.

Practice is necessary before one can become adept in retinoscopy. It is necessary to remember that the *central portion of the cornea* is the part used for vision ordinarily with pupil of natural size; hence it is important, in estimating the state of refraction when the pupil is dilated, to direct one's attention to the shadow when it crosses the center of the cornea, and to disregard its behavior elsewhere, since the curvature of the cornea at its periphery is somewhat different from that of the center.

This difference in the refraction of light in these two different parts of the cornea accounts for confusing shadows sometimes seen with the retinoscopic examination. One such difficulty is the occurrence of *"scissors movement,"* when two shadows will be seen to move toward or away from each other like the opening and closing of the blades of a pair of scissors; in such cases the examiner should correct the more intense shadow in the visual zone (the central part) of the cornea and disregard the other.

In irregular astigmatism the application of retinoscopy is difficult since there will be conflicting shadows moving irregularly in various directions; such astigmatism cannot be corrected by any lens or combination of lenses, although the wear-

ing of these may result in some improvement in vision.

In conical cornea there is a bright central illumination moving against the mirror; this movement of the light is rapid at the periphery and slow at the center; on this account it appears to spin around a point corresponding to the apex of the cone, situated at or just below the center of the cornea.

The results obtained with retinoscopy will be found to approximate those of the subjective test. In very young children and in unintelligent individuals whose answers cannot be depended upon, the retinoscopic findings may have to be used as a basis for the prescription for glasses. But in those whose cooperation can be relied upon, *the subjective test should be used to check the retinoscopic results*; this often will lead to slight corrections in the strength of lenses and in the axis of cylinders.

The Ophthalmometer (Keratometer) is an instrument used for the objective determination of the principal meridians and the amount of *corneal astigmatism*. It does not register the total amount of astigmatism, since the latter is influenced by changes in the lens. It may be of service when used in connection with other tests; but its principal use is in estimating *corneal astigmatism* after removal of the lens for cataract (*aphakia*). One model of the keratometer (Fig. 20-20) measures the dioptic power and the axes of the two principal meridians with one setting of the instrument. After accurate focusing, the image of a circular target is projected upon the cornea. The axis of astigmatism as well as the dioptric powers of the two principal meridians are indicated upon drums placed on the side of the instrument when the corneal image shows coincidence of certain signs reflected from the target (Fig. 20-21).

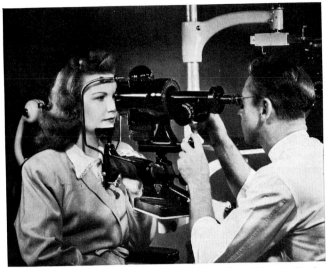

Fig. 20-20. The keratometer with circular targets (Bausch and Lomb Optical Company).

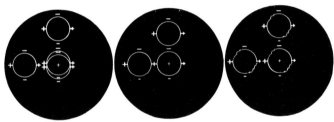

Fig. 20-21. Appearance of mire images: *left*, when instrument is slightly out of focus; *center*, when perfect focus, correct axis and power are recorded; *right*, showing distortion caused by an irregular corneal surface.

The Prescription for Glasses

The preceding description of the various tests employed to detect and measure errors of refraction comprises the methods which may be used. In many instances it will not be necessary to make use of all of them.

Although there are exceptions, it often is possible to conclude the entire examination at one visit, if the patient is willing to spend the time necessary to conclude both manifest and cycloplegic examinations.

In persons in the forties and beyond, glasses can be prescribed after a comparatively short visit. But if both manifest and cycloplegic examinations are made, we must count on detaining the patient for a considerable time.

Some ophthalmologists direct the patient to return for a *postcycloplegic* examination. This may be necessary in some instances in which results have been unsatisfactory because contradictory or inconclusive, but in many cases the prescription for glasses can be given at once, based upon a comparison of the manifest and the static examinations.

The *rules which apply to the selection of glasses* for the different varieties of errors of refraction have been given in the paragraphs describing the treatment suitable for each of such refractive errors.

Eyeglasses, Spectacles, Protective Glasses and Aids to Poor Vision

Adjustment. Much of the comfort and relief which lenses bring depends upon the skill with which the glasses are fitted to the face. The lenses must be supported in their frames in such a manner that the distance between their geometric centers corresponds to the interval between the centers of the pupils (interpupillary distance).

If the glasses are to be worn constantly, the level of the geometrical center of the lenses should be slightly *below the center* of the pupils, and the lenses should be *tilted* so that their surfaces form an angle of about 15° with the plane of the face. If worn for distance only, the level of the lenses should be the same and the tilting about 10°. If worn for near work only, the lenses should be lower, decentered inward slightly, inclined about 20°. In every case the glasses should be worn as *near the eyes* as possible, just avoiding the lashes.

In cases of *astigmatism,* it is necessary that the *axis of the cylinder remain constant,* as prescribed. Because of this the lenses should be mounted in frames which are rigid and will not permit the lenses to turn.

Lenses usually are made of crown glass. *Periscopic* (toric) lenses are preferred, since these give better definition of the peripheral parts of the field when the eyes are moved from side to side; although such lenses give a perfect focus only when the central portion is brought in the line of vision, as a matter of fact one instinctively uses only this portion by unconsciously moving the head. Special lenses are manufactured in which every part gives an equally perfect focus and thus a wider field of perfect optical effect; such lenses are known by the trade names, Orthogon and Tillyer.

Nonshatterable lenses have a thin lamina of colorless celluloid interposed between two layers of glass, are as perfect optically as ordinary lenses and wear almost equally well.

Hardened lenses have been exposed to a process similar to that used in tempering steel; such lenses are extremely hard and resistant to impact and breakage; they serve as important protection to the eyes in the goggles worn by workmen who are subject to eye injuries from accidents resulting from pieces of ordinary broken lenses and from chips of metal loosened by hammer and chisel. The protection is much greater than is supplied by nonshatterable glass.

Unbreakable lenses are made of plastic material, are moulded from highly polished metal or glass dies, do not change color or warp with wear, weigh less than half of an equivalent glass lens, soften only with great heat (158° F.) and will burn only when exposed to a free flame; such lenses cost twice as much and scratch much more easily than glass lenses.

Cylinders generally are ground with two curved surfaces, the cylinder corresponding to the outer surface. *Spherocylinders* usually have both the cylindrical and spherical curves ground on the outer surface, the inner being deeply concave; this gives an enlarged field and reduces the weight and thickness of the lens.

Bifocal Lenses (Figs. 20-22 to 20-25) obviate the necessity of constantly changing from distance to reading glasses and back again; they consist of an upper portion of one focus, and a lower part of another, and are used principally in cases of *presbyopia associated with ametropia,* the lower portion being used for reading and near work, and the upper for distance. Oval or circular glass wafers representing

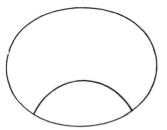

FIG. 20-22. Bifocal lens (oval reading segment).

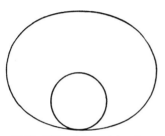

FIG. 20-23. Bifocal lens (circular reading segment).

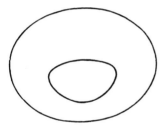

FIG.20-24. Bifocal lens.

The wearer of bifocals often complains of blurred view of objects on the ground, for instance the steps in going downstairs, since he is then looking through the reading segment. Bifocal lenses are obtainable which obviate this difficulty; in these the upper, lower and lateral portions of the lens are adapted for distance vision, and a square, circle or oval in the lower central part has the focus necessary for reading (Figs. 20-24 and 20-25).

Trifocal Lenses, giving correction for distance, intermediate and near vision, have been developed; these are useful in certain individuals who require good vision in these ranges.

Recumbent spectacles occasionally are used; they are provided with prisms which reflect the rays, so that the page of a book resting upon the chest of an invalid who is compelled to remain in a supine position can be read with the eyes directed upward; this obviates the strain from extreme downward direction of the eyes, or the discomfort to the arms when reading matter is held above the level of the face. They can be worn over existing spectacles or fitted with the wearer's own reading correction.

the presbyopic correction formerly were cemented to the lower portion of the distance glass; but these have been supplanted by bifocal lenses in one piece; the latter are of two kinds: (1) the *fused bifocal*, in which the small reading segment, made of flint glass, is fused into the lower hollowed portion of the larger distance lens (crown glass); the increased strength of the smaller lens depends upon the higher refractive index of flint glass; (2) the *one-piece bifocal*, in which both distance and near correction are ground on a single piece of crown glass in toric form.

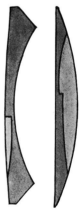

FIG. 20-25. Section of bifocal lens: *left*, convex; *right*, concave.

Protective Glasses. These are of two kinds: (1) to prevent the discomfort and ill effects of *excessive light* and (2) to guard against eye injury in industrial occupations, especially from *foreign bodies*.

Excessive light. Many persons are hypersensitive to bright light, not only if eye strain exists and requires proper glasses, or when conjunctivitis is present and calls for local treatment, but also with apparently normal eyes. These individuals are more comfortable if they wear lenses made of glass of special chemical composition, which reduces the intensity of the visible rays. Such special lenses relieve *glare*; the ones most frequently used are Crooke's and Cruxite No. 1, having a faint gray tint, and Soft-Lite No. 1, of a slightly pinkish hue. Recently a third variety, Polaroid glass, has been introduced with glare-eliminating claims. Deeper shades of Crooke's, Cruxite, Calobar or Rayban are prescribed to guard against very brilliant light such as is experienced in the tropics or caused by the reflection from snow, etc.

In many diseases of the cornea, uvea and retina the eyes must be protected from light by *smoked glasses* worn alone or over the distance lenses ordinarily used; the shade of these is designated by numbers, 1 being the lightest and 6 the darkest; Nos. 4 and 5 are the ones usually prescribed if in ordinary smoked glass, and No. 4 if in Crooke's, Cruxite or Calobar glass. If the patient wears distance glasses, the tinted or smoked lenses can be added conveniently in "hook-on" frames which can be attached or removed easily from the glasses habitually worn. Amber glass also is used for the same purpose, though less frequently; such colored glass is known by trade names, Noviol,

Chlorophyll, Euphos, etc. Blue glass is not suitable. With very intense light, such as is experienced with electric welding, deeply colored glasses are worn, often in the form of a plate of red glass covering a similar plate of green or blue.

Protection glasses. *Injuries* to the eye constitute the most serious of all nonfatal accidents in industrial occupations and are responsible for a considerable proportion of blindness. The majority of such injuries result from *flying chips of metal* loosened by hammer and chisel. Hence the importance of guarding eyes exposed to such hazards with *goggles*; these should be light in weight, provided for replacement of scratched or damaged glass, and have wire mesh side protection; the glass should be of the *hardened* variety. Lenses made of hardened glass or of the nonshatterable variety are useful not only for insertion in goggles worn by workmen in certain industries, but also in sports such as baseball, basketball, tennis, etc., and sometimes even for lively children. For sports and at times for children, if expense and the necessity of more frequent renewal on account of scratching are no objections, the plastic variety of lenses has advantages.

Magnifying glasses are useful when vision is reduced to such an extent that reading is impossible with ordinary glasses. These should be of horizontal cylindrical form and mounted upon a stand which steadies the glass at its focal distance and permits the perception of one or more lines of print, thus facilitating reading.

Telescopic spectacles are sometimes of value in high myopes and others handicapped with poor vision.

Contact lenses are described in connection with conical cornea.

21

Disturbances of Motility of the Eye

Anatomy and Physiology

The eyeball is moved by six muscles, the *extrinsic muscles*, consisting of the four rectus muscles and the two obliques; these arise from the wall of the orbit and are inserted into the sclera.

The recti (*medial, lateral, superior, inferior*) arise from the circumference of the optic foramen at the apex of the orbit, run forward, surrounding the optic nerve and posterior portion of the eyeball, and are inserted into the sclera by means of flattened tendons about 10 mm. wide (Fig. 21-1).

The lines of insertion of these muscles are not equidistant from the cornea, but have somewhat the form of a spiral. The insertion of the medial rectus is 5 mm., the inferior rectus 6 mm., the lateral rectus 7 mm., and the superior rectus 8 mm. from the cornea.

The superior oblique arises from the border of the optic foramen, runs forward to the upper and inner angle of the orbit, at the anterior extremity of which it passes through a fibrous pulley, the trochlea; it then continues outward and backward, passing beneath the superior rectus, and is inserted into the upper part of the sclera behind the equator.

The inferior oblique arises from the superior maxillary bone at the inner portion of the lower border of the orbit, passes backward and outward below the inferior rectus and is inserted into the outer part of the sclera behind the equator.

The muscles are ensheathed by the fascia of the orbit, which covers the sclera as *Tenon's capsule*, and sends prolongations to the walls of the orbit which serve to fix the eyeball in its place. These prolongations are most prominent upon the internal and external recti muscles; they serve to restrain the excursions of the eyeball and are known as "*check ligaments.*"

Nerve supply. The *third* nerve (oculomotor) supplies all the muscles except the lateral rectus, innervated by the *sixth* (abducens), and the superior oblique, which is supplied by the *fourth* (trochlearis). The nuclei for these three nerves are found in the floor of the fourth ventricle.

Action of the Muscles. The six extrinsic muscles serve to rotate the eyeball around a *vertical, horizontal and anteroposterior axis,* the center of rotation corresponding approximately to the center of the eyeball, and the movements being free in all directions, like a ball-and-socket joint. The movements which take place about the vertical axis are *adduction* (toward the nose) and *abduction* (toward the temple); about the horizontal axis, *elevation* and *depression,* and about the anteroposterior axis, wheel rotation or *torsion,* causing the upper end of the vertical meridian to be inclined inward (*intorsion*) or outward (*extorsion*). Except in the case of the medial and lateral recti, which adduct and abduct the eyeball respectively, each muscle has a main action and also subsidiary actions.

The main actions of the superior and inferior recti and the subsidiary actions of the obliques increase as the eyeball is abducted; the main action of the obliques and the subsidiary actions of the superior

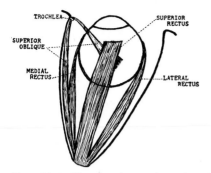

FIG. 21-1. Sketch of muscles of right orbit seen from above.

and inferior recti increase as the eyeball is adducted.

The Field of Action of a muscle is that direction of gaze in which its main action is greatest. In every movement of the eyes *several muscles of each eye act at the same time*; but on moving them in any of the six cardinal directions of gaze (see below), there is always *one muscle of each eye acting predominantly in that direction* (Fig. 21-2); this is the muscle in whose field of action the eye is placed. Table 21-1, based on Duane, gives the field of action of the various muscles.

Both eyes always move simultaneously (*associated movements*), regulated by centers of association which innervate certain muscles or groups of muscles of the two eyes simultaneously. The associated or

TABLE 21-1

Field of Action of the Various Muscles of the Eye (after Duane)

Eyes Directed to:*	Muscle Predominantly Acting	
	Right	Left
Right	R. lateral rectus	L. medial rectus
Left	R. medial rectus	L. lateral rectus
Up and right	R. superior rectus	L. inferior oblique
Up and left	R. inferior oblique	L. superior rectus
Down and right	R. inferior rectus	L. superior oblique
Down and left	R. superior oblique	L. inferior rectus

* The cardinal directions of gaze.

conjugate movements occur either in the same direction, with the *visual lines parallel*, or with the lines inclined toward each other (*convergence*) or away from each other (*divergence*). Defects in the associated movements of the eyes result from lesions above the motor nuclei. Involvement below this level affects individual ocular muscles.

The Field of Fixation corresponds to the *limits* of movement of the eyeball in *different directions*, without moving the

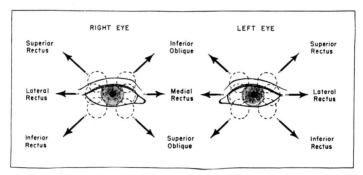

FIG. 21-2. Diagram showing the muscles acting predominantly in the six cardinal directions of gaze.

head. It is best estimated by the perimeter (Fig. 3-5). The patient's head is fixed so that the eye under examination is opposite the center of the instrument, and the other eye is covered. A short word printed with small test letters is moved along the arc of the perimeter, from the periphery to the center, until the patient can name the word, using the eye alone and not moving the head. The field of fixation in the normal eye is about 45° upward, inward and outward, and about 60° downward. A special instrument (Stevens' tropometer) may be used for the determination of the rotations of the eyes.

Binocular Vision and Diplopia. Under ordinary conditions, both eyes are concerned in the action of vision, and are involuntarily adjusted, so that the image of an object is focused on the macula of each eye. The two images then are fused into a single mental perception. This faculty constitutes *binocular single vision*, and is controlled by the sense of *fusion*, the origin of the impulse being the fusion center of the brain.

Fusion is divided into three grades: (1) simultaneous macular perception, (2) simultaneous vision with fusion and (3) fusion with depth perception (stereoscopic vision).

When images fall on symmetrical points of the two retinae, a single visual sensation is produced (*binocular single vision*). When the visual lines of the two eyes are not directed toward the same object, *i.e.*, when one eye deviates, *diplopia or double images* result, unless the image of the deviating eye is suppressed. The diplopia is proportional to the amount of deviation. The image which corresponds to the eye which "fixes" the object is distinct, because it lies at the macula; the image of the deviating eye is less distinct, because it is perceived by a peripheral part of the retina.

Objects situated to the right of the point of fixation throw their images to the left of the macula; those placed to the left of the point of fixation form images to the right of the macula. In the same manner objects above or below the point of fixation cast their images below or above the macula, respectively. By reversing this process the situation of an object is determined by placing it at the extremity of an imaginary line drawn from the retinal image through the nodal point; this process is known as *projection,* and is learned by experience. It permits judgment of the relative positions of objects; an object which forms its image to the right of the macula is situated to our left; one which throws its image below the macula is situated above, etc.

If an eye is deflected, an object situated straight ahead will form its image on either side of the macula and, following out this process of projection, it will be referred to the opposite side of the outside world.

Diplopia is said to be *homonymous* when the false image is on the same side as the deviating eye, and *crossed* when it is on the opposite side. When the two images are level, the diplopia is known as *horizontal*; when displaced vertically, the diplopia is called *vertical*.

In Figure 21-3 the right eye is turned in, and diplopia results. The patient sees a true image with the left eye, forming at the macula and referred to its proper place, *TI*. In the right eye on account of the deviation inward, the image is thrown upon the retina to the left of the macula and consequently is projected to the right, at *FI*. The image of the right eye being to the right of the image of the left eye, the case is one of *homonymous diplopia.*

In Figure 21-4, the right eye turns out and diplopia results. The image of the candle lies on the macula in the left eye and is referred to its correct position; a true image is seen at *TI*. In the right eye, because of its outward deviation, the image

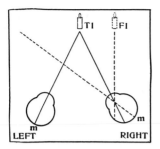

FIG. 21-3. Deviation of the right eye inward; homonymous diplopia. *TI*, True image; *FI*, false image; *m*, macula.

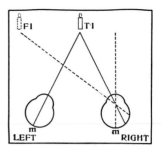

FIG. 21-4. Deviation of the right eye outward; crossed diplopia. *TI*, True image; *FI*, false image; *m*, macula.

falls to the right of the macula and is consequently projected to the left, at *FI*. The images having crossed in their relative positions, that of the right being seen to the left of the image of the left eye, the case is one of *crossed diplopia*.

Double images also may be produced without any deviation by placing a *prism* in front of the eyes. The prism will deflect the rays so that instead of falling upon the macula, they reach the retina to one side of it.

Varieties of Ocular Deviations. A deviation may be *paralytic* or *nonparalytic*. In *paralysis*, the deviation is due to a loss of function of one or more of the ocular muscles; the paralysis may be *complete* or *partial* (paresis). *Nonparalytic* (*concomitant*) deviations are produced by anomalies of the power of convergence and of divergence. In these cases the amount and character of the deviation do not vary in different directions of gaze. Deviations may be *manifest* or *latent*. *Strabismus* (*squint* or *heterotropia*) is a *manifest* deviation in which binocular fixation is impossible. Fixation is maintained with one eye or the other but never with both at the same time. *Heterophoria* is a condition in which the eyes have a constant *tendency* to deviate, but are forced into simultaneous fixation by muscular effort prompted by the desire for binocular single vision. Ordinarily the de-

viation is not apparent; hence it is said to be *latent*. There is no sharp distinction between heterophoria and squint; frequently a heterophoria progresses until the patient is no longer able to overcome the deviation and it then becomes manifest (squint).

Paralysis of the Ocular Muscles

Symptoms. *Limitation of movement* of the eye in the field of action of the paralyzed muscle is complete or nearly so in paralysis, but less obvious in paresis. It can be detected when the patient keeps his head fixed and tries to follow with his eyes an object moved in the six cardinal directions of gaze (excursion test). In some instances the limitation of movement may be so slight that the diagnosis must be made from the nature of the diplopia.

Deviation. When the eyes are turned in the field of action of the paralyzed muscle, the sound eye will be directed properly, but the affected eye will lag. The deviation generally is apparent, but becomes greater the farther the eyes are moved in the field of action of the paralyzed muscle. When the eyes are turned in any direction in which the paralyzed muscle does not have to participate, there is no squint.

The deflection of the squinting eye, known as the *primary deviation*, always is in the direction opposite to the normal action of the paralyzed muscle. If the affected eye fixes an object and the sound eye is covered, the latter will squint in a corresponding direction much more than the affected eye; this deflection of the sound eye is known as the *secondary deviation*. The secondary deviation is greater than the primary because the strong impulse of innervation required to enable the paralyzed eye to fix, being simultaneously transmitted to the associated muscle of the sound eye, produces overaction of this muscle, hence a greater amount of squint. This is an important point in distinguishing between paralytic and nonparalytic (concomitant) squint; in the latter, the primary and secondary deviations are equal.

Diplopia occurs in the *field of action of the paralyzed muscle* and becomes greater as the eyes are moved into this field. The presence or absence of diplopia, the relative position of the double images and the increase or diminution of the distance between them in the nine main directions of gaze form the more important means of diagnosing an ocular muscle paralysis (Figs. 21-5 to 21-10).

Head tilting (ocular torticollis). The patient usually turns his head in the direction of action of the paralyzed muscle. The oblique position of the head is a suggestive but not a diagnostic sign.

False projection. The paralyzed eye does not see objects in their correct location. The false projection is due to greatly increased innervation, conveyed to the nerve supplying the paralyzed muscle in an effort to force it to act; this gives the patient an erroneous idea of the position of the eye. It can be demonstrated by closing the patient's sound eye and telling him to point quickly at an object in front of him; the finger will be directed to the side of the object corresponding to the field of action of the paralyzed muscle.

Vertigo, nausea and uncertain gait are frequent symptoms due to diplopia and false projection; they are relieved by closing one eye.

Diagnosis. Limitation of movement, deviation and diplopia are the three important symptoms of ocular paralysis. All of these symptoms increase in the field of action of the paralyzed muscle. In paretic cases, in which the limitation of motion and squint are slight in amount, the behavior of the diplopia is most important.

Method of testing for diplopia. The patient is seated facing a wall at a distance of 30 inches from it. A *red glass* is placed before the right eye, and the head and body are kept still. A small electric light (May electric ophthalmoscope with the lens disk removed) or a lighted candle is moved in the nine directions of gaze and the nature and amount of diplopia in each field are recorded. The data required are (1) in which direction of gaze there is single vision and in which diplopia; (2) whether the diplopia is homonymous, crossed, vertical or mixed; (3) whether the diplopia increases in any direction of gaze. A rule which is helpful in interpretation of diplopia is: The image of the paralyzed eye always lies on the side toward which the diplopia increases, and the diplopia always increases in the field of action of the paralyzed muscle. By knowing the direction in which the diplopia increases and which is the affected eye, it is possible to determine the particular muscle involved. The diplopia field can be most satisfactorily determined by the use of the special tangent plane of Duane.

After paralysis of an extraocular muscle has lasted a long time, the symptoms become less characteristic. Diplopia disappears because the image of the paralyzed eye is *suppressed* and faulty projection is corrected by newly acquired experience; *contracture* of the antagonist of the affected muscle increases the squint.

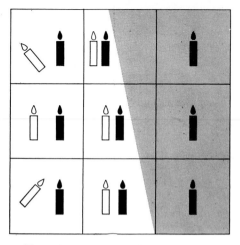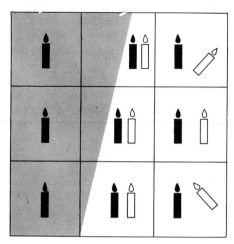

FIG. 21-5. Paralysis of the external rectus. The *black candle* is the fixation object and the *outlined candle* represents the position of the false image as seen by the patient. *Left,* left eye; *right,* right eye.

When one muscle only is paralyzed, the diagnosis is easy, but when several muscles are involved, it sometimes is difficult to determine the exact combination.

Varieties of Ocular Paralysis. One muscle may be involved or several muscles may be affected. Paralysis of the lateral rectus is the most common acquired paralysis of a single muscle; less frequently the superior oblique or one of the muscles supplied by the third nerve is affected. Combined paralysis of some or all of the four muscles supplied by the third nerve is exceedingly common.

Paralysis of the lateral (external) rectus. There are limitation of movement outward, convergent squint and homonymous diplopia. All of these symptoms increase as the affected eye is abducted (Fig. 21-5). The images are on the same level; the lateral separation increases as the paralyzed eye attempts to move out. The head is turned to the side of the affected muscle.

Paralysis of the medial (internal) rectus. There are limitation of movement inward, divergent squint and crossed diplopia (Fig. 21-6). All of these symptoms

increase as the affected eye is abducted. The images are on the same level; the lateral separation increases as the paralyzed eye attempts to move in. The head is turned to the side of the affected muscle.

Paralysis of the superior rectus. There are limitation of movement upward (most evident in the upper outer field), vertical squint and mixed diplopia (Fig. 21-7). The diplopia is mainly vertical but usually also is slightly crossed. The image of the paralyzed eye is higher and the vertical separation of the images increases as the affected eye attempts to move up and out; the intorsion of the false image and the crossed diplopia increase in the upper nasal field.

Paralysis of the inferior rectus. There are limitation of movement downward (most obvious in the lower outer field), vertical squint and mixed diplopia (Fig. 21-8). The diplopia is mainly vertical but usually is also crossed. The image of the paralyzed eye is lower and the vertical separation of the images increases as the affected eye attempts to move down and out; the extorsion of the false image

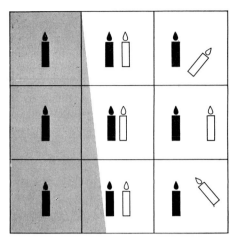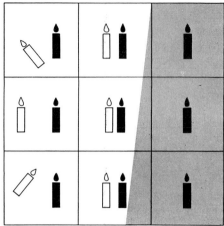

FIG. 21-6. Paralysis of the internal rectus. The *black candle* is the fixation object and the *outlined candle* represents the position of the false image as seen by the patient. *Left,* left eye; *right,* right eye.

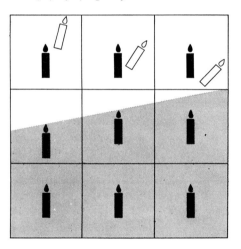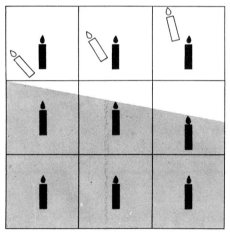

FIG. 21-7. Paralysis of the superior rectus. The *black candle* is the fixation object and the *outlined candle* represents the position of the false image as seen by the patient. *Left,* left eye; *right,* right eye.

and crossed diplopia increase in the lower nasal field.

Paralysis of the superior oblique. There are limitation of movement downward (most apparent in the lower nasal field), vertical squint and mixed diplopia (Fig. 21-9). The diplopia is chiefly vertical but usually is also homonymous. The image of the paralyzed eye is lower and the vertical separation of the images increases in its lower nasal field; the intorsion of the false image and homonymous diplopia increase in its lower temporal field. There is head tilt to the side opposite the affected eye.

Paralysis of the inferior oblique.

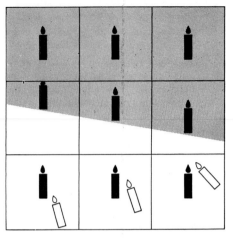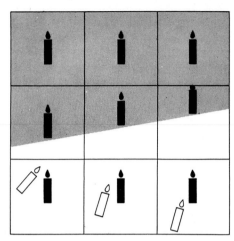

FIG. 21-8. Paralysis of the inferior rectus. The *black candle* is the fixation object and the *outlined candle* represents the position of the false image as seen by the patient. *Left,* left eye; *right*, right eye.

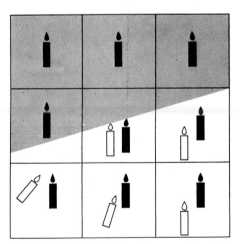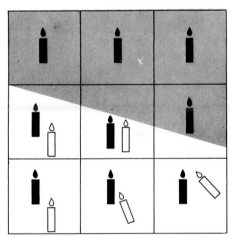

FIG. 21-9. Paralysis of the superior oblique. The *black candle* is the fixation object and the *outlined candle* represents the position of the false image as seen by the patient. *Left,* left eye; *right*, right eye.

There are limitation of movement upward (most evident in the upper nasal field), vertical squint and mixed diplopia (Fig. 21-10). The diplopia is mainly vertical but usually is homonymous. The image of the paralyzed eye is higher and the vertical separation of the images increases in its upper nasal field; the extorsion of the false image and homonymous diplopia increase in its upper temporal field.

Paralysis of the Third Nerve. With complete paralysis of this nerve there is *ptosis*; the *eyeball is almost immobile,* the limitation of motion being upward, inward and slightly downward; the eye *deviates outward* and somewhat down-

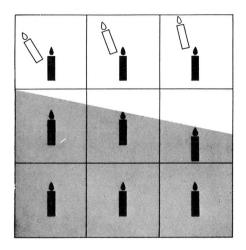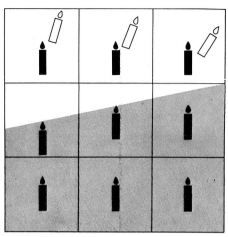

FIG. 21-10. Paralysis of the inferior oblique. The *black candle* is the fixation object and the *outlined candle* represents the position of the false image as seen by the patient. *Left*, left eye; *right*, right eye.

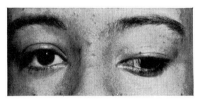

FIG. 21-11. Left oculomotor paralysis.

ward (Fig. 21-11), with the upper end of the vertical meridian inclined inward, especially on looking downward; the face is directed upward and toward the sound side, and the head is inclined to the shoulder of the paralyzed side. There is slight exophthalmos owing to paralysis of the three recti which normally draw the eyeball backward; the *pupil* is *dilated* and is *immobile*; *accommodation* is *paralyzed*; there is crossed *diplopia*—the false image is higher, and its upper end inclined toward the paralyzed side.

Paralysis of the third nerve is *common*; it is often incomplete, two or three of the muscles being affected. It may be associated with paralysis of other nerves.

When all the muscles of one eye are

paralyzed, including the iris and ciliary body, the condition is known as *total ophthalmoplegia*.

When all the external muscles of the eyeball are paralyzed, but not the iris and ciliary body, the condition is known as *external ophthalmoplegia*. This variety is more common than total ophthalmoplegia. The nuclei for the sphincter pupillae and ciliary muscle are separate; thus they often escape involvement by the lesions affecting the origin of the extraocular muscles; this form is generally of central (nuclear) origin.

Paralysis limited to the sphincter pupillae and the ciliary muscle is known as *internal ophthalmoplegia*; it may be *partial* or *complete*. It is observed most commonly, and then only temporarily, after the use of mydriatics and cycloplegics employed for examination of the fundus, estimation of errors of refraction and treatment of certain ocular affections. It occurs sometimes after *diphtheria*. Other causes are *contusions* of the eyeball, and less frequently *syphilis*, diabetes and cerebral disease. The symptoms are *loss* of the power of *accommodation,* and *dilatation* of the *pupil.* The *prognosis* often is good, especially when the affection is due to diphtheria or syphilis; in traumatic cases, the condition often is permanent. *Treatment* calls for removal of the cause. In syphilis, specific treatment is indicated; in postdiphtheritic paralysis, strychnine is given. Locally, miotics (pilocarpine or eserine) are employed; these may relieve the symptoms temporarily by producing spasm of accommodation; the alternate contraction and relaxation of the ciliary muscle often stimulates it to action. In traumatic cases, complete ocular rest is indicated. If the paralysis of accommodation is permanent, convex lenses may be prescribed for close work.

Etiology. The lesions causing paralysis may be situated anywhere in the course of the nerve tract, from the cerebral cortex to the muscle. According to its site, the lesion is distinguished as *central* or *peripheral.*

Central lesions may be situated in the *cortical* centers, *association* centers, *nuclei* of origin or the fibers which connect these centers. Lesions occurring above the nuclei do not produce an individual muscle paralysis but a paralysis of the conjugate movements (*conjugate paralysis*). *Nuclear* paralysis usually involves more than one muscle and may be bilateral.

Peripheral lesions occur either between the exit from the brain and entrance into the orbit (*basilar* paralysis) or in the orbit (*orbital* paralysis). Peripheral lesions are unilateral and usually complete.

The nature of the lesion. The lesion may be a neighboring exudation, hemorrhage, periostitis, tumor, injury or vascular change, causing compression or inflammation of the nerves. A common cause is *aneurysm*; next in frequency come *head trauma, vascular changes* (hemorrhage, occlusion), *neoplasm* and *syphilis.* Muscle paralyses occur in various central nervous

system diseases (tabes, encephalitis, general paralysis, disseminated sclerosis, etc.); after acute infectious diseases (diphtheria, influenza, etc.); in acute poisonings (alcohol, ptomaine, botulism, etc.); in diabetes and in exophthalmic goiter.

Course. The onset may be sudden or gradual. The course always is *chronic* and even in favorable cases, 6 weeks or more are required to effect a cure. *Relapses* are common. The prognosis depends upon the cause. After paralysis has existed for a long time the prognosis becomes less favorable on account of secondary changes (atrophy of the paralyzed muscle and contraction of the antagonist).

Treatment should be *directed to the cause.* In syphilis, energetic specific treatment is indicated; in diphtheria, strychnine; and in obscure cases potassium iodide is sometimes used.

Symptomatic treatment consists in relief of the diplopia. Prisms are rarely successful because even in slight paralysis the diplopia changes in amount in whatever direction the eye is moved. The only satisfactory way to avoid double vision is to *occlude one eye* by a patch or by a ground glass in a spectacle frame. The sound eye usually is occluded in order to hasten recovery or to prevent contracture.

If the condition persists for a long time in spite of all treatment, and if the paralysis seems incurable, *operative treatment* is indicated. This consists in a resection or advancement of the paralyzed muscle, combined, in many cases, with a tenotomy or recession of the antagonist; the results of this operation often are disappointing but the cosmetic improvement may be satisfactory.

Spasm of the Ocular Muscles is due to excessive innervation; it may be primary or secondary. *Primary spasm* is rare; it may be produced by meningeal or by reflex irritation. *Secondary spasm* is common and occurs with paralysis of one of the ocular muscles, producing excessive movement in the field of action of the spastic muscle causing deviation of the eye. It appears frequently in the direct antagonist of a paralyzed muscle, *e.g.*, spasm of the internal rectus following paralysis of the external rectus of the same eye. When the paralyzed eye is used for fixation, there often is a secondary spasmodic deviation of the *other* eye caused by spasm of the associate of the paralyzed muscle. The most common example of this type of deviation occurs in paralysis of the superior rectus followed by a spasm of the inferior oblique of the other eye. Treatment of secondary spasms is operative, *i.e.*, tenotomy or recession to weaken the action of the overactive muscle.

Congenital Paralyses are common, often being due to structural defects in the muscles themselves; the *superior rectus* is most frequently involved. Congenital fibrosis of the external rectus (*retraction syndrome* or *Duane's syndrome*) shows itself in inability to abduct the eye together with slight enophthalmos on abduction; the eyes may be straight in the primary position, or there may be a convergent squint; in the latter case, operation for cosmetic effect may be needed.

CONCOMITANT STRABISMUS

Concomitant strabismus (*concomitant squint or heterotropia*) is a *manifest deviation* from parallelism of the two eyes; these maintain the same faulty relationship of axes in every direction in which they are turned. The power of the different muscles of the two eyes usually is normal, and the squinting eye follows the other in all its movements, always deviating from the correct position to the same extent. The eye which is directed toward the object looked at is known as the *fixing eye*, the other as the *squinting eye*.

Concomitant strabismus differs from heterophoria, which is a latent deviation. It is distinguished from paralytic squint by presenting a *normal range of movement* of each eye and the *same deviation* in all parts of the visual field, while in paralysis the deviation is present only in the field of action of the paralyzed muscle and there is limitation of movement in a certain direction. In concomitant squint the *primary and secondary deviations are equal*, while in paralytic squint the secondary deviation is greater than the primary. Diplopia, a prominent symptom in paralytic squint, is seldom present in concomitant squint.

Varieties. Concomitant squint may be (1) *constant*, if present all the time; (2) *intermittent*, if under the same visual conditions it is present sometimes and absent at others; (3) *periodic*, if greater for near than for distance, and *vice versa*; (4) *continuous*, if equal in amount for both distance and near; (5) *monocular*, when one eye constantly deviates, the other being used habitually for fixation; (6) *alternating*, when the patient fixes with either eye indifferently, or one eye fixes for distance and the other for near.

According to the *direction of deviation*, concomitant squint is classified into (1) *convergent* strabismus (internal squint, esotropia); (2) *divergent* strabismus (external squint, exotropia); (3) *vertical* strabismus (strabismus sursum vergens, when upward; and deorsum vergens, when downward; hypertropia, right or left, according to the higher eye).

Diagnosis. This usually can be made by inspection, but in slight cases this cannot be depended upon. The *binocular uncovering test* affords a simple method of differentiating between a heterophoria and a squint: The patient fixes a test object and one eye is alternately covered and uncovered, leaving the other uncovered all the time. In heterophoria, when one eye is covered it deviates, and on removal of the screen it swings back into place to take up fixation with the other eye which has remained fixing; movement occurs only in the eye covered and uncovered. If the deviation is a squint and the squinting eye is covered and uncovered, no movement of either eye occurs; but when the fixing eye is covered and uncovered both eyes move.

The Measurement of Squint. The amount of deviation present can be measured (1) by the screen test, (2) by the perimeter and (3) by the corneal reflex test.

The screen test cannot be used where there is loss of power of fixation in one eye; in all others it is the most accurate method. With the patient fixing an object, a card is placed before one eye and then passed quickly to and fro from one eye to the other. The card is so passed that the patient has no chance to fix with both eyes at the same time but must alternate his fixation. Each eye when covered deviates, and when uncovered turns back into the fixing position. A prism (apex in for internal squint, apex out for external squint) of sufficient strength to abolish this movement of correction represents the exact amount of deviation present. This test usually is made both at 20 feet and at 13 inches, and the amount of deviation at both distances is recorded.

The perimeter (Fig. 3-5) gives the *angular measurement* of squint. The patient is seated with the *squinting eye* in the center of the instrument and is directed to fix with both eyes a distant object placed in the median line. A lighted candle or small electric lamp now is moved along the inside of the arc from the center outward until its reflection on the cornea is seen in the center of the pupil of the squinting eye; the number of degrees on the arc at this point indicates the angle of strabismus.

The corneal reflection test also measures the amount of squint in degrees of arc. The patient looks at a lighted candle held 1 foot in front of the eyes. The examiner, placed directly behind the light, observes the position of its reflection on the cornea of the squinting eye. If it is opposite the pupillary margin it indicates a deviation of approximately 15 degrees. If the reflex is at the margin of the cornea, it represents a squint of approximately 45 degrees. When the reflex lies in other positions, the angle of the deviation may be estimated by the rule that every millimeter of displacement of the reflex from the center of the cornea represents approximately 7 degrees of arc of squint.

Symptoms. The *disfigurement* is the symptom which usually leads the patient to consult an oculist. There is *no diplopia* except in the very early stages, the double images soon disappearing owing to a psychic process of *suppression* of the image of the squinting eye. There usually is *diminution in the acuity of vision* of the deviating eye (except in alternating squint). This may or may not have existed prior to the development of strabismus; in either case, it increases with the duration of the squint from disuse (*amblyopia ex anopsia*), and may become severe. There are no asthenopic symptoms.

Etiology. Concomitant squint results from abnormal supranuclear innervation, leading to *disproportion in strength between the power of convergence and the power of divergence.* To converge the eyes there must be simultaneous and equal contraction of both internal recti, causing equal movement inward of each eye. Divergence is effected largely through a relaxation of both internal recti, although some contraction of the external recti occurs. Divergence and convergence oppose each other; an overaction of one of them leads to a subsequent weakening of the other and *vice versa.*

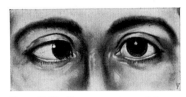

FIG. 21-12. Convergent strabismus.

Most concomitant squints start as an anomaly of one of these powers, but both soon become involved. A *disturbance in the normal balance* between convergence and divergence may be accommodative or nonaccommodative in origin.

The *accommodative squints* are those in which the normal relation between convergence and accommodation has been disturbed by *errors of refraction.*

The *nonaccommodative* cases comprise those with anisometropia, impaired vision in one eye from various causes and deficiency of the fusion faculty.

A congenital *defect of the fusion* faculty is believed to be important in causing squint; this faculty develops early and is complete before the sixth year; it forms a desire for binocular single vision which keeps the eyes straight. If congenitally absent, defective, late or imperfect in development, any disturbance of the motor coordinations, which preserve the normal relative directions of the eyes, will cause a squint.

In many cases, the retinal image formed at the macula of the fixing eye is associated with the image formed in an extramacular area of the retina of the squinting eye (*abnormal retinal correspondence,* binocular false projection, retinal incongruity). This is the more likely if the onset of squint is early and the angle large.

Convergent Concomitant Strabismus

In this form of squint (esotropia) there is *deviation inward* of the visual line of one eye (Fig. 21-12). It generally is asso-

ciated with *hyperopia*, with or without hyperopic astigmatism; rarely it occurs in myopia and in emmetropia. It usually commences in *early life*, between the *first and fourth years*, when the child begins to use his accommodation for near objects, such as toys and pictures; rarely it is congenital. At first the squint may be noticed only at times (periodic), with near vision, or when there is interference with the general health; but it is apt to become constant for both near and distant vision; occasionally it disappears at about the age of puberty.

The *acuteness of vision* in the squinting eye often presents considerable *reduction*, and there may be severe *amblyopia*, acquired *from disuse* of the squinting eye.

Development. A child who is hyperopic must use some accommodation for distance and more for near vision. *Accommodation and convergence* being *associated*, he must increase his convergence with increase of accommodation. In looking at a near object, the stimulus to converge not only corresponds to the amount present in the emmetrope, but includes an additional and abnormal amount called for by the extra accommodation required to compensate for his hyperopia. At first the child shows a spasmodic esophoria for near, owing to the overestimation of convergence; little by little the deviation increases until binocular fixation for near is impossible and he develops a squint at close range, along with which will be a slight esophoria for distance; then as time goes on, the deviation becomes manifest for both distance and near; in other words he develops a secondary weakening of his power of divergence. Exceptionally an esotropia begins as a primary squint for distance, due to a divergence insufficiency, with the later development of secondary excess of convergence.

Treatment comprises (1) optical—the correction of refractive errors by glasses,

(2) exercise of the squinting eye by occluding or atropinizing its fellow, (3) developing the fusion sense and (4) operation.

Nonoperative Treatment. The *error of refraction* should be estimated under *homatropine or atropine*, and convex *glasses* correcting very nearly the total hyperopia (also the astigmatism, if present) prescribed for *constant wear*. In slight cases, especially if periodic, this sometimes effects a cure. Glasses may be worn by infants or children of any age. It is sometimes advisable to keep the eyes atropinized for a week when the glasses first are worn. Bifocals may be useful in some cases of accommodative strabismus.

If very defective, vision of the squinting eye must be improved before nonsurgical treatment can be employed. The fixing eye must be *fully and continuously occluded* by a patch, bandage or attachment to the spectacle; this compels the squinting eye to fix, prevents amblyopia from disuse and tends to restore the sight of the deviating eye. However, the visual acuity must be tested in each eye every month, not only to determine improvement in the defective eye but also to prevent the development of an "occlusion" amblyopia in the occluded eye. Another plan, though less desirable, is to instil 1 drop of 0.5 per cent atropine into the fixing eye every morning, so as to encourage the use of the squinting eye for near vision. With either type of treatment, special activity such as cutting out objects along outlines or use of coloring books should be arranged to stimulate visual activity in the "open" eye.

Training of *binocular vision* aims at encouraging *the use of the two eyes at the same time,* thereby overcoming the habit of suppression of the image of one eye. The desire for the simultaneous use of both eyes then is used to *exercise the muscles* which can keep the eyes straight. In favorable cases this treatment alone may correct the squint.

It is important to use exercises which will hold the child's attention, and to vary them often in order to interest and amuse.

The instruments used are the stereoscope, the amblyoscope, the cheiroscope and the synoptophore.

The stereoscope is of value only for *home use* in the later stages of orthoptic training if the child has acquired true binocular projection.

The amblyoscope consists of two brass tubes joined by a hinge, each provided with a mirror and a convex lens. The two halves of the instrument can be brought together to suit a convergence up to 60°, or separated to suit a divergence of 30°. Vertical adjustments also can be made. Each tube is lighted by a separate electric lamp, the brilliancy of which can be regulated by a rheostat, thus increasing or diminishing the illumination of either of the *object slides*. The latter consist of pictures drawn on translucent celluloid squares and are of three classes: (1) those which do not require any blending of the images but only *simultaneous vision* of dissimilar objects with the two eyes (Fig. 21-13, for example); (2) devices of the second class (*e.g.*, Fig. 21-14), which require *true fusion* of images in order that the full picture may be seen; (3) devices such as are shown in Figure 21-15, which can only be appreciated by persons who have a *sense of perspective*.

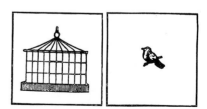

Fig. 21-13. Object slides used for orthoptic training (first degree, to encourage binocular perception).

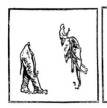 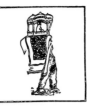

Fig. 21-14. Object slides used for orthoptic training (second degree, to encourage true fusion).

 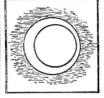

Fig. 21-15. Object slides used for orthoptic training (third degree, to encourage the sense of perspective).

The first step in the treatment is to *overcome the suppression of the image seen by the deviating eye.* The instrument is adjusted to the angle of the squint, and exercises are begun by showing pictures of the first group, to stimulate simultaneous perception. The illumination of the picture before the deviating eye is increased and the relative brilliancy of the lights adjusted until the objects on both sides are seen simultaneously; the bird is made to go into the cage and out again by slightly moving the two sides of the instrument. If projection has been found to be false, this has to be corrected first by special exercises. Many similar devices are shown until the symptom of suppression is entirely overcome under all conditions of illumination. The child next is taught to *fuse images* by using slides from the second group, and then is encouraged to keep them fused over as wide a range of movement (abduction and adduction) as possible. When the range or amplitude of fusion has been sufficiently increased, the

sense of *perspective* is developed by slides from group 3.

If good amplitude of fusion has been obtained there will be a strong tendency to binocular single vision. This tendency will be sufficient to overcome a small deviation or a deviation which has been approximately corrected by operation.

The cheiroscope is an instrument with which a test object (picture), reflected by means of a mirror so as to be seen by the sound eye, is projected by the other eye to a drawing board, where it is translated by tracing with a pencil guided by the hand. The hand, being directed by the eye under treatment, arouses interest of the defective eye, and coordination of the two eyes is effected by this effort of the hand.

The synoptophore (Fig. 21-16) is an elaborate development of the amblyoscope which has the advantage that the trainer has an unimpeded view of the patient's eyes; the position of the corneal reflexes given by the separate lights in each tube of the instrument can be watched and the *true position of the eyes observed*; this is impossible with the amblyoscope. One thus can determine whether the child is fixing the pictures with each macula (*true binocular projection*) or whether he is seeing the picture opposite the squinting eye with another part of the retina adjacent to the macula (*binocular false projection* or retinal incongruity).

The *most favorable age* for training is between 3 and 6 years; beyond the age of 7 years satisfactory results are rare. Good monocular fixation in the squinting eye is essential. If the child is old enough to be tested, the visual acuity should not be less than 20/60 with correcting glasses.

Orthoptic training requires much *time and patience* and the selection of *suitable cases.* The exercises often are delegated to experts who have been trained or to clinics equipped for this purpose. Such

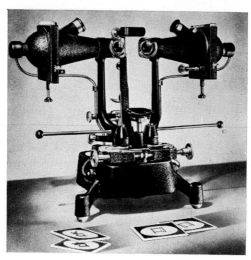

FIG. 21-16. The synoptophore.

training is of value in determining the selection of suitable cases for early operation.

The methods of training described above also may be used for treatment of *heterophoria* and in the slighter examples of paresis of ocular muscles.

Nonoperative treatment is successful in a fair proportion of cases of convergent concomitant squint *if used sufficiently early*. The earlier such treatment is begun, the better the results; after the sixth year it usually is not effective.

Operative Treatment. If nonoperative measures do not greatly improve or overcome the deviation after a thorough trial for 1 year, *operation* is indicated.

The production of binocular and stereoscopic vision is much more likely to follow early operation, and orthoptic exercises can be given much more successfully if the deviation is removed at an early age. Furthermore, a most important reason for early operation is the *unfavorable psychologic effect* that the disfigurement has upon the child. Any imperfect result of early operation can be repaired at a subsequent operation.

The operations used are *recession* (retroplacement) of the medial rectus or *advancement, resection* or *tucking* of the lateral rectus, or a combination of these procedures.

The choice of operation depends upon the amount of squint present for distance and for near, the lateral excursions for both eyes and the near point of convergence. *Careful examination* is necessary before deciding this question. As a rule, advancement (or resection) of one or both lateral rectus muscles, with or without recession of the medial rectus, is the operation of choice. If the squint is greater than 30 degrees and present for both distance and near, a combination of the two operations is indicated. In the infrequent cases in which the squint is present only for near, recession of the internal rectus is required; when the squint exists only for distance, an advancement or resection of the external rectus is called for. In some patients with alternating esotropia, a bilateral recession of the medial rectus may be indicated. These operations are done first on the squinting eye and subsequently, if necessary, on the other eye;

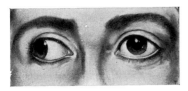

FIG. 21-17. Divergent strabismus.

they may be done on both eyes at the same time. The rules above presuppose that the patient is wearing full correction.

Divergent Concomitant Strabismus

This form of squint (exotropia) exists when one eye fixes an object and the other *deviates outward* (Fig. 21-17). It usually is associated with *myopia*, but may occur with hyperopia. It occurs frequently after the *loss of useful vision in one eye*, the sight of the other eye remaining good; here the incentive to converge is destroyed. It sometimes occurs after tenotomies performed for the cure of internal squint. Divergent strabismus usually does not become manifest in early childhood, but usually *develops in youth* or early adult life. It is much less frequent than convergent squint.

Development. These cases start as either (1) insufficiency of convergence or (2) excess of divergence.

Some cases of concomitant divergent strabismus start as a *weakness of convergence* due to myopia. In nearsightedness, little or no accommodation is needed for near vision; consequently there is an habitual deficiency of the stimulus for convergence; this power, therefore, weakens and the patient has a deviation at close range but none at distance; then there is a gradual increase in the amount of deviation until it is present at all distances.

On the other hand, *divergence excess* is common as a primary condition, and as such at first shows a divergence only at distance, but as time goes on the power of convergence weakens and the deviation persists for both distance and near. This type of deviation is found independently of the refractive error, which usually is low in amount and hyperopic in character.

Treatment. The *full correction* of any existing myopia is indicated; this will correct those cases due to an uncorrected myopia, where the deviation is still periodic. *Operation* is required in all other cases. *Recession of the lateral rectus* is the operation of choice where the deviation is present only at distance; this can be done on one eye or on both, according to the amount of deviation present. In all cases where the converging power is severely weakened, an *advancement* (or resection) of one or both medial recti should be done. A deviation which is continuous and equal in amount both at 20 feet and at 13 inches should have a combination of these operations performed on one or both eyes.

Heterophoria

Heterophoria is a *latent deviation* in which the eyes have a *constant tendency to deviate* and do so when one eye is covered. This deviation is *overcome by muscular effort* because of the strong desire to maintain binocular single vision. In concomitant strabismus the deviation is manifest. As the same etiologic factors produce both conditions, heterophoria and concomitant squint are differentiated solely by the patient's ability to overcome the deviation. A deviation therefore may be a heterophoria on one examination and a squint on the next.

Varieties. When a normal person fixes an object, both eyes are directed at that object under all conditions. This condition of perfect muscle balance is known as *orthophoria*. The varieties of imperfect muscle balance (heterophoria) are (1) *exophoria*, a tendency to deviate *outward*; (2) *esophoria*, a tendency to deviate *inward*; (3) *hyperphoria*, a tendency of one eye to deviate *upward—right* hyperphoria when the right eye tends to deviate upward, *left* hyperphoria when the left eye tends to deviate upward; this variety may be associated with exophoria or esophoria; (4) *cyclophoria*, a tendency of the vertical meridian of one eye to deviate from the vertical position.

Tests. Some of the tests are used both at 20 feet and at 13 inches, since the state of muscular balance or imbalance at both of these distances must be known to make a definite diagnosis.

A candle flame or a small electric light is a satisfactory test object. When the eyes are in a state of *perfect balance*, there is orthophoria for distance (1° to 2° of either esophoria or exophoria also are considered normal), a normal prism divergence, a slight exophoria (2° to 4°) for near, a normal near point of convergence and normal motility in all fields.

The *amount* of heterophoria present for both distance and near can be determined satisfactorily by the use of (1) the screen and parallax test (the cover test), (2) the Maddox rod and (3) the phorometer.

The screen and parallax test. This is a combination of the objective screen test and the subjective parallax test. It is done exactly as described on p. 333, except that in addition to the observer observing the direction in which the eyes move, the patient reports the *direction of the movement of the test object*. A *prism* of sufficient strength to abolish all movement of both the test object and the eye represents the exact amount of deviation. This combined test is very accurate; deflection of 0.5° can be measured by it.

The Maddox rod (Fig. 21-18) consists of one or more pieces of colorless or red glass rod set in a hard rubber disk, so as to fit into the trial frame. It converts

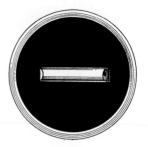

Fig. 21-18. Maddox rod.

the image of the flame perceived by one eye into a long streak of light, so that there remains no desire to fuse it with the image of the other eye. Any strong convex cylinder answers the same purpose. The line is always at right angles to the axis of the rod.

The Maddox rod is placed in the *horizontal* plane before the right eye, converting its image of the candle flame into a vertical streak. If *orthophoria* is present, this streak appears to pass directly through the image seen with the other eye (Fig. 21-19, *left*). If the line of light appears to the left of the flame, there is crossed diplopia, indicating *exophoria* (Fig. 21-19, *center*); if to the right of the flame, there is homonymous diplopia, indicating *esophoria* (Fig. 21-19, *right*). The amount of heterophoria is measured by the prism, base in or out, which serves to displace the streak until it runs directly through the flame.

The rod then is placed in the *vertical* plane before the right eye, converting the image of this eye into a horizontal line of light, which will pass through the image of the left eye (Fig. 21-20, *left*) if *orthophoria* prevails. If the line is below the image of the flame seen with the left eye, there is *right hyperphoria* (Fig. 21-20, *right*); if above, there is *left hyperphoria* (Fig. 21-20, *center*). The degree of hyperphoria is measured by the prism, base up or down, which causes the light streak to pass directly through the flame.

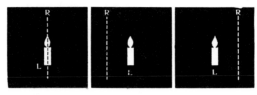

Fig. 21-19. The Maddox rod test. *Left*, in orthophoria; *center*, in exophoria; *right*, in esophoria.

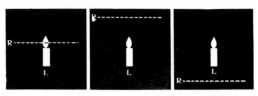

Fig. 21-20. The Maddox rod test. *Left*, in orthophoria; *center*, in left hyperphoria; *right*, in right hyperphoria.

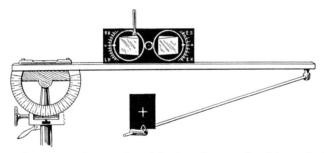

Fig. 21-21. The phorometer (base and upright have been omitted from the illustration).

The phorometer (Fig. 21-21) consists of a pair of 5° or 6° prisms which are placed with their bases up and down so as to produce vertical diplopia; if the double images do not appear one exactly over the other, there is exophoria or esophoria; by rotation of the prisms, the images can be brought into vertical alignment, and the degree of rotation required, which can be read off on an attached arc, indicates the amount of exophoria or esophoria. Hyperphoria is determined in a similar manner, the prisms being placed with their bases in. The test object for near is a small metal plate, in the center of which is a small cross with perforation.

The near point of convergence is determined by moving a fine test object (small white-headed pin) up to the eyes to determine the nearest point at which, with maximum effort, convergence can be maintained. This point should not be more than 75 mm. from the anterior focal plane of the eye (the plane on which spectacles are worn). Any persistent remoteness of the near point of convergence denotes a weakness of that power.

In addition to determining the amount of heterophoria for distance and near, it is important to measure the amount of prism the eyes can overcome. *Prism divergence* (*abduction*) is the ability to overcome prisms base in while looking at a distant object; the normal limits of this power are from 4° to 9°; it is constant and gives reliable information of the diverging power. *Prism convergence (abduction)* is the ability to overcome prisms base out; it is variable in amount and is of value only when repeated tests show a subnormal power; the normal limits are from 15° to 40°. The *rotary prism* (Fig. 21-22) is a convenient instrument for measuring these powers.

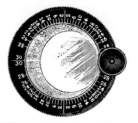

FIG. 21-22. The rotary prism.

Symptoms. In slight degrees of heterophoria very often there are no symptoms whatever. In greater degrees, the symptoms of *muscular asthenopia* occur: headaches, pain in the eyes, indistinctness or "running together" of print, heavy and uncomfortable sensations referred to the eyelids, diplopia, nausea and vertigo. These asthenopic symptoms are the result of the *strain* imposed upon the muscles in overcoming the deviation. There frequently are periods of clear vision with strain, alternating with periods of diplopia with confused vision. Head tilting (ocular torticollis) may occur as a result of the patient's endeavor to correct diplopia, particularly if it is vertical. These symptoms may be more severe on close use of the eyes, or on looking at distant objects, depending upon the cause of the heterophoria. A characteristic feature of the symptoms due to muscular trouble is their disappearance on the closure of one eye. Neurasthenia and disturbances of digestion and nutrition may be the result of the muscular imbalance in predisposed individuals.

Etiology. Heterophoria may be *refractive* or *nonrefractive in origin*.

An *error of refraction* is a frequent cause for a disturbance of the normal relationship between accommodation and convergence. For example, a hyperope has to use an abnormally great amount of accommodation to maintain clear vision; thus his power of convergence is constantly overstimulated and esophoria re-

sults; conversely, a myope uses too little accommodation and is likely to develop exophoria.

Heterophoria of *nonrefractive* origin is common, since all the cases due to a primary dysfunction (overactivity or underactivity) of the power of divergence are not influenced by the state of refraction; it is equally true that many cases of weakness of convergence result from nonrefractive causes. Heterophoria frequently is seen in neurasthenia, hysteria, anemia and focal infections, and in persons who are debilitated from any cause whatever; it also is found in perfectly healthy individuals. Occasionally an anatomic defect of one of the external muscles is responsible for the deviation.

Treatment consists in correction of the error of refraction, attention to the general health, prism exercises, the wearing of prisms and, as a last resort, operation. *Correction of the refractive error* is of the greatest importance, and frequently is curative, though some cases are uninfluenced by glasses. An esophoria due to a *convergence excess, i.e.,* one which is greatest in amount at close range, usually is corrected by the constant use of the full hyperopic and astigmatic correction; if myopia is present it should be undercorrected. A *convergence insufficiency* causing an exophoria for near range calls for a full correction of the myopia and an undercorrection of the hyperopia. An exophoria or an esophoria due to a *divergence* anomaly, *i.e.,* greater for distance, is not materially influenced by the correction of a refractive error.

Attention to the general health is a necessary and valuable adjunct to local treatment, especially in neurasthenic and debilitated individuals who show a high degree of exophoria at close range and a very remote near point of convergence, with no refractive error to account for the deviation.

Prism exercises are used chiefly in *exophoria* due to a nonaccommodative weakness of convergence. Here the patient looks at a lighted candle, a prism base out is placed before one eye and the two images are fused into one; after a few seconds the prism is removed. Starting with a weak prism (5°), the strength is gradually increased until the patient can overcome at least a 50° prism base out. This exercise is used at either 20 feet or 13 inches, or at both distances. It is continued for several minutes two or three times a day and must be persisted in for several weeks to give results. In esophoria and hyperphoria prism exercises are not satisfactory.

Prisms for wear may be used to correct deviations of low degree; the apex always is placed in the direction in which the eye turns. They are most satisfactory in hyperphoria when limited to the amount present in the lower field. In esophoria and exophoria, prisms constantly worn tend to increase the deviation and are not generally advisable; in selected cases they may give temporary relief.

If glasses are worn, the effect of a prism may be obtained by *decentering*—that is, displacing the optical center so that it no longer corresponds to the geometric center of the lens. *Decentering a convex lens in*, or a *concave lens out*, produces the effect of a *prism* with its *base toward the nose*; decentering a convex lens up or a concave lens down gives the effect of a prism with its base up. A lens of 1.00 D. must be decentered 8.7 mm. to produce the effect of a prism of 1°. To calculate the amount of decentering necessary to produce a certain prismatic effect, multiply 8.7 by the value of the prism, and divide the result by the strength of the lens in diopters. For example, a +4.00 D. lens ◯ prism of 2°, base in, equals (8.7 × 2)/4 or 4.3 mm.; such a lens should be decentered inward 4.3 mm. in order to have the added effect of a prism of 2° base in.

Operation, if used in carefully chosen cases, gives satisfactory results, but is not indicated until one is certain that no other measures will suffice. Its success depends entirely upon a correct diagnosis of the underlying conditions producing the heterophoria. In exophoria due to divergence excess, the best results are obtained by a *recession* of the external rectus.

Operation. The operations used to correct muscular deviations are (1) *tenotomy and recession*, intended to weaken a muscle, and (2) *advancement, resection and tucking*, designed to strengthen a muscle.

Tenotomy rarely is performed except upon the inferior oblique and superior oblique muscles.

Tenotomy of the inferior oblique is indicated in spasm of the inferior oblique, either secondary to paresis or paralysis of the opposite superior rectus, or in the rare primary cases; it is also performed on an eye affected with incurable paralysis of the superior oblique. A small incision is made with scissors in the medial portion of the lower conjunctival fornix, and the dissection is continued to the floor of the orbit. A muscle hook is passed into the opening at the lateral end of the incision, and pushed back in contact with the floor of the orbit; then the inferior oblique muscle is engaged by sweeping the hook nasally. Gentle traction causes up-

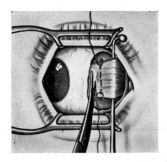 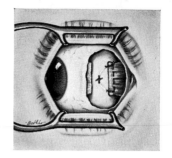

Fig. 21-23. Recession of medial rectus muscle. *Left,* the tendon being severed; *right,* the tendon sutured to sclera behind stump.

ward movement of the eyeball if the muscle has been secured. The muscle is drawn forward and isolated from surrounding tissue; it then is cut between two clamps so as to effect a myotomy or myectomy. The conjunctival incision is closed with one or two gut or silk sutures, and an adhesive dressing is applied for 2 days.

Tenotomy or tenectomy of the superior oblique muscle may be employed for the treatment of hypertropia associated with overaction of this muscle. The superior oblique tendon is reached through the conjunctiva on the nasal side of the superior rectus muscle. The reflected tendon of the superior oblique muscle and its sheath are engaged on a muscle hook. The tendon sheath is opened and the tendon is severed or a portion resected, depending upon the effect desired. The conjunctiva is closed by means of one or two gut sutures.

Recession generally is used now in the surgical treatment of squint. It preserves the effects of tenotomy and adds an element of *precision and safety* lacking in tenotomy. This operation consists of tenotomy and *suturing the severed muscle to the sclera* at a selected point back of its original attachment.

Technique. Recession of the internal rectus is performed as follows: A vertical incision of the conjunctiva 7 to 8 mm. in length is made about 1 mm. in front of the semilunar fold; the conjunctiva is dissected away, completely exposing Tenon's capsule and the underlying muscle. Tenon's capsule is opened by buttonholing about 3 mm. above and well behind the insertion of the muscle; a squint hook is inserted through this opening and swept behind the muscle and the capsule is opened at a corresponding point below. With the scissors, horizontal incisions are carried backward from the openings in the capsule both above and below, dividing lateral attachments, and in this way isolating the muscle. Its tendon then is transfixed with two double-armed (Fig. 21-23, *left*) gut sutures, and cut from its insertion. The sutures are passed through the outer layer of the sclera at a point posterior to the insertion, which previously has been decided upon. The sutures are tied (Fig. 21-23, *right*), the conjunctival incision is closed with interrupted gut sutures and a firm adhesive dressing is applied for 24 hours.

The procedure with the other rectus muscles is the same, with allowances for the variations in the distance from the limbus at which different muscles are inserted.

The amount of recession is determined by the operator after measurement of the squint. The internal rectus should never be recessed more than 5 mm. from the insertion of the muscle, and rarely so much.

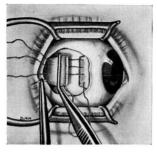 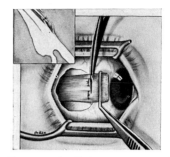

FIG. 21-24. Resection of lateral rectus muscle (Lancaster). *Left*, sutures are being passed through muscle behind forceps; *right*, sutures are tied and muscle is being excised.

Recession of the inferior oblique at its insertion is being employed for spasm of this muscle.

Advancement and Resection of an Ocular Muscle. The term advancement may be applied in a general sense to any operation designed to increase the action of an ocular muscle. There are three varieties: (1) *advancement*, which brings the attachment of the muscle further forward, (2) *resection*, in which a piece of the muscle is cut out, thus shortening the muscle, and (3) *muscle tucking*, in which a permanent fold is made in the muscle and the latter thus is shortened.

Advancement. In slight deviations it will be sufficient to advance the muscle without receding its opponent; for squints of greater degree, it is best to include a recession upon the opposing muscle. Many methods of advancement have been designed. A simple procedure comprises exposure and isolation of the muscle tendon as described under the recession operation; advancement forceps grasp the tendon which is severed from its insertion; two double-armed gut sutures are passed through the cut end of the muscle and through the outer scleral fibers anterior to the muscle stump and tied; the conjunctival incision is closed with interrupted or continuous gut sutures. The immediate effect is the permanent result, and overcorrection is not necessary. The operated eye is dressed for 24 hours.

Resection. One of the best of the muscle-shortening operations is that devised by Lancaster. Local anesthesia may be sufficient, but general anesthesia is preferred, especially in children and nervous individuals.

A vertical incision is made in the conjunctiva along the insertion of the muscle. At the upper and lower ends of the wound an opening is made into the tissue anterior to the sclera, through which a strabismus hook is passed upward beneath the muscle. With the muscle held taut it is carefully freed from surrounding tissues. One blade of the advancement forceps is inserted under the muscle and the forceps is clamped on the tendon about 3 mm. from its insertion; the tendon should be thoroughly spread out on the clamp before it is closed; it is divided 1 mm. from its insertion, leaving a stump.

Two double-armed gut sutures are then passed through the muscle at the desired distance behind the cut end (Fig. 21-24, *left*). The clamp is brought forward and the sutures are tightened and tied. The portion of muscle distal to the sutures is excised (Fig. 21-24, *right*). The conjunctiva is closed with interrupted gut sutures and a firm adhesive dressing applied for 24 hours.

Tendon tucking. Many operations for producing permanent folding of the muscles have been advocated. The muscle and tendon are exposed and freed from all attachments to the sclera, and then a portion of the muscle is folded upon itself, often by means of a specially constructed double or triple hook; the folds of tendon are then sewn together with catgut, and thus a permanent shortening of the muscle is produced.

Nystagmus

Nystagmus is a short, rapid, involuntary *oscillation* of the eyeball, usually affecting *both* eyes and associated with *imperfect vision;* it may be *congenital* or *acquired.* The movements most frequently are from side to side (*lateral nystagmus*) or around the anteroposterior axis (*rotary nystagmus*), sometimes up and down (*vertical nystagmus*). There may be a combination of the lateral or vertical with the rotary movements (*mixed nystagmus*). The oscillations are similar in kind, duration and frequency in the two eyes. They may be constant or present or exaggerated only when the eyes are turned in certain directions. The patient as a rule is *not inconvenienced* by the existence of this condition, but when it commences in adult life there may be much annoyance from the apparent movement of objects.

Most cases exist from *infancy*, and depend upon diminution in the acuteness of vision or *amblyopia* as a result of opacities of the media, intraocular diseases, albinism and other congenital anomalies, and severe errors of refraction; in such instances the affection is due to defective vision, which prevents the infant or child from learning to fix properly.

In adults it may develop with many *cerebral affections*, especially disseminated sclerosis, disease of the cerebellum and Friedreich's disease. It is found in miners (*miner's nystagmus*); in these cases it is due to defective illumination and strain and exhaustion of the ocular muscles, because the eyes must be turned in unnatural directions, especially when predisposed by errors of refraction. It occurs also in labyrinthine irritation and disease (*labyrinthine nystagmus*).

The usual infantile cases are *not amenable to treatment*, though the condition sometimes decreases with advancing years; the *correction of errors of refraction* may be of some benefit. Miner's nystagmus generally disappears when the patient gives up this kind of work, and the labyrinthine variety ceases after the cause has been removed.

22

Ocular Therapeutics
General Rules for Eye Operations

The eye being a very delicate and sensitive organ, it becomes necessary, in applying various therapeutic resources, to limit the strength of local applications and to observe care in the manner in which such remedies are applied. However the eye offers a unique opportunity for the observation and study of the effects of a wide variety of drugs such as parasympathetic stimulants or blocking agents, sympathetic stimulants or adrenergic blocking agents, acute bacterial, acute fungal and acute viral agents as well as acute inflammatory drugs and a large number of other drugs used either for the treatment of ocular or general disease. Also because of the variety of tissues and cells in the eye a number of different toxic effects of drugs may be observed in different portions of the eye.

Treatment of disease of the eye may be divided into (1) *constitutional* and (2) *local* measures.

Constitutional forms of therapy frequently are prescribed and often exercise great influence on the progress of ocular disease. Many systemic disorders present ocular manifestations, and an important part of the treatment of the latter consists in general medication intended to correct the constitutional disturbance. Syphilis, tuberculosis, anemia and other general diseases give rise to eye symptoms and diseases which will yield only after proper *general treatment*. Some ocular diseases are dependent upon a lowering of the general health, for which appropriate treatment is indicated. *Rest in bed* often is absolutely necessary for

the effective control of some of the acute affections of the deeper structures of the eye. Thus it is evident that the patient's general condition, cannot be disregarded in the treatment of ocular diseases.

Local. Drugs intended for local use are most frequently dissolved in *water,* physiologic salt solution, an aqueous buffer vehicle or a buffer solution containing a compound such as methyl cellulose or polyvinyl alcohol which increases the viscosity of the drops. Some drugs are prepared for local use in oily solutions or suspensions, in ointment, as fine powder or in solid form. Occasionally drugs in aqueous or buffer solutions are injected under the conjunctiva or into the anterior chamber; however, because of the intense inflammatory reactions these injections usually induce, other methods of enhancing local absorption of the medication are preferred. These include the application of a surface tension reducing agent simultaneously or a minute or two before applying the medication, placing the drug under a contact lens, placing saturated pledgets of cotton in the fornix for 5 or 10 minutes and adding drops of the medicine every minute during this treatment, or by the use of iontophoresis.

For treatment of lesions of the lid, lid margin and conjunctiva the medication may be applied in any vehicle but when the cornea is injured or ulcerated or when there has been a penetrating wound of the globe oily solutions and ointments are to be avoided because of the delay and interference with healing they produce.

Topical solutions may be uncomfortable

346

and irritating unless the hydrogen ion concentration lies within a range of pH 6.5 to pH 8.5 and the tonicity of the solution is close to that of tears which have a tonicity equivalent to a 1.4 per cent saline solution.

Topical and local medications for use on the eye should be sterile and in addition should contain a preservative which will maintain sterility. Preparation of sterile eye solutions is difficult unless proper equipment is available. For this reason local pharmacists increasingly have come to depend upon the large drug manufacturers to supply prepackaged sterile ophthalmic preparations which meet the standards set by the pharmacopoeia and the Food and Drug Administration.

Cleansing and Irrigating Solutions

Solutions of this sort are employed for *flushing* the conjunctival sac and *removing secretions.* They should be *bland,* and used *lukewarm.* They are allowed to run between the lids from a wad of *absorbent cotton,* from an *eye dropper* (two or three dropperfuls), poured out very conveniently by means of the *undine* (Fig. 22-1), with a soft-rubber bulb syringe or with an eye irrigator.

The cleansing and protective solutions used most frequently are: *sodium chloride* in 1.4 per cent solution (isotonic with the tears); *alkaline eye drops; mercuric chloride* from 1:10,000 to 1:6,000; *methyl cellulose* in 0.5 to 1 per cent solution.

Methyl Cellulose solution, instilled into the conjunctival sac every hour or two, protects the cornea from drying in keratoconjunctivitis sicca, lagophthalmos and after operations for ptosis. However, because of its viscosity it remains on the conjunctiva longer than aqueous solutions; therefore it also is useful as a vehicle for medications.

Alkaline Eye Drops. An excellent eye wash is:

℞ Sodii bicarbonat.	1.00 (gr. xv)
Sodii biborat.	1.00 (gr. xv)
Sodii chloridi	1.00 (gr. xv)
Glycerini	4.00 (ℨ i)
Aquae filtrat.	250.00 (ℨ viii)

M.S. Eye wash.

This solution will be found very useful for general and free use in the various forms of conjunctivitis and for washing out the eyes following exposure to wind and dust.

Patients often find it refreshing and useful to wash out the conjunctival sac upon arising and when retiring, or after exposure to wind and dust, and then prefer to make the solution themselves. In such cases, the following directions can be given for preparing the eye wash at home:

"Take a moderately heaped teaspoonful *each* of bicarbonate of soda, of borax, and of table salt; dissolve these in one quart of boiled water; add a teaspoonful of glycerine, and filter."

Before using any eye wash, the lashes should be cleansed with cotton wet with the solution.

When flushing the conjunctival sac, the escaping fluid may be caught much more neatly than with a pus basin, by a roll of

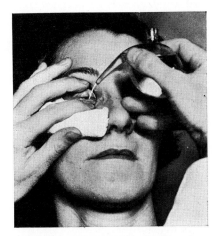

FIG. 22-1. Method of irrigating the eye with a solution poured from an undine.

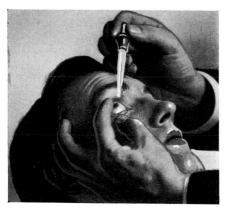

FIG. 22-2. Method of instilling drops by means of an eye dropper.

Cellucotton (cellulose) pressed against the cheek below the lower lid (Fig. 22-1); this wood pulp product resembles absorbent cotton in texture, is cheap and is much more absorbent than ordinary cotton.

A simple and equally effective solution is a 1 per cent aqueous solution of *monohydrated sodium carbonate*. It is especially valuable in dissolving stringy mucoid secretions, such as occur in vernal conjunctivitis.

Stimulating and Astringent Remedies

The remedies of this class used most frequently are zinc sulfate, camphor, silver nitrate, copper sulfate, yellow oxide of mercury and ammoniated mercury. They are used chiefly in various forms of *conjunctivitis*. Most of these remedies are employed in *watery solution*. Such solutions are prescribed in *small quantity;* 1 or 2 drops are allowed to fall upon the everted lower lid from an eye dropper (Fig. 22-2); the latter must not touch the lids or lashes, since such contact might infect the liquid contained in the bottle to which the dropper is returned.

Zinc Sulfate is used very often in chronic forms of conjunctivitis:

℞ Zinci sulf.   0.03 (gr. ss)
   Acidi borici   0.15 (gr. iiss)
   Aquae destill.   15.0 (℥ ss)
M.S. Two drops in each eye twice a day.

℞ Zinci sulf.   0.03 (gr. ss)
   Aqua camphor.   0.30 (M. v)
   Aquae destill.   15.0 (℥ ss)
M.S. Eye drops.

Camphor. Though feebly soluble in water, aqua camphorae is stimulating and astringent, and often is incorporated in collyriums.

Yellow Oxide of Mercury, insoluble in water, is employed in an *ointment* made with petrolatum, cold cream or lanolin (1 to 3 per cent) when a strong irritant is indicated.

Ammoniated Mercury, a white, insoluble powder, is prescribed as a 3, 5 or 10 per cent ointment in the treatment of blepharitis marginalis, particularly of the seborrheic variety.

Occasionally persons are allergic to all mercury compounds and then the local use causes undue, often severe, conjunctival reaction with swelling and inflammation of the lids; in such cases their use is contraindicated. Pigmentation of the skin of the eyelids may follow prolonged use of ointments containing mercury compounds.

Ointments intended for home use are available in *collapsible metal tubes*; the patient is directed to pull down the lower lid, place the uncovered opening of the tube upon the everted conjunctiva, press out a small portion of the ointment and then to close the lids before withdrawing the point of the tube; otherwise the ointment will be withdrawn with removal of the tube.

Disinfectants and Cauterants

True disinfectants (capable of destroying germs) cannot be instilled into the conjunctival sac without injury to the cornea; they are, however, applied to *circumscribed* areas, the excess being washed off with water. Some of the remedies classified under this head, though not strictly speaking true disinfectants in the strength used, have an inhibitory action upon the growth of micro-organisms and thus act as *practical disinfectants.* Those used most commonly in connection with the eye are mercuric chloride, Metaphen, carbolic acid, tincture of iodine, trichloracetic acid, silver nitrate, Argyrol, Protargol, iodoform, ethylhydrocupreine, the thermophore and the cautery.

Mercuric Chloride (corrosive sublimate) is used occasionally in the treatment of resistant forms of conjunctivitis. It may be used safely in 1:5000 solution; when stronger, it injuries the cornea, and consequently must be limited to the everted lids, and the excess carefully washed off.

Corrosive sublimate is used in 1:3000 *ointment;* this salve is bland, antiseptic and useful at times in various forms of conjunctivitis, ulcers of the cornea and phylctenular affections, serving to keep the conjunctival sac filled with a weak disinfectant and to prevent adhesion of the lid margins overnight.

Metaphen, an organic mercury derivative, comes from the manufacturer in 1:500 solution and is diluted with distilled water. It then is suitable for use as drops or irrigating solution in the treatment of purulent and other forms of *conjunctivitis.*

Carbolic Acid, Pure, and Trichloracetic Acid, Pure, are sometimes applied to *infected ulcers* of the cornea.

Tincture of Iodine is a useful remedy in the treatment of infective and dendritic *ulcers* of the cornea.

Silver Nitrate, always dissolved in *distilled water,* is an astringent in weak solution (0.02 to 0.04 per cent) but is an anti-septic and a cauterizing agent in stronger solutions (0.5 to 10.0 per cent). The stronger solutions are applied with a moistened, but not dripping, applicator to the skin, the lid margins or the anesthetized conjunctiva. It produces coagulation of the superficial cells. This material should be removed either mechanically or by irrigation a few minutes after it has formed and loosened.

Silver nitrate in 1 per cent or 2 per cent aqueous solution, or silver acetate in 1 per cent aqueous solution, may be used in the Credé method of prophylaxis against gonorrheal ophthalmia in the newborn. Solutions of silver nitrate spoil upon contact with organic matter; the brush or cotton applicator should not be dipped into the bottle, but some of the solution should be poured into a small vessel for each use. Silver solutions, when used for any length of time, may permanently *stain* the conjunctiva (*argyrosis,* Plate 12*B*); hence their use should be restricted to a *limited period.*

Copper Sulfate ("bluestone") is used as a 0.1 to 0.125 per cent aqueous solution, 0.5 to 1.0 per cent glycerine solution or 0.25 to 0.5 per cent ointment for the treatment of fungus infections and trachoma.

Argyrol, an *organic salt of silver* used in 5 to 25 per cent watery solution, is employed in the hospital but should never be prescribed for use by the patient at home. It is penetrating, not precipitated by albuminous fluids, and is *devoid of the irritating qualities* of silver nitrate, but it may leave a brown spot on the cornea when ulceration exists. Its solutions must be *freshly prepared* once a week and kept in dark bottles. Argyrol has moderate broad germicidal activity and is used frequently preliminary to irrigation of the conjunctiva, for complete removal of the brownish color indicates thorough mechanical cleansing of the conjunctiva. It is especially valuable, for this reason, just prior to intraocular surgery.

Permanent brown or purplish *staining* of the bulbar and palpebral conjunctiva, especially the lower part (*argyrosis*, Plate 12B), often is seen after frequent instillation and long continued home use of all silver salts; this may follow from the common habit of using Argyrol as a panacea for all eye affections. For these reasons, it should never be given to patients and its home use should be avoided. Disfigurement from argyrosis can be removed or lessened by subconjunctival injections of ferricyanidethiosulfate solution.

Protargol (5 to 25 per cent) and other organic silver salts known by trade names (Neo-Silvol) have properties similar to Argyrol.

Ethylhydrocupreine (Optochin), a derivative of quinine, is used in *pneumococcus* ulcer in 1 per cent solution.

The Thermophore, an instrument with which a high degree of electrically generated heat can be controlled, is useful in all forms of *corneal ulcers*, but especially in the infected variety. The head of the instrument is applied directly to the ulcer, after local anesthesia, and kept there at a temperature which may be varied according to indication; with hypopyon keratitis this should be 155° F. for 1 minute. It also is of benefit in marginal chalazia.

The Electrocautery occasionally is used to limit the spread of *corneal ulcers*, by destroying the infecting micro-organisms, and also occasionally in conical cornea when contact lenses fail.

Mydriatics and Cycloplegics

Mydriatics are remedies which produce *dilatation of the pupil; cycloplegics* are agents which cause *paralysis of the ciliary muscle* and of accommodation. Practically,

these terms are *interchangeable*, since, with few exceptions, mydriatics also produce paralysis of the ciliary muscle.

The commonly employed cycloplegics are *atropine*, scopolamine and *homatropine*. The agents used to *dilate the pupil*, with practically no action on the ciliary muscle, are *cocaine, Euphthalmine, Paredrine, Benzedrine* and *ephedrine*.

Indications. Atropine, scopolamine or one of the other cycloplegics is used (1) to paralyze accommodation in estimating the state of refraction and (2) in various diseases of the cornea, inflammatory diseases of the iris and ciliary body, and after certain operations to dilate the pupil to prevent adhesions and to put the iris and ciliary body at rest to overcome photophobia and the pain of movement of the inflamed iris and ciliary body.

Atropine Sulfate, the alkaloid of belladonna, is a parasympatholytic drug and is used in small children in 0.5 per cent solution or ointment, in older children and adults in 1 per cent solution and occasionally in deeply pigmented individuals in 2 per cent aqueous solution.

The paralytic effect of atropine on the sphincter of the pupil and the ciliary muscle reaches its maximum 1 hour after instillation upon the cornea, remains at a maximum for a short time and then subsides slowly over the course of 1 week. Repeated doses tend to prolong the maximum effect. Thus in young children 0.5 per cent solution or ointment usually is administered three times a day for 3 days with the last drop instilled 1 hour prior to refraction. In older children and adults, the drops may be used as frequently as five times in the 24 hours preceding the refraction, or 1 drop every 5 minutes for three times after a preliminary drop of a surface active agent such as 5 per cent cocaine hydrochloride, 1 per cent Paredrine hydrobromide or 1 per cent Benzedrine sulfate. For prolonged cycloplegia in corneal or anterior uveal disease, 0.5 or 1 per cent solution may be used once, twice or three times a day.

Atropine is *contraindicated in glaucoma* and in persons who have a tendency to this disease. Therefore the ocular tension should be tested in persons over 35 years of age before instilling atropine or any other cycloplegic.

Atropine poisoning. In susceptible individuals, atropine may cause *general toxic symptoms*: dryness of the throat, flushing of the face, headache, vomiting, quick pulse, cutaneous eruption, excitability and even delirium. *The antidote is morphine.* In such cases, absorption occurs from the nasopharyngeal mucosa after passage through the nasolacrimal passages, in addition to that from the conjunctiva.

Thus pressure should be applied over the lacrimal sac for 2 minutes after each instillation, or in especially susceptible individuals another cycloplegic should be used.

Atropine irritation may result in chronic conjunctivitis of either a follicular or a papillary variety after prolonged use of the drug, and a high percentage of patients develop contact sensitivity of the conjunctiva and skin of the lids after prolonged or repeated use.

Scopolamine Hydrobromide is another parasympatholytic agent closely related to atropine which is used for the same purposes or as a substitute in individuals who have become sensitive to atropine. Scopolamine usually is prescribed as 0.2 per cent drops or ointment. It has a span of activity of 3 to 4 days increased to 5 days by repeated instillations. This is somewhat shorter than the action of atropine. It is less likely to result in sensitization of a patient on prolonged use than is atropine. However it produces general toxic symptoms in susceptible individuals or in patients in whom there is excessive absorption. They

consist of dryness of the mouth, flushing, excitement and delusions.

Homatropine Hydrobromide also a parasympatholytic drug resembles atropine, but is *weaker*. It is used as a 5 per cent solution for refraction in adults, and sometimes as a substitute for atropine or scopolamine when a more transient effect is desired. The cycloplegic action lasts only 48 hours. *Paredrine* hydrobromide (1 per cent) or *Benzedrine* sulfate (1 per cent) is sometimes used in conjunction with homatropine to enhance the cycloplegic effects of the latter.

Cyclopentolate Hydrochloride (Cyclogyl) another parasympatholytic agent has a shorter span of activity (18 to 24 hours) than homatropine but at its height of activity is almost as effective. It is used as a 0.5 or 1.0 per cent solution.

Tropicamide (Mydriacyl) is a newer and an even shorter acting parasympatholytic agent since its effects wear off in 6 to 8 hours.

Euphthalmine (Eucatropine) is useful for dilating the pupil for *ophthalmoscopic* examination; 1 or 2 drops of a 5 per cent solution cause mydriasis in 30 minutes, and the effects pass off within 2 hours. It has but a feeble action upon accommodation and rarely causes increase in tension.

Paredrine Hydrobromide, a sympathomimetic agent is used in a 1 per cent aqueous solution not only to enhance the effects of other cycloplegics, but is valuable for dilating the pupil for *ophthalmoscopic* examination. One drop causes satisfactory mydriasis in 30 minutes.

Benzedrine sulfate is another mydriatic having the same properties as Paredrine.

Cocaine Hydrochloride because of its sympathomimetic action often is used for *moderate dilatation* of the pupil for *opthalmoscopic* examination . One or 2 drops of a 5 per cent solution cause sufficient dilatation in 30 minutes and produce insignificant interference with accommodation; the effects disappear within an hour. Cocaine dilates the pupil moderately by peripheral stimulation of the sympathetic nerve endings.

Phenylephrine Hydrochloride (Neo-Synephrine), a synthetic substitute for epinephrine and a sympathomimetic drug has an excellent mydriatic effect in 10 per cent solution or emulsion.

Ephedrine in 5 per cent aqueous solution of the hydrochloride or sulfate resembles Adrenalin in physiologic action; a drop of this solution dilates the pupil in 40 minutes, without affecting accommodation; it constricts the conjunctival blood vessels; intraocular tension is either uninfluenced or may be lowered slightly. Mydriasis lasts half an hour.

Miotics

Miotics diminish the size of the pupil producing tonic contraction of the sphincter and the ciliary muscle and reduce intraocular pressure. They accomplish these actions either as cholinergic stimulating agents (acetylcholine, methacholine, carbamylcholine, pilocarpine) or as cholinesterase inhibiting agents (physostigmine, neostigmine, edrophonium chloride, demecarium bromide, echothiopate iodide, diisopropyl fluorophosphate).

Cholinergic Stimulating Agents. Acetylcholine has no action on application to the external eye but is used occasionally in 1:5000 dilution for direct application to the iris in surgical procedures to constrict the pupil.

Methacholine (Mecholyl) is used in the treatment of glaucoma occasionally as drops of a 10 to 25 per cent aqueous solution in conjunction with an anticholinesterase agent. It also is used diagnostically in suspected cases of tonic pupil (Adie's syndrome). A 2.5 per cent solution will cause rapid constriction of a tonic pupil but will not affect a normal pupil.

Carbamylcholine (Carbachol) is not absorbed unless a wetting agent is applied to the cornea before or simultaneously. Thus a 1.5 to 3 per cent solution of Carbachol in 1:5000 solution of benzalkonium chloride is used as an alternative to other miotic drugs in the treatment of glaucoma. Its duration of action is 6 to 8 hours.

Pilocarpine a direct acting cholinergic drug, unlike Carbachol, is absorbed adequately on application to the cornea to produce miosis, increase facility of outflow of the aqueous humor, lower intraocular pressure, and to increase accommodation. It is used in 1, 2, 3, 4, and 6 per cent solutions but should be used in the weakest concentration that will be adequately effective. It usually is instilled one to four times per day. Its duration of action is 6 hours or slightly more.

Cholinesterase Inhibiting Agents. Physostigmine (eserine), the first miotic used to treat glaucoma has been replaced by longer acting drugs because of its tendency on prolonged use to cause conjunctival irritation, sensitivity reactions, and rubeosis iridis. It is still used in acute situations in 0.5 to 1 per cent solution. Its duration of action is approximately 6 hours.

Neostigmine (Prostigmin), a synthetic analogue of physostigmine is poorly absorbed through the cornea and requires the application of a drop of a 5 per cent solution every 4 to 6 hours. Thus it is seldom used.

Demecarium bromide (Humorsol) is a long acting potent cholinesterase inhibiting agent which produces intense miosis in a dosage of 1 drop of a 0.25 per cent solution every 12 to 72 hours.

Echothiopate iodide (phospholine iodide) another potent and long acting intense miotic, is used every 12 hours as a 0.06 to 0.25 per cent aqueous solution. It also increases the facility of outflow of aqueous humor and causes intense contraction, even spasm at times, of the ciliary muscle.

Both echothiopate iodide and diisopropyl fluorophosphate are contraindicated for use in patients with angle closure glaucoma, Parkinson's disease, bronchial asthma, gastrointestinal spasm, vascular hypertension and myocardial infarction.

Diisopropyl fluorophosphate (DFP, Floropryl) a long acting potent oil soluble anticholinesterase which was originally developed as a war gas produces intense miosis for 24 hours following the instillation of a drop of a 0.025 to 0.1 per cent solution. It is inactivated by water so users must be careful not to contaminate the medication with tears or other aqueous solutions.

Osmotic Agents

Mannitol is a higher alcohol derived by reduction from fructose. It is not metabolized significantly, does not enter the eye significantly but is excreted by filtration through the renal glomeruli and is not reabsorbed by the tubules and carries water with it. When given in a 20 per cent solution intravenously it causes a fall in intraocular pressure within an hour, which persists for approximately 4 hours. The dosage is 1.0 to 3.0 gm. per kilogram, usually 500 ml. of a 20 per cent solution. In addition to diuresis the patient may complain of headache.

Urea when administered intravenously in a dosage of 1.0 to 1.5 gm. per kilogram of body weight in a 30 per cent solution in 10 per cent invert sugar at a rate of 60 drops per minute will produce a fall in intraocular pressure in approximately 30 minutes and lasts for 4 to 5 hours. The drug causes a great reduction in intracranial pressure as well as in ocular tension along with a copious diuresis. The patient frequently has a severe headache and may experience nausea and vomiting. Renal impairment and previous brain damage are contraindications to this therapy.

Glycerol (glycerin, trihydroxypropane) is a sweet oily fluid which when given orally as a 50 per cent solution diluted with cold lemon juice or orange juice in a dosage of 1.0 to 1.5 gm. per kilogram of body weight produces a decrease in intraocular pressure within 30 to 45 minutes and lasts 4 to 5 hours. The drug produces moderate diuresis and moderate diarrhea but few if any other side effects.

Carbonic Anhydrase Inhibitors

Certain of the carbonic anhydrase inhibitors decrease the production of aqueous humor and a concomitant reduction in intraocular pressure without correlated diuresis.

Acetazolamide (Diamox) the first and most widely used of these drugs in ophthalmology produces a 50 to 60 per cent reduction in aqueous humor production. It may be given intravenously in 250 to 500 mg. doses in emergencies, or it may be given orally in 125 to 500 mg. doses in the adult and 62.5 mg. doses in the infant. It becomes effective in 1 hour and lasts for 6 hours; therefore for uniform control of intraocular pressure the drug should be given every 6 hours. It is valuable in acute primary and secondary glaucomas and as short term preoperative medication to delay glaucoma surgery until the eye is in a more favorable condition. Insignificant side effects are common but serious ones occur occasionally. They include paraesthesia with numbness and tingling in the extremities, anorexia, myopia, sodium and potassium depletion, renal lithiasis, aplastic anemia and exfoliative dermatitis. Any of these, however, may necessitate a trial of another carbonic anhydrase inhibitor.

Dichlorphenamide (Daranide) may be given in oral doses of 25 to 75 mg. every 6 hours.

Ethoxzolamide (Cardrase) is given in an oral dose of 125 mg. every 6 hours.

Methozolamide (Neptazane) may be given in an oral dosage of 50 to 100 mg. every 6 hours.

Cardiac Glycosides

The cardiac glycosides because of their inhibition of sodium and potassium adenosine triphosphatase which enters into the production of aqueous humor were thought to be of possible use in the treatment of glaucoma. However the results on trial at present have not shown them to be effective enough for general use.

Topical Anesthetics

Cocaine Hydrochloride in 5 per cent solution is the most commonly used remedy for producing local anesthesia of the conjunctiva, cornea and iris during *operations* upon the eye; it acts by paralyzing the terminal filaments of the fifth nerve. It serves as a *temporary* anodyne in corneal and iritic affections, and as a *mydriatic* for ophthalmoscopic examinations. Combined with mydriatics and cycloplegics, it enhances the action of these agents. Cocaine produces a local vasoconstriction and lowers intraocular pressure slightly; it has a tendency to cause *desiccation with desquamation of the corneal epithelium;* hence after instillation the patient should be directed to keep the lids closed. For the same reason it should not be used for any length of time, and it is unwise to prescribe cocaine for home use.

One drop of 5 per cent solution with a second drop after a few minutes is sufficient to anesthetize the cornea for the removal of foreign bodies; for this purpose the synthetic substitutes, described below, are superior; for more penetrating effects, such as required in operations, cocaine or its substitutes are instilled five times, at intervals of 2 minutes. Solutions of cocaine *do not keep well,* and should be prepared freshly when used for operations.

Cocaine Substitutes. A number of *synthetic* substitutes for cocaine have come into common use, especially in the *office* and for minor operations; these have many *advantages* over cocaine. They are not narcotics and consequently do not come under the restrictions of the Harrison Narcotic Act. Cocaine remains the choice in the operating room, but the most popular substitutes for cocaine for surface anesthesia are Nupercaine, Pontocaine, proparacaine hydrochloride (Ophthaine, Ophthetic) and benoxinate hydrochloride (Dorsacaine). With all cocaine substitutes, there is encountered an occasional instance of allergic local reaction in the form of severe swelling and redness of the conjunctiva and lids.

Local Anesthetics

Procaine hydrochloride (Novocain) was the anesthetic of choice for *hypodermic* use in lid and lacrimal sac operations and injection anesthesia in general. It generally is used in 2 per cent solution combined with Adrenalin chloride, 1:20,000. *Such solutions should be freshly prepared,* or else *sterile ampoules* should be employed.

Lidocaine (Xylocaine) in a 2 per cent solution has proved more popular recently because it produces more prolonged anesthesia more rapidly than procaine hydrochloride.

Antibacterial Agents

Sulfonamide Compounds (sulfanilamide, sulfathiazole, sulfadiazine, sulfacetamide, sulfapyridine) have revolutionized the treatment of many ocular infections. The action of these agents is *bacteriostatic* rather than bactericidal; none of the typical viruses is affected, but a group of atypical viruses is sulfonamide-sensitive.

Sulfonamide derivatives are used with excellent results in trachoma, inclusion conjunctivitis, gonorrheal ophthalmia, Streptococcus pseudomembranous conjunctivitis, pneumococcic and streptococcic corneal ulcer and in staphylococcic blepharoconjunctivitis; favorable results have been observed following their use in purulent endophthalmitis, panophthalmitis and orbital cellulitis; there has been no benefit in sympathetic ophthalmia, tularemia, ocular tuberculosis and syphilis.

The compounds of the sulfonamide group are given *by mouth* for systemic effect, or *topically*; for oral therapy *sulfadiazine* has a slight advantage on account of a lower toxicity. The *dose* for oral administration depends upon the age and weight of the patient; effective response to this chemotherapeutic agent is attained when the concentration reaches a level of 5 to 10 mg. per 100 cc. of blood; the amount required to maintain this level averages 0.1 gm. per kilogram of body weight, given in divided doses every 4 to 6 hours; the *initial dose* is 4.0 gm. and *maintenance doses* 1.0 gm. every 4 hours for the first 24 hours, and then 1.0 gm. every 6 hours, with modifications according to determinations of the level in the blood.

Mild *toxic reactions* from oral administration are frequent, dangerous ones rare. The patient should be seen daily and the drug discontinued at the onset of *toxic manifestations* (fever, rash, jaundice, hemolytic anemia and granulocytopenia). *Laboratory checks* are indicated; these include blood counts, determination of the level in the blood and examination of the urine; the latter should be kept neutral or alkaline to prevent formation of renal calculi, the most alarming complication. A previous toxic reaction is a contraindication to oral administration.

Oral therapy *should not be used in minor affections* which do not warrant the risk of toxic reactions.

Locally these drugs are used in solution (10 to 30 per cent solution of sodium sulfacetamide), in powder (sulfathiazole preferred), in ointment (5 per cent sulfathiazole or sulfadiazine, 10 per cent sodium sulfacetamide) or in emulsion or jelly. When powder is selected, the crystals must be broken up and the powder sifted. When local sensitivity is encountered, the drug must be discontinued.

Antibiotics have an important place in the treatment of ocular infections. However, in general they should be reserved for serious infectious processes caused by organisms specifically sensitive to the antibiotic.

Penicillin is most effective against the Gram-negative cocci, the treponemas, the Gram-positive rods and the Gram-positive cocci, with the exception of staphylococci. It is ineffective against the Gram-negative rods, Rickettsia, fungi and viruses.

Because of the increasing frequency of the development of allergy to penicillin, it should be reserved for the treatment of syphilis, gonorrhea and only the most severe infections caused by other susceptible agents. It should be given orally or parenterally and never used topically in ocular infections.

Some of the new synthetic penicillin compounds give promise of effectiveness against additional agents, but have yet to be proved.

Streptomycin is especially valuable in the treatment of tularemia and bubonic plague as well as enterococcal infections, Brucella infections and tuberculous infections, and is of occasional value in the treatment of gonorrheal, Pseudomonas and staphylococcic infections. However, it must be controlled carefully because of its tendency to damage hearing and equilibrium.

The tetracycline antibiotics, Aureomycin, Terramycin and Achromycin, are especially valuable in the treatment of rickettsial infections, psittacosis, lymphogranuloma venereum, trachoma, inclusion blennorhea, Brucella infections and granuloma inguinale, and are useful in a wide variety of Gram-negative rod infections as well as amebiasis.

Chloramphenicol has a broad spectrum of activity against bacteria and Rickettsia but because of its serious and frequently fatal toxic depression of the bone marrow, it should be used only in the most serious infections and then only if a safer antibiotic is not adequate.

Erythromycin is often useful for treatment of staphylococcic, streptococcic or pneumococcic infections but is of no value in Gram-negative rod infections.

Both polymyxin B and colistin are especially effective against *Pseudomonas aeruginosa* infections and often are effective against colon and paracolon bacillus infections as well as Aerobacter and Klebsiella infections. However, they are quite toxic but are effective on topical application, so are useful by this method of treatment of corneal ulcers.

Bacitracin, tyrothricin and neomycin also are highly toxic but are effective on topical application to a wide variety of bacteria. Therefore, when severe local infections caused by susceptible bacteria require antibiotic therapy, one or all of these three agents are the drugs of choice.

Amphotericin B, a recently developed drug, is used both topically and intravenously for the treatment of fungus infections. However, its usefulness is limited both by its narrow spectrum and by its toxicity.

A form of *toxic conjunctivitis* has been reported occasionally from the topical use of antibiotics. The conjunctival reaction has an abrupt onset, with lacrimation, negative cultures, basophilic granules in the conjunctival scrapings, the tendency to pseudomembranes and necrosis, and redness and edema of the eyelids.

Isoniazid is a potent inhibitor of the tubercle bacillus derived from nicotinic acid. It penetrates the blood aqueous barrier well and thus is useful in the treatment of ocular as well as general tuberculosis either alone or in combination with p-aminosalicylic acid. The usual dosage of isoniazid is 100 mg. three times a day for 3 or 4 days with a gradual reduction to 50 mg. twice a day for a long period even up to a year. Toxic effects of isoniazid include drowsiness, vertigo, muscular twitching, ataxia and at times toxic neuritis. Pyroxidine (vitamin B_6) given in 10- to 15-mg. doses daily will prevent most of these side effects. The lower dosages after the first week also reduce the probability of side effects.

p-Aminosalicyclic acid usually is prescribed along with isoniazid to reduce the probability of the organisms developing resistance to the medications. It is given in doses of 2 to 4 gm. three times a day. Streptomycin also may be used as an adjuvant in severe infections.

Antiviral Agents

Idoxyuridine (IDU, 5-Iodo-2-deoxyuridine) an antimetabolite inhibits the utilization of thymidic acid in the synthesis of DNA. It has been reported to inhibit bacteria, herpes simplex virus, vaccinia virus and some tumor cells in tissue culture. In ophthalmology a 0.1 per cent aqueous solution is used in a dosage of 1 drop every hour or 2 hours for several days then descreased gradually as healing occurs in dendritic keratitis and vaccinal keratitis. It is moderately effective in epithelial lesions but has little or no effect on stromal lesions.

Cytosine Arabinoside inhibits the metabolism of cytosine similar to the effect of IDU on thymidic acid. It also has antiviral activity but it has a greater toxic effect on normal corneal cells; therefore its use has been limited to the treatment of IDU resistant infections.

Antimalarial Agent

Pyramethamine (Daraprim) is a synthetic antimalarial agent and folic acid antagonist which has been found to be effective against intracellular dividing forms of the Toxoplasma parasite. It is used in combination with one of the sulfonamides (p. 362) and with folinic acid. Blood counts should be made twice weekly during periods of treatment.

Other Therapeutic Measures

Adrenalin (Suprarenin, epinephrine), the active principle of the *suprarenal gland,* comes in 1:1,000 aqueous solution of the chloride, which can be diluted with normal saline. Instillation of solutions from 1:10,000 to 1:1,000 causes *blanching* of the conjunctival blood vessels. It is used in operations to control bleeding, and in association with topical and local anesthetics to delay their absorption and prolong their action. However it penetrates the cornea poorly. Thus by topical application a 1:1000 concentration is ineffective in dilating the pupil except in cases in which the sympathetic fibers to the dilator pupillae have been interrupted. It does dilate the pupil, however, when injected subconjunctivally.

In stronger concentrations epinephrine and its levo analogues are used as primary drugs or as adjuncts to other glaucoma therapeutic agents (miotics and carbonic anhydrase inhibitors) in the treatment of open angle gluacoma. These drugs reduce intraocular pressure both by decreasing aqueous humor production and by improving outflow. The commonly used preparations are epinephrine 1 per cent, epinephrine bitartrate 2 per cent, epinephrine hydrochloride 2 per cent and phenylephrine hydrochloride 1, 2.5 and 10 per cent.

These preparations should be used with caution in patients with hypertensive cardiovascular disease. Also their prolonged use may lead to the deposition of dark brown or black pigment granules in the conjunctiva or cornea.

Cortisone and ACTH. The adrenal glands produce several hormones which are concerned with fluid and electrolyte metabolism (mineralocorticoids), with the development of sex characteristics (androgens) and with the metabolism of fat, carbohydrate and protein as well as control of inflammatory and immune processes (glucocorticoids). The latter group is especially significant in ophthalmic practice because of their ability to control inflammation and exudation. They do not act on the cause of the disease but only on the reaction of the tissues to allergic, toxic and physical trauma. These agents are most useful as topical applications in allergic and in noninfectious inflammatory diseases of the external eye and in acute anterior uveitis. Treatment of posterior uveitis, pseudotumor of the orbit, and optic neuritis is more effective by oral or parenteral administration of the drugs.

Topical applications of drops, suspensions, or ointments usually range from 0.5 to 2.5 per cent concentration (cortisone, hydrocortisone, prednisolone, dexamethasone). They may be administered as often as every hour during the acute phase but should be reduced in frequency as rapidly as possible compatible with improvement of the lesion for topical application of any of these preparations four times a day or more for 3 to 8 weeks is likely to produce increased resistance to outflow of aqueous humor and increased intraocular pressure in one-third or more of patients. In prolonged use posterior subcapsular cataracts may develop.

Oral administration varies with the

steroid preparation and may be administered every 4 hours, or by a single dose in the morning every 48 hours equivalent to the 2-day dosage when given four times a day. The latter method seems to be fully as effective and much less likely to produce side effects than the four times a day regimen. However the dosage should be decreased as rapidly as possible and discontinued as soon as feasible. Contraindications to oral corticosteroid therapy include diabetes mellitus, peptic ulcer, renal disease, cardiovascular disorders, arrested tuberculosis, thrombophlebitis, osteoporosis and generalized infections not satisfactorily controlled by drug therapy. Prolonged oral or parenteral steroid therapy may be responsible for the development of posterior subcapsular cataracts and occasionally may cause increased intraocular pressure.

Both oral and topical steroid therapy are contraindicated in acute virus infections especially herpes simplex infections, in fungus infections and in acute bacterial infections of the eye. Both topical and general administration of steroids cause some delay in wound healing; however, this has not posed a serious problem in ocular surgery.

ACTH. The administration of ACTH (adrenocorticotropic hormone produced by the anterior lobe of the pituitary gland) stimulates the adrenal cortex to produce corticosteroids, therefore produces the same effect as the administration of the glucocorticoids. ACTH must be given parenterally and the adrenal cortex must be functioning. Since prolonged administration of the glucocorticoids tend to suppress the function of the adrenal cortex, ACTH frequently is employed to stimulate adrenal function while the steroid dosage is being decreased and for a while after the steroids have been discontinued. ACTH may be used for the treatment of the same problems for which the steroids are used but because of the need for parenteral administration, the topical or oral steroids generally are preferred.

The usual dosage of ACTH is 10 USP units four times a day or 40 USP units of the purified gel form daily. In severe situations larger doses may be given for a few days but should be reduced as rapidly as possible.

In addition to the side effects of the glucocorticoids ACTH is more likely to cause vascular hypertension and hirsutism.

The contraindications are the same as for the steroids.

Fluorescein, an orange-red powder, is used in 2 per cent aqueous solution (with sodium bicarbonate, 3 per cent added) to detect *abrasions, infiltrations and ulcers* of the cornea and to define the limits of such lesions. A drop of solution is instilled into the conjunctival sac and after a few minutes the excess is washed off with water; a green stain indicates loss or infiltration of corneal epithelium.

Because of the frequency of contamination of fluorescein solutions by *Pseudomonas aeruginosa* they are seldom used now. Instead specially prepared sterile packages each containing a sterile strip of filter paper impregnated with fluorescein dye or sterile singe dose containers are used.

Fluorescein for intravenous use (Fluorescite) is prepared as a sterile 5 per cent solution of sodium fluorescein and packaged in 10-ml. vials for use in evaluation of lesions of the uvea, retina and optic nerve. Normally the dye appears in the arterioles of the fundus approximately 9 seconds after intravenous injection in the arm. Then it is seen in both the arterioles and veins for a second or two before disappearing from the arterioles and finally disappearing from the veins. It is especially valuable in the study of vascular lesions but it is being found useful in differentiating a number of ocular lesions (Figs. 11-4, 11-5 and 11-6).

Merbromin (Mercurochrome) 2 per cent aqueous solution may be used instead of fluorescein but does not stain the lesion as well.

Rose Bengal in 1 per cent aqueous solution also is used for staining the cornea but tends to irritate and stain normal epithelium unless its application is followed immediately by careful irrigation. It is especially valuable for staining the filaments which are characteristically seen in keratoconjunctivitis sicca.

Methylene Blue 1 per cent aqueous solution like rose bengal is more irritating to the eye than fluorescein but is especially useful in delimiting the extent of loosened epithelium around a corneal lesion such as a dendritic figure.

Vaccines and Sera are valuable agents in suitable cases of ocular disease, vaccines more often than sera. *Staphylococcal* vaccine is used chiefly in the treatment of recurrent hordeola and occasionally in ulcerative blepharitis. *Autogenous* vaccines, prepared from cultures made from the focus of infection, such as tonsils, teeth, sinuses, prostate, etc., are sometimes of advantage in the treatment of corneal ulcers, hordeola, iritis and uveitis, especially when such a focus of infection cannot be removed.

Sera are not used often in ophthalmic therapeutics. Diphtheria *antitoxin* is valuable in the rare cases of diphtheritic conjunctivitis (2000 to 3000 units). *Antitetanus* serum (1500 units) is indicated in lacerating injuries of the lids and orbit.

Tuberculin is used in tuberculous eye affections, sometimes with very good results. It is used both for diagnosis and treatment.

For *diagnostic* purposes successive intradermal injections of 0.001, 0.01 and 0.1 mg. of *old tuberculin* (O.T.) are given until a positive local or focal reaction is obtained. General reactions sometimes occur but are undesirable. The *local reaction* shows itself in redness, induration and swelling at the site of injection; the *focal reaction* produces an *increase in the ocular manifestations* and is a valuable indication of the tuberculous nature of the affection; a *general reaction* usually occurs in addition to a local and a focal reaction and consists of fever, sometimes associated with chills and exacerbation of all tuberculous foci.

The *intradermal test* not only is valuable for diagnosis but also furnishes information as to the relative sensitiveness of the patient to tuberculin and thus gives an indication of the size of the initial injection if it is decided to use the remedy for therapeutic purposes.

Von Pirquet's test is useful only in young children; it is inconclusive in adults unless a negative reaction is obtained.

For *treatment*, old tuberculin (O.T.) is generally employed, but other preparations (T.R., B.E., B.F.) are sometimes used. The initial dose usually is 0.00001 mg.; the injections are repeated every fourth day and the dose increased to 0.0001 mg.; then 0.0001 mg. is added to each successive dose until 0.001 mg. is reached; then 0.001 mg. is added with each dose until 0.01 is reached; then 0.01 mg. is added until 0.1 is the dose; this is then increased by 0.1 mg. for each injection until finally 1.0 mg. is given. The course of treatment occupies *many months*. Convenient serial dilutions are prepared by a number of manufacturing laboratories. Care must be taken to avoid a reaction, and the dose reduced if a reaction occurs. *Children must be given very much less than adults.* Tuberculin treatment is used in periphlebitis retinae, tuberculous iritis, iridocyclitis, choroiditis, episcleritis, scleritis and sclerosing keratitis; less frequently in phlyctenular affections and rarer forms of ocular tuberculosis. *It is contraindicated if the patient has active tuberculosis elsewhere in the body.*

Sometimes tuberculin is employed, with good results, in ocular disease in which the clinical signs point to tuberculosis, and yet no positive tuberculin reaction has been obtained; in these cases the tuberculin may act as foreign protein.

Nonspecific Protein Therapy is used often in the treatment of ocular diseases with much benefit. The agent generally used for this purpose is typhoid H antigen.

Typhoid H antigen is injected intravenously in adults. The initial dose varies from 5 to 50 million organisms, depending upon the effect desired. For mild stimulation of the defense mechanisms of the patient, 5 million organisms are given daily or every other day for several injections. For greater stimulation, 25 to 50 million organisms are given initially and, depending upon the reaction obtained, the second dose is doubled or tripled in order to obtain a comparable or better reaction. Each subsequent dose is determined in the same manner. In children, because of the instability of the temperature-regulating mechanism, intravenous typhoid therapy is *not* used; however, stimulation of the defense mechanism may be produced by intramuscular injections of typhoid vaccine in 0.5-cc. doses increasing to 2.0-cc. doses.

The *indications* for the use of foreign protein comprise infected corneal ulcers, severe iritis and iridcyoclitis, scleritis and sympathetic ophthalmitis; the results are often very gratifying.

Heat. *Hot, moist compresses* are prescribed in affections of the *cornea, iris, ciliary body, sclera and orbit,* and also to hasten the formation of pus and to relieve pain in hordeola, incipient chalazia, lacrimal abscess and panophthalmitis. They are applied by means of flannel, gauze or washrag, wrung out of water as hot as can be borne (115° F.), placed upon the closed lids and renewed every minute for at least 15 minutes several times a day.

Cold. *Cold compresses* are used in inflammatory affections of the *conjunctiva.* Strips of lint, gauze or similar material are folded to make pads of four thicknesses, about 2 inches square, moistened and cooled upon a block of ice; they are laid upon the closed lids and changed as soon as they become warm. Ice should never be applied directly to the lids.

Electricity is used occasionally in ocular therapeutics, in the form of the *electrocautery* for corneal ulcer and conical cornea, in the form of *diathermy* and *electrolysis* in operations for detachment of the retina, and in the removal of distorted lashes and small tumors of the lids.

Radium is used in epithelioma, severe forms of vernal conjunctivitis and for destroying hemangiomas of the lids and conjunctiva. Radon seeds buried in the growth have been employed in the treatment of intraocular and orbital tumors.

X-rays are used in the treatment of conditions similar to those for which radium is employed, and, in addition, in multiple doses for the treatment of retinoblastoma, and for irradiation of the orbit after the removal of eyeballs containing malignant growths and after exenteration of the orbit. All forms of treatment making use of radium or x-rays must be employed by an expert who will select the proper dosage and make use of suitable protection of the eyes so as to prevent cataract.

Grenz Rays (superficially acting rays between ultraviolet and x-rays) are used with varying success in superficial lesions of the cornea, such as ulcers and infiltrations, especially catarrhal ulcers and superficial punctate keratitis, and also in episcleritis and scleritis.

Ultraviolet Light Therapy ("artificial sunlight") is used occasionally in *tubercu-*

lous diseases of the eye, *phlyctenular* keratitis, scleritis, sclerosing keratitis and dendritic keratitis. General irradiation of the body is effected by a mercury vapor, a carbon arc lamp or the Alpine sun lamp, and local therapy, by focusing the rays on the lesion through the addition of a screen and a quartz applicator.

Massage is employed for reducing tension in *glaucoma* and in the treatment of *blepharitis*. In glaucoma, massage is used both in unoperated cases and especially after operation in which filtration is not satisfactory; pressure is made and released by a finger of each hand placed upon the upper lid, causing a weak indentation of the globe, not enough to cause pain, repeated about 20 times, 3 times a day. In blepharitis the edges of the lids are cleansed and then massaged with a small ball of absorbent cotton after applying some ointment such as sulfathiazole, 5 per cent, or yellow oxide of mercury.

Protective Measures of various sorts are applied to the eye to insure *rest*, to keep out *light*, air, wind and dust, to supply *warmth* and to give *support*. Various kinds of glasses intended to *subdue light* are frequently ordered; the colors generally used are varying shades of Crooke's, Cruxite, Calobar, Rayban, smoke or amber. Goggles and nonshatterable glasses are worn by workmen engaged in stone-cutting, metal work and similar occupations. *Black patches* are made use of to keep out light, to hold dressings in place or when imperfect protection is sufficient; these should always be curved and never flat. The application of eye *dressings* is described later (Figs. 22-5 and 22-6).

TOXIC EFFECTS OF DRUGS ON THE EYE

Aconite, a drug which is almost obsolete because of its toxicity, produced yellowish green vision, mydriasis, cycloplegia and transient blurring of vision frequently.

Adrenal Steroids. Administration of the glucosteroids by oral or parenteral routes in the treatment of general diseases by suppressing the defense mechanism render the eye more susceptible to infection to bacteria, fungi and viruses. They are especially likely to activate latent or quiescent herpes simplex lesions, particularly dendritic keratitis. Prolonged general treatment may cause cataracts and glaucoma at times, although the latter occurs more frequently after local applications to the eye.

Alcohol. *Ethyl alcohol* accentuates a phoria or tropia which existed prior to drinking thus in the average individual produces a diplopia by changing the physiologic esophoria into a temporary esotropia. In so called tobacco-alcohol amblyopia, the essential lesion is due to a nutritional deficiency due to decreased food intake in a chronic user of alcohol and tobacco.

Methyl alcohol on the other hand will produce a primary optic atrophy in those individuals who survive the general toxic reaction.

Aminopyrine (Pyramidon) an antipyretic and analgesic has been reported to cause transitory diplopia occasionally in children.

Amphetamine (Benzedrine) a synthetic central nervous system stimulant may cause dilatation of the pupils and slight blurring of near vision. It improves the reactivity of the pupil to light in approximately half of patients with Argyll-Robertson pupil.

Antihistamines. The antihistamines have a strong tendency to produce sensitivity reactions especially on topical application and dryness of the mucous membranes on prolonged use. Diphenhydramine (Benadryl) and prophenpyridamine (Trimeton) occasionally cause slight dilatation of the pupils and impairment of accommodation.

Antiinfective Agents. *Chloramphenicol* after prolonged treatment, particularly of cystic fibrosis, has been reported to cause optic neuritis or retrobulbar neuritis. When the drug is stopped early the changes usually are reversible but some have gone on to optic atrophy.

Isoniazid given in large doses for any length of time may produce optic neuritis and optic atrophy.

Streptomycin after long administration may cause xanthopsia, central scotomas for blue, nerve fiber bundle scotomas, bilateral optic neuritis with central scotomas, or altitudinal hemianopsia, all of which are transitory. However, rarely, optic atrophy and blindness may occur.

Sulfonamides most commonly affect the eye by the production of an acute myopia affecting both eyes but disappears rapidly on stopping the drug. Sulfathiazole may produce conjunctivitis and episcleritis by general administration of the usual dosages but this too is transitory when the drug is stopped. Some of the newer and long acting sulfonamides have produced an erythema multiforme type skin reaction associated with conjunctivitis, photophobia and discharge with changes developing in the conjunctiva resembling pemphigoid. Occasionally retinal hemorrhages and rarely toxic amblyopia and optic atrophy may occur.

Antimalarial Drugs. *Quinine,* in large and prolonged dosage, may cause a degenerative change in the retina, sometimes simulating primary pigmentary degeneration of the retina, night blindness, constriction of the visual fields and optic atrophy. Some individuals are more susceptible to these effects and may react to very small doses.

Chloroquine (Aralen) and its derivatives, hydroxy chloroquine (Plaquenil) amodiaquin (Camoquin) are used in the treatment of malaria, amebiasis, rheumatoid arthritis, lupus erythematosis, polymorphus light eruption, bronchial asthma and infectious mononucleosis as well as malaria. They may produce visual symptoms consisting of blurred vision, aching eyes, momentary difficulty in focusing the eyes, colored haloes and lights, photophobia and nausea. In 30 to 70 per cent of patients the drug or its metabolic products are deposited as fine greenish yellow pigment deposits in the corneal epithelium. They may be diffuse or in whorl or curvilinear arrangement. These changes tend to occur after large doses but may appear as early as 2 to 3 weeks after treatment begins. They usually disappear in 2 to 3 months after treatment is stopped. A more serious and permanent change is a pigmentary retinopathy which may occur in 0.1 to 3.0 per cent of patients on prolonged therapy usually of higher doses. An abnormal granular appearance of the macula is followed by the deposition of pigment granules and patches of depigmentation. Edema of the macula may precede or accompany the granular changes. The macular changes are bilateral and symmetrical. In some patients more extensive changes occur in the retina accompanied by general attenuation of the arterioles and later pallor of the disk. The retinal changes are not reversible therefore patients on prolonged treatment should have repeated ocular examinations and the drug should be discontinued with the earliest signs of retinal change.

Antiperspirants or deodorants are most likely to get into the conjunctiva and cornea in spray form. They cause transitory irritation and at times fine superficial epithelial keratitis and mild anterior uveitis without permanent damage.

Antipyrine (phenazone) an analgesic and antipyretic frequently causes sensitivity reactions about the eyes, characterized by swelling of the lids, dermatitis, conjunctivitis and, in rare cases, keratitis. Transient amblyopia lasting up to 8 days has been observed in a few patients following excessive doses.

Arsenicals used in the treatment of syphilis usually are organic compounds. The older ones, *p*- or *m*-arsanilic acid, sodium arsanilate (Atoxyl, Soamin), sodium acetylarsenilate (Arsacetin), N-acetyl-4-hydroxy-*m*-arsanilic acid (Acetarsone, Spirocid, Stovarsol, Acetylarsan) sodium methylacetyl aminophenylarsonate (Orsudan) and sodium *N*-carbamoylmethyl arsanilate (tryparsamide) have induced optic neuritis with rapidly constricting fields, loss of central vision and optic atrophy. Inorganic arsenicals by contact or by systemic absorption from arsenical dusts such as arsenic trioxide and copper acetoarsenite (Paris green) used commercially and agriculturally produce an itching burning type of conjunctivitis with hyperemia, chemosis, photophobia and tearing.

Aspirin (acetyl salicylic acid) rarely has caused ocular toxic effects. It may cause allergic conjunctivitis and keratitis but does not cause permanent damage. In excessive dosage decreased intraocular pressure may occur with acidosis but the pressure returns to normal as the acidosis clears.

Atropine, a widely used parasympatholytic agent may cause toxic reactions from topical application to the eye or from general absorption. The ocular action of the drug consists of mydriasis and cycloplegia whether it is applied topically or given orally or parenterally. In patients with narrow angles dilatation of pupil may be associated with increased intraocular pressure thus atropine and its derivatives must be administered to glaucoma patients with caution. In severe systemic atropine intoxication, visual hallucinations, disorientation, excitement, skin flushing and fever are common. Sensitivity reaction is common after prolonged topical use of atropine. Other parasympatholytic agents which have toxic effects similar to atropine, several of which are used for gastrointestinal lesions, include: belladonna, Cantil, chlorisondamine chloride, Darbid, Darstine, diphemanil methylsulfate, Esyntin, ethopropazine, isopropamide, methantheline bromide (Banthine), scopolamine, tetraethanolammonium hydroxide and valethamate bromide.

Barbiturates may be responsible for either acute or chronic poisoning. In both cases the pupils may be affected, but irregularly, many patients showing hippus and sluggish reaction to light; however, mydriasis and miosis occur with approximately equal frequency. Transitory nystagmus, weakness of convergence and weakness of individual ocular muscles also occur in either acute or chronic poisoning. Bilateral temporary diminished vision, xanthopsia (yellow vision) or chloropsia (green vision), and even blindness have been observed in the period of recovery from barbital or phenobarbital induced coma.

Bromides in excessive dosage may cause enlargement of the pupils which react poorly to light and in accommodation. Rarely miosis and diplopia have been observed. Patients may complain of blurring vision, apparent waviness or movement of objects, change in apparent size of objects, visual hallucinations, disturbances in color perception and rarely photophobia.

Busulfan used orally in the treatment of chronic granulocytic leukemia may cause cataracts resembling those induced by radiation.

Cannabis (marihuana, Indian hemp, hashish) induces transient mydriasis, impairment of accommodation, diplopia, visual hallucinations and disturbances of color vision.

Carbon dioxide asphyxiation may cause temporary proptosis, mydriasis, yellow vision or temporary blindness.

Carbonic anhydrase inhibitors, acetozolamide (Diamox) dichlorphenamide (Daranide) ethoxzolamide (Cardrase) and methazolamide (Neptazane) may cause transient myopia in conjunction with other side effects.

Chloral hydrate may cause transitory swelling of the lids, ptosis, hyperemia and chemosis of the conjunctiva and tearing in moderate doses but in excessive dosage may cause mydriasis, diminution in convergence and transient diminution of vision.

Chlorothiazide (Diuril) may cause xanthopsis (yellow vision).

Chrysarobin used in the treatment of psoriasis may cause conjunctivitis and keratitis by direct contact or by systemic absorption.

Curare, curarine and tubocurarine, alkaloid muscle relaxants administered systemically may cause weakness of convergence, diplopia, and nystagmus. Topical application apparently is ineffective.

Digitalis or its derivatives long have been known to produce reversible disturbances in vision. These include flickering of light, light colored objects appear bright and dazzling as if covered with snow, objects may appear to have blue colored borders, or all objects may appear yellow, orange or green. Rarely visual acuity may be decreased sometimes accompanied by bilateral central scotomas.

Diphenylhydantoin (Dilantin, Epanutin) rarely may cause transient amblyopia diplopia, nystagmus, ptosis, visual and auditory hallucinations.

Ergot poisoning from ingestion of the parasitic fungus has been reported to cause diplopia, scintillating scotomas, nystagmus and cataracts. In rare instances, ergot containing medications have produced cyclopegia, slight hyperopia, slight edema of the retina, narrowing of the arterioles, bilateral diminution in vision or blindness. Most of these are reversible.

Gold administered systemically in the prolonged treatment of arthritis and tuberculosis has been observed to accumulate in the corneal stroma as fine distinct tiny gold to violet colored granules without disturbance of vision and without irritation.

Insulin in overdosages produces hypoglycemia associated with temporary mydriasis, strabismus and diplopia.

Lysergic acid diethylamide (LSD 25), an ergot derivative, in addition to mental disturbances produces visual hallucinations and an elevation in the visual threshold.

Meperidine (Demerol, Pethadine, Dolantin) in excessive dosage may produce either miosis or mydriasis.

Mephenesin (Myanesin, Tolserol), an antispasmotic muscle relaxant, following intravenous administration may produce nystagmus, and diplopia along with weakness, dizziness and muscular incoordination.

Mescaline causes visual hallucinations, with great disturbance in the appearance of form and color of a temporary character.

Methsuximide (Celontin) may cause diplopia or blurring of vision drowsiness and ataxia.

Methyl Salicylate (Wintergreen Oil) in excessive dosage may cause dimness of vision (15 per cent of cases) xanthopsia and disturbances of accommodation.

Morphine rarely produces toxic affects on the eyes. Miosis occurs with the usual doses. In fatal overdoses the miosis may persist or may be replaced by mydriasis just before death. Withdrawal symptoms in addicts include excessive tearing, irregularity of the pupils, paresis of accommodation, blurring of vision, occasional diplopia and rarely amblyopia.

Oil of Chenopodium may cause temporary diminution of vision and mydriasis.

Phenolphthalein may cause edema of the eyelids and subconjunctival hemorrhage, in association with diffuse skin reaction.

Phenylbutazone (Butazolidin) has been reported to cause conjunctival chemosis and pseudomembranous conjuctivitis.

Phthalofyne (Whipcide), an anthelmintic, in 10 per cent of patients receiving 100 to 200 mg. per kilogram and in all patients receiving more than 200 mg. per kilogram of body weight orally have shown conjunctival irritation and a diffuse keratitis associated with pain and photophobia. In some instances dense opacities of the cornea developed in 24 hours but all of these have cleared completely in 7 to 21 days.

Sodium Salicylate after ingestion of 8 to 20 gm. in the course of a few days usually causes visual disturbance, progressing to blindness in a few hours and lasting for several to 24 hours, followed by a slow return to normal.

Santonin, an anthelmintic especially useful against Ascaris, in excessive dosage produces disturbances in vision and color vision. Objects appear to be seen through yellow or yellow green filters. Bright objects appear yellowish green but dark surfaces may appear violet. The violet sensation may persist with the eyes closed. In addition the pupils may be dilated and react poorly to light, the patient complaining of photopsia (flashing of light) and persistent after-images. Rarely visual loss to complete blindness has occurred as a transitory phenomenon.

Silver Salts when ingested over a period of time will produce an argyrosis of the skin which also involves the conjunctiva and cornea. Similar but more severe deposition of silver in the conjunctiva and cornea may follow topical applications of the salts.

Strychnine poisoning is sometimes accompanied by mydriasis, proptosis and deviations of the eyes. Blindness may occur rarely.

Trimethadione (Tridione), an anticonvulsant used in the treatment of petit mal and psychomotor epilepsy, commonly causes an altered sensitivity of the eyes to light in adolescent and adult patients but rarely in children. The patient experiences intense glare in bright light associated with an apparent fading of colors. Light adaptation is greatly delayed. In subdued illumination the patient is comfortable and vision normal. These symptoms disappear gradually after the drug is stopped.

Tranquilizing Agents. The minor tranquilizing agents used in the treatment of anxiety and tension of psychoneurotic or psychosomatic disorders produce no eye problems. These include meprobamate, phenaglycodol, chlordiazepoxide, diazepam and hydroxyzine.

The phenothiazine derivatives used in the treatment of psychoses are selectively stored in retinal and uveal pigment and may produce retinal damage. These drugs include chlorpromazine, promazine, triflupromazine, fluphenazine, perphenazine, prochlorphenazine, prochlorperazine, trifluperazine and thioridazine. Retinal damage is directly related to dosage and duration of treatment. The patients complain of visual loss and night blindness. This is followed or accompanied by pigment degeneration of the retina which begins usually as a fine deposit in the macula but later these change to large clumps of pigment. The retinal arterioles become narrow along their entire course. Some individuals seem more susceptible than the majority.

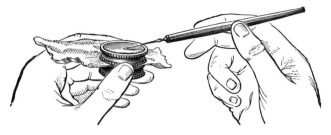

Fig. 22-3. Drum used to test the cutting edges of eye instruments.

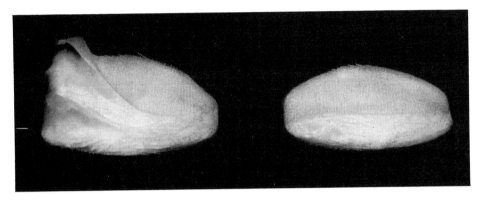

Fig. 22-4. A satisfactory pad for an eye dressing (*right*) consists of a layer of absorbent cotton between two layers of gauze as shown by the opened pad on the *left*.

Vitamin A in excessive dosage for several weeks to several months causes weakness of the extraocular muscles, diplopia, increased intracranial pressure with papilledema and peripapillary hemorrhages with enlargement of the blind spots on visual field examination.

Vitamin D in excessive dosage causes calcification of the conjunctiva and cornea. The cornea usually develops a band-shaped keratopathy but may develop a diffuse calcification.

GENERAL CONSIDERATION OF OPERATIONS

The rules of *asepsis and antisepsis* which govern general surgery are also indicated in ophthalmic operations, except that *strong solutions of germicides are not tolerated* by the eye. In other respects, the preparations connected with an operation are similar to those employed by the general surgeon.

Preparation of the Patient. The patient should be in good physical condition but old age, nephritis, and diabetes are not contraindications; however, such patients require special care.

It is imperative to examine the conjunctiva and the lacrimal region before deciding to operate upon the eyeball, especially if the eyeball is to be opened, as in iridectomy and cataract extraction. The presence of *purulent* or *mucopurulent* secretion renders such an operation extremely hazardous, on account of the danger of *infection.* In such cases the conjunctival or lacrimal affection first must be cured by appropriate treatment. A *culture of the conjunctival secretion* should be made in every case in which an incision into the globe is required; in cases of doubt, it is well to dress the eye for 24 hours and then to examine and make cultures from it.

Preparation of the Hands of the Operator comprises thorough scrubbing with soap and warm water and immersion in alcohol. Rubber gloves are worn by most operators.

Preparation of Instruments. *Blunt instruments* should be cleaned and polished, *boiled* in 1 per cent solution of soda, *rinsed* with sterile water and then allowed to dry in sterilized gauze until ready for use. They also may be sterilized by autoclave or in the hot air sterilizer.

Previous to sterilizing, the cutting qualities of *sharp instruments* should be tested upon thin kid stretched in the testing drum (Fig. 22-3). *Knives* with delicate cutting edges (such as cataract knives, keratomes, knife needles and cystotomes) are cleansed carefully and sterilized in a hot air sterilizer; throughout this preparation great

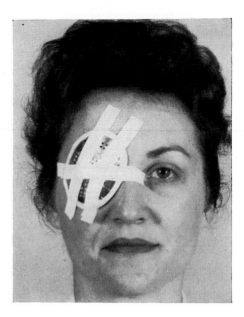

FIG. 22-6. Dressing covered by perforated metal shield to protect the eye from bumps or pressure. The metal shield, which usually is used following intraocular surgery or wounds of the globe, is shaped to rest against the bones of the face but not against the dressing.

care must be taken not to injure the point or edge.

Position of the Patient. The patient should lie on a narrow *operating table.* If for any reason it is desirable to operate with the patient in his bed, the head of the latter must be sufficiently low not to interfere with the operator. An operating chair will answer for minor operations. Good *daylight* is sometimes employed for operations upon the lids, but in operations upon the globe, especially cataract extraction, iridectomy and the like, *artificial illumination* is required, the light being condensed upon the field of operation by a large condensing lens or, better, by means of an *electric projection lamp.* Most operating rooms are equipped for using projected electric light for *all* operations.

Preparation of the Region of Oper-

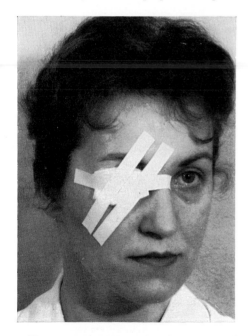

FIG. 22-5. Simple eye dressing. The pad is placed under the brow and held in place by three pieces of narrow adhesive tape.

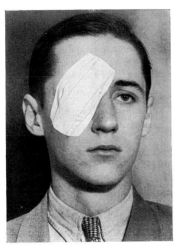

Fig. 22-7. A moderate pressure dressing may be obtained when desired by use of several eye pads snugly covered by several strips of tape.

ation. The eyelids, including the lashes, brow and the surrounding skin, should be cleansed thoroughly with soap and warm water, and then washed with 70 per cent alcohol; many operators have the eye prepared on the morning of the operation, and then covered by a sterile gauze dressing, which is not disturbed until the operation. The conjunctival sac is flushed with a large quantity of warm saline or boric acid solution preceding the operation; then the lashes and lid margins are painted with 3 per cent iodine, and wiped off with 70 per cent alcohol.

Anesthesia. In the majority of operations on the eyes of adults, local anesthesia is adequate. A dose of phenobarbital or other barbiturate given ½ hour before operation allays nervousness and reduces reactions to the local anesthetic.

Surface anesthesia of the conjunctiva and cornea is obtained by the instillation of 1 drop of 5 per cent cocaine at 2-minute intervals for five doses, the lids being kept closed in the intervals.

Retrobulbar injection of 1 cc. of 2 per cent Novocain containing 1:20,000 Adrenalin made in the vicinity of the ciliary ganglion renders operation upon the globe painless, even to cutting of the iris.

Block anesthesia of the sensory nerves supplying the lids and face is obtained by injecting 2 per cent Novocain containing 1:20,000 Adrenalin at their points of emergence from the orbit or bony canals. Also akinesia of the facial (seventh) nerve is made by a similar injection at the point where it crosses the ramus of the mandible.

In children, in apprehensive adults and in extensive operations on the lids and orbit, general anesthesia is used.

Cleansing Solutions. In the course of

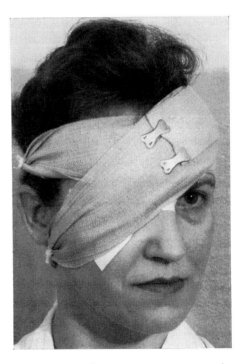

Fig. 22-8. Greater pressure may be obtained by application of an elastic roller bandage over a moderate pressure dressing. Additional pressure may be secured by tying the bandage above and below the ear as illustrated.

operations upon the eyeball, it is necessary to cleanse the field of operation and to *irrigate* the cornea frequently to prevent desiccation. For this purpose a 1.4 per cent solution of sodium chloride, which is isotonic with tears, is preferred. It is applied by an irrigator, an undine, a rubber ear syringe or an eye dropper.

Dressings vary little with the nature of the operation. Usually a dressing made of two layers of gauze enclosing a thin layer of absorbent cotton (Fig. 22-4) is fastened to the face and brow by three narrow strips of adhesive tape (Fig. 22-5). When

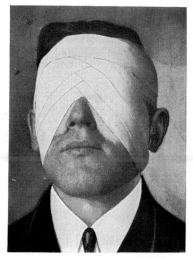

FIG. 22-9. Binocular bandage.

protection of the globe from pressure or rubbing, etc. is required, a Fox metal shield bent so as to rest upon the bony portions of the brow, cheek and nose without touching the underlying dressing is taped in place as shown in Figure 22-6.

In some situations a pressure dressing may be required and is obtained by adding folded gauze sponges over the regular eye dressing and applying adhesive tape as shown in Figure 22-7. Additional pressure may be added by use of a roller bandage 1½ inches wide and 5 to 7 yards long (Figs. 22-8 and 22-9).

The monocular bandage (Fig. 22-8) is applied as follows: Begin at the temple of the affected eye (right, for example); make one turn around the forehead; then on the second round pass across the occiput, below the right ear and obliquely across the right eye; thereafter these turns are alternated in the same way three or four times.

The binocular bandage (Fig. 22-9). Begin at the temple, the right, for example; make a full turn around the forehead and continue to the left temple, then obliquely across the occiput, below the right ear, across the right eye; around the upper occipital region, above the right ear, downward over the left eye, below left ear, across the occiput; below the right ear, across the right eye, and alternate in this manner for three or four turns.

23

The Ocular Manifestations of General Diseases

Ocular involvement occurs in the course of and as a part of the morbid process or as a complication of many diseases affecting the body as a whole or a particular system such as the cardiovascular system, the endocrine system or the nervous system. Ocular signs and symptoms frequently are the first manifestations of some of these diseases, thus alerting the ophthalmologist to the need of referring the patient for a general examination. At other times the ocular signs, in their evolution and course of resolution, are significant prognostic signs of the general disease.

Diseases of the Blood and Reticuloendothelial System

Anemia, Either Primary or Secondary (simple, pernicious, secondary or chlorosis) is manifest by pallor of the conjunctiva, pearly white sclera, pale fundus and disk, and by retinal vessels which are pale, tortuous and slightly broader than normal. Occasionally retinal hemorrhages of all types, and rarely preretinal hemorrhages, retinal edema or neuroretinal edema, occur and may be followed by optic atrophy.

Anemia of the Sickle Cell Type is manifest by small aneurysm-like dilatations of the conjunctival vessels which tend to disappear with heat, even that of the slit lamp. However, more characteristic are the venous thromboses and hemorrhages which occur in the peripheral vessels first, then become more numerous, with extensive retinal hemorrhage, neovascularization and later proliferative retinopathy. These manifestations occur in sickle cell anemia of the SS-, SC-, SD- and S-thalassemia types.

Cryoglobulinemia is a condition which, as the result of exposure to cold, results in sludging of the blood of the conjunctival vessels, and at times in the retina, producing venous occlusions, retinal edema and hemorrhages and in severe cases edema of the nervehead and occlusion of the central retinal vein.

Hemophilia predisposes to profuse hemorrhages or to prolonged and sometimes serious bleeding even after minor injury; thus injuries to the eye and adnexa are included. Hemorrhages into and from the lids, conjunctiva and orbit may be persistent, and hyphema and hemorrhage into the retina or vitreous may follow seemingly trivial injuries.

Hemorrhage, either of the sudden massive type or of the repeated severe type, may be associated with little or no changes in the eyes, or may be accompanied by severe visual changes and permanent loss of vision in both eyes. The fundus may be pale with slight constriction of the vessels, or the changes may resemble those of occlusion of the central retinal artery with greatly constricted vessels and a cherry-red spot in the macula surrounded by a pale or milky edema of the perimacular region. The patient may lose vision in both eyes suddenly, immediately or shortly after the hemorrhage, or the visual loss may be delayed for several weeks, but in either case optic atrophy follows in many patients and approximately half of them never regain their vision.

Retinal hemorrhages seldom occur in

this acute form of anemia, but may develop later if a chronic secondary anemia ensues.

In Polycythemia, either primary or secondary, the general color of the fundus is dusky red or cyanotic and the retinal veins are dilated, darker than normal and, because of constrictions at the arteriovenous crossings, may resemble a string of sausages. The arteries usually remain normal. In polycythemia vera, hemorrhages of all types may occur as well as retinal edema and, rarely, neuroretinal edema. Hemorrhages and edema occur only rarely in secondary polycythemia.

Hodgkin's Disease, a disease of the reticuloendothelial system of unknown cause, frequently is associated with typical lymphomatous lesions of the lids, lacrimal glands and orbit. The ocular lesion may be primary but, when the lacrimal gland is involved, there may be similar involvement of the salivary glands, as well as the preauricular and cervical lymph nodes, producing Mikulicz's syndrome. Other causes of Mikulicz's syndrome, however, include inflammatory diseases (such as uveoparotid fever of Heerfordt, mumps, tuberculosis, syphilis and sarcoidosis), leukemia, lymphosarcoma and benign lymphoid hyperplasia.

Eosinophilic Granuloma is a benign destructive process which usually involves a single bone of the skull, vertebrae or long bones in children and young adults. In exceptional cases, an orbital bone, especially the upper temporal rim, is involved. A soft mass at the upper outer rim causes swelling of the lids which, on examination by x-ray, shows a bony erosion. On excision the soft, friable lesion is composed of large numbers of eosinophils and reticulum cells, some of which usually contain lipids.

Hand-Schüller-Christian Disease, a disorder closely related to or a variant of eosinophilic granuloma, affects children and young adults by a characteristic triad of signs and symptoms: (1) sharply defined or punched-out defects on x-rays of the skull, (2) unilateral or bilateral exophthalmos and (3) pituitary dysfunction, particularly diabetes insipidus. Pathologically the lesions are similar to those of eosinophilic granuloma, but they show more lipid-laden histiocytes and the tissue shows a high content of cholesterol, cholesterol esters and neutral fat, and with time the lesion shows considerable fibrosis and inflammatory reaction. The destructive proliferative lesions may involve any organ of the body.

Letterer-Siwe Disease is the most serious of the reticuloendothelioses, affecting infants and very young children by a rapidly progressive and fatal course. It usually begins acutely: fever, ecchymosis, anemia and enlargement of the lymph nodes and spleen. The bones and other tissues, including the eyes and orbit, occasionally are infiltrated by large mononuclear cells containing little or no demonstrable lipid (nonlipoid histiocytosis).

Leukemia of all types produces ocular signs and symptoms which are the same for all types. Some of the ocular signs are due to the associated anemia, but the leukemic manifestations may occur in either the leukemic or the aleukemic phase of the disease; once established, some, if not all, usually persist thereafter.

Edema, hemorrhages and nodular infiltrations occur in the lids and orbit. Rarely, in a child, a nodular, tumor-like, infiltrative lesion which has a peculiar greenish color involves the orbit, producing an exophthalmos. Because of the color, the tumor is called a chloroma.

The early changes in the fundus are pallor due to the anemia and occasionally hemorrhages. However, the veins become dilated and tortuous, early in the disease, and show numerous constrictions so they resemble a string of sausages. Later the arteries as well as the veins become dilated and they both become pale, yellowish red in color and difficult to distinguish from each other. The hemorrhages increase in number and are of all types except punctate, but the characteristic ones are spindle-shaped, moderately large and have yellowish white centers. In some instances, leukemic infiltrations, which are yellowish white, round or oval elevated lesions, one-fourth to one-half the diameter of the disk, are visible between the hemorrhages.

Lymphoma may involve the lids or the conjunctiva. There usually is symmetrical involvement of the lids by smooth nodules of infiltration associated with smooth pink or fleshy elevations of the conjunctiva, frequently involving the caruncles or fornices, and sometimes the orbit. They usually are benign and are not accompanied by a disturbance of the blood. In some instances, especially in children, they may accompany or may be followed by acute leukemia; however, the two types usually can be differentiated histologically in that the benign type is a reactive lymphoid hyperplasia, whereas the other contains immature malignant blood cells.

Macroglobulinemia, a disease characterized by an increase in the serum proteins of high molecular weight, like cryoglobulinemia, may cause sludging in the conjunctival and retinal vessels, hemorrhages, venous occlusions, edema, neuroretinal edema, occlusion of the central retinal vein, vitreous hemorrhage and subsequently secondary glaucoma.

Methemoglobinemia, either congenital or acquired, may produce generalized cyanosis, which includes the conjunctiva, without associated cardiac or respiratory signs or symptoms.

Purpura often is accompanied by petechial hemorrhages in the skin of the lids and conjunctiva, hyphema, which may occur repeatedly, and also retinal hemorrhages. Occasionally hemorrhages occur in the orbit.

Blood Transfusion Reactions commonly produce retinal hemorrhages which clear, leaving little or no visual disturbance; however, at times temporary blindness occurs without significant ocular signs.

Diseases of the Cardiovascular System

Aortic Insufficiency due to the great difference between systolic and diastolic pressures causes pulsation in the retinal arteries. Other conditions having a large pulse pressure also may produce pulsation of the retinal arteries. These are heart block; Graves' disease (hyperthyroidism) and occasionally high fevers. Glaucoma also, at times, may produce pulsation of the arteries on the disk, but in this case the mechanism is compression of the artery in diastole by the increased intraocular pressure.

Aneurysm of the Aorta, by irritation of the cervical sympathetics, may give rise to mydriasis and widening of the palpebral fissure or, by paralysis of the cervical sympathetics, may produce miosis, slight ptosis and apparent or slight enophthalmos, Horner's syndrome. Other mechanisms for the production of Horner's syndrome include tumors or abscess of the neck or cervical rib, and occasionally lesions of the apex of the lung.

Aneurysm of the Cerebral Arteries, especially those involving the internal carotid and occasionally those involving the middle cerebral and basilar arteries, may cause pain in the eye, oculomotor palsies and visual field defects.

Arteriovenous Aneurysm involving the internal carotid artery and the cavernous sinus produces congestion of the vessels of the conjunctiva, orbit and retina; pulsating proptosis; bruit which can be heard over eye and forehead associated with rumbling noises heard by the patient; edema of the lids; and sometimes papilledema and loss of vision (Chap. 16).

Arteriosclerosis and Hypertension, in addition to the characteristic changes in the retinal vessels described in Chapter 10, may be responsible for hemorrhages in the lids, conjunctiva and orbit, and at times may cause ocular signs and symptoms by the production of thrombotic or hemorrhagic lesions in the central nervous system.

Buerger's Disease or thromboangiitis obliterans rarely may cause visual field defects of the hemianopic type as a result of thrombosis of an intracranial vessel or occlusion of the central vein or of the central retinal artery.

Coarctation of the Aorta is associated with corkscrew tortuosity and serpentine pulsation of the retinal arterioles, especially in the perimacular region.

Coronary Occlusion, an atheromatous disease, may be accompanied by atheromatous changes in the central retinal artery, but since these usually occur in the optic nerve at or behind the lamina cribrosa, they are seldom visible. Therefore diminution in size of, or obstruction of, the central retinal artery may occur along with other manifestations of hypertension and arteriosclerosis in patients with coronary disease.

Endocarditis, of either the acute or the subacute variety, may produce ocular lesions but they seldom are observed in the rare but rapidly fatal acute form of the disease. In the much more frequent subacute form, showers of petechial hemorrhages involve the conjunctiva and retina along with the skin and mucous membranes. However, in the retina, in addition to the hemorrhages which may be round or flame-shaped, white round or oval spots which may at times have some hemorrhage around or partly around

them (Roth's spots) develop, especially in the perimacular region and around the disk. Roth's spots are small septic infarcts of very small arterioles or capillaries and must be distinguished from cotton wool patches which occur in hypertensive arteriosclerotic-nephritic retinopathy and from the white-centered hemorrhages of leukemic retinopathy, either of which they may resemble at times. Embolic occlusion of an arteriole or the central retinal artery may occur at times.

Heart Disease, particularly of the congenital types of the cyanotic group, including the tetralogy of Fallot, tricuspid stenosis and atresia, single ventricle with pulmonary stenosis, Eisenmenger's complex, transposition of the great vessels, truncus arteriosus, severe ventricular septal defects and interauricular septal defects, produces cyanosis of the conjunctiva, associated with cyanosis and tortuosity of the retinal veins. In cardiac insufficiency, dependent edema may involve the eyelids, especially upon rising in the morning.

Intracranial Hemorrhage from trauma or vascular disease may give rise to a variety of ocular manifestations depending upon the location of the hemorrhage in the brain or meninges, upon its effect in raising the intracranial pressure and also upon involvement of the optic pathways or oculomotor areas. For example, subarachnoid hemorrhage frequently is associated with hemorrhage in or on the optic disk, and basilar skull fracture not infrequently is followed by hemorrhage appearing in the lower lids 24 to 48 hours after the injury.

Pulseless Disease (Takayasu's disease) causes patients to complain of recurrent episodes of blurring of vision which last longer and longer, especially on suddenly rising to an erect posture. Ophthalmoscopic examination reveals arteriovenous anastomoses, hemorrhages and transudates. The arterioles cease to carry blood with slight pressure on the globe. Frequently optic atrophy results.

Raynaud's Disease may be accompanied by spasm of the retinal artery or arterioles.

Thrombosis of the Cavernous Sinus produces engorgement of the veins of the orbit and lids, resulting in edema of the lids and orbit and in papilledema. Exophthalmos accompanies the orbital edema.

Diseases of the Kidneys

Nephritis presents many ocular manifestations. Edema often is present in the lids, and also may show itself in the conjunctiva (chemosis). Nephritic retinopathy is common, occurring most frequently with the chronic varieties of renal disease, but liable to complicate the nephritis of scarlatina and pregnancy. Detachment of the retina may occur in toxemia of pregnancy. During an attack of uremia, rapid loss of vision (uremic amaurosis) may occur without ophthalmoscopic changes; in this condition the pupils are apt to be moderately dilated.

Diseases of the Nervous System

Diseases which affect the central nervous system may affect the eyes, since the retina is a specialized part of the central nervous system and the optic nerve may be considered as a nerve fiber tract. Particulars regarding the condition of the optic nerves, the pupils, the eye muscles, the acuteness of vision and the fields of vision are of great value.

Chorea. True chorea does not cause ocular anomalies. Patients with "habit chorea" or "habit spasm," having choreic movements of the muscles of the lids and of the face and neck, often suffer from errors of refraction, less frequently from heterophoria; the relief of these errors occasionally effects a cure.

Coma. Objective examination of the eyes may give important data in all forms of coma. If dependent upon organic brain disease there may be papilledema, mydriasis and deviation of the eyes. If due to cerebral hemorrhage there may be miosis, inequality of the pupils and conjugate deviation. With increased intracranial pressure, there may be dilated pupils. If uremia, nephritic retinopathy may be found. When alcoholic, there may be dilatation of the pupils and pareses of external ocular muscles. If due to poisoning by opium or similar drugs, there will be extreme miosis.

Epilepsy. The seizure frequently begins with a visual aura: flashes of light, colored sensations and hemianopic or complete loss of vision. During the attack, there may be narrowing of the retinal arteries, the pupils generally are dilated and the light reflex is lost, and there often is spasm of the extrinsic ocular muscles causing conjugate lateral deviation of the eyes. After the seizure, there are distention of the retinal veins, often alterations in size of the pupils and sometimes temporary concentric contraction of the field and reduction in vision. Not very often, but certainly in some cases, epilepsy is made worse by eye strain, and the number and severity of attacks are reduced by the wearing of proper glasses.

Hysteria sometimes is responsible for a great variety of ocular symptoms, the principal ones being diminution in the acuteness of vision (amblyopia and even blindness), spiral contraction of the field of vision for form and colors, therefore becoming smaller with each repeated examination. Reversal in the relative size of the color fields frequently occurs. Other ocular manifestations in hysteria are scotoma, hemianopsia, photophobia, blepharospasm and monocular diplopia. The pupillary reflexes and the ophthalmoscopic appearances are normal. The ocular manifestations almost always are referred to one eye.

Neurasthenia is often accompanied by pain in or around the eyes, or headache, usually aggravated upon close work. In many cases these symptoms depend upon errors of refraction or heterophoria which in healthy individuals would give rise to no discomfort. In some cases glasses are ineffective or give only partial relief; then the asthenopia is regarded as "neurasthenic" and is considered a neurosis dependent upon a general asthenic condition of the system.

Encephalitis Lethargica frequently presents as an early symptom paralysis or paresis of the third nerve of one or both sides, giving rise to ptosis, strabismus, diplopia and pupillary disturbances; sometimes the fourth or sixth nerve is involved. Nystagmus is common. Changes in the fundi (hemorrhages, papilledema) occur, but are rather uncommon.

Friedreich's Disease rarely has any ocular disturbance except a peculiar pseudonystagmus consisting of irregular twitchings when the eyes are fixed upon a moving object in the horizontal direction. Ocular palsies, optic neuritis and Argyll-Robertson pupils occur rarely.

Headache is a common symptom of disease of the central nervous system and should always prompt a careful examination of the eyes. Errors of refraction are common causes of headache and neuralgia; not infrequently we find anomalies of the extrinsic ocular muscles; less often, uncorrected presbyopia and accommodation weakness are found to be responsible for head pains. The error of refraction which is most commonly responsible is astigmatism, less often hyperopia; the amount of astigmatism may be very moderate, even 0.25 or 0.50 D. The site of the pain varies, but is often supraorbital and frontal. We often find that the glasses required to cure headaches in individuals who were debilitated are no longer necessary when the system has regained its normal tone after a vacation.

Migraine. This affection, thought to depend upon some disturbance in the circulation of the cerebral cortex, is characterized by periodic or irregular attacks commencing with blurring of vision with or without scintillating scotoma, often more or less hemianopic in character. After a period varying from several minutes to half an hour, vision again becomes normal; then a very severe headache develops, accompanied often by nausea and vomiting, and followed by marked general depression. The attacks often are aggravated by eye strain; in such cases the seizures sometimes are made less severe, though rarely prevented, by correction of errors of refraction or of heterophoria.

Hydrocephalus often is accompanied by optic nerve atrophy and by ocular muscle palsies; less frequently papilledema is found.

Meningitis often presents optic neuritis, abnormalities of the pupils and palsies or spasms of the ocular muscles, causing deviations. These ocular manifestations are seen most frequently in tuberculous meningitis, in which variety tubercles of the choroid frequently are found.

Myasthenia Gravis is almost always accompanied by bilateral ptosis and weakness of the orbicularis; the ptosis increases with fatigue and is always least evident in the morning and most prominent in the evening. In many cases there also is partial or complete ophthalmoplegia externa, but the intrinsic muscles are not affected. Nystagmoid movements may be present but are not common.

Myelitis infrequently is accompanied by optic neuritis, retrobulbar in type, causing intense pain in the orbit and brow.

Syphilis of the Central Nervous System includes syphilitic arachnoiditis, general paresis and tabes.

Syphilitic archnoiditis may result in the formation of bands which compress the optic nerves or chiasm, producing visual field changes and optic atrophy.

General paresis. The subjects of this disease often present inequality and irregularity of the pupils, also miosis, and less frequently mydriasis. There commonly is impairment or loss of the light reflex (Argyll-Robertson pupil); later there is added partial or complete loss of reaction to accommodation. Sometimes atrophy of the optic nerve with reduction in the acuteness of vision and restriction of the field is observed. Palsies of the third, fourth and sixth nerves may occur.

Tabes is accompanied by many ocular signs. The Argyll-Robertson pupil, in which the reaction to light is lost, while that of convergence and accommodation is preserved, is present in the great majority of cases and usually exists on both sides. A deviation from circular shape, inequality and contraction of the pupil (miosis) are very common; much less frequently mydriasis is present, but it is then very often associated with blindness. Atrophy of the optic nerve occurs often as an early sign, is progressive and generally leads to blindness; with this change in the optic nerve there are reduction in the acuteness of vision and concentric contraction of the field. Ocular palsies are very common; they often occur early in the disease, involve the third and sixth nerves, rarely the fourth, appear suddenly in many instances, are generally transient and are accompanied by diplopia and ptosis if the third nerve is involved. Epiphora sometimes is observed; also uncoordinated movements of the eyeballs.

Multiple Sclerosis presents numerous ocular manifestations; the latter are found in fully one-half of the cases. Retrobulbar neuritis is very common and causes irregular peripheral contraction of the field of vision and a central or paracentral scotoma, relative or absolute; later there is incomplete optic nerve atrophy, unilateral or bilateral, evidenced by pallor of the temporal portion of the disk. Nystagmus is a frequent symptom. There are also partial paralyses of the extraocular muscles, giving rise to diplopia.

Tumor of the Brain (Including Abscess) gives rise to papilledema in most cases, generally bilateral. There may be palsies of ocular muscles and alterations in the field of vision. The characteristics of these changes are a great aid in localization. Tumors of the occipital and temporal lobes produce homonymous defects of the visual fields.

Neoplasms involving the optic nerve may give rise to optic atrophy of the simple (primary) type.

Diseases of the Endocrine Glands

Adrenal Glands. Pheochromocytoma of the adrenal gland may occur at any age, producing either a paroxysmal or a sustained hypertension. Either of these may produce ocular signs of hypertension (Chap. 10). These consist of transitory or sustained visual disturbances, retinal hemorrhages, edema, edema residues, neuroretinal edema and changes in the vessels themselves, including focal or generalized arteriolar spasms, crossing phenomena and, in the sustained hypertensive cases, copper wire reflex, perivascular sheathing and silver wire phenomenon.

Addison's disease, a primary insufficiency of the adrenal cortex, produces increased pigmentation throughout the body and causes increased pigmentation of the skin of the lids and at times of the conjunctiva and uvea.

Pituitary Gland. *Tumors of the pituitary gland* cause impairment of vision consisting of varying degrees of bitemporal field defects and partial to complete optic atrophy. The visual field defect depends upon the relationship of the growth to the optic pathways, so at times may be irregular, or there may be central and paracentral scotomas, but generally the defect begins in the superior temporal quadrant (Fig. 23-1), extends into the inferior temporal quadrant, the inferior nasal quadrant and, finally, the superior nasal quadrant (Fig. 23-2). One eye usually shows a greater field defect and maintains this difference through the course of the disease. Recovery following surgical removal or irradiation therapy of the tumor frequently is accompanied by recovery of part or all of the visual field. The defect disappears in the reverse order of its appearance. The field defect develops insidiously and at times may be quite extensive before interfering with visual acuity. The patient tends to bump

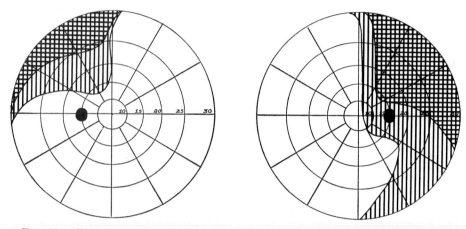

FIG. 23-1. Bjerrum screen visual field in bitemporal hemianopsia, showing greater involvement of the right than of the left field.

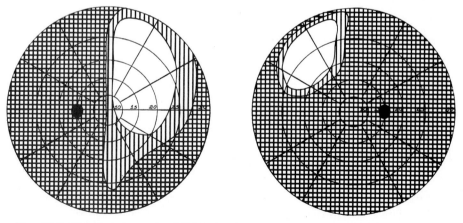

FIG. 23-2. Bjerrum screen visual field, showing later stage of development of bitemporal hemianopsia than is shown in Figure 23-1.

into things he "does not see" to either side.

Papilledema rarely is associated with pituitary tumor, the visual field loss being accompanied by pallor of the disks and eventually by optic atrophy unless the tumor is removed or controlled by irradiation therapy. Suprasellar tumors, on the other hand, may cause papilledema as well as bitemporal hemianopsia. Tumors of the pituitary which produce these signs commonly are eosinophil or chromophil adenoma and neutrophil or chromophobe adenoma and, rarely, basophil adenoma.

Thyroid Gland. *Thyroid deficiency* resulting in myxedema and cretinism gives rise to ocular signs consisting of noninflammatory edema of the eyelids and thinning of the brows early in the course of the affection. At times punctate opacities, visible only with biomicroscopic magnification, may develop in the lens and slowly progress to complete cataract formation.

Thyroid hyperactivity, or thyrotoxicosis, is associated with the development of exophthalmos, Graves' disease.

The thyrotoxic symptoms due to the excess production of thyroxine by a hyperplastic or hyperactive thyroid gland consist of heat intolerance, sweating, tremor, especially of the hands, muscle weakness, rapid irregular pulse, weight loss in spite of increased appetite, increased metabolic rate and nervousness.

Exophthalmos probably is due to some factor other than the excess production of thyroxine. Although responsible for most of the ocular manifestations of Graves' disease, exophthalmos is neither the first nor the only ocular sign.

Even before measurable exophthalmos can be demonstrated, the palpebral fissures are widened, the frequency of blinking of the lids is diminished and the upper lid does not move downward normally (lid lag) when the eye is turned downward. These signs, while characteristic of Graves' disease, also are seen in exophthalmic ophthalmoplegia and probably result from increased tone in the sympathetic nervous system. They affect both eyes.

However, the ocular signs in Graves' disease include (1) widening of the palpebral fissure or retraction of the upper lid (Dalrymple's sign), (2) diminished frequency of blinking (Stellwag's sign), (3) upper lid lag (Graefe's sign), (4) fullness of the upper lid and puffiness of both the lids (Enroth's sign), (5) jerky or cogwheel movement of the upper lid on looking downward (Boston's sign), (6) difficulty in everting the upper lid (Gifford's sign), (7) pigmentation of the upper lid (Jellinek's sign), (8) spastic retraction of the upper lid in addition to the usual widening of the palpebral fissure (Kocher's sign), (9) more rapid elevation of the upper lid in looking upward, or globe lag (Kocher's sign), (10) lag of lower lid on looking upward (Griffith's sign), (11) tremor of the closed lids (Rosenbach's sign), (12) weakness of convergence (Möbius' sign), (13) inability to maintain lateral rotation of the eyes (Suker's sign), (14) partial or complete paresis of one or more extraocular muscles (Ballet's sign), (15) jerky consensual pupillary reaction (Cowen's sign) and (16) rapid and wide dilatation of the pupils with weak solution of Adrenalin (Löwy's sign). The four most characteristic are retraction of the upper lid, lid lag, fullness of the upper lid and limitation of ocular movements, especially weakness of convergence. Congestion and chemosis of the conjunctiva, constant findings in proptosis and exophthalmos of any extent, usually develop in Graves' disease and exophthalmic ophthalmoplegia before the exophthalmos. In fact, beginning or intensification of congestion over the lateral rectus muscle insertion usually precedes and foreshadows increase in exophthalmos (Dunphy's sign).

Exophthalmos in Graves' disease usually is bilateral but frequently begins in one eye and continues to be greater in that eye throughout the course of the disease. Treatment and control of the thyrotoxicosis may or may not control the exophthalmos; however, when it increases to the degree that the lids cannot protect the eyes properly, local measures must be taken to prevent the development of exposure keratitis, corneal ulceration and their sequelae. Temporarily, protective condensation shields may be made for the patient or lateral tarsorraphy may be made. This is an operation which shortens and narrows the palpebral fissure by closing the lids for a short distance at the lateral end of the palpebral fissure and does not cause a great disturbance in the appearance of the patient. Should this not be adequate, a decompression of the orbit must be accomplished. The most effective and least disturbing method is removal of the lateral bony wall and, if necessary, part of the temporal muscle.

Exophthalmic ophthalmoplegia is a term used to describe the progressive exophthalmos which occurs in the euthyroid state or after thyrotoxicosis has been controlled, although sometimes it is used erroneously to describe any type of endocrine exophthalmos. In this disease, suppression of thyroid activity only increases the exophthalmos; therefore desiccated thyroid or other medications which inhibit pituitary activity are administered, and the eyes are observed and treated to prevent exposure and drying.

Parathyroid Glands. *Parathyroid deficiency* results in alteration of calcium metabolism and may lead to the formation of zonular or parathyroidea priva cataract (see Chap. 12).

Pancreas. Ocular manifestations of *diabetes mellitus* include alterations in vi-sion due to transitory changes in the refractive state of the eye after the blood sugar has remained over 250 mg. for a prolonged period, or as the result of quick reduction and control of the blood sugar level below 150 mg. after it has been elevated for some time. In either case, the change is temporary and the eyes return to their usual refractive state after the blood sugar has been controlled for 1 week to 10 days. Distinctive and pathognomonic cataracts of either a snowstorm variety or a subcapsular plaque-like type occur in children. Cataracts also may occur in adults, or the senile variety of cataracts may be hastened because of poor control, but they are not sufficiently different to be distinguishable as diabetes-induced changes. In addition to the retinal changes (described in detail in Chap. 10), which consist of microaneurysms, retinal hemorrhages of the punctate variety early but later of any type, edema residues and crystalline deposits in the retina, venous aneurysmal-like dilatations, venous obstructions, including obstruction of the central retinal vein, vitreous hemorrhage and proliferative retinopathy, secondary glaucoma may follow occlusion of the central retinal vein and vitreous hemorrhage. Rubeosis of the iris develops as a result of changes in the vessels of the iris and more or less atrophy of the stroma of the iris. In addition, arteriosclerotic changes develop in the diabetic patient and frequently contribute to the ocular lesions. Less frequently, paresis of one or more of the extraocular muscles and paralysis of accommodation occur. Optic neuritis and retrobulbar neuritis rarely occur, but may be coincidental or due only in part to diabetes.

Lipemia retinalis is a rare manifestation of diabetes mellitus especially likely to occur in young individuals who have exercised little or very poor efforts at control and are either in coma or on the verge of it (Chap. 10). Lipemia, however, occurs in a number of other conditions without visible evidence of it in the retina, or with it in rare situations. An exact explanation for the difference has not been found.

Metabolic Disorders

Amyloidosis may be primary or secondary to such diseases as tuberculosis, leprosy, bronchiestasis, osteomyelitis and neoplasms. In either case, it may cause the deposition of yellow colloid material under the palpebral or bulbar conjunctiva and in some instances may cause paresis of the extraocular muscles and hemorrhagic retinopathy.

Cystinosis (Fanconi or de Toni-Lignac-Fanconi syndrome), in addition to depositing cystine in the reticuloendothelial cells, lymph nodes, spleen, bone marrow and liver, is characterized by the deposition of crystals in the conjunctiva and cornea associated with photophobia. The crystals appear as minute shiny dots and are seen best with the biomicroscope.

Galactosemia, a metabolic disorder manifest shortly after birth by vomiting, diarrhea and weight loss caused by the infant's inability to convert galactose to glucose, is associated with the development of changes in the lens which are reversible if the infant is taken off galactose-containing foods early enough; otherwise this may progress to the development of cataracts.

Gaucher's Disease, a familial metabolic disorder of cerebroside storage in the reticuloendothelial cells, especially of the spleen and liver, may produce yellow pigmentation of the lids and yellow or yellowish brown deposits in the conjunctiva and sclera, especially in the portions exposed with the lids open.

Gout, a disturbance in purine metabolism, frequently hereditary, is responsible at times for episcleritis, scleritis and iritis.

Hepatolenticular   Degeneration (Wilson's disease), a familial disease of adolescents and young adults, is characterized by degeneration of the lenticular nuclei, nodular cirrhosis of the liver and incoordination and tremors of the extremities, thought to result from abnormal copper metabolism; it is associated with a ring of greenish, brown or golden brown discoloration of the posterior peripheral portion of the cornea. This pigmentation, the Kayser-Fleischer ring, is pathognomonic.

Ochronosis (alkaptonuria) is a metabolic disorder in which homogentisic acid, a degradation product of tyrosine and phenylalanine, is not broken down but is deposited in tissues, giving rise to melanosis, especially in cartilage, joint capsules, the skin of the lids, the conjunctiva and the sclera. Brown deposits are especially likely to develop between the insertion of the recti and the cornea.

Porphyria is an abnormality of blood pigment metabolism in which excessive amounts of porphyrins are found in the blood and urine and which is associated with light sensitivity in the congenital and chronic forms of the disease. Bullae or vesicles occur on the skin of the lids. Vesicular conjunctivitis which may be followed by symblepharon may be associated with vesicular keratitis leading to vascularization and scarring, and occasionally with ulcers of the sclera followed by staphylomas. Occasionally there may be hemorrhagic retinopathy, optic atrophy and muscle palsies.

Xanthomatosis, a disorder probably of metabolism of lipids and fats leading to deposition of these substances in flat or slightly elevated plaques in the skin especially of the eyelids (xanthoma), occurs in middle-aged and elderly individuals without apparent disease at times. Xanthomas occur frequently in diabetics, in whom the lesion is called "xanthoma diabeticorum."

The Connective Tissue Diseases

Cranial Arteritis, a chronic inflammatory disease of the arteries of elderly persons, has a predilection for the temporal arteries but can be widespread through the body. It affects the arteries of the anterior portion of the optic nerve in approximately half of the cases. Usually after a period of pain, tenderness and swelling of the temporal artery, but occasionally without it, the patient suddenly loses part or all of the vision of one eye and the other is affected similarly within a few weeks in almost half of the cases, frequently ending in total blindness. Ophthalmoscopic examination discloses changes similar to those of occlusion of the central retinal artery: narrow vessels, edema of the retina, especially in the perimacular region, occasionally some hemorrhages and cotton wool patches. This is followed by pallor of the disk as optic atrophy develops.

Periarteritis Nodosa, a widespread disease of the arteries, frequently produces renal damage and hypertension which in turn produce any or all of the manifestations of hypertensive disease in the eye (Chap. 10). The retinal and uveal blood vessels rarely exhibit the typical lesions, but they may become large enough to be recognized ophthalmoscopically.

Dermatomyositis, a rare systemic disease characterized by inflammatory and degenerative changes in the skin and muscles, may have an insidious or abrupt onset with fever, bright erythema of the skin and painful swollen muscles. The lid may be the primary site of involvement. Swelling of the lids, brawny and purplish red, spreads onto the face and ears or may remain patchy and symmetrical, but is followed by atrophy and pigmentation.

The extraocular muscles may be involved, resulting in nystagmus or palsies and occasionally exophthalmos. Conjunctivitis, iritis and hemorrhagic retinopathy with cotton wool patches occur rarely.

Scleroderma, a disease characterized by diffuse or localized alteration of the connective tissue, may produce thickening of the skin of the lids and brows and occasionally is associated with iritis and cataracts.

Lupus Erythematosus, in the acute form, with fever, leukopenia, splenomegaly, arthralgias and nephritis, produces a purplish butterfly type of eruption of the skin of the cheeks and across the nose which may spread to involve the skin of the lids and onto the conjunctiva. There may be localized or nodular inflammatory lesions of the choroid and hemorrhagic retinopathy with cotton wool patches, perivascular sheathing, arterial occlusions and papilledema. There also may be nystagmus and extraocular muscle palsies, probably from central nervous system involvement. In the chronic form, ocular involvement is limited to the lids and conjunctiva.

Diseases of the Bones and Joints

Arthritis frequently is associated with inflammatory diseases of the uveal tract and, less commonly, Tenon's capsule, episclera, sclera and conjunctiva.

Rheumatoid Arthritis, a disease of unknown cause affecting many joints, in general affects women between the ages of 25 and 50 about 2 or 3 times as often as men. Younger individuals with acute arthritis of this type may develop scleromalacia perforans, a chronic inflammatory lesion of the episclera and sclera with associated uveitis which may result in staphylomas or perforation of the globe. The lesions are likely to be recurrent. In patients who are considerably older at the onset of the joint disturbances, scleromalacia is not likely to occur, but keratoconjunctivitis sicca (Sjögren's syndrome) may precede or accompany the arthritis.

Rheumatoid Spondylitis (ankylosing spondylitis, Marie-Strümpell disease), a form of adult rheumatoid arthritis causing chronic progressive disease of the small joints of the spine, reverses the sex ratio, affecting young adult males in a ratio of approximately 9:1. This disorder is frequently associated with recurrent iritis, which may lead to posterior synechia formation, secondary glaucoma and cataracts if not controlled.

Juvenile Rheumatoid Arthritis (Still's disease), a polyarthritic lesion affecting children and involving growing joints, thus more likely to produce deformities but otherwise similar to adult rheumatoid arthritis, may cause anterior uveitis of a chronic nature leading to posterior synechiae, cataracts and secondary glaucoma unless adequately controlled. In half of the children with ocular lesions a band-shaped opacity develops in the cornea and eventually leads to repeated bouts of superficial corneal ulceration and may end with degeneration of the globe.

Gonococcal Arthritis, an acute monarticular arthritis usually affecting the knee or elbow and usually associated with an active or recently active gonorrheal urethritis, may be associated with a unilateral or rarely bilateral gonorrheal iritis, occasionally a tenonitis and rarely a metastatic conjunctivitis.

The iritis is acute and plastic in character. A large amount of fibrin passes into and becomes clotted in the anterior chamber so there is no circulation of the aqueous. Posterior synechiae tend to form quickly between the posterior surface of the iris and lens, and an inflammatory membrane may develop across the lens, occluding the pupillary opening. Because of this, treatment must be prompt and, in addition to treatment of the infection with penicillin intramuscularly and sulfonamides orally, the pupil must be dilated and the ciliary body put at rest by the establishment of complete cycloplegia. Fever therapy produced either by foreign protein injections intravenously or by fever cabinet therapy is the most effective method of causing contraction of the clot and re-establishing circulation in the anterior chamber. Before penicillin and sulfonamide therapy were available, these episodes were likely to be recurrent, but with adequate therapy there should be no recurrences except with newly acquired urethral infections.

Gonorrheal tenonitis may occur alone or in association with iritis or metastatic conjunctivitis with a similar relationship to gonorrheal arthritis. The conjunctiva is chemotic, the globe is slightly proptosed and movement of the globe is painful and limited.

Metastatic gonorrheal conjunctivitis is a purulent type in which the organisms cannot be demonstrated in the secretions or on the epithelial cells of the conjunctiva. They have been demonstrated in the subconjunctival tissue by biopsy; however, this is not advisable. Diagnosis of all three of these ocular lesions depends upon the history, relationship to urethritis and arthritis, demonstration of positive cultures from the bloodstream and the acute joint and rapid response to treatment.

Tuberculous Arthritis and Bone Disease in children is especially likely to be followed by tuberculous periphlebitis or uveitis several years after the bone or joint lesion has healed, and occurs only rarely during the active phase. Treatment is palliative to the eye, including cycloplegic rest, with general treatment of tuberculosis.

Gargoylism (dysostosis multiplex, Hurler's disease) is characterized by a large head with wide separation of the orbits and a broad flat nose, in a dwarf. In about 75 per cent of cases, the patient's cornea is cloudy because of fine gray dots visible with biomicroscopic magnification in the middle and posterior portions of the stroma.

Morquio's disease and Morquio-Ullrich's disease, similar types of dwarfism but without the gargoylism, also show corneal clouding similar to that of Hurler's disease.

Arachnodactyly (Marfan's syndrome), a hereditary and familial disorder charac-terized by long thin fingers and toes and long extremities, generally shows miosis and congenital subluxation of the lenses which at times may be associated with in-creased depth of the anterior chamber, iridodonesis and poor vision.

Brachymorphia Spherophakia Syndrome (Marchesani syndrome) is a he-reditary and familial disorder character-ized by short, stocky individuals with short stubby fingers, poorly developed zonules and excessively curved subluxated lenses, which frequently progress to dis-location of the lens or glaucoma or both.

GENERAL INFECTIOUS DISEASES

Ocular involvement or ocular signs are of frequent occurrence in general or sys-temic infectious processes. Since the gen-eral symptomatology, course and treat-ment of these diseases fall in the province of the internist, only the ocular signs, symptoms and involvement are discussed here. The strictly ocular infections have been discussed elsewhere in this book.

Bacterial Infections

Brucellosis may be associated with acute or chronic iritis, iridocyclitis, uve-itis, chorioretinitis and occasionally optic neuritis. Chronic nodular uveitis probably is the most frequent.

Cholera, as a result of the great de-hydration and malnutrition, produces shrinkage of the orbital contents so the eyeballs are shrunken in the orbit and the lids have a bluish appearance. The cornea frequently becomes dull, infiltrated and ulcerated. Subconjunctival hemorrhages occur and occasionally cataracts develop rapidly.

Diphtheria, in addition to the produc-tion of membranous, purulent or occa-sionally simple catarrhal conjunctivitis in association with diphtheria of the upper respiratory passages, may cause paralysis of one or more of the extraocular muscles, usually the external rectus, and paralysis of accommodation in the period after the acute stage of the disease has passed. Oc-casionally optic neuritis occurs.

Erysipelas may spread to and involve the lids and orbit, resulting in abscess or gangrene and sloughing of the skin. When the disease extends into the orbit it causes orbital cellulitis, thrombosis of the retinal veins, optic neuritis and atrophy of the optic nerve. It can lead to cavernous sinus thrombosis.

Glanders may produce a unilateral or, very rarely, a bilateral nodular type of conjunctivitis associated with regional lymphadenopathy.

Gonorrhea. See page 382.

Infectious Mononucleosis may be ac-companied at its onset by an acute or sub-acute conjunctivitis. Rarely dacryoadeni-tis, dacryocystitis, episcleritis, retinal periphlebitis, papilledema or optic neuritis, nystagmus, extraocular muscle palsies and visual field defects may develop in the course of the disease.

Influenza nearly always is accompa-nied by acute catarrhal conjunctivitis, but in addition there may be pain in and back of the eyes and rarely corneal ulcers, paresis of the extraocular muscles, retro-bulbar neuritis, optic neuritis, optic atrophy and orbital cellulitis. In the post-infectious period of depression and weakness, asthenopia and weakness of accommodation may be observed.

Leprosy produces nodular lesions of the brow and occasionally of the lids, with loss of the hairs of the brow beginning in the external part, episcleritis, avascular keratitis, keratitis with pannus, keratitis with interstitial vascularization or keratitis with both pannus and interstitial vascularization, all of which are pathognomonic of the disease. In addition, iritis or iridocyclitis of an acute simple variety or a chronic nodular variety may occur. As complications, secondary glaucoma and cataract may develop, but the disease seldom if ever involves the posterior portion of the eye and optic nerve. Miliary lepromas or "pearls" develop in the subconjunctival tissue especially near the limbus, in the cornea and in the iris in the course of the disease in many patients. They also develop in the ciliary body and have been observed to appear and disappear in the retina, probably on the internal surface of the retina, but they probably were formed anteriorly, broke free and were carried to the retina by chance movement rather than having actually developed in the retina.

Lymphogranuloma Inguinale may produce an ulceronodular lesion of the conjunctiva associated with regional lymphadenopathy rarely. The cornea may be involved in the course of the conjunctival disease.

Meningitis, caused by *Neisseria meningitidis*, rarely may begin with an acute purulent conjunctivitis as its portal of entry, or more commonly the conjunctivitis occurs simultaneously with the onset or in the course of the general disease. Vitreous abscess and endophthalmitis were frequent complications of the process before the advent of the sulfonamide drugs. Other sequelae which formerly were

more prevalent include paresis of the extraocular muscles, ptosis, nystagmus, abnormalities of the pupils, retinal hemorrhage, optic neuritis and optic atrophy.

Pneumonia also was frequently a cause of vitreous abscess and endophthalmitis before the advent of the sulfonamide drugs, but now exists only as a rare and exceptional cause.

Relapsing Fever is a descriptive diagnosis of a clinical condition which may be caused by a large number of different bacteria varying with the locality of the patient. However, a number of these infectious processes may be accompanied by conjunctivitis at the onset or during the course of the disease, and many of them may cause iritis, iridocyclitis or uveitis, and rarely panophthalmitis, optic atrophy and paralysis of the extraocular muscles.

Scarlet Fever is frequently accompanied by acute catarrhal conjunctivitis and rarely corneal ulceration. These lesions are more likely to occur in the convalescent stage. When the disease is complicated by nephritis, acute hemorrhagic edematous retinopathy with cotton wool patches and sometimes neuroretinopathy also may occur.

Septicemia and Pyemia may cause retinal hemorrhages, septic infarcts (Roth's spots as described under subacute bacterial endocarditis), embolic obstruction of arterioles and venules, endophthalmitis or panophthalmitis.

Syphilis is frequently the cause of ocular disease. Congenital syphilis may be manifest by a secondary rash on the lids, rarely, or more commonly syphilitic chorioretinitis with or without interstitial keratitis. Acquired syphilis may begin as a primary lesion on the lids or conjunctiva rarely. Secondary rashes almost always involve the lids and frequently produce iritis. In the later stages choroiditis is more likely to occur. In the tertiary stage gummas may occur in the iris, ciliary body, periosteum and orbital wall. Optic neuritis may occur. Also in the tertiary stage paralysis and paresis of the extraocular and intraocular muscles are common (also see below).

Tetanus may begin with spasms of the orbicularis or extraocular muscles following wounds about the head and orbit.

Tuberculosis, rarely, may begin from exogenous infection of a wound of the conjunctiva or lids, and rarely primary infection may occur in the lacrimal sac; however, these are quite infrequent and the majority of tuberculous lesions of the eye and adnexa are secondary. These lesions include tuberculous dacryoadenitis, periostitis and dacryocystitis, but the more common lesions are tuberculous uveitis, which may involve the anterior or posterior uvea, and periphlebitis retinae (Eale's disease). Anterior tuberculous uveitis also may cause parenchymatous keratitis (tuberculous interstitial keratitis), or scleritis and scleratizing keratitis.

Phlyctenular conjunctivitis and keratitis are the result of tuberculous infection and the development of sensitivity to tuberculin.

Tularemia produces an ulceroglandular conjunctivitis as a result of contamination of the conjunctiva with infectious material from animals and, rarely, bloodsucking insects such as the tick.

Typhoid Fever may produce conjunctivitis; retinopathy, with edema, hemorrhages, septic infarcts (Roth's spots) and neuroretinal edema; optic neuritis; metastatic choroiditis and iritis; and occasionally temporary paresis of the extraocular muscles, particularly the lateral rectus.

Whooping Cough often causes subconjunctival hemorrhages as a result of the severe paroxysms of coughing. Occasionally such an extravasation takes place in the lid, and rarely it involves the orbit, producing serious damage.

Yellow Fever in its early stage produces congestion of the conjunctiva, later modified by the addition of a yellowish discoloration. Retinal hemorrhages as well as subconjunctival hemorrhages also occur.

Weil's Disease produces yellowish discoloration and infection of the conjunctiva, subconjunctival hemorrhages and occasionally uveitis.

Fungus Diseases

Fungus diseases are becoming increasingly important in all aspects of medicine. In ophthalmology there has been an increase in the number of primary infections of ocular tissues as well as an increase in the number of generalized fungus infections with ocular manifestations.

Mucormycosis, occurring as a general or central nervous system infection in diabetic patients, has extended into or become localized in the orbit, producing proptosis as a result of a chronic inflammation of the orbital tissues.

Rickettsial Infections

Rickettsial Diseases include *typhus fever, scrub typhus* (tsutsugamushi fever) and *Rocky Mountain spotted fever*. The principal ocular lesions in these diseases are subconjunctival hemorrhages, hemorrhagic edematous retinopathy, perivasculitis and cotton wool patches and hemorrhagic edematous uveitis. Optic neuritis and occasionally extraocular muscle palsies occur in typhus fever, and corneal ulcers, especially of the lower portion, may occur occasionally during convalescence.

In scrub typhus a hemorrhagic eschar may form at the site of the mite bite, which occasionally may be located on the lids.

Virus Infections

Chicken Pox (varicella) produces vesicular lesions on the lids, and usually there is some conjunctival irritation. At times there may be more intense bulbar and circumcorneal injection associated with photophobia but no visible lesion of the cornea or iritis. In other patients, however, severe iritis and optic neuritis may occur.

Herpes Zoster, which is caused by the same virus as chicken pox, may affect the ophthalmic division of the fifth cranial nerve, producing the typical vesicular skin lesions without other ocular involvement, but vesicular lesions of the conjunctiva and cornea, deep or diskiform keratitis, severe and prolonged anterior uveitis and transitory extraocular muscle palsies may occur. When corneal lesions develop they usually result in considerable scarring and loss of vision.

Measles (rubeola) may be diagnosed at times by the appearance of spots resembling Koplik's spots on the caruncle or semilunar fold as early as 2 days before they occur in the mouth. Conjunctival injection and superficial punctate epithelial keratitis visible only with biomicroscopic magnification appear in the coryzal stage of the infection and frequently persist through the course of the disease. Optic neuritis may occur rarely. Secondary bacterial infection of the conjunctiva and cornea occurs occasionally and may lead to serious lesions and sequelae.

Squint often is said by patients to have developed while a child had measles; however, the cause and effect relationship is not so simple and may be mere coincidence or no more than accentuation of a pre-existing weakness by the general debility of the disease.

Rubella (German measles) has little effect on the eyes of the patient but can produce serious developmental defects in babies whose mothers contract the disease during the first trimester of pregnancy. These consist of bilateral congenital cataracts, congenital defects of the heart, teeth, ears and other organs and mental retardation. Many of the babies are small, poorly nourished and die early from bronchopneumonia. However, since there is an approximately 100 per cent probability of serious defects being present at birth in mothers who have rubella during the first 2 months of pregnancy and a 50 per cent probability during the third month, it is important to expose girls to rubella before the childbearing age, for unfortunately the disease frequently is so slight that the mother may remember it only in retrospect when considering the tragic results after delivery. Otherwise serious consideration should be given to termination of a pregnancy complicated by rubella in the first trimester.

Mumps or epidemic parotitis most commonly produces a dacryoadenitis which may become suppurative as an ocular manifestation of the infection. However, occasionally keratitis with considerable photophobia occurs but usually clears without scarring or vascularization. Paralysis of accommodation, paresis of one or more of the extraocular muscles and optic neuritis may occur rarely.

Vaccinia may effect the eyelids by accidental inoculation, by accidental transfer of the vaccine from the site of inoculation to the lids by the patient after the inoculation, or by the localization of the virus in a pre-existing break in the skin of the lids or a pre-existing dermal lesion during the period of viremia, which ordinarily is between 2 and 6 days following inoculation. Lesions on the lid run the same usual course of vesicle, pustule, crust and scar as the lesion at the site of inoculation, but scarring frequently is less severe. However, care must be taken to prevent spread or contamination of the conjunctiva and especially the cornea, for a severe keratitis resulting in dense scarring and vascularization usually follows if it is involved. Because of the tendency for the virus to localize in pre-existing lesions during the period of viremia, persons with lid, lid margin, conjunctival or corneal lesions should not be vaccinated until the lesion has healed.

Variola always involves the lids with typical lesions, but at times these may become severe, resulting in destructive gangrenous lesions. Ordinarily the conjunctiva and cornea are not involved, but care must be taken to prevent crusts of the lid lesions falling into the conjunctiva and inoculating it or the cornea. As in vaccinia, severe keratitis of a diskiform type usually develops and produces severe scarring and eventually heavy vascularization. Occasionally ulceration and perforation of the cornea may occur and, if the eye is saved, a staphyloma ensues.

Miscellaneous Diseases and Conditions

Consanguinity of Parentage tends to accentuate ocular abnormalities in the offspring, especially retinitis pigmentosa and congenital ocular malformations.

Ear. Congestion of the papilla and papilledema are frequently observed in sinus thrombosis complicating mastoiditis. Abducens paralysis and trigeminal neuralgia may accompany infection of the petrous pyramid as a sequela of otitis media (Gradenigo's syndrome). Nystagmus is common in affections of the labyrinth and vestibular pathways.

Nose and Throat. The communication between the nose and the conjunctival sac by means of the lacrimal duct, in part, explains the frequent occurrence of ocular symptoms and affections as a result of nasal disease. Often in coryza there is conjunctival congestion or acute catarrhal conjunctivitis with severe lacrimation. In hay fever these conditions also are very annoying, with itching. Conjunctivitis, blepharitis and phlyctenular affections may complicate chronic rhinitis; in addition, the nasal swelling may obstruct the lower end of the lacrimal duct and produce stenosis, dacryocystitis and lacrimal abscess. The lacrimal duct may be the means of conveying infective material from the nose to the conjunctival sac, and thus explain the occurrence of corneal ulcer. Adenoids may be associated with catarrhal or follicular conjunctivitis, epiphora and asthenopia.

Diseases of the Accessory Sinuses may be responsible for many ocular symptoms and diseases, among which are orbital periostitis and cellulitis, exophthalmos, paresis or paralysis of the ocular muscles, asthenopia, changes in the visual fields including scotomas and increase in size of the blind spot, choroiditis, optic neuritis, neuroretinitis, retrobulbar neuritis and optic atrophy.

Teeth. The occurrence of ocular symptoms and diseases dependent upon dental disease is not rare, and in such cases it is common to have the ocular symptoms disappear and the ocular disease improve when the offending tooth is extracted. Such symptoms include conjunctival congestion, photophobia, epiphora, asthenopia, amblyopia and weakness of accommodation. Iritis, keratitis, cyclitis and choroiditis may be dependent upon oral sepsis.

Stomach and Intestines. Chronic affections of these organs may cause ocular symptoms by interfering with nutrition and reducing the general tone of the individual; thus asthenopia, weakness of accommodation and heterophoria are found frequently. Absorption of toxic material from the gastrointestinal tract may give rise to intraocular inflammation. The loss of much blood from gastric or intestinal hemorrhage may cause amblyopia with anemia of the retina without other ophthalmoscopic changes, or with subsequent optic nerve atrophy. Straining associated with constipation may result in subconjunctival, retinal and vitreous hemorrhage.

Liver. Diseases of the liver may cause ocular symptoms such as asthenopia and weakness of accommodation as a result of general loss in strength. In jaundice, the yellowish discoloration of the sclera and of the conjunctiva is one of the earliest signs.

Menstruation. Ocular diseases often show an exacerbation at the menstrual period, and asthenopic symptoms and weakness of accommodation sometimes are observed at this time. Vicarious menstruation is represented occasionally by subconjunctival, vitreous or retinal hemorrhage.

Parturition is accompanied by danger to the eyes of the child: Conjunctival infection may give rise to ophthalmia neonatorum; the use of forceps during delivery has resulted in bruising of the lids, injury to the cornea, orbital hemorrhage causing exophthalmos, and even rupture of the eyeball. Birth trauma may cause ocular palsies and hemorrhages; the latter are common. If the mother has lost much blood, she may have amblyopia with or without subsequent optic nerve atrophy. Puerperal infection may result in metastatic choroiditis or in panophthalmitis with loss of the eye. Parturition rarely may be followed also by optic neuritis, atrophy of the optic nerve, retrobulbar neuritis, retinal hemorrhages and embolism of the central artery of the retina.

Lactation, if prolonged and causing impairment of the mother's health, may be responsible for paresis of accommodation and asthenopic symptoms.

Poisons and Intoxications may cause ocular symptoms and disease, especially retrobulbar neuritis (less often neuroretinitis and optic nerve atrophy) resulting from poisoning by alcohol, tobacco, wood alcohol, chloral, iodoform, lead, arsenic compounds, bisulfide of carbon, nitrobenzol, thallium acetate and aniline. Cataract may follow poisoning by naphthalene and the use of dinitrophenol for reducing purposes.

Vitamin Deficiency. Vitamin A deficiency may result in defective dark adaptation and in the night blindness of keratomalacia. Lack of vitamin B_1 may cause toxic amblyopia or optic neuritis. Deficiency of vitamin B_2 (riboflavin) may be followed by corneal vascularization. The subjects of rickets sometimes present zonular cataract and interstitial keratitis. Scurvy is accompanied by subconjunctival, palpebral, retinal and occasionally orbital hemorrhages.

Vertigo (ocular), with or without nausea, often is dependent upon refractive errors or heterophoria or may be due to pareses of extraocular muscles.

Appendix

Ocular Requirements for Driving and for Admission to the Army, Navy, Marine Corps, Air Force and Coast Guard of the United States

VISUAL STANDARDS FOR OPERATING MOTOR VEHICLES

The large number of accidents and deaths caused by motor vehicles has called attention to the necessity of limiting the drivers of such conveyances to those possessing a sufficient degree of visual efficiency. A committee of the Section on Ophthalmology of the American Medical Association gave this subject serious consideration for many years, formulated a schedule of minimum visual requirements and advised its adoption by licensing boards; this has been approved by the American Medical Association.

These standards are the following:

A. For an unlimited license:
1. Visual acuity with or without glasses of 20/40 in one eye and 20/200 in the other.
2. A form field of not less than 45 degrees in all meridians from the point of fixation.
3. The presence of binocular single vision.
4. Ability to distinguish red, green and yellow.
5. Night blindness not to be present.
6. Glasses, when required, must be worn while driving, and those employed in public transportation be provided with an extra pair.

B. Visual standards for limited license:
1. Visual acuity of not less than 20/65 in the better eye.
2. Field vision of not less than 60 degrees horizontally and 50 degrees vertically from point of fixation in one eye.
3. Diplopia not to be present.
4. Glasses to be worn when prescribed.
5. Coordination of eye, mind and muscle to be fully adequate to meet the practical visual road tests.
6. A limited license not to be issued to those employed in public transportation.

C. Renewals, retesting and re-examinations:
1. Renewals of license to be issued at least every third year. The applicant shall with each renewal make a declaration that he knows of no visual defect which had developed during the past year.
2. Retesting of acuity to be made at least every 6 years.
3. If any visual defects have developed, an examination by an ophthalmologist, and the report thereof, to be required before reissuing the licence.
4. License to state thereon the specific limitation for driving.

OCULAR REQUIREMENTS FOR THE U. S. ARMY

A. Causes for Rejection for Appointment, Enlistment, and Induction

a. Lids
1. Blepharitis, chronic more than mild. Cases of acute blepharitis will be rejected until cured.
2. Blepharospasm.

389

3. Dacryocystitis, acute or chronic.
4. Destruction of the lids, complete or extensive, sufficient to impair protection of the eye from exposure.
5. Disfiguring cicatrices and adhesions of the eyelids to each other or to the eyeball.
6. Growth or tumor of the eyelid other than small early basal cell tumors of the eyelid, which can be cured by treatment, and small nonprogressive asymptomatic benign lesions.
7. Marked inversion or eversion of the eyelids sufficient to cause unsightly appearance or watering of eyes (entropion or ectropion).
8. Lagophthalmos.
9. Ptosis interfering with vision.
10. Trichiasis, severe.

b. Conjunctiva
1. Conjunctivitis, chronic, including vernal catarrh and trachoma. Individuals with acute conjunctivitis are unacceptable until the condition is cured.
6. Pterygium
   a) Pterygium recurring after three operative procedures.
   b) Pterygium encroaching on the cornea in excess of 3 mm. or interfering with vision.

c. Cornea
1. Dystrophy, corneal, of any type including keratoconus of any degree.
2. Keratitis, acute or chronic.
3. Ulcer, corneal; history of recurrent ulcers or corneal abrasions (including herpetic ulcers).
4. Vascularization or opacification of the cornea from any cause which interferes with visual function or is progressive.

d. Uveal tract: Inflammation of the uveal tract except healed traumatic choroiditis.

e. Retina
1. Angiomatoses, phakomatoses, retinal cysts, and other congenito-hereditary conditions that impair visual function.
2. Degenerations of the retina to include macular cysts, holes, and other degenerations (hereditary or acquired degenerative changes) and other conditions affecting the macula. All types of pigmentary degenerations (primary and secondary).
3. Detachment of the retina or history of surgery for same.
4. Inflammation of the retina (retinitis or other inflammatory conditions of the retina to include Coat's disease, diabetic retinopathy, Eales' disease, and retinitis proliferans).

f. Optic nerve
1. Congenito-hereditary conditions of the optic nerve or any other central nervous system pathology affecting the efficient function of the optic nerve.
2. Optic neuritis, neuroretinitis, or secondary optic atrophy resulting therefrom or documented history of attacks of retrobulbar neuritis.
3. Optic atrophy (primary or secondary).
4. Papilledema.

g. Lens
1. Aphakia (unilateral or bilateral).
2. Dislocation, partial or complete, of a lens.
3. Opacities of the lens which interfere with vision or which are considered to be progressive.

h. Ocular mobility and motility
1. Diplopia, documented, constant

or intermittent from any cause or of any degree interfering with visual function (*i.e.*, may suppress).

2. Diplopia, monocular, documented, interfering with visual function.
3. Nystagmus, with both eyes fixing, congenital or acquired.
4. Strabismus of 40 prism diopters or more, uncorrectable by lenses to less than 40 diopters.
5. Strabismus of any degree accompanied by documented diplopia.
6. Strabismus, surgery for the correction of, within the preceding 6 months.

i. Miscellaneous defects and diseases
1. Abnormal conditions of the eye or visual fields due to diseases of the central nervous system.
2. Absence of an eye.
3. Asthenopia, severe.
4. Exophthalmos, unilateral and bilateral.
5. Glaucoma, primary and secondary.
6. Hemianopsia of any type.
7. Loss of normal pupillary reflex reactions to light or accomodation to distance or Adie's syndrome.
8. Loss of visual fields due to organic disease.
9. Night blindness associated with objective disease of the eye. Verified congenital night blindness.
10. Residuals of old contusions, lacerations, penetrations, etc., which impair visual function required for satisfactory performance of military duty.
11. Retain intraocular foreign body.
12. Tumors.
13. Any organic disease of the eye

or adnexa not specified above which threatens continuity of vision or impairment of visual function.

j. Distant visual acuity: Distant visual acuity of any degree which does not correct to at least one of the following:
1. 20/40 in one eye and 20/70 in the other eye.
2. 20/30 in one eye and 20/100 in the other eye.
3. 20/20 in one eye and 20/400 in the other eye.

k. Near visual acuity: Near visual acuity of any degree which does not correct to at least J.6 in the better eye.

l. Refractive error: Any degree of refractive error in spherical equivalent of over −8.00 or +8.00; or if ordinary spectacles cause discomfort by reason of ghost images, prismatic displacement, etc.; or if an ophthalmologic consultation reveals a condition which is disqualifying.

m. Contact lens: Complicated cases requiring contact lens for adequate correction of vision as keratoconus, corneal scars, and irregular astigmatism.

B. Causes of Medical Unfitness for further Military Service

a. Active eye disease or any progressive organic eye disease regardless of the stage of activity, resistant to treatment which affects the distant visual acuity or visual field of an eye to any degree when:
1. The distant visual acuity in the unaffected eye cannot be corrected to 20/40 or better, or
2. The diameter of the visual field in the unaffected eye is less than 20 degrees.

b. Aphakia, bilateral.

c. Atrophy of optic nerve due to disease.

d. Chronic congestive (closed angle) glaucoma or chronic noncongestive (open angle) glaucoma if well established with demonstrable changes in the optic disk or visual fields.

e. Congenital and developmental defects do not *per se*, render the individual medically unfit.

f. Degenerations: When visual loss exceeds the limits shown below or when vision is correctable only by the use of contact lenses, or other special corrective devices (telescopic lenses, etc.).

g. Diseases and infections of the eye. When chronic, more than mildly symptomatic, progressive, and resistant to treatment after a reasonable period.

h. Ocular manifestations of endocrine or metabolic disorders do not in themselves, render the individual medically unfit. However the residuals or complications thereof or the underlying disease may render medically unfit.

i. Residuals or complications of injury to the eye which are progressive or which bring vision below the criteria in paragraphs k through q.

j. Retina, detachment of:

  1. Unilateral.

    a) When vision in the better eye cannot be corrected to at least 20/40,

    b) When the visual field in the better eye is constricted to less than 20° in diameter,

    c) When uncorrectable diplopia exists, or

    d) When the detachment is the result of documented organic progressive disease or new growth, regardless of the condition of the better eye.

  2. Bilateral. Regardless of etiology or results of corrective surgery.

k. Aniseikonia. Subjective eye discomfort, neurologic symptoms, sensations of motion sickness and other gastrointestinal disturbances, functional disturbances and difficulties in form sense, and not corrected by iseikonic lenses.

l. Binocular diplopia. Not correctable by surgery, and which is severe, constant, and in zone less than 20° from the primary position.

m. Hemianopsia. Of any type, if bilateral, permanent, and based on an organic defect. Those due to a functional neurosis and those due to transitory conditions, such as periodic migraine are not considered to render an individual unfit.

n. Loss of an eye.

o. Night blindness: Of such a degree that the individual requires assistance in any travel at night.

p. Visual acuity which cannot be corrected to at least 20/40 in the better eye.

q. Visual field; bilateral concentric constriction to less than 20°.

C. **Causes of Medical Unfitness for Flying Duty Classes 1, 1A, 2 and 3 are Listed in Paragraph Aa through Ai, plus the following:**

a. Asthenopia of any degree.

b. Chorioretinitis or substantiated history thereof.

c. Coloboma of the choroid or iris.

d. Epiphora.

e. Inflammation of the uveal tract; acute, chronic, or recurrent.

f. Pterygium which encroaches on the cornea more than 1 mm. or is progressive, as evidenced by marked vascularity or a thick elevated head.

g. Trachoma unless healed without cicatrices.

h. Class 1.

1. Color vision

    a) Five or more errors in reading the 14 test plates of the Pseudoisochromatic Plate Set (Federal stock No. 6515-299-8186), or

    b) Four or more errors in reading the 17 test plates of the Pseudoisochromatic Plate Set (Federal stock No. 6515-388-6606) or

    c) Rescinded.

2. Depth perception

    a) Any error in lines B, C, or D when using the Machine Vision Tester.

    b) Any error with Verhoeff Stereometer when used in lieu of a) above or when examinee fails a).

3. Distant visual acuity uncorrected, less than 20/20 in each eye.

4. Field of vision

    a) Any demonstrable scotoma, other than physiologic.

    b) Contraction of the field for form of 15° or more in any meridian.

5. Near visual acuity, uncorrected, less than 20/20 (J.1) in each eye.

6. Night vision: Failure to pass test when indicated by history of night blindness.

7. Ocular motility

    a) Any diplopia or suppression in the red lens test which develops within 20 inches from the center of the screen in any of the six cardinal directions.

    b) Esophoria greater than 10 prism diopters.

    c) Exophoria greater than 5 prism diopters.

    d) Hyperphoria greater than 1 prism diopter.

    e) Heterotropia, any degree.

8. Power of accommodation of less than minimum for age.

9. Refractive error

    a) Astigmatism in excess of 0.75 diopter.

    b) Hyperopia in excess of 1.75 diopter in any meridian.

    c) Myopia in excess of 0.25 diopter in any meridian.

i. Class 1A. Same as Class 1 except as listed below.

1. Distant visual acuity. Uncorrected less than 20/50 in each eye or not correctable to 20/20 in each eye.

2. Near visual acuity

    a) Individuals under age 35: Uncorrected less than 20/20 (J.1) in each eye.

    b) Individuals age 35 or over: Uncorrected, less than 20/50 or not correctable to 20/20 in each eye.

3. Refractive error

    a) Astigmatism greater than 0.75 diopter.

    b) Hyperopia

        1) Individuals under age 35: Greater than 1.75 diopter in any meridian.

        2) Individuals age 35 or over: Greater than 2.00 diopters in any meridian

    c) Myopia greater than 0.75 diopter in any meridian.

j. Class 2. Same as Class 1 except as listed below:

1. Color vision

    a) Five or more errors in reading the 14 test plates of the Pseudoisochromatic Plate Set

(Federal stock No. 6515-388-6606), or

b) Four or more errors in reading the 17 test plates of the Pseudoisochromatic Plate Set (Federal stock No. 6515-388-6606), or

c) Failure to pass the Farnsworth Lantern Test when used in lieu of a) or b) above.

2. Distant visual acuity

a) Control tower operators: Uncorrected less than 20/50 in each eye or not correctable to 20/20 in each eye.

b) Rescinded.

c) Pilots: Uncorrected less than 20/100 in each eye or not correctable to 20/20 in each eye.

3. Field of vision: Scotoma, other than physiologic unless the pathologic process is healed and which will in no way interfere with flying efficiency or the well being of the individual.

4. Near visual acuity. Uncorrected less than 20/100 (J.16) in each eye or not correctable to 20/20 in each eye.

5. Ocular motility

a) Hyperphoria greater than 1.5 prism diopters.

b) Failure of the Red Lens Test (suppression or diplopia within 20 inches from the center of the screen in any of the six cardinal directions) until a complete evaluation by a certified ophthalmologist has been forwarded to The Surgeon General for review.

6. Refractive error: No maximum limits prescribed.

k. Class 3

1. Color vision: Same as Class 2 j. 1. above.

2. Distant visual acuity: Uncor-

rected, less than 20/200 in each eye, not correctable to 20/20 in each eye.

3. Near visual acuity, field of vision, night vision, depth perception, power of accommodation, ocular motility: Same as Class 2.

D. Causes of Medical Unfitness for U. S. Military Academy

a. 1. Any acute or chronic disease of the eye or adnexa.

b. Any disfiguring or incapacitating abnormality.

c. Ocular mobility and motility.

1. Esophoria of over 15 prism diopters.

2. Exophoria of over 10 prism diopters.

3. Hyperphoria of over 2 prism diopters.

4. Strabismus of any degree.

d. Color blindness: Inability to distinguish and identify without confusion the color of an object, substance, material or light that is uniformly colored a vivid red or vivid green.

e. Visual acuity: Distant visual acuity which does not correct to at least 20/20 in each eye.

f. Refractive error

1. Anisometropia: Over 3.50 diopters.

2. Astigmatism: All types over 3.00 diopters.

3. Hyperopia: Over 5.50 diopters in any meridian.

4. Myopia: Over 5.50 diopters in any meridian.

OCULAR REQUIREMENTS FOR THE U. S. NAVY AND MARINE CORPS

(1) Applicants for Enlistment

Distant visual acuity of any degree which will correct to at least 20/40 in one eye and 20/70 in the other; or

20/30 in one eye and 20/100 in the other; or 20/20 in one eye and 20/400 in the other.

(2) Candidates for Commission

(a) Navy Line: Minimum acuity of 20/40 in each eye correctable to 20/20 with standard lenses. Must have normal color perception.

(b) Staff: Minimum acuity of 20/100 in each eye correctable to 20/20 in each with standard lenses.

(c) Naval Academy: Minimum acuity of 20/20 in each eye, unaided by lenses. Must have normal color perception.

(d) Commission in the Marine Corps: Minimum acuity of 20/40 in each eye correctable to 20/20 with standard lenses.

(3) Any Acute or Chronic Pathologic Condition of the eye is cause of rejection; this applies to all applicants and candidates.

OCULAR REQUIREMENTS FOR THE U. S. AIR FORCE

Eye

a. Enlistment—Causes for Rejection

(1) Lids

(a) Trichiasis.

(b) Destruction of the lids sufficient to impair protection of the eye from exposure.

(c) Disfiguring cicatrices and adhesions of the lids to each other or to the eyeball.

(d) Blepharitis, chronic, unless it is the opinion of the examiner that it is sufficiently mild in degree to interfere in no way with performance of duty.

(e) Blepharospasm.

(f) Ptosis interfering with vision.

(g) Inversion or eversion of the eyelids.

(h) Lagophthalmos.

(i) Growth or tumor of the eyelid other than asymptomatic, nonprogressive, small benign lesions.

(j) Dacryocystitis, acute or chronic.

(k) Epiphora.

(2) Conjunctiva

(a) Conjunctivitis, acute until recovered.

(b) Conjunctivitis, chronic, including vernal catarrh.

(c) Trachoma unless healed without cicatrices.

(d) Zerophthalmia.

(e) Pterygium which encroaches on the cornea more than 1 mm. or is progressive, as evidenced by marked vascularity or a thick, elevated head.

(3) Cornea

(a) Keratitis, acute or chronic.

(b) Corneal ulcer or history of recurrent ulcers.

(c) Vascularization or opacification of the cornea from any cause which interferes with visual function or is progressive.

(d) Corneal dystrophy of any type including keratoconus of any degree.

(4) Uveal Tract. Inflammation of the uveal tract (iris, ciliary body or choroid), acute, chronic, or recurrent.

(5) Retina

(a) Detachment of the retina or history of treatment for same.

(b) Degenerations of the retina to include macular diseases, macular cysts, holes and other degenerations (hereditary or acquired) affecting the macula; pigmentary degenerations (primary and secondary).

(c) Retinitis.

(d) Chorioretinitis, unless healed, considered unlikely to recur and not interfering significantly with visual function.

(6) Optic Nerve

(a) Optic neuritis, neuroretinitis, or documented history of retrobulbar neuritis.

(b) Optic atrophy.

(c) Papilledema.

(7) Lens

(a) Aphakia (unilateral or bilateral).

(b) Dislocation of a lens, partial or complete.

(c) Opacities of the lens which are considered to be progressive, or which interfere in any way with vision.

(8) Miscellaneous Defects and Diseases

(a) Asthenopia, if more than moderate.

(b) Glaucoma, primary or secondary.

(c) Tumor of the eye.

(d) Tumor of the orbit.

(e) Exophthalmos.

(f) Nystagmus.

(g) Diplopia.

(h) Hemianopsia.

(i) Loss of normal pupillary reflex.

(j) Retained-intraocular foreign body.

(k) Heterotropia greater than 15 degrees (26 prism diopters). Heterotropia of 15 degrees or less is acceptable when it is not due to underlying ocular or neurologic disease, and is not progressive.

(l) Any organic disease of the eye or adnexa not specified above which threatens continuity of vision or impairment of visual function.

b. Commission—Causes for Rejection. Same as "a" and "f".

c. Air Force Academy—Causes for Rejection. Same as "a" and "f".

d. Flying Class III—Causes for Rejection. Same as "a" and "f".

e. Flying Class II—Causes for Rejection. Same as "a" and "f", except that each condition must be individually evaluated with regard to severity, prognosis, and importance in relation to continued flying duties.

f. Flying Classes I and IA—Causes for Rejection. Same as "a". In addition:

(1) History of chorioretinitis.

(2) Heterotropia.

(3) History of glaucoma, primary or secondary.

(4) History of uveitis.

(5) History of optic neuritis.

Refraction

a. Enlistment—Causes for Rejection

(1) Refractive error of more than +8.00 or −8.00 in any meridian or if ordinary spectacles cause discomfort by reason of ghost images, prismatic displacement, etc.; or ophthalmologic consultation reveals a disqualifying condition.

(2) Complicated cases which can only be corrected by contact lenses.

b. Commission—Causes for Rejection

(1) Total hyperopia greater than 5.50 diopters in any one meridian.

(2) Total myopia greater than 5.50 diopters in any one meridian.

(3) Astigmatism—all types over 3.00 diopters.

(4) Anisometropia greater than 3.50 diopters.

(5) For exceptional cases, see paragraph 19 h.

c. Air Force Academy—Causes for Rejection

(1) Total hyperopia greater than 1.75 diopters in any one meridian.

(2) Total myopia greater than 0.25 diopter in any one meridian.

(3) Astigmatism greater than 0.75 diopter.

(4) On recommendation of the Superintendent, United States Air Force Academy, waiver of the above standards may be granted up to, but not exceeding +3.00 or −3.00 diopters.

d. Flying Class III—Causes for Rejection. Same as "b".

e. Flying Class II—Causes for Rejection. Requires individual evaluation.

f. Flying Class I—Causes for Rejection

(1) Total hyperopia greater than 1.75 diopters in any one meridian.

(2) Total myopia greater than 0.25 diopter in any one meridian.

(3) Astigmatism greater than 0.75 diopter.

g. Flying Class IA—Causes for Rejection. No standards.

Distance Vision

The actual possession of suitable glasses by an individual is not required for his acceptance under the following standards.

a. Acceptable for Enlistment

(1) Physical Profile Classification 1. Minimum vision of 20/70 in each eye correctable with glasses to 20/20 in one eye and 20/30 in the other, provided the defective vision is not due to active or progressive organic disease.

(2) Physical Profile Classification 2. Minimum vision of 20/400 in each eye correctable with glasses to 20/40 in each eye, provided the defective vision is not due to active or progressive organic disease.

(3) Physical Profile Classification 3. Vision correctable to 20/40 in one eye and 20/70 in the other, or 20/30 in one eye and 20/100 in the other, or 20/20 in one eye and 20/400 in the other, provided the defective vision is not due to active or progressive organic disease.

b. Enlistment—Causes for Rejection: Vision less than "a (3)".

c. Commission—Causes for Rejection

(1) Uncorrected. Vision less than 20/400 in each eye.

(2) Corrected. Vision less than 20/30 in one eye and 20/40 in the other.

d. Air Force Academy—Causes for Rejection

(1) Uncorrected. Vision less than 20/20 in each eye.

(2) On recommendation of the Superintendent, U. S. Air Force Academy, waiver may be granted up to, but not exceeding uncorrected distance vision of 20/200 correctable to 20/20.

e. Flying Class III—Causes for Rejection

(1) Uncorrected. Vision less than 20/400 in each eye.

(2) Corrected. Vision less than 20/20 in one eye and 20/30 in the other.

f. Flying Class II—Causes for Rejection

(1) Uncorrected. Vision less than 20/50 in each eye.

(2) Corrected. Vision less than 20/20 in each eye.

g. Flying Class IA—Causes for Rejection

(1) Uncorrected. Vision less than 20/50 in each eye.

(2) Corrected. Vision less than 20/20 in each eye.

h. Flying Class I—Causes for Rejection

(1) Uncorrected. Vision less than 20/20 in each eye.

Near Vision

a. Enlistment—Causes for Rejection

(1) Uncorrected. No standards.

(2) Corrected. Vision less than 20/40 in the better eye.

b. Commission—Causes for Rejection
   (1) Uncorrected. No standards.
   (2) Corrected. Vision less than 20/20 in one eye and 20/40 in the other.

c. Air Force Academy—Causes for Rejection
   (1) Uncorrected. Vision less than 20/20 in each eye.
   (2) On recommendation of the Superintendent, U. S. Air Force Academy, waiver may be granted up to, but not exceeding near vision of 20/200 correctable to 20/20.

d. Flying Class III—Causes for Rejection
   (1) Uncorrected. No standards.
   (2) Corrected. Vision less than 20/20 in one eye and 20/30 in the other.

e. Flying Class II—Causes for Rejection
   (1) Uncorrected. Vision less than 20/50 in each eye.
   (2) Corrected. Vision less than 20/20 in each eye.

f. Flying Class I and IA—Causes for Rejection
   (1) Uncorrected. Vision less than 20/20 in each eye.

Field of Vision

a. Enlistment—Causes for Rejection. Defects which interfere significantly with binocular vision function.

b. Commission—Causes for Rejection. Same as "a".

c. Air Force Academy—Causes for Rejection. Same as "e".

d. Flying, Classes II and III—Causes for Rejection
   (1) Contraction of the field of 15° or more in any meridian, unless the contraction is the result of an anatomic conformation of the examinee's face.

(2) Scotoma due to an active pathologic process.

(3) Scotoma, the result of a healed lesion, unless after full investigation it is the opinion of the examiner that it will interfere in no way with the flying efficiency and well being of the examinee.

e. Flying, Classes I and IA—Causes for Rejection
   (1) Contraction of the field of 15° or more in any meridian, unless the contraction is the result of an anatomic conformation of the examinee's face.
   (2) Any demonstrable scotoma other than physiologic.

Color Vision

a. Enlistment—Causes for Rejection. Impaired color perception is not disqualifying for enlistment. However, normal color vision is a prerequisite to many Air Force specialties. When color vision is found to be impaired, the degree of impairment will be noted on SF 88 (VTA-CTT Score).

b. Commission—Causes for Rejection. Same as "a".

c. Air Force Academy—Causes for Rejection
   (1) Same as "e".
   (2) On recomendation of the Superintendent, U. S. Air Force Academy, waiver may be granted for deficient color vision provided the VTA-CTT Score is not below 34.

d. Flying, Classes II and III—Causes for Rejection. Five or more incorrect responses, including failures to make responses in reading the 14 test charts of the standard color vision test set unless the individual makes a score of 50 or better using the color threshold tester (grade 1). Applicants for the designation of flight medical officer must pass the color vision test (VTS-CV).

e. Flying Classes I and IA—Causes for Rejection. Five or more incorrect responses, including failures to make responses in reading the 14 test charts of the standard color vision test set (VTS-CV).

Night Vision

a. Enlistment—Causes for Rejection
   (1) Verified congenital night blindness.
   (2) Night blindness associated with objective disease of the eye.
b. Commission—Causes for Rejection. Same as "a".
c. Air Force Academy—Causes for Rejection: Same as "d".
d. Flying Classes I, IA, II and III—Causes for Rejection. Unsatisfactory visual efficiency.

Depth Perception

a. Enlistment, Commission and Flying Class III—Causes for Rejection. No standards.
b. Air Force Academy—Causes for Rejection
   (1) Same as "c".
   (2) On recommendation of the Superintendent, U. S. Air Force Academy, this requirement may be waived.
c. Flying Classes I, IA, and II—Causes for Rejection
   (1) An error in group B, C, or D using the VTA-ND.
   (2) Using the Verhoeff depth perception apparatus (DPA-V), any error in eight presentations during first trial, or in second and third trials.
   (3) Average error greater than 30

mm. using the Howard-Dolman apparatus (DPA-HD).

Heterophoria, Heterotropia and Ocular Motility

a. Enlistment—Causes for Rejection: Heterotropia of more than 15 degrees (26 prism diopters).
b. Commission—Causes for Rejection
   (1) Esophoria. Greater than 15 prism diopters.
   (2) Exophoria. Greater than 8 prism diopters.
   (3) Hyperphoria. Greater than 2 prism diopters.
   (4) Heterotropia.
c. Air Force Academy—Causes for Rejection
   (1) Same as "F".
   (2) On recommendation of the Superintendent, U. S. Air Force Academy, this requirement may be waived to "b" above.
d. Flying Class III—Causes for Rejection: Same as "b".
e. Flying Class II—Causes for Rejection
   (1) Esophoria. Greater than 10 prism diopters.
   (2) Exophoria. Greater than 5 prism diopters.
   (3) Hyperphoria. Greater than 1.5 prism diopters.
   (4) Point of convergence (Pc) greater than 70 mm.
   (5) Heterotropia.
f. Flying Class I and IA—Causes for Rejection
   (1) Esophoria. Greater than 10 prism diopters.
   (2) Exophoria. Greater than 5 prism diopters.
   (3) Hyperphoria. Greater than 1 prism diopter.
   (4) Point of convergence (Pc) greater than 70 mm.
   (5) Heterotropia.

Red Lens Test

a. Enlistment, Commission, Flying Classes II and III—Causes for Rejection. No standards.

b. Air Force Academy. Flying Classes I and IA—Causes for Rejection. Any diplopia or suppression in the red lens test which develops within 20 inches of the center of the screen in any of the six cardinal directions is considered a failure. However, failure of the red lens test in the absence of other eye defects or related disease will not necessarily be disqualifying for flying training. Such cases will be seen in consultation by a qualified ophthalmologist and the results will be sent for decision to the Surgeon, USAF Academy, in the case of AFA applicants, or to the Surgeon, Air University, in the case of AFROTC applicants for flying training, or to the Surgeon Air Training Command, in the case of flying training applicants other than AFROTC.

Near Point of Accommodation

a. Enlistment, Commission, and Flying Class III—Causes for Rejection. No standards.

b. Air Force Academy—Causes for Rejection.
   (1) Same as "c".
   (2) On recommendation of the Superintendent, U. S. Air Force Academy, this requirement may be waived.

c. Flying Classes I and II—Causes for Rejection. Near point of accommodation less than the minimum for age.

d. Flying Class IA—Causes for Rejection. When Flying Class I standards for visual acuity are not fulfilled: Near point of accommodation less than the normal mean value for age.

Intraocular Tension

a. Routine determination of intraocular tension by tonometry is performed only in those individuals age 40 or over. Tonometry is also performed when the medical history or physical examination is suggestive of abnormal intraocular pressure. Examinees with tensions as follows must be referred to a qualified ophthalmologist for consultation:
   (1) Two or more current determinations of 22 mm. Hg or higher.
   (2) One or more determinations of 25 mm. Hg or higher.
   (3) A difference of more than 4 mm. between right and left eyes.

b. When ophthalmologic consultation results in a diagnosis of glaucoma, any type, or the need for medication, (either topical or systemic) to control intraocular tension the condition is disqualifying for all categories. For personnel who are required to meet medical standards for flying, after an effective therapeutic regime has been established, if the flight surgeon and ophthalmologist agree that there are no apparent aeromedical reasons to justify continued suspension from flying duties, the flyer may be referred to an Aviation Medicine Consultation center for evaluation. Upon the favorable recommendation of the Aeromedical Evaluation Service and with the approval of the Surgeon General, some of these patients may be returned to flying status with waiver. It must be emphasized that therapy must be effective and completely free of adverse side effects. Patients who require systemic medication will not be considered for return to flying duties.

c. For personnel who are required to meet Medical Standards for flying, a

"Preglaucoma" group may be identified. This group will include those flying personnel whose intraocular pressure exceeds the limits in "a" above but who have no visual field defect or optic disk changes and whose pressure is below 30 mm. Members of this group may be granted a waiver for retention on flying duty by HQ USAF provided they are followed at three month intervals by an ophthalmologist. A decrement in visual fields, changes in the optic disk, or elevation of the tonometer reading to, or above 30 mm. will require institution of therapy and immediate removal from flying duty.

OCULAR REQUIREMENTS FOR THE U. S. COAST GUARD

Disqualification Conditions for All Personnel

1. **Conjunctiva**
   a. *Conjunctivitis.* Chronic conjunctivitis including vernal catarrh and trachoma.
   b. *Pterygium*
      (1) Pterygium recurring after three operative procedures.
      (2) Pterygium encroaching on the cornea.
   c. *Xerophthalmia.*

2. **Cornea**
   a. *Dystrophy.* Corneal dystrophy of any type including keratoconus of any degree.
   b. *Keratitis.* Acute or chronic keratitis.
   c. *Staphyloma.*
   d. *Ulcer.* Corneal ulcer; history of recurrent ulcers or corneal abrasions (including herpetic ulcers).
   e. *Vascularization.* Vascularization or opacification of the cornea from any cause which interferes with visual function or is progressive.

3. **Iris or Pupils**
   a. *Coloboma.* Extensive coloboma of the choroid or iris, absence of pigment (albino), glaucoma, iritis, or extensive or progressive choroiditis of any degree.
   b. *Irregularities.* Irregularities in the form of the iris, or anterior or posterior synechia sufficient to reduce the visual acuity below the standard.
   c. *Reactions.* Loss of normal pupillary reflex reactions to light or accommodation to distance or Adie's syndrome.

4. **Lens**
   a. *Aphakia.* Unilateral or bilateral aphakia.
   b. *Dislocation.* Partial or complete dislocation of a lens.
   c. *Opacities.* Opacities of the lens or its capsule which interfere with vision or which are considered to be progressive; or progressive cataract of any degree.

5. **Lids**
   a. *Destruction.* Complete or extensive destruction of the lids sufficient to impair protection of the eye from exposure; disfiguring cicatrices and adhesions of the lids to each other or to the eyeball.
   b. *Epiphora.* Epiphora, chronic dacryocystitis, or lachrymal fistula.
   c. *Inversion.* Inversion or eversion of the eyelids sufficient to cause unsightly appearance or watering of eyes (entropion or ectropion).
   d. *Lagophthalmos*
   e. *Trichiasis.* Trichiasis, ptosis, blepharospasm, or chronic blepharitis.
   f. *Tumor.* Growth or tumor of the eyelid other than small nonprogressive asymptomatic benign lesions.

6. **Optic Nerve**
   a. *Atrophy.* Optic atrophy (primary or secondary).
   b. *Neuritis.* Optic neuritis, neuroretinitis,

or secondary optic atrophy resulting therefrom; or history of attacks of retrobulbar neuritis.

c. *Papilledema*

d. *Pathology.* Congenito-hereditary conditions of the optic nerve or any other central nervous system pathology affecting the efficient function of the optic nerve.

7. Retina

a. *Angiomatoses.* Angiomatoses, phakomatoses, retinal cysts, and other congenito-hereditary conditions that impair visual function.

b. *Degenerations.* Degenerations of the retina to include macular diseases, macular cysts, holes, and other degenerations (hereditary or acquired) affecting the macular pigmentary degenerations (primary and secondary).

c. *Detachment.* Detachment of the retina or history of surgery for same.

d. *Inflammation.* Inflammation of the retina (retinitis or other inflammatory conditions of the retina to include Coat's disease, diabetic retinopathy, Eales' disease, and retinitis proliferans).

8. Uveal Tract. Inflammation of the uveal tract except healed traumatic choroiditis.

9. Miscellaneous Eye Defects and Diseases

a. *Abnormalities.* Abnormal conditions of the eye due to diseases of the central nervous system. Abnormal condition of the eye due to disease of the brain. Any disfiguring or incapacitating abnormality, or acute or chronic disease of either eye.

b. *Absence.* Absence or disorganization of either eye.

c. *Asthenopia*

d. *Exophthalmos.* Unilateral or bilateral exophthalmos.

e. *Foreign Body.* Retained intraocular foreign body.

f. *Glaucoma.* Primary or secondary glaucoma.

g. *Hemianopsia.* Hemianopsia of any type.

h. *Organic Disease.* Any organic disease of the eye or adnexa not specified herein which threatens continuity of vision or impairment of visual function.

i. *Residuals.* Residuals of old contusions, lacerations, penetrations, etc., which impair visual function required for satisfactory performance of military duty.

j. *Visual Field.* Abnormal condition of the visual field due to diseases of the central nervous system. Loss of visual fields due to organic disease. Contraction of visual field, "tunnel vision".

Disqualifying Conditions of Ocular Motility

1. Diplopia. Constant or intermittent from any cause or of any degree interfering with visual function. Monocular diplopia interfering with visual function.

2. Nystagmus. Pronounced nystagmus, or with both eyes fixing, congenital or acquired.

3. Strabismus. Well-marked strabismus or lack of continuous and complete third degree binocular fusion. Strabismus of any degree accompanied by diplopia. Surgery for the correction of strabismus within the preceding 6 months.

Near Vision

Testing of near vision is not usually required unless medically indicated. Testing is done with Jaeger's test types.

Heterophoria

Except for aviation personnel, special tests for heterophoria are not required unless medically indicated.

Accommodation

Except for aviation personnel, special tests for accommodation are not required unless medically indicated.

Color Vision

Color blindness complete or partial, is cause for disqualification of all categories of personnel except applicants for enlistment in, and enlisted members of the Coast Guard Reserve, and women (both officers and enlisted) of the Coast Guard Reserve. However, color perception tests shall be administered to these reservists and recorded in order that the results may be available in the event an individual is considered for assignment to training, or to duties, or for a specialized rate requiring color perception.

Depth Perception

Except for aviation personnel, special tests for depth perception are not required unless medically indicated.

Field of Vision

Except for aviation personnel, special tests for field of vision are not required unless medically indicated.

Night Vision

A test for night vision (dark adaptation) is not required unless indicated for medical or special reasons.

Red Lens Test

Except for aviation personnel, the red lens test is not required unless diplopia (double images) is suspected.

Intraocular Tension

Intraocular tension should be ascertained each time an eye refraction is to be performed.

U. S. COAST GUARD MINIMUM DISTANT VISUAL ACUITY REQUIREMENTS

Category	Vision
A. Aviation Personnel	
1. Candidate for flight training...................	20/20 uncorrected.
2. Pilot, Class 1, Service Group I................	20/30 uncorrected.
3. Pilot, Class 1, Service Group II...............	20/50 uncorrected; when less than 20/30 in either eye must be corrective to 20/20 each eye.
4. Pilot, Class 1, Service Group III..............	20/100 uncorrected; when less than 20/30 in either eye must be corrective to 20/20 each eye.
5. Aviation Observer (under 50)..................	Same as A.3.
6. Aviation Observer (over 50)...................	Same as A.4.
7. Technical Observer...........................	Corrective to 20/30.
8. Candidate for Flight Surgeon or Aviation Medical Examiner.............................	20/100 uncorrected; corrective to 20/20.
9. Designated Flight Surgeon or Aviation Medical Examiner.............................	Corrective to 20/30.
10. Candidate for Aircrewman....................	Same as A.3.
11. Designated Aircrewman......................	Same as A.4.
B. General Duty Male Officers & Candidates	
1. Officers (commissioned or warrant) in the USCG or USCGR.........................	Corrective to 20/30.
2. Appointment in USCG of Licensed Officers of the U. S. Merchant Marine......................	20/50 uncorrected; corrective to 20/30.
3. Direct Commission in the USCGR..............	20/100 uncorrected; corrective to 20/30.
4. Cadet Candidate for Academy.................	20/30 uncorrected; corrective to 20/20.
5. Precommissioning of Cadets...................	20/100 uncorrected; corrective to 20/20.
6. OCS Candidates..............................	20/50 uncorrected; corrective to 20/30.
7. Precommissioning of Officer Candidates..........	Same as B.6.
C. Enlisted Male Personnel	
1. Original Enlistment USCG (less musicians and Ex-Service Personnel)........................	20/100 uncorrected; corrected to 20/30 one eye, and 20/40 other eye.
2. Original Enlistment USCG (musicians and Ex-Service Personnel only)......................	Corrective to 20/30 one eye, and 20/40 other eye.
3. Reenlistment or Enlisted Personnel USCG........	Corrective to 20/30 one eye, and 20/40 other eye.

U. S. COAST GUARD MINIMUM DISTANT VISUAL ACUITY REQUIREMENTS—*Continued*

Category	Vision
C. Enlisted Male Personnel—*Continued*	
4. Original Enlistment USCGR....................	Corrective to at least 20/40 one eye & 20/70 other, or 20/30 one eye & 20/100 other, or 20/20 one eye & 20/400 other eye.
5. Reenlistment or Enlisted Personnel USCGR......	Same as C.4.
D. Female Personnel	
1. Officer and Enlisted Personnel in USCGR........	20/200 uncorrected; corrective to 20/30.

Index